Essential Radiology for Sports Medicine

Philip Robinson
Editor

Essential Radiology for Sports Medicine

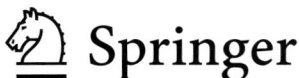

Editor
Philip Robinson, FRCR
Department of Radiology
Leeds Teaching Hospitals
Leeds, UK
p.robinson@leedsth.nhs.uk

ISBN 978-1-4419-5972-0   e-ISBN 978-1-4419-5973-7
DOI 10.1007/978-1-4419-5973-7
Springer New York Dordrecht Heidelberg London

Library of Congress Control Number: 2010927879

© Springer Science+Business Media, LLC 2010
All rights reserved. This work may not be translated or copied in whole or in part without the written permission of the publisher (Springer Science+Business Media, LLC, 233 Spring Street, New York, NY 10013, USA), except for brief excerpts in connection with reviews or scholarly analysis. Use in connection with any form of information storage and retrieval, electronic adaptation, computer software, or by similar or dissimilar methodology now known or hereafter developed is forbidden.
The use in this publication of trade names, trademarks, service marks, and similar terms, even if they are not identified as such, is not to be taken as an expression of opinion as to whether or not they are subject to proprietary rights.
While the advice and information in this book are believed to be true and accurate at the date of going to press, neither the authors nor the editors nor the publisher can accept any legal responsibility for any errors or omissions that may be made. The publisher makes no warranty, express or implied, with respect to the material contained herein.

Printed on acid-free paper

Springer is part of Springer Science+Business Media (www.springer.com)

For my parents, Peter and Anwen, and my family Oonagh, Eve, Ted and Roddy for their constant love, support and belief

Preface

Imaging plays an increasingly vital role in the management of athletes aiding diagnosis, injury grading and prognosis, as well as guiding therapy. These processes apply equally to elite and recreational athletes young and old.

I have always found that understanding the relevance of imaging findings is easier when accompanied by knowledge of the anatomy, biomechanics and pathological processes involved in injury formation. This textbook has been developed with both radiologists and sports clinicians in mind and aims to bring all these processes together and illustrate the spectrum of injury and associated clinical features for specific anatomical areas. Internationally recognized musculoskeletal experts have contributed chapters which provide an imaging and clinical overview of the most relevant joint, bone and soft tissue athletic injuries. There is guidance for the reader on why specific injuries occur, how to identify the optimal imaging evaluation and how to interpret the subsequent imaging findings. Acute and overuse injuries are discussed as well as the premature degenerative processes that occur in athletes.

State-of-the-art imaging techniques and findings are presented including the use of musculoskeletal ultrasound, conventional MR imaging and MR arthrography. Therapeutic image-guided intervention using fluoroscopy, CT, and ultrasound is also discussed. This balance of techniques should allow a clinician whose practice focuses on one particular modality to become aware not only of that technique's abilities but other modalities and their capabilities and limitations.

Leeds, UK   Philip Robinson

Contents

1. **Knee Injuries** 1
   Melanie A. Hopper and Andrew J. Grainger

2. **Hip, Pelvis and Groin Injuries** 29
   Philip Robinson

3. **Ankle and Foot Injuries** 49
   Ne Siang Chew, Justin Lee, Mark Davies, and Jeremiah Healy

4. **Osseous Stress Injury in Athletes** 89
   Melanie A. Hopper and Philip Robinson

5. **Shoulder Injuries** 103
   Andrew J. Grainger and Phillip F.J. Tirman

6. **Elbow Injuries** 127
   Kenneth S. Lee, Michael J. Tuite, and Humberto G. Rosas

7. **Hand and Wrist Injuries** 143
   Philip J. O'Connor

8. **Postoperative Imaging in Sports Medicine** 173
   Ali Naraghi and Lawrence M. White

9. **Muscle Injury and Complications** 199
   Abhijit Datir and David A. Connell

10. **Sports-Related Disorders of the Spine and Sacrum** 217
    Rob Campbell and Andrew Dunn

11. **Ultrasound-Guided Sports Intervention** 241
    Philip J. O'Connor

Index 251

Contributors

Rob Campbell, FRCR
Department of Radiology, Royal Liverpool University Hospital, Liverpool, UK

Ne Siang Chew, MRCP, FRCR
Department of Radiology, Chelsea and Westminster Hospital, London, UK

David A. Connell, FRANZCR
Department of Radiology, Royal National Orthopedic Hospital, Stanmore, UK

Abhijit Datir, MD, FRCR
Department of Radiology, Royal National Orthopedic Hospital, Stanmore, UK

Mark Davies, MS, FRCS
London Foot and Ankle Center, Hospital of St. John and St. Elizabeth, London, UK

Andrew Dunn, FRCR
Department of Radiology, Royal Liverpool University Hospital, Liverpool, UK

Andrew J. Grainger, MRCP, FRCR
Department of Radiology, Chapel Allerton Hospital, Leeds Teaching Hospitals, Leeds, UK

Jeremiah Healy, MA, MRCP, FRCR, FFSEM
Department of Radiology, Chelsea and Westminster Hospital, London, UK;
London Foot and Ankle Center, Hospital of St. John and St. Elizabeth, London, UK

Melanie A. Hopper, FRCR
Department of Radiology, Leeds Teaching Hospitals, Leeds, UK

Justin Lee, MBBS, MRCS, FRCR
Department of Radiology, Chelsea and Westminster Hospital, London, UK;
London Foot and Ankle Center, Hospital of St. John and St. Elizabeth, London, UK

Kenneth S. Lee, MD
Department of Radiology, University of Wisconsin Hospitals and Clinics,
University of Wisconsin School of Medicine and Public Health, Madison, WI, USA

Ali Naraghi, FRCR
Department of Medical Imaging, Toronto Western Hospital, University of Toronto, Toronto, ON, Canada

Philip J. O'Connor, MRCP, FRCR, FFSEM(UK)
Department of Musculoskeletal Radiology, Leeds Teaching Hospitals, Leeds, UK

Philip Robinson, FRCR
Department of Musculoskeletal Radiology, Chapel Allerton Hospital,
Leeds Teaching Hospitals, Leeds, UK

Humberto G. Rosas, MD
Department of Radiology, University of Wisconsin Hospitals and Clinics,
University of Wisconsin School of Medicine and Public Health, Madison, WI, USA

Phillip F.J. Tirman, MD
Norcal Division, MRI Department, Radnet, Inc., Walnut Creek, CA, USA

Michael J. Tuite, MD
Department of Radiology, University of Wisconsin Hospitals and Clinics,
University of Wisconsin School of Medicine and Public Health, Madison, WI, USA

Lawrence M. White, MD
Department of Medical Imaging, Mount Sinai Hospital, University of Toronto,
Toronto, ON, Canada

Chapter 1
Knee Injuries

Melanie A. Hopper and Andrew J. Grainger

Introduction

The knee is vulnerable to a wide variety of acute and chronic injuries sustained during sporting activity. Acute knee injuries most frequently involve the bone, menisci, articular cartilage and ligaments. They are particularly common in sports involving twisting movements and sudden changes of direction. Examples include soccer and rugby, skiing, basketball and volleyball. The knee transmits considerable forces and repetitive injury particularly to the cartilage and tendons is common, especially in sports involving running and jumping.

Anatomy

The knee comprises two joints, the tibiofemoral joint, with its medial and lateral compartments, and the patellofemoral joint. The menisci and ligaments are fundamental to the maintenance of joint stability.

Menisci

The fibrocartilaginous medial and lateral menisci have distinct morphology reflected in their imaging appearances. The medial meniscus is U shaped and larger than the more C-shaped lateral meniscus. Both menisci are triangular in cross-section with a 3–5 mm high peripheral rim, tapering to a thin free edge centrally. They comprise anterior and posterior horns separated by the meniscal body. The anterior horn of the medial meniscus is smaller than the posterior horn whereas the lateral meniscus is more uniform in shape. Both the medial and lateral menisci are firmly attached to the underlying tibia by anterior and posterior root ligaments (Fig. 1.1).

A number of ligaments are associated with the meniscal attachments and although they are very variable it is important to be aware of these and their potential to mimic meniscal injury on magnetic resonance (MR) imaging. They can be identified as meniscal ligaments by following their course on consecutive image slices between recognised points of origin and insertion. The transverse intermeniscal ligament links the anterior horns and may be seen as a fibrous band traversing Hoffa's fat pad. Posteriorly, the lateral meniscus may attach to the medial femoral condyle via the anterior and posterior meniscofemoral ligaments, the ligaments of Humphrey and Wrisberg, respectively. Frequently, one of the two ligaments is more prominent and most usually on MR imaging only one ligament is seen [1] (Fig. 1.2).

Ligaments have also been recognised passing from the anterior horn of one meniscus to the posterior horn of the opposite meniscus. These oblique intermeniscal ligaments are uncommon and are named after the meniscus of their posterior attachment [2].

The medial meniscus is firmly attached to the joint capsule and to the deep fibres of the medial collateral ligament via the meniscotibial and meniscofemoral ligaments making it less mobile than the lateral and more prone to injury. The lateral meniscus is more loosely attached to the capsule except posterolaterally where the inferior and superior popliteomeniscal fascicles extend from the lateral meniscus around the popliteus tendon attaching to the adjacent joint capsule. This connection allows the popliteus to pull the lateral meniscus posteriorly during knee flexion preventing meniscal entrapment. In this region, the appearance of the popliteus tendon separated from the meniscus by a thin line of fluid can mimic tearing of the posterior horn (Fig. 1.3a).

Although the medial meniscus has no direct muscle attachment, it is likely that indirect attachment to the semimembranosus muscle provides retraction of its posterior horn during knee movement.

In the foetus the menisci have intrinsic vessels, but from birth there is rapid restriction of blood supply so that by early adulthood only the outer third of a meniscus retains vascularity. This has important implications to the surgeon contemplating the viability of meniscal repair procedures.

Andrew J. Grainger (✉)
Department of Radiology, Leeds Teaching Hospitals, Leeds, UK
e-mail: andrew.grainger@leedsth.nhs.uk

Cruciate Ligaments

The cruciate ligaments are intra-capsular but extrasynovial. The anterior cruciate ligament (ACL) is on average 4 cm long and 1 cm wide and arises from the medial aspect of the lateral femoral condyle. Proximally it runs parallel to the roof of the intercondylar notch fanning out to insert onto the anterior tibial eminence. The ACL comprises two functional bundles or units. The anteromedial (AM) bundle is smaller and more tightly packed than the posterolateral (PL) fibres. During knee flexion the AM fibres are taut; the larger PL bundle comes under tension in extension and provides the main resistance to hyperextension.

The posterior cruciate ligament (PCL) is thicker and stronger than the ACL and has a more robust blood supply. It takes its origin from the lateral aspect of the medial femoral condyle inserting into a small depression on the posterior aspect of the tibia. Again the ligament has two functional bundles of fibres. The anterolateral (AL) bundle is taut in knee flexion; the posteromedial (PM) fibre bundle becomes tight during knee extension.

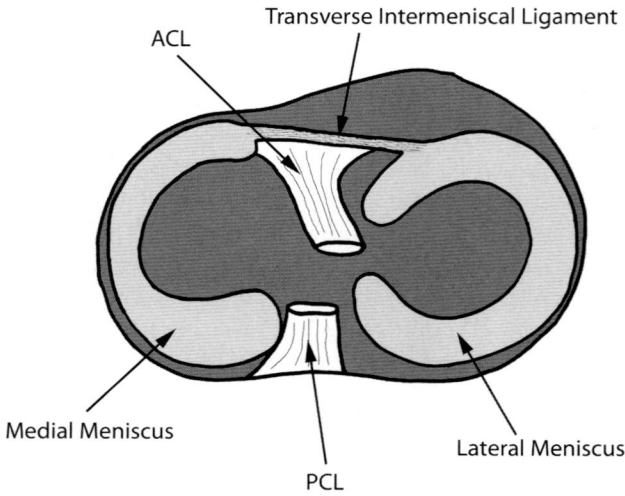

Fig. 1.1 Diagram showing the arrangement of meniscal attachments on the tibial plateau and their relationship to the cruciate ligament insertions. Note the medial meniscus has a "U"-shaped configuration while the lateral meniscus has a tighter "C" shape. The posterior horn of the medial meniscus is larger than the anterior horn in contrast to the lateral meniscus where the two horns are of similar size. Note also the transverse intermeniscal ligament

The Collateral Ligaments and Posterior Corners

The medial and lateral ligament complexes are functionally and anatomically complex and are essential for knee stability.

The medial stabilising structures of the knee have a layered configuration first described by Warren and Marshall [3]. Deep crural and sartorial fascia provides the most superficial of the three layers. The middle layer is composed of the superficial medial collateral ligament (MCL). The deepest layer structures are the deep MCL, the patellomeniscal ligament and the posteromedial capsule.

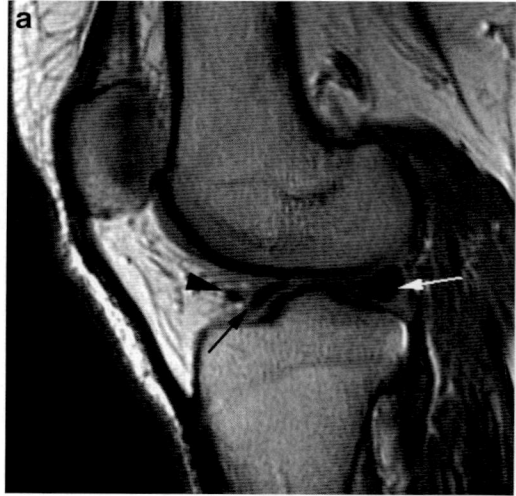 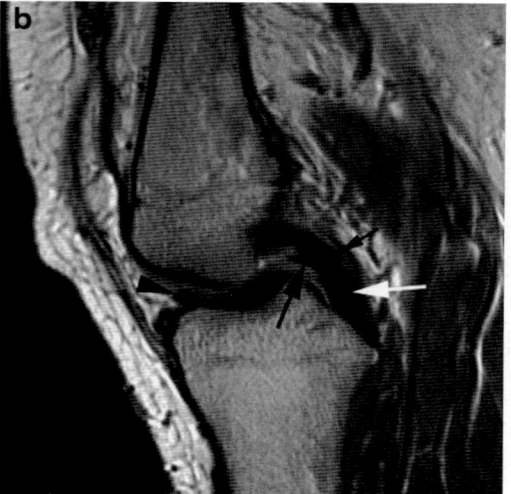

Fig. 1.2 Normal meniscal ligaments. Proton density sagittal images. (**a**) This section passes through the anterior (*black arrow*) and posterior (*white arrow*) horns of the lateral meniscus. The anterior intermeniscal ligament (*arrowhead*) is seen as a separate structure adjacent to the anterior horn of the meniscus. (**b**) This section is taken closer to the midline than **a** and passes through the intercondylar notch. The PCL is seen (*white arrow*). Anterior to it is seen the anterior meniscofemoral ligament of Humphrey (*large black arrow*) while posteriorly a rather smaller posterior meniscofemoral ligament of Wrisberg is seen (*small black arrow*). Anteriorly, the intermeniscal ligament seen in A continues across the midline (*arrowhead*)

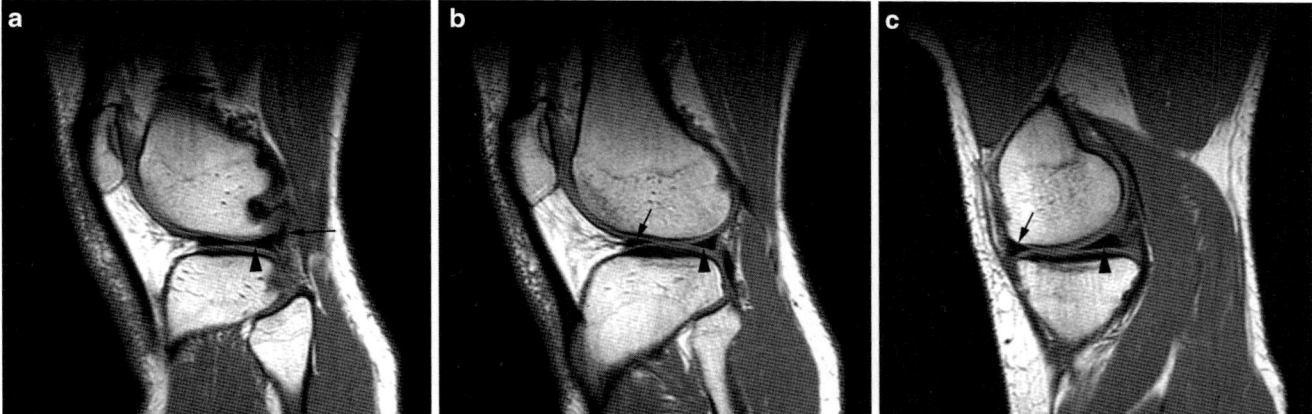

Fig. 1.3 Normal meniscal anatomy. Sagittal T1-weighted images. (**a**) This section passes through the far lateral aspect of the lateral meniscus which shows the classic "bow tie" configuration at this point (*arrowhead*). The popliteus tendon is seen passing posteriorly adjacent to the posterior aspect of the meniscus (*arrow*). (**b**) This section is more medial than **a** and passes through the anterior (*arrow*) and posterior (*arrowhead*) horns of the lateral meniscus. Note that the two horns are of similar size. (**c**) This image passes through the anterior (*arrow*) and posterior (*arrowhead*) horns of the medial meniscus. In contrast to the lateral meniscus the posterior horn is larger than the anterior

At its anterior aspect the superficial MCL runs from the medial femoral condyle to the medial aspect of the proximal tibia, attaching approximately 6 cm below the joint line. Posteriorly, fibres of the superficial MCL extend obliquely from the adductor tubercle to form the posterior oblique ligament (POL). The deep MCL attaches to the medial meniscus and comprises meniscofemoral and meniscotibial (coronary ligament) components. A bursa may exist between the superficial and deep MCL. Dynamic stabilisation for the medial aspect of the knee joint comes from the semimembranosus complex, the medial quadriceps and the pes anserinus muscle tendon units.

At the anterolateral corner of the knee the iliotibial band (ITB) attaches to Gerdys tubercle and provides stabilisation along with the joint capsule. Behind the ITB the tendon of biceps femoris inserts onto the lateral margin of the fibula head as a conjoined tendon with the lateral collateral ligament (LCL) which originates from the lateral femoral condyle. The LCL is one of the structures of the posterolateral corner, also referred to as the arcuate complex, an important knee stabiliser. The other ligaments and muscles involved in the posterolateral corner include popliteus, the arcuate ligament, the lateral head of gastrocnemius, the fabellofibular ligament and the popliteofibular ligament.

The popliteus tendon is intra-articular as it passes from the lateral femoral condyle between the LCL and the lateral meniscus through the popliteal hiatus where the arcuate ligament lies on its superficial aspect. At this point it leaves the joint and the popliteus muscle belly attaches to the posteromedial proximal tibia. Fibres extend from the popliteus to the lateral meniscus (the popliteomeniscal ligament) and to the styloid process of the fibula (the popliteofibular ligament). The arcuate ligament is Y-shaped. From the posterior joint capsule the medial limb runs superficial to popliteus before blending with the oblique popliteal ligament, the lateral limb runs from the capsule laterally over the popliteus tendon and muscle to insert on the posterior aspect of the fibula head. 20% of the population have a fabella as an ossicle within the lateral head of gastrocnemius, when the fabella is present the fabellofibular ligament passes from the lateral femoral condyle to the fabella and onto the styloid process of the fibula.

The Menisci

Meniscal injury is common, particularly in the athletic population and meniscal tears represent the most frequent reason for knee arthroscopy. Signs and symptoms of meniscal injury are unreliable but a history of mechanical problems such as locking or giving way is suggestive. Although many clinical tests have been described, no single test has been shown to be specific and sensitive in the assessment of meniscal pathology. Joint line tenderness is thought to have the closest correlation [4].

Imaging

MR imaging is the imaging modality of choice for imaging meniscal injury with a reported diagnostic accuracy of between 90 and 95% [5]. A brief discussion later in the chapter will be given with regard to other modalities.

Magnetic Resonance Imaging

Short echo time sequences (conventional spin echo T1, PD or gradient echo) are the most sensitive at demonstrating linear meniscal tears and form the basis of MR imaging protocols. T2 sequences, with a longer echo time are less sensitive but more specific. There is controversy as to the role of fast spin echo (FSE) in meniscal evaluation. Several studies report comparable accuracy with conventional spin echo when an echo train length of 4 to 5 is used in addition to faster data acquisition [6, 7]. Other authors determine that the blurring inherent in short TE FSE sequences can obscure a tear or render it less conspicuous [8, 9].

Normal Meniscus

The normal meniscus is low signal on all sequences due to its fibrocartilaginous structure. In sagittal plane both menisci have a "bow-tie" appearance peripherally on at least two consecutive images. The anterior and posterior horns of the lateral meniscus are approximately the same size, whereas the posterior horn of the medial meniscus is roughly twice the size of the anterior horn (Fig. 1.3). These normal features are important to recognise as subtle abnormalities can represent a meniscal tear (Fig. 1.4).

Discoid Meniscus

A discoid meniscus can range from a complete disc to a circular ring and affects the lateral meniscus significantly more frequently than the medial. With a reported incidence of 4.5% a discoid meniscus should be asymptomatic unless torn [10]. There is an increased incidence of tears in a lateral discoid meniscus [10].

On MR imaging the typical finding is of a complete "bow-tie" on three or more contiguous sagittal images, the discoid nature of the meniscus can usually also be appreciated on coronal imaging (Fig. 1.5).

Persistent Meniscal Vascularisation

In the majority of adults only the outer third of the meniscus retains a vascular supply. In a small number of people meniscal vessels persist into adulthood, causing intra-substance high T2-weighted (T2w) signal which may be misinterpreted as meniscal degeneration. The altered signal does not extend to an articular surface and so should not be confused for a meniscal tear.

Classification and MR Imaging Appearances of Tears

Two key features should be looked for when examining the menisci for possible tear. First, signal abnormalities within the normally low signal meniscus and second, alterations in meniscal morphology.

MR imaging meniscal signal abnormalities correlate well with pathology [11] (Table 1.1). Grade 1 signal change seen as globular high signal is not clinically significant and

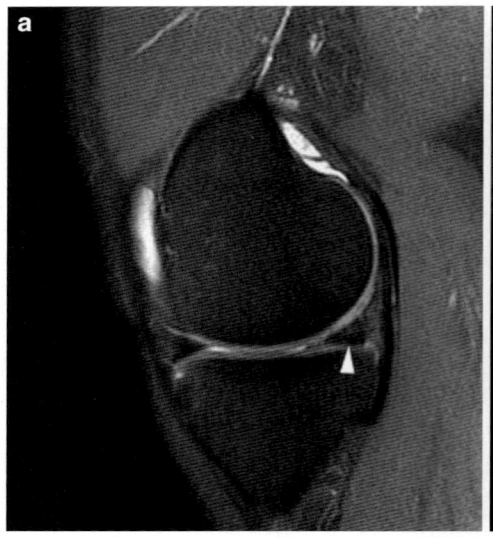
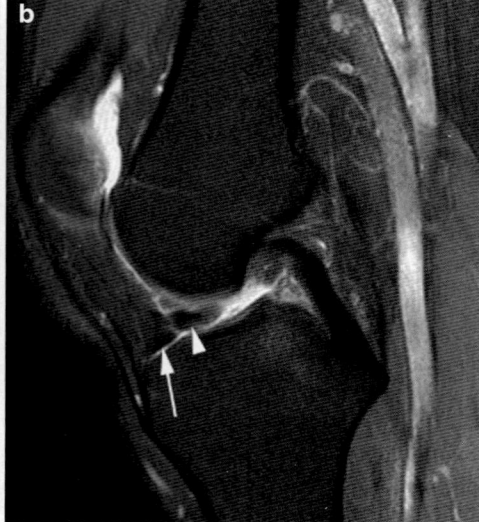

Fig. 1.4 Displaced tear of the medial meniscus. Sagittal proton density images with fat saturation. (**a**) This section passes through the anterior and posterior horns of the medial meniscus. Although no tear is evident the posterior horn (*arrowhead*) should be larger than the anterior but in this case looks to be of similar size. (**b**) This section passes through the intercondylar notch and is lateral to **a**. The cause of the small posterior horn is identified. The meniscus has torn and a fragment of the posterior horn has flipped anteriorly (*arrowhead*) to lie adjacent to the root of the anterior horn (*arrow*)

Fig. 1.5 Discoid meniscus. (**a–c**) Proton density sagittal images with fat saturation. The lateral meniscus has a "bow tie" configuration on multiple slices suggesting a discoid meniscus (*arrowheads*). (**d**) Coronal proton density fat-suppressed imaging. This section passes through the mid-plane of the lateral joint compartment and confirms the discoid meniscus (*arrowhead*)

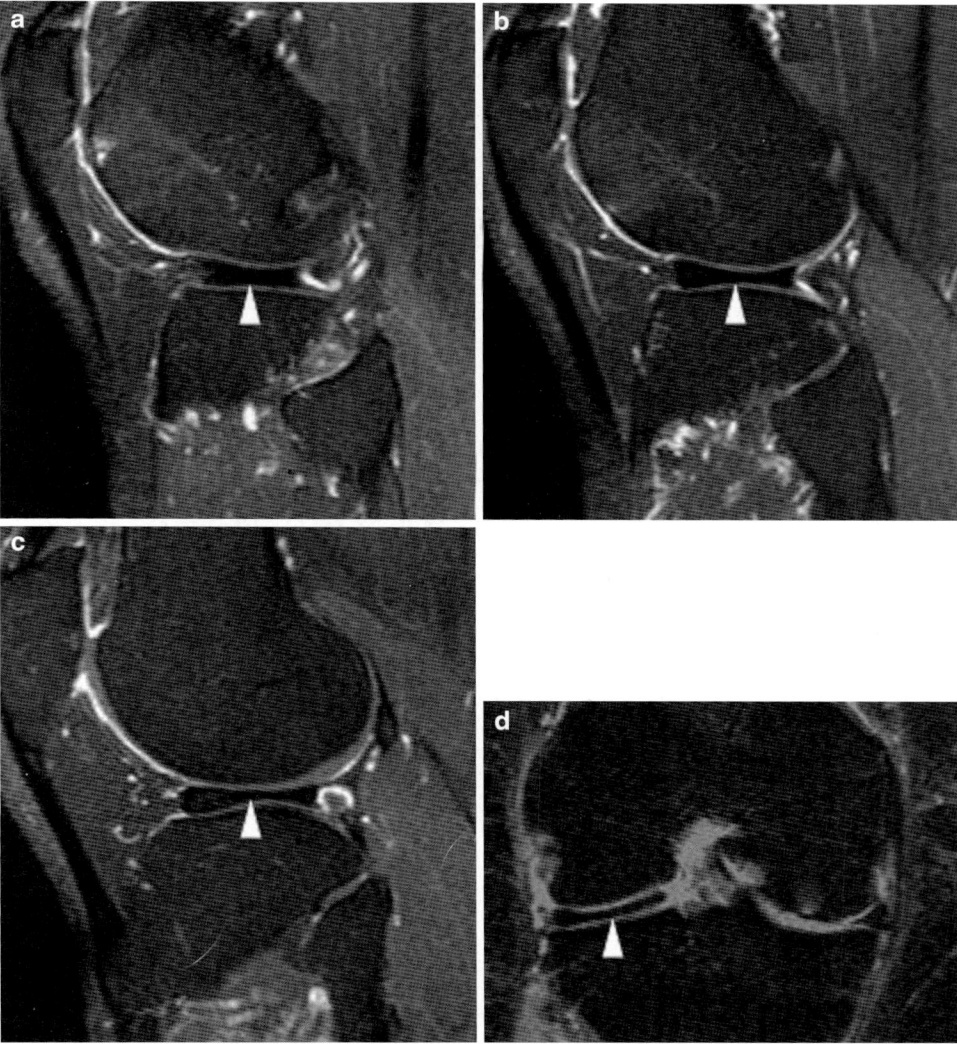

Table 1.1 MRI classification of meniscal tears

Grade 0	Normal
Grade 1	Globular intra-substance intermediate signal not extending to an articular surface
Grade 2	Linear intra-substance intermediate signal not extending to an articular surface
Grade 3	Intermediate signal extending to an articular surface
Grade 3a	Intermediate signal reaches 1 articular surface
Grade 3b	Intermediate signal reaches both articular surfaces

is seen in asymptomatic athletes. Grade 2 meniscal changes represent part of a continuum of changes occurring in meniscal degeneration. It is seen as linear high signal within the meniscal substance and is typically asymptomatic occurring most frequently in the posterior horn of the medial meniscus (Fig. 1.6). High/intermediate signal within a meniscus that extends to one or both articular surfaces represents a meniscal tear and is termed a Grade 3 abnormality (Fig. 1.7). Only grade 3 signal abnormalities represent a meniscal tear and Grade 1 and 2 abnormalities are not prognostic for Grade 3 change [12].

In addition to the signal characteristics within a meniscus, it is vital to assess meniscal morphology in order to recognise displaced or absent meniscal tissue.

Tear Orientation

Meniscal tears can be subdivided according to their orientation.

1. Horizontal tears are parallel to the tibial articular surface.
2. Longitudinal tears are vertically oriented and extend along the circumferential axis of the meniscus.

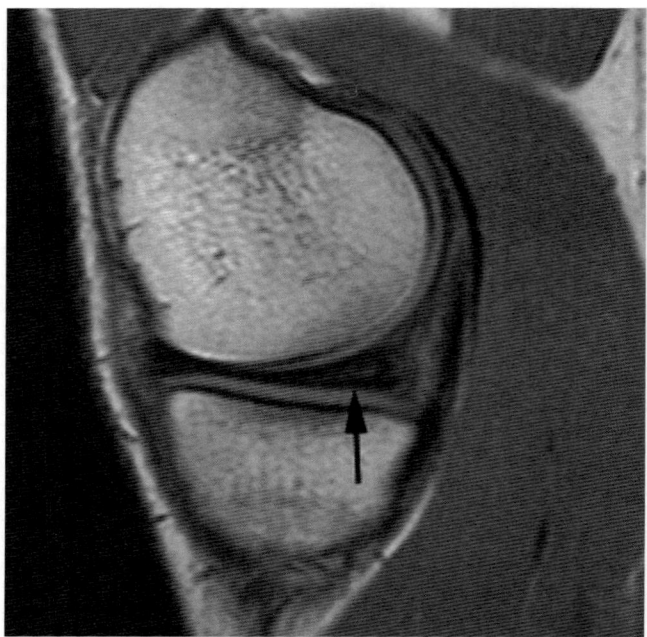

Fig. 1.6 Type 2 intra-meniscal signal change. Sagittal proton density image. The posterior horn of the medial meniscus is seen to contain linear increased signal. This does not contact the articular surface of the meniscus and represents type 2 signal change in the meniscus in keeping with intra-substance degeneration. No tear is shown

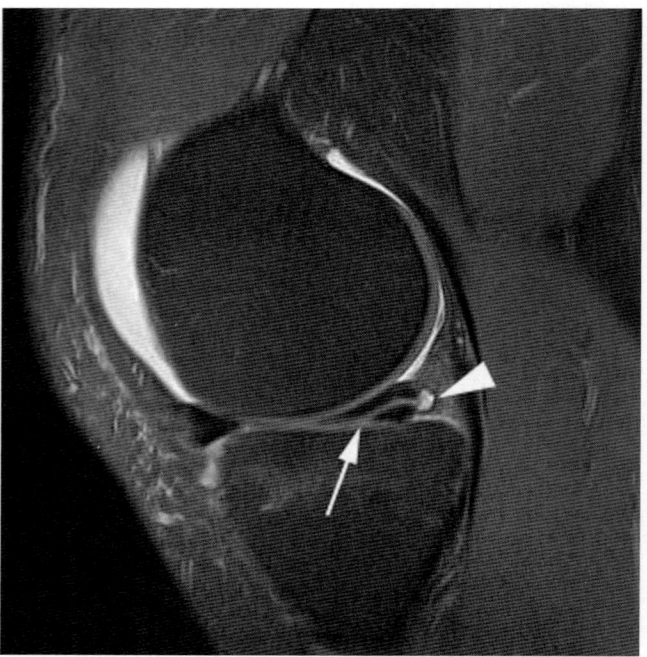

Fig. 1.7 Horizontal meniscal tear with small meniscal cyst. Sagittal proton density image with fat saturation. Linear high signal is seen extending horizontally to the inferior surface of the posterior horn of the medial meniscus (*arrow*) in keeping with a horizontal tear. A small parameniscal cyst (*arrowhead*) has formed at the outer edge of the meniscus

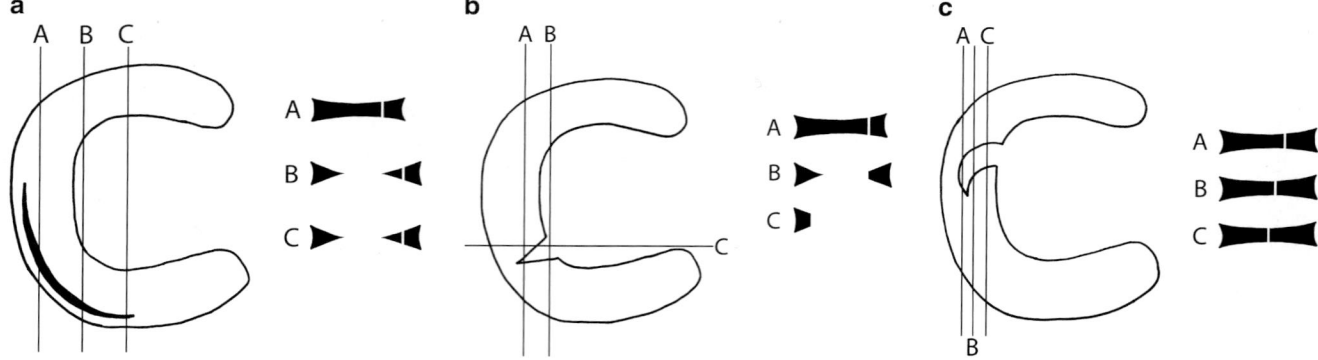

Fig. 1.8 Diagrams demonstrating the appearance of different meniscal tears on sections taken through the tear. (**a**) Peripheral longitudinal tear. (**b**) Radial tear. (**c**) Parrot beak tear

3. Radial tears are also vertically orientated but propagate perpendicular to the main meniscal axis.
4. Complex tears consist of components of two or more configurations.

Horizontal Tears

Tears running parallel to the tibial articular surface are also known as cleavage or horizontal tears. These tears may disrupt the superior or inferior surface of the meniscus, extending for a variable length into the substance of the meniscus (Fig. 1.7).

Longitudinal Tears

Typically longitudinal tears occur peripherally within the meniscus. Undisplaced peripheral longitudinal tears are characterised by abnormal high signal in the meniscus extending to both superior and inferior articular surfaces of the meniscus (Figs. 1.8a and 1.9). Displacement of the central meniscal fragment may occur and is referred to as a bucket handle tear; these are usually acute and represent approximately 10% of all meniscal tears [13]. The fragment usually displaces into the intercondylar notch. The sensitivity of MR imaging for the detection of bucket handle tears is less than that for other meniscal lesions [14]. Use of a coronal STIR sequence has been reported to significantly increase detection rates [15] and the authors find a coronal fat-suppressed PD or T2 sequence similarly helpful (Fig. 1.10). Several signs have been described to aid in the diagnosis of bucket handle tears (Table 1.2). In the sagittal plane, loss of the normal peripheral bow-tie configuration, or an inadequate number of bow-ties, suggests some of the meniscus is missing and should prompt further evaluation to identify displaced meniscal material. A double posterior cruciate ligament (PCL) sign has been described with bucket handle tears of the medial meniscus, the fragment lies in front of the PCL and is readily recognisable on sagittal imaging (Fig. 1.10b). Bucket handle tears of the lateral meniscus are associated with pseudo-tears of the anterior cruciate ligament as the meniscal fragment may lie just lateral to the ACL suggesting a tear (Fig. 1.11). Instead of displacing centrally into the intercondylar notch the meniscal fragment may flip anteriorly giving the appearance of a large anterior horn, the so-called flipped meniscus sign [13] (Fig. 1.4).

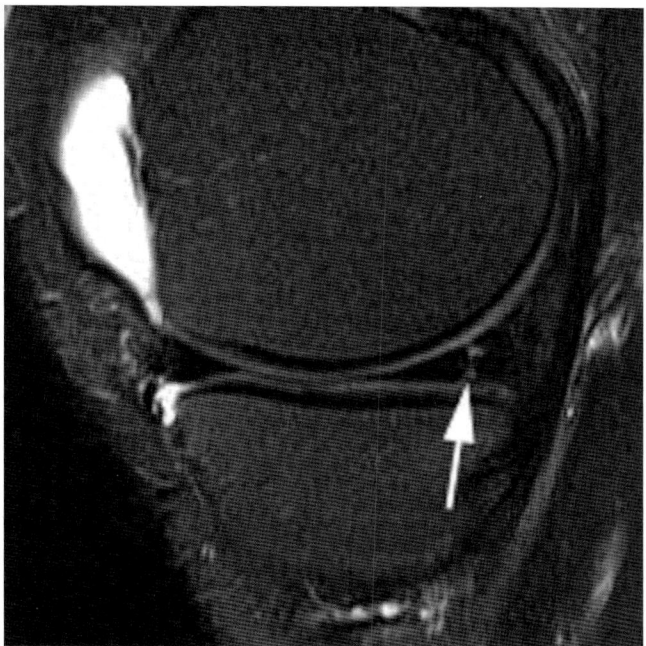

Fig. 1.9 Peripheral longitudinal meniscal tear. Sagittal proton density image with fat saturation. There is linear high signal extending from the superior to the inferior surface of the posterior horn of the medial meniscus (*arrow*). This represents a peripheral longitudinal tear

Table 1.2 Imaging findings in bucket handle tears

- Absent bow-ties
- Fragment in the intercondylar notch
- Double PCL sign
- ACL pseudo-tear
- Flipped meniscus

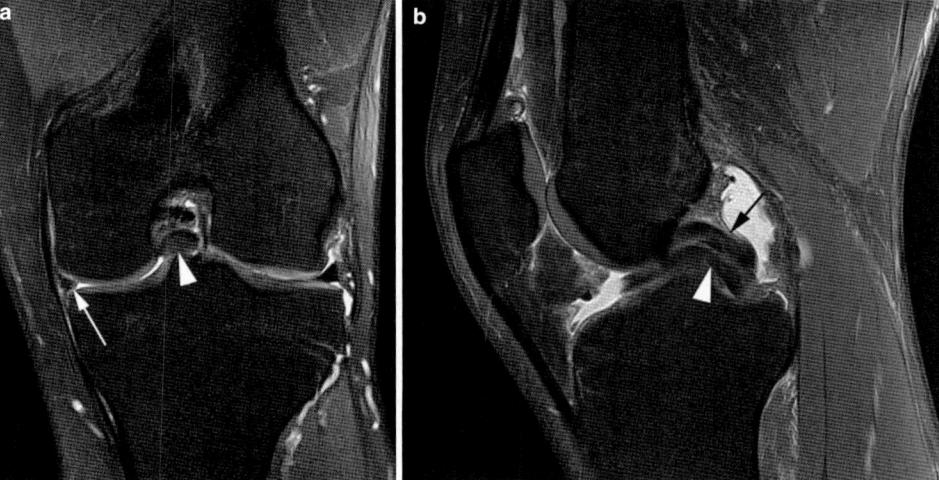

Fig. 1.10 Bucket handle meniscal tear with double PCL sign. Coronal (**a**) and sagittal (**b**) proton density images with fat saturation. (**a**) There is a bucket handle tear of the medial meniscus. The displaced meniscal material is seen in the intercondylar notch (*arrowhead*) while the body of the medial meniscus (*arrow*) is too small compared with the lateral meniscus. (**b**) The displaced meniscal material (*arrowhead*) lies in the intercondylar notch alongside the PCL (*arrow*) giving the impression of a double PCL, a characteristic sign

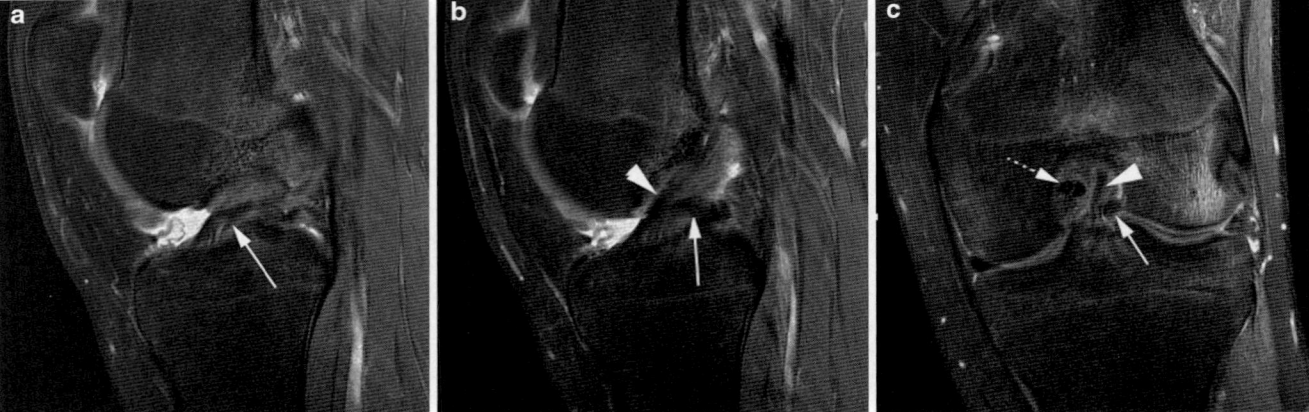

Fig. 1.11 Bucket handle meniscal tear with ACL pseudo-tear. Sagittal (**a** and **b**) and coronal (**c**) proton density images with fat saturation. (**a**) There is an abnormal appearance in the intercondylar notch (*arrow*) which was initially thought to represent a torn ACL. (**b**) The adjacent sagittal slice in fact confirms the ACL to be intact (*arrowhead*) but abnormal material is seen adjacent to the ACL in the intercondylar notch (*arrow*). (**c**) The coronal image confirms a bucket handle tear of the lateral meniscus with the displaced meniscal material (*arrow*) lying adjacent to the ACL (*arrowhead*). The PCL (*broken arrow*) is also seen in the intercondylar notch. The body of the lateral meniscus has an abnormal appearance as a result of the tear and there is extensive marrow oedema seen in the lateral femoral condyle

Table 1.3 Imaging findings in radial tears

- Truncated triangle
- Cleft sign
- Marching cleft
- Ghost meniscus

Radial Tears

Radial tears are purely vertical, orientated at 90° to the meniscal surface (Fig. 1.8b). The majority involve the posterior horns and bodies of the menisci [16]. MR imaging findings depend upon the position of the radial tear and four imaging signs have been described (Table 1.3). On sagittal and coronal images a radial tear can truncate the normal triangular shape of the meniscal horns (Fig. 1.12). A linear vertical cleft of high signal within the meniscus may also be evident (Fig. 1.13). Depending on position of the tear this may be present over successive images as the tear extends peripherally (Fig. 1.8c). When a radial tear is orientated in the plane of an image the meniscal signal may not be apparent, typically volume averaging causes a triangle of high signal not representative of the normal meniscus, termed the ghost meniscus (Fig. 1.12b).

Radial tears can have a more oblique orientation with respect to the main meniscal axis when they may be termed parrot beak tears. This subset of radial tears is unstable as they are prone to displacement of the meniscal fragment.

Meniscocapsular and Meniscal Root Injury

Tears may occur at the meniscal attachment to the joint capsule (meniscocapsular injury) or attachment to the tibia (meniscal root injury) (Fig. 1.14). When evaluating the MR imaging scan, it is important to follow the meniscus down to its tibial attachments to ensure they are intact. On MR imaging, meniscocapsular separation is seen as an increased distance between the capsule and the outer meniscal border and fluid is seen to separate the structures. It has been pointed out that these signs have a relatively high false-positive rate [17].

Meniscal Imaging with Other Modalities

Conventional Radiography

Although not able to demonstrate meniscal pathology, plain radiography remains a useful initial investigation following knee trauma. While suspected fracture is a clear indication, plain radiographs may also demonstrate loose bodies, chondrocalcinosis and other degenerative changes which may mimic meniscal symptoms.

Ultrasound

Ultrasonography (US) has low sensitivity and specificity in the diagnosis of meniscal tears and is generally not helpful in the assessment of acute meniscal trauma. The normal meniscus can be identified at the joint line as a triangular hypoechoic structure. However, the deeper components of the meniscus including the intra-articular free edge are not visualised. Meniscal tears are seen on US when they are peripheral and posterior. They typically appear as fluid-filled

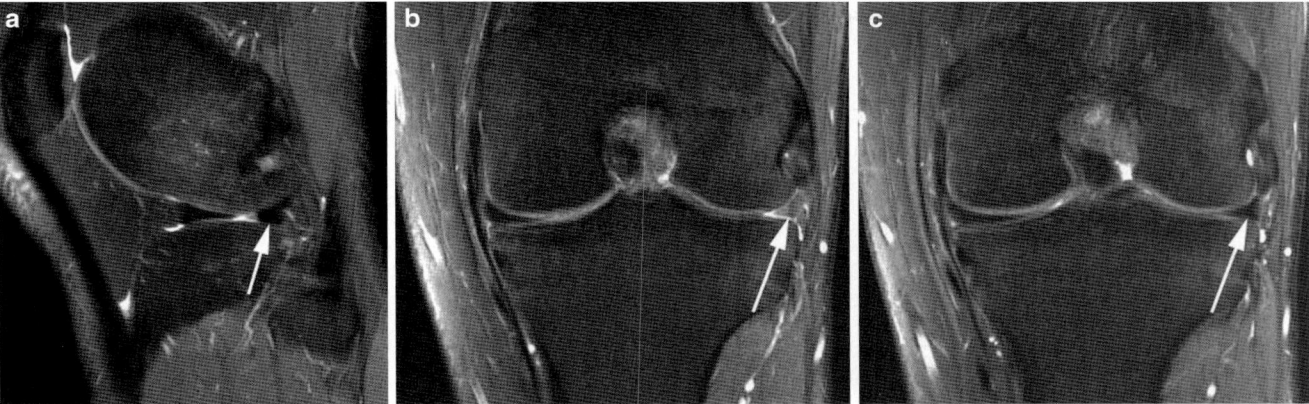

Fig. 1.12 Radial tear of meniscus. Sagittal (**a**) and coronal (**b** and **c**) proton density images with fat saturation. (**a**) There is truncation of the posterior horn of the lateral meniscus (*arrow*) in keeping with a radial tear. (**b**) This coronal image passes through the tear and the lateral meniscus appears as a "ghost" meniscus as a result (*arrow*). (**c**) The next slice posterior to **b** shows the normal appearance of the lateral meniscus adjacent to the tear (*arrow*)

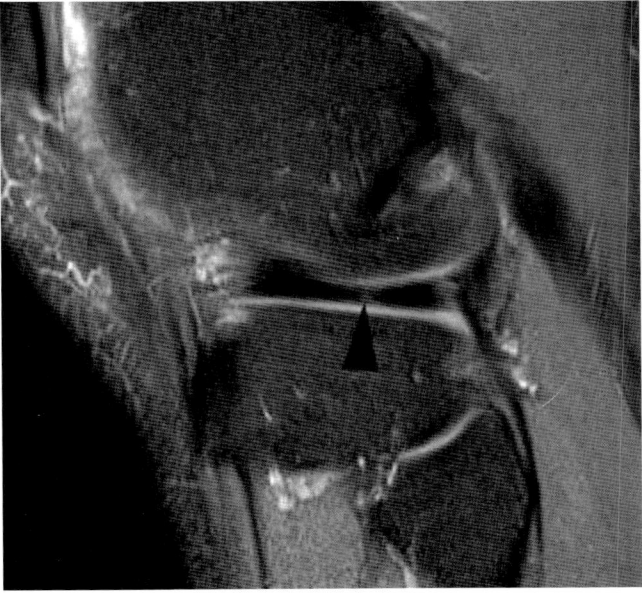

Fig. 1.13 Radial tear of meniscus. Sagittal proton density image with fat saturation. There is a radial tear seen as a vertical intermediate to high signal line passing through the "bow-tie" of the lateral meniscus

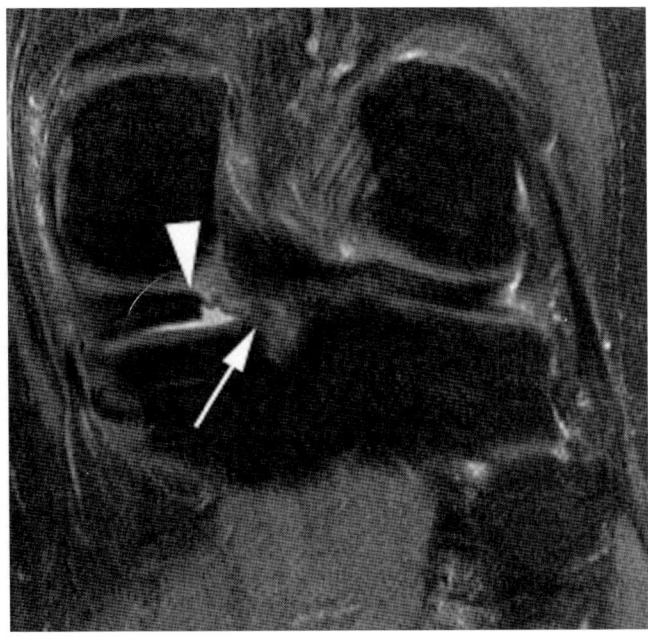

Fig. 1.14 Meniscal root tear. Coronal proton density image with fat saturation. There is a tear of the meniscal root of the posterior horn of the medial meniscus. The meniscal root shows abnormal increased signal (*arrow*). There is truncation of the posterior horn of the meniscus (*arrowhead*)

clefts within the meniscus. US has a role in the assessment of meniscal cysts, see later discussion.

Conventional and CT Arthrography

Conventional arthrography of the knee was once the imaging modality of choice for meniscal injury. It has now been superseded by cross-sectional imaging modalities. While MR imaging remains the first-line imaging modality of choice, CT arthrography can be useful in patients where MR imaging is contraindicated and may have a role in the investigation of the post-operative meniscus.

Meniscal Cysts

Meniscal cysts are relatively common and can either be contained within the substance of the meniscus or extend into the soft tissue structures surrounding the meniscus. They are usually associated with a meniscal tear and this should always be sought when a cyst is identified (Fig. 1.15). Although US is unreliable for meniscal tears, it is possible to evaluate parameniscal and peripheral intra-meniscal cysts

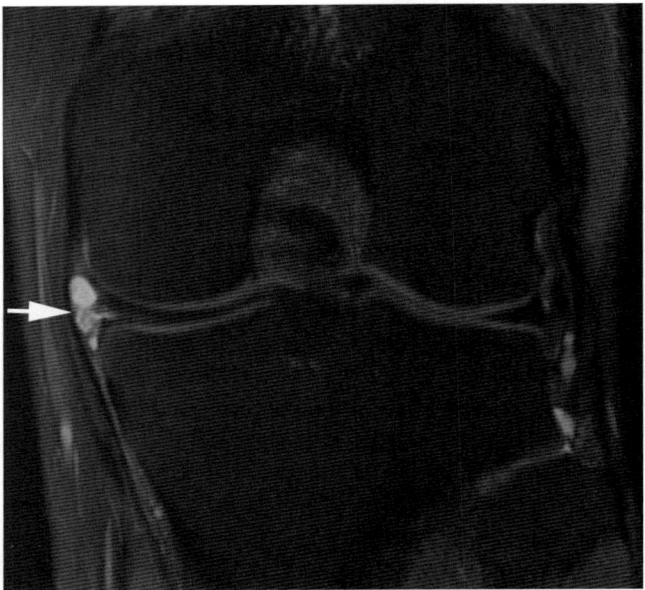

Fig. 1.15 Parameniscal cyst. Coronal proton density image with fat saturation. There is a parameniscal cyst (*arrow*) confined deep to the MCL arising from a, partly seen, horizontal tear in the meniscus

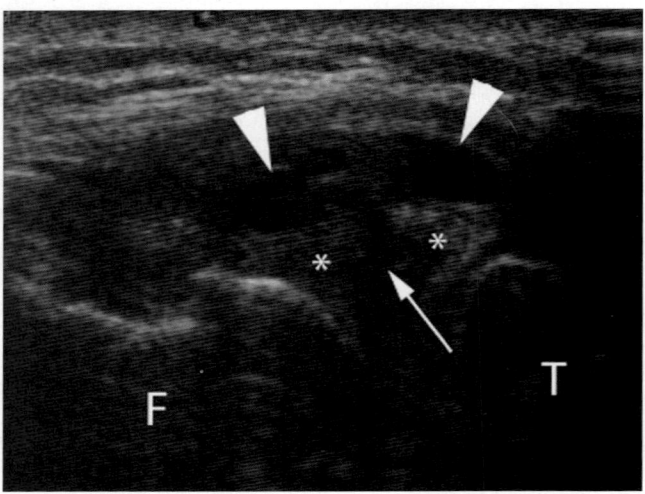

Fig. 1.16 Parameniscal cyst. Longitudinal ultrasound across the lateral knee joint line. There is a complex cystic structure in the lateral knee joint line (*arrowheads*) which arises from a horizontal tear (*arrow*) in the lateral meniscus (*). *F* lateral femoral condyle; *T* lateral tibial plateau

using sonography (Fig. 1.16). These are seen as encapsulated fluid-filled structures that are usually hypo- or anechoic.

The Post-operative Meniscus (also see Chapter 8)

Advances in meniscal surgery, together with an increasing desire for maximal meniscal preservation have generated a marked increase in the number of MR scans in patients who have undergone meniscal repair or partial resection and who have recurrent or persisting knee pain. Assessment of the menisci in this group provides new challenges as the usual criteria followed to diagnose a meniscal tear do not apply at the site of previous surgery. Despite this, for most authors, conventional MR imaging remains the modality of choice [18]. In the majority of cases, if less than 25% of the meniscus has been resected the usual diagnostic criteria may be applied. However, with more extensive resection these criteria become increasingly unreliable [19].

Abnormal signal may persist at the site of previous surgery for several years and is routinely evident for up to 12 months [20]. Partial resection of unstable meniscal material may result in adjacent intra-substance high signal now extending to an articular surface, giving the false appearance of a tear. Subsequent to a successful primary meniscal repair, evolving granulation tissue is evident for 6–12 months as increased short TE signal extending to the articular surface [20]. Assessment of meniscal morphology will also be unreliable, apparently absent tissue, blunting or truncation of the expected meniscal contour may all represent post-operative findings. The most specific sign of a recurrent tear is fluid signal tracking to the articular surface of the meniscus, although this has a sensitivity of only 60% [20].

The limitations of conventional MR imaging in the evaluation of the post-operative meniscus has prompted the use of both direct and indirect MR arthrography in this group. Strict diagnostic criteria are suggested and a tear should only be diagnosed when a displaced fragment is seen or when contrast enters the meniscal substance [21] (Fig. 1.17). MR arthrography has not been shown to be of additional benefit when there has been less than 25% meniscal resection [21].

CT arthrographic imaging of the post-operative meniscus is little studied but has been shown to have a likely comparable accuracy to direct MR arthrography [22].

The Cruciate Ligaments

The integrity of the cruciate ligaments is fundamental to the stability of the knee joint and their disruption represents a potentially career ending injury to the professional athlete. Injury is frequently accompanied by damage to other structures of the knee including the menisci, osteochondral surfaces, collateral ligaments and posterolateral and posteromedial corner structures.

Injury Grading

Cruciate ligament injury is graded from I to III (Table 1.4), Grade III injuries are complete tears while the lower-grade injuries represent partial tears or ligamentous sprains. Partial tears of the ACL frequently involve the AM bundle

1 Knee Injuries

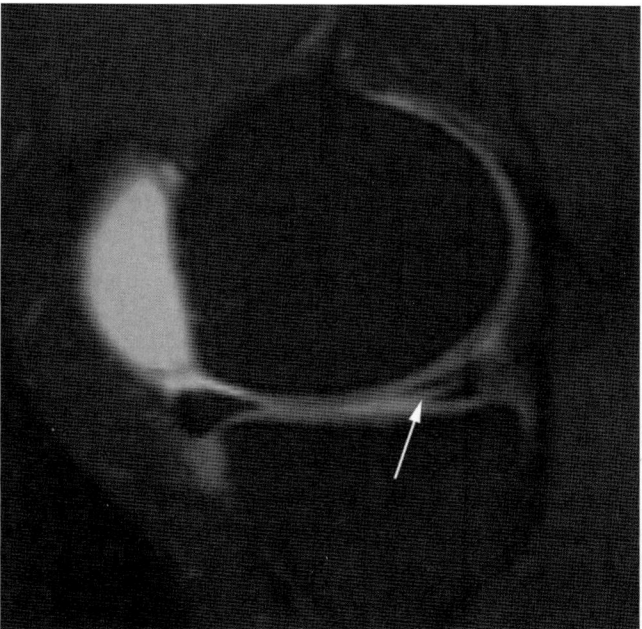

Fig. 1.17 Recurrent meniscal tear on MR arthrography. MR arthrogram: sagittal T1-weighted image with fat saturation following intra-articular gadolinium. The patient has previously undergone a partial medial meniscectomy. The MR arthrogram shows high signal contrast tracking into a recurrent horizontal tear in the residual posterior horn of the meniscus (*arrow*)

Table 1.4 Ligament injury grading

I	Intraligamentous injury without change in ligament length
II	Intraligamentous injury with increase in ligament length
III	Complete ligamentous disruption

and are important to recognise as they have a poor ability to heal and may progress to complete tears.

Imaging

MR imaging is the imaging modality of choice for diagnosing knee ligament injury. Not only does it readily identify the ligament disruption but it is also able to show concomitant injury to the menisci, collateral ligaments and posterolateral and posteromedial corner complexes.

Conventional Radiographs and CT

In the acute situation the presence of an effusion or lipohaemarthrosis raises suspicion of a significant knee injury. Disruption of cruciate function may occur as a result of avulsion of the ligament from the tibia and in this case the avulsion fragment may be demonstrated (Fig. 1.18). This is particularly common in children and adolescents.

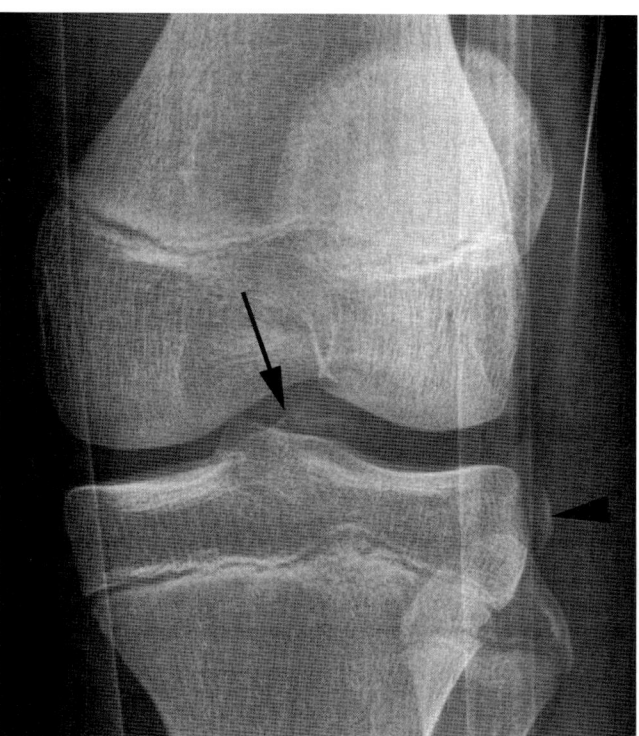

Fig. 1.18 ACL avulsion fracture with Segond fracture. AP radiograph. There is an avulsion fracture at the insertion of the ACL (*arrow*) This is associated with a Segond fracture from the lateral rim of the tibia (*arrowhead*). The artefact on the image is due to a knee splint worn by the patient

The Segond fracture, an avulsion from the lateral tibial rim, is a highly specific finding for anterior cruciate ligament injury and will be discussed further below.

MR Imaging

Plane Selection

The cruciate ligaments run obliquely to the normal orthogonal planes. In an attempt to obtain sections along the line of the ACL, sagittal imaging of the knee joint is generally carried out with around 20° of internal rotation relative to the true sagittal plane. However, it is important to recognise that cruciate ligament injury is often better assessed on the axial and coronal images and imaging in all three planes is desirable.

Normal MR Imaging Appearances

The cruciate ligaments have low signal on all sequences, but the ACL contains linear areas of fat and connective tissue between fascicles, seen as intermediate/high signal interposed between fibres (Fig. 1.19a). Although, it is not generally possible to differentiate the two ACL bundles on sagittal sequences they can be distinguished on other imaging planes (Fig. 1.19b, c).

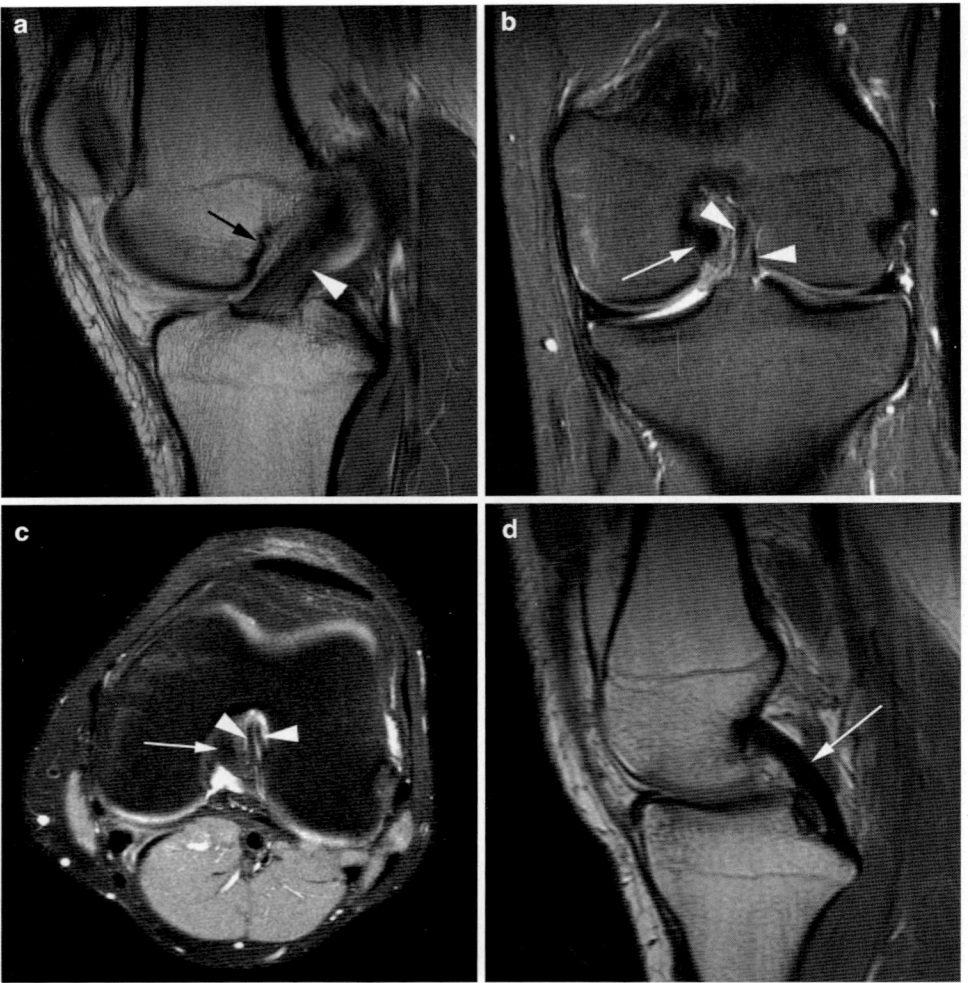

Fig. 1.19 Normal ACL and PCL. Sagittal proton density (**a** and **d**), coronal (**b**) and axial (**c**) proton density images with fat saturation. (**a**) Normal ACL (*arrowhead*). Blumensaat's line representing the roof of the intercondylar notch is also seen (*arrow*). Note how the course of the ACL parallels the line. (**b** and **c**) On coronal and axial imaging the two component bundles of the ACL can be appreciated (*arrowheads*). The PCL is also seen in the intercondylar notch (*arrow*). (**d**) Normal PCL (*arrow*). The PCL has a homogenous low signal appearance in contrast to the appearances of the ACL (compare with **a**)

The PCL appears as a homogenous low signal cord like bundle (Fig. 1.19d). As described previously, the meniscofemoral ligaments where present pass anterior and/or posterior to the ligament. Magic angle artefact may cause some signal variation in the proximal third of the PCL on gradient echo and short TE imaging.

Anterior Cruciate Ligament Tears

Mechanism of Injury

In sports activity the majority of ACL injuries occur as a result of non-contact trauma. High-risk sports include downhill skiing, soccer, gymnastics and lacrosse. The ACL is at particular risk during landing, twisting and deceleration, particularly when the knee is in near full extension. The classic mechanism is seen in downhill skiing where the skier falls forward catching the inside edge of the ski forcing the tibia to externally rotate in valgus stress. Seen also in other sports this mechanism characteristically causes lateral compartment contusion and is associated with meniscal and posterolateral capsular injury. In soccer, most ACL injuries occur due to hyperextension caused by force to the anterior tibia with the foot planted, a typical tackling injury. Associated meniscal and PCL injuries are common. Clip injuries, seen particularly in American football cause ACL injury during pure valgus stress to a partly flexed knee, a high proportion have MCL and/or meniscal injury.

MR Imaging

The primary signs of an ACL tear are alterations of the signal characteristics and morphology of the ligament (Table 1.5). It is important to assess ligament continuity and signal using all three planes. Loss of continuity or abnormal intra-substance signal are accurate signs of tear (Fig. 1.20). The roof of the intercondylar notch, also known as Blumensaat's line closely parallels the course of the normal ACL (Fig. 1.19a). Loss of the normal parallel configuration, as the torn ACL sags away from the roof of the notch is a sensitive sign of a tear (Fig. 1.21). Chronic ACL tears may result in atrophy of the ACL so that no residual tissue is discernable.

Secondary signs are useful but their absence does not exclude an ACL tear (Table 1.5). Anterior tibial translation is seen less often in athletes with ACL rupture due to increased musculature, but when evident it is an indirect indicator of ACL deficiency. On sagittal images normally a vertical line from the posterolateral femoral condyle should intersect the posterolateral tibial plateau when the ACL is intact. Anterior

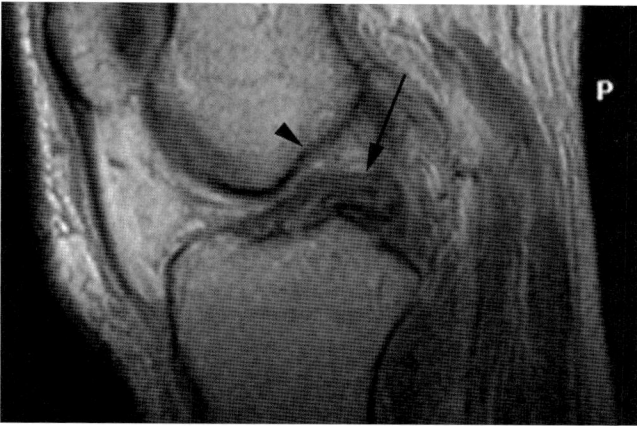

Fig. 1.21 ACL tear. Sagittal proton density image. The anterior margin of the ACL (*arrow*) is no longer parallel to the roof of the intercondylar notch (*arrowhead*)

translation may also cause buckling or hooking of the PCL as long as it is intact. Impaction of the posterior tibia on the lateral femoral condyle results in corresponding bone contusions which are valuable secondary signs of ACL rupture (Fig. 1.22). A fracture of the lateral tibial rim, termed a Segond fracture, although an infrequent finding, has a very high association with ACL injury. These may be difficult to appreciate on MR imaging due to their small size and surrounding oedema [23] (Figs. 1.18 and 1.22).

Partial tears are suggested by focal signal abnormality in an otherwise apparently intact ligament, or kinking or buckling of the ligament. It may be possible to identify loss of a single bundle on coronal or axial sequences (Fig. 1.23).

Associated injury is frequently seen with both full and partial thickness ACL disruption. Up to 70% of high-grade ACL injuries are accompanied by meniscal pathology and PCL and MCL tears are also common. Posterolateral corner injury is important to identify as it is thought to represent the most common cause of failed ACL repair [24].

Table 1.5 MRI features of ACL tear

Primary	Secondary
Ligament discontinuity	Anterior tibial translation
Abnormal ligament course	Lateral compartment bony contusion
Abnormal ligament signal characteristic	Posteromedial tibial plateau contusion
	Segond fracture

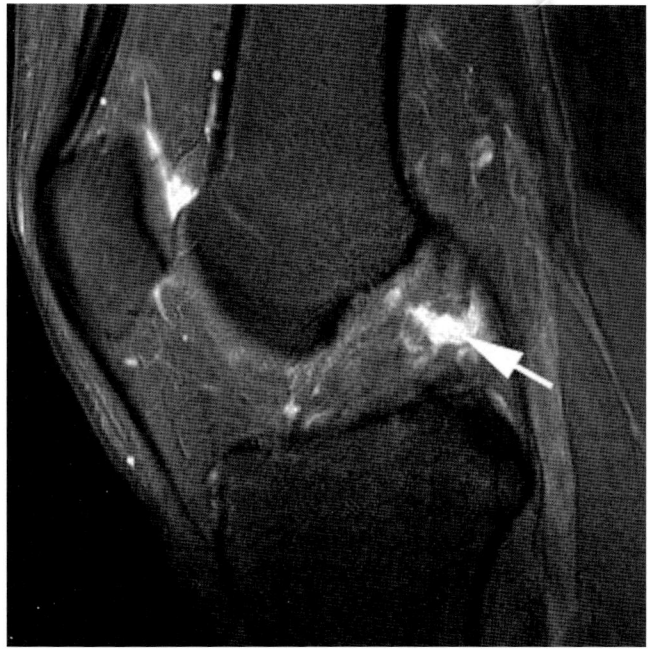

Fig. 1.20 ACL tear. Sagittal T2-weighted image with fat saturation. The normal morphology of the ACL has been lost and a high signal tear is seen through its substance (*arrow*)

Posterior Cruciate Ligament Tears

The PCL has higher tensile strength enabling it to resist force more readily than the ACL and it is injured considerably less frequently. The majority of PCL tears occur in association with ACL tears. Unlike the ACL, PCL injury is most often seen in contact sport although a high percentage occur in track and field events and soccer. In the general population the dashboard injury is the most common mechanism with force applied to the anterior tibia. In sport this is replicated by a fall onto a flexed knee. As with the ACL, acute complete tears show replacement of normal fibre structure by amorphous high signal intensity (Fig. 1.24).

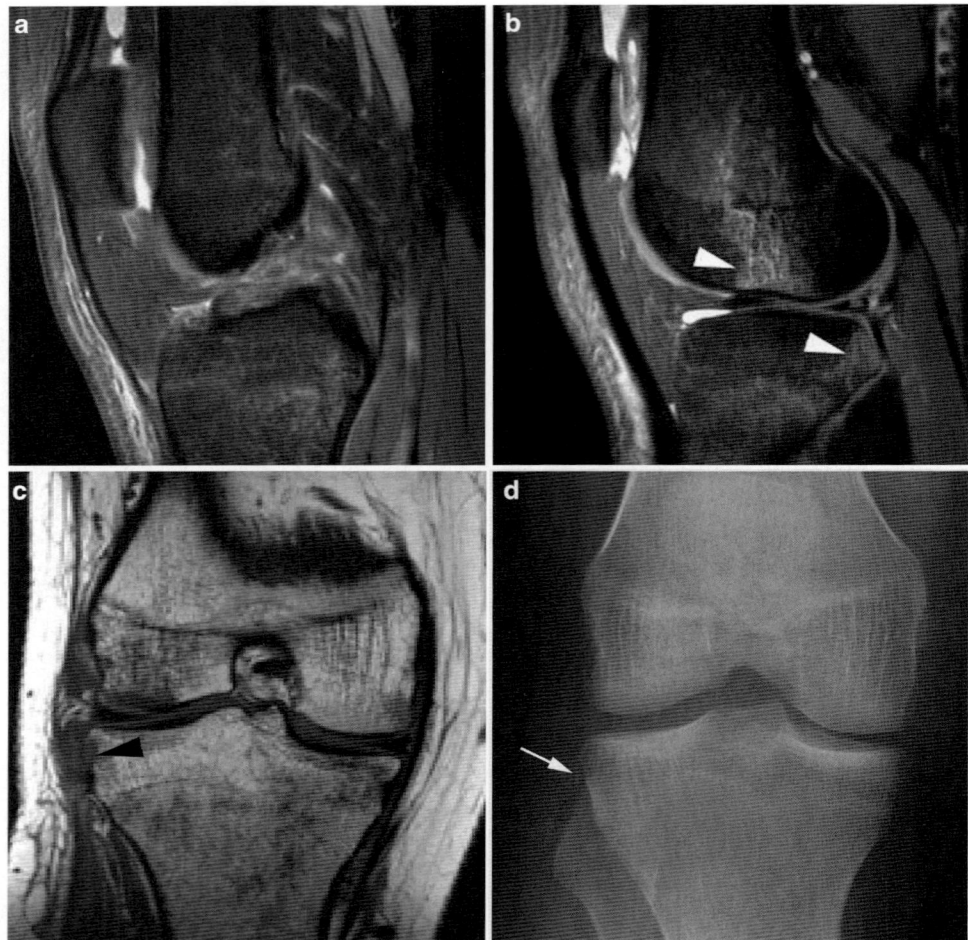

Fig. 1.22 ACL tear with bone bruise and Segond fracture. Sagittal proton density with fat saturation (**a** and **b**) and coronal T1 (**c**) images and AP radiograph (**d**). (**a**) There is a full thickness ACL tear with no visible normal ACL material. The intercondylar notch is filled with debris. (**b**) This section is taken through the lateral joint compartment. It shows the characteristic, associated bone bruise pattern involving the central aspect of the lateral femoral condyle and posterior aspect of the tibial plateau (*arrowheads*). There is also a tear of the posterior horn of the lateral meniscus. (**c** and **d**) Although there is evidence of soft tissue damage to the lateral aspect of the knee and there looks to be a bone defect in the lateral tibial epiphyses (*arrowhead*) the Segond avulsion fracture is not as clearly shown as it is on the plain film (*arrow*)

With incomplete tears, partial ligament continuity is evident. Partial tears are more common than complete rupture on MR imaging [25].

Associated injuries include meniscal tears although this is less common than is seen with ACL tears. Conversely collateral ligament injury is seen more frequently with PCL than with ACL injuries [25]. Bony injury is variably reported but is more likely when the PCL injury is not isolated and particularly involves the anterior aspect of the knee joint [25].

A high percentage of PCL tears are associated with injury to the posterolateral corner. This may be minor without clinical instability but it is vital to identify those with more significant trauma since, as with the ACL, failure to repair the posterolateral corner at the time of ligamentous repair leads to a significantly higher rate of surgical failure [25]. While many surgeons advocate non-operative management of an isolated PCL tear, this is less certain in the athletic population.

Post-operative Imaging (also see Chapter 8)

The ACL is most usually repaired with autologous graft, and patellar tendon and hamstring grafts have been most frequently used. Immediately following surgery grafts are avascular with low signal intensity lasting for several weeks. Over time, the graft becomes enveloped by synovial tissue causing increased signal within the graft. Finally, by 2 years the graft undergoes ligamentisation and gains signal intensity similar to that of normal ACL [26].

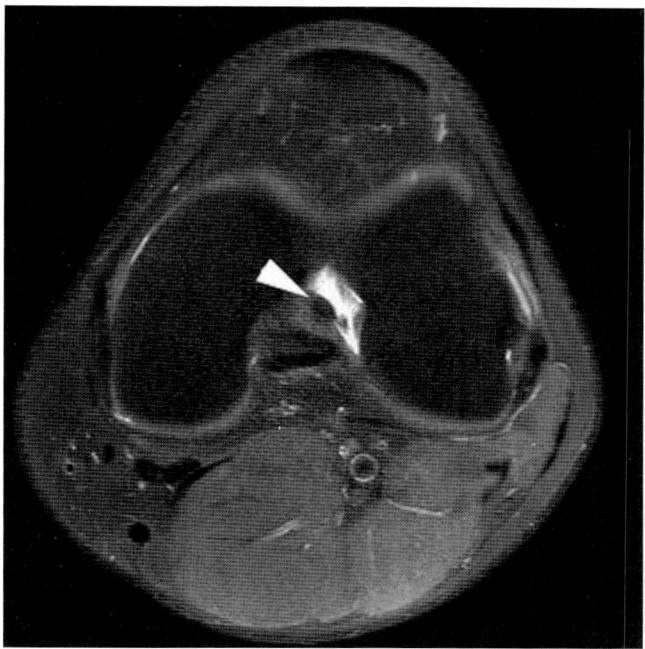

Fig. 1.23 Partial thickness ACL tear. Axial proton density with fat saturation image: Partial thickness tear of the ACL. Fluid seen in the lateral aspect of the intercondylar notch is at the site of the disrupted posterolateral bundle which itself is not visualised. The anteromedial bundle is seen to be intact (*arrowhead*)

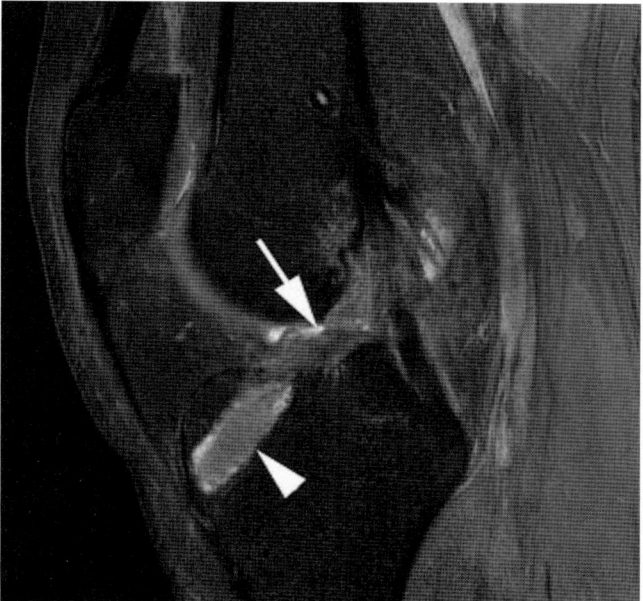

Fig. 1.25 ACL graft disruption. Sagittal PD image. There is complete disruption of the ACL graft. The tibial tunnel (*arrowhead*) is seen to lie anterior to the intercondylar notch roof (*arrow*)

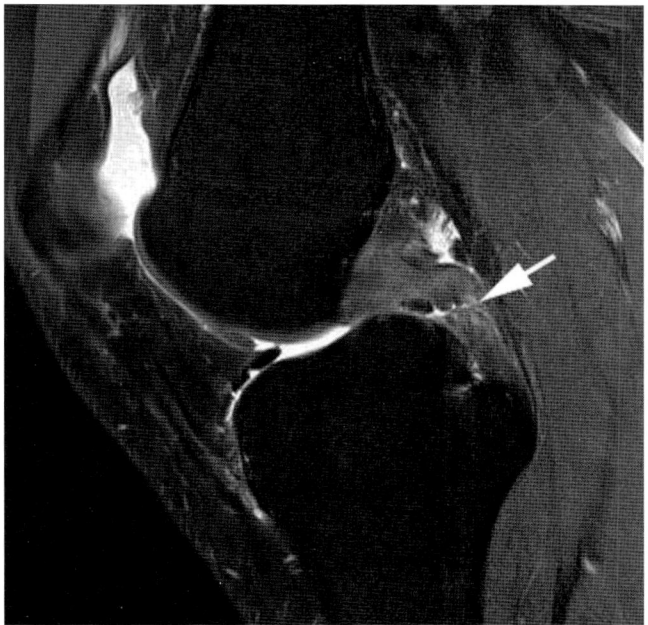

Fig. 1.24 PCL tear. Sagittal T2-weighted image. The PCL shows diffusely abnormal signal with a discontinuity (*arrow*). The appearances are of a full thickness PCL tear

MR imaging allows assessment of the autologous graft donor site and other internal knee structures as well as the graft. Femoral and tibial tunnel position can be accurately evaluated using plain radiography. Position of the femoral tunnel is crucial in maintaining graft tension and length throughout knee movement. An anteriorly placed femoral tunnel is one of the most common errors of graft placement and results in knee instability. Incorrect positioning of the tibial tunnel is also important to recognise; if the tunnel is too anterior it places the graft at risk of impingement against the intercondylar roof, eventually leading to graft breakdown (Fig. 1.25). When correctly positioned, lateral radiographs will show the tibial tunnel to be posterior and parallel to the slope of the intercondylar roof. Tunnel expansion occurs more commonly in hamstring graft repairs but thus far has not been shown to result in clinical instability in the short term [27]. Arthrofibrosis, the formation of a fibrous tissue anterior to the ACL graft that acts to mechanically impede extension, is a recognised complication of ACL reconstruction. MR imaging provides information on graft integrity and can identify such changes.

Cruciate Ganglion Cysts

Ganglia of the ACL are rare, seen in around 1.3% of knee MR studies, and ganglion cysts of the PCL are even less frequent [28]. The aetiology of cruciate ganglia is uncertain but is likely to be related to previous trauma. Their appearance can be variable ranging from locules of fluid interspersed between ligament fibres to well-defined cysts adjacent to the ligament (Fig. 1.26). Although the majority are asymptomatic, a small number of patients experience pain, usually activity related and in this situation the ganglion cyst can be treated successfully at arthroscopy.

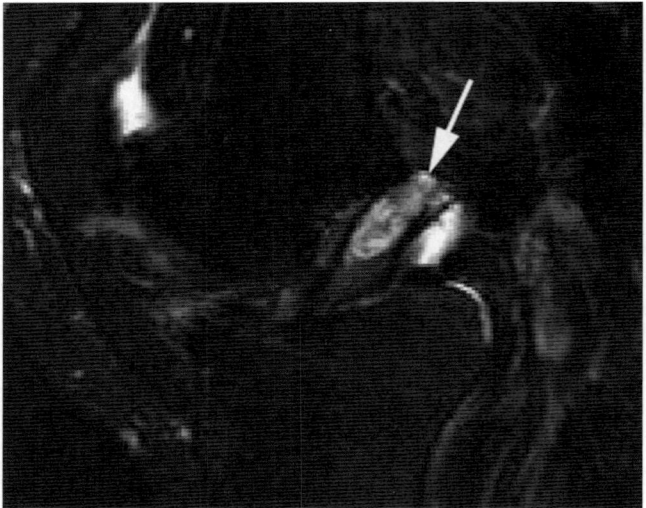

Fig. 1.26 ACL ganglion cyst. Sagittal T2-weighted image. There is a complex cystic structure seen within the substance of the ACL representing a ganglion cyst (*arrow*)

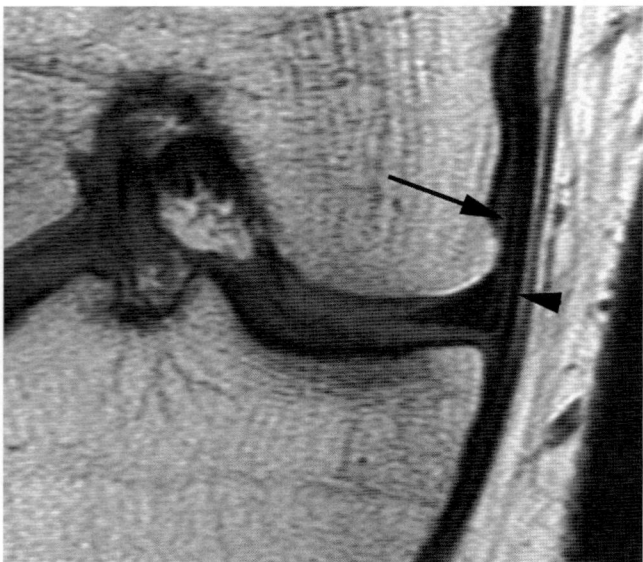

Fig. 1.27 Normal MCL. Coronal T1-weighted image: Both superficial (*arrowhead*) and deep meniscofemoral (*arrow*) components of the MCL are demonstrated as low signal lines

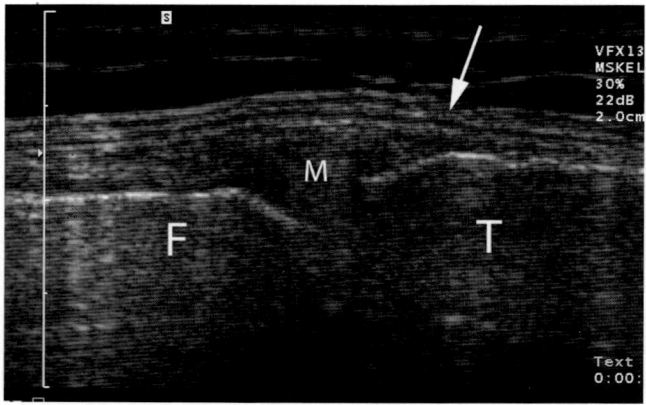

Fig. 1.28 Normal MCL. Longitudinal US across the medial joint line: The MCL is seen as a trilaminar structure (*arrow*). In this patient the medial meniscus (M) is partially extruded from the joint line. *F* medial femoral condyle; *T* medial tibial plateau

Collateral Ligaments and Posterior Corner Injuries

The collateral ligaments are superficial structures and are readily visible at US. However, MR imaging remains the primary imaging modality of choice allowing the identification of concomitant injury to other structures such as the cruciate ligaments and menisci not seen at US.

Normal Imaging Appearances

The superficial MCL is typically seen on coronal imaging as a low signal band between 8 and 11 cm in length. Coronal imaging will demonstrate the meniscofemoral and meniscotibial components of the deep MCL as well as the intervening MCL bursa. Axial and medial sagittal images are more useful in evaluation of the oblique popliteal ligament and the adjacent pes anserine tendons (Fig. 1.27).

The MCL is seen as a trilaminar structure on ultrasound comprising the superficial and deep layers separated by a thin layer of connective tissue (Fig. 1.28).

The LCL runs obliquely and so is not usually seen in its entirety on a single coronal MR image. The axial plane and peripheral sagittal images are particularly useful in evaluation of the posterolateral corner; however, these anatomically variable structures may be difficult to fully visualise and some authors propose an oblique coronal sequence to better demonstrate the arcuate, fabellofibular and popliteofibular ligaments [29]. In practise, the LCL and popliteus tendons are readily identified with conventional imaging and more detailed imaging of the posterolateral corner is rarely necessary (Fig. 1.29).

Ultrasound identifies the iliotibial band and LCL as linear structures. It is able to demonstrate the popliteus tendon at its insertion but the structure becomes harder to follow as it passes distally and deeper.

Medial Collateral Complex

The fibres of the deep MCL are relatively weak and are the first to tear following injury which results from valgus stress; these fibres do not significantly contribute to joint stability and so most MCL tears do not cause instability [30].

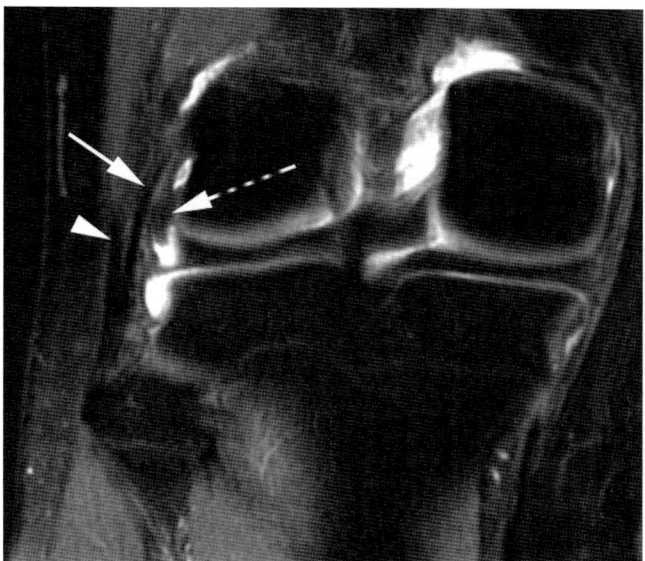

Fig. 1.29 Normal lateral structures. Coronal T2-weighted image with fat saturation. Parts of the distal biceps femoris tendon (*arrowhead*), lateral collateral ligament (*arrow*) and popliteus tendon (*dotted arrow*) are demonstrated. Note how the lateral collateral ligament and biceps tendon combine to form a conjoint tendon

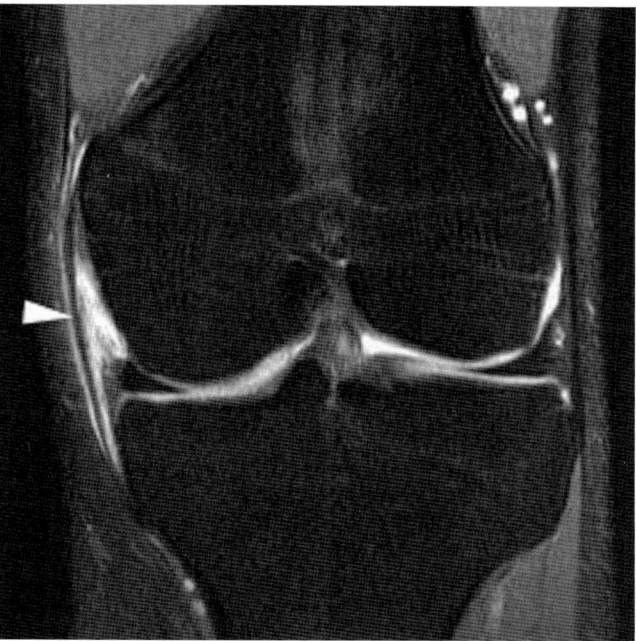

Fig. 1.30 Grade 2 MCL tear. Coronal proton density image with fat saturation. Although the superficial fibres of the MCL are intact (*arrowhead*), they are surrounded by high signal oedema and haemorrhage and there is disruption of the deep components of the MCL. The meniscotibial ligament is seen to be intact but there is disruption of the meniscofemoral ligament

Isolated MCL tears are common but associated ACL injury is frequently encountered, particularly with higher grade MCL tears. PCL and meniscal injury may also be seen.

Subcutaneous oedema seen as irregular fluid signal within the superficial fat adjacent to the MCL may be evident in grade I MCL injury and is most conspicuous using fat-suppressed T2-weighted sequences. Grade II tears demonstrate intra-substance signal abnormality as well as surrounding oedema and haemorrhage including fluid in the MCL bursa, fascial oedema has been reported as the most sensitive finding in grade II MCL injury [30] (Fig. 1.30). In addition, partial ligament discontinuity may be seen. Complete tears of the MCL constitute grade III injury but may be difficult to distinguish from high-grade partial tears. Disruption of the MCL can also be seen with ultrasound and a dynamic assessment of the ligament can help distinguish the grade 3 from a severe grade 2 injury.

Ossification occurring within the MCL, referred to as Pelligrini–Stieda disease, may be seen as a sequelae of trauma and is readily visualised on plain films, US and MR imaging.

Lateral Collateral Complex and Posterolateral Corner

Injury to the LCL occurs less frequently than to the MCL and unlike the MCL, isolated tears are rare. Tears of the LCL occur due to varus stress and the posterolateral structures are at risk in hyperextension with external rotation. Posterolateral corner injuries are typically seen in complex knee trauma combined with cruciate, medial ligamentous, capsular and meniscal injury. Undiagnosed posterolateral corner trauma is increasingly recognised as a cause of chronic instability, pain and early degenerative changes and has a deleterious effect on cruciate repair [31].

Lower-grade injuries are seen on MR imaging as oedema and haemorrhage around the LCL which may be thickened or lax. Ligament discontinuity indicates a grade 3 injury (Fig. 1.31). Avulsion of the attachments of the conjoined tendon of biceps femoris and the LCL and posterolateral structures to the fibular head can be seen on MR imaging and plain radiography (Fig. 1.32). It is known as the arcuate sign and signifies a significant injury. As previously noted, avulsion fractures of the lateral tibial rim, referred to as Segond fractures, have a strong association with concomitant ACL tears.

Injuries to popliteus and the other posterolateral corner structures are more conspicuous on fat-suppressed axial and sagittal imaging. Increased signal intensity within the popliteus muscle and tendon indicates injury to these structures. Isolated popliteus tears do occur but are rare and typically there is involvement of the other posterolateral ligaments (Fig. 1.31). As the popliteus tendon is intra-articular care should be taken not misinterpret extension of fluid from the knee joint around the popliteus as an injury to the popliteus or posterior corner.

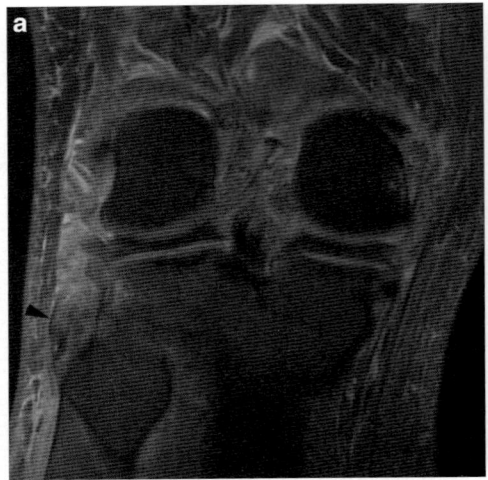 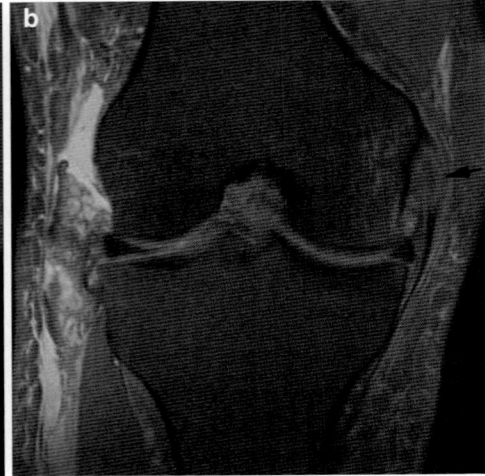

Fig. 1.31 Complex LCL and Posterolateral corner disruption with ACL tear. Coronal proton density weighted images with fat saturation. (**a**) There is extensive, abnormal, increased signal over the lateral aspect of the joint with full thickness disruption of the LCL and popliteus tendon. The residual stump of the conjoint tendon is visible with abnormal increased signal at its insertion into the fibular head (*arrowhead*). (**b**) A more anterior section shows further disruption of the lateral capsular tissues. The intercondylar notch is filled with amorphous tissue reflecting the ACL and PCL disruption sustained by this patient. There is also evidence of MCL disruption (*arrow*)

Tendinopathy and Overuse Injuries

Given the fundamental role the knee plays in many sporting activities it is little wonder that it is susceptible to a variety of overuse injuries. Generally, these result from repetitive microtrauma or abnormal joint mechanics and imaging has an important role to play in their diagnosis and on occasional treatment.

Patellar Tendinopathy

The patellar tendon is a vital component of the extensor mechanism extending from the patella to the tibial tuberosity. Its shadow may be seen on plain films but ultrasound and MR imaging prove the mainstay for imaging this superficial structure.

Although the patellar tendon is often considered to originate from the lower pole and anterior aspect of the patella, anatomical studies show that a component of the patellar tendon represents a direct extension, over the anterior aspect of the patella, of the deeper fibres of the rectus femoris component of the quadriceps tendon [32]. This direct continuation of fibres can be appreciated on ultrasound.

The patellar tendon is a large tendon with a ribbon-like shape, being relatively thin in the sagittal plane (typically 3 to 4 mm) but with considerable axial width which increases more proximally closer to the patellar attachment. The normal tendon should not exceed 7 mm in sagittal diameter. Anteriorly, the tendon is covered with subcutaneous fat and the pre-patella bursa, while

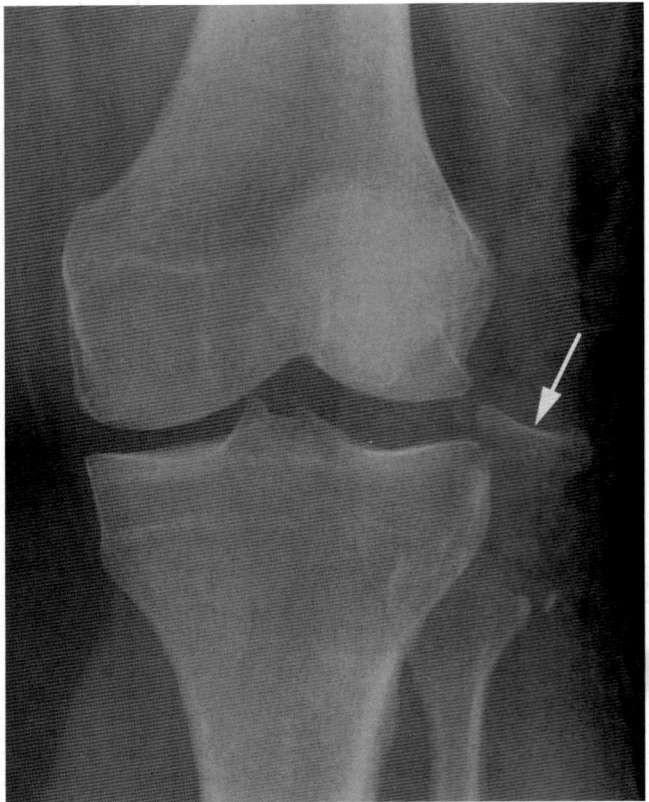

Fig. 1.32 Arcuate sign. AP radiograph. There is an avulsion fracture from the fibular head (*arrow*) representing an avulsion of the LCL and distal biceps tendon. This is a marker for a significant knee injury

its deep surface is in contact with Hoffa's fat pad. It does not have a tendon sheath but is surrounded by a paratenon composed of vascularised connective and adipose tissue.

Conventional MR imaging shows the patellar tendon to be of low signal on all sequences. Ultrasound is able to provide high-resolution imaging of the patellar tendon given its superficial location. It is best seen when taut, achieved by examining the tendon with the knee in around 30° of flexion.

Patellar tendinopathy represents chronic degeneration of the patellar tendon at its insertion into the lower pole of the patellar. It is thought to be the result of chronic micro-trauma and maybe associated with micro-tearing of the tendon. As its alternative name of "Jumpers Knee" suggests it is relatively common in sports involving jumping, and is also seen in athletes who sprint or cycle. It usually presents with anterior knee pain classically localised to the lower pole of the patella. The condition is readily diagnosed on both ultrasound and MR imaging.

On MR imaging the patellar tendon is best studied on sagittal and axial imaging. In patellar tendinopathy thickening of the tendon is seen at the site of disease and this is associated with intermediate to high signal change seen on all sequences. The fact that the signal change is also seen on T2 imaging is useful in distinguishing tendinopathy from the magic angle effect which will only be visible on short TE sequences. The signal change seen on T2 imaging is usually intermediate; when high signal change is seen on this sequence it indicates cystic degeneration or partial thickness tearing. The deep margin of the patellar tendon may become indistinct at the site of tendinopathy and there may be oedematous change in the adjacent Hoffa's fat pad (Fig. 1.33).

Classically, the area of abnormality is extremely focal involving only a portion of the cross-sectional area of the tendon, most commonly the medial portion [33].

Ultrasound demonstrates discrete thickening of the patellar tendon at the site of tendinopathy (Fig. 1.34). The involved tendon will show a loss of the normal fibrillar structure seen on ultrasound with low reflective change present. The area of abnormal tendon may show neovascularisation when examined with colour or power Doppler. Although ultrasound examination of the tendon is normally undertaken with the knee in 30° of flexion, vascularity is best demonstrated with the knee

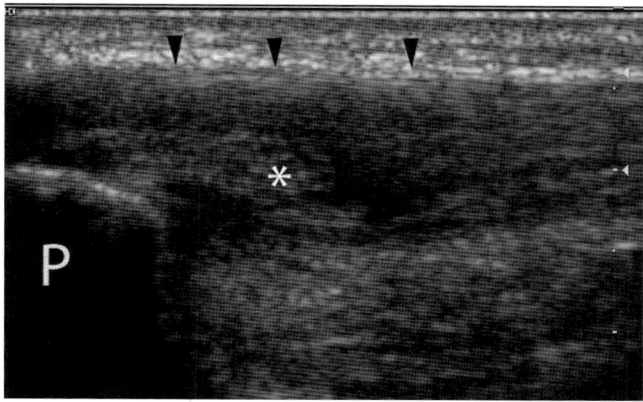

Fig. 1.34 Patellar tendinopathy (jumper's knee). Longitudinal US over the proximal patellar tendon. The deep fibres of the patellar tendon (*) have lost their normal striated appearance with a heterogenous amorphous appearance. Areas of very low reflectivity are seen within the tendon (either side of *) and are likely to represent intra-substance tearing. Note the normal appearance of the most superficial fibres (*arrowheads*) as seen in Fig. 1.33. *P* lower pole of the patella

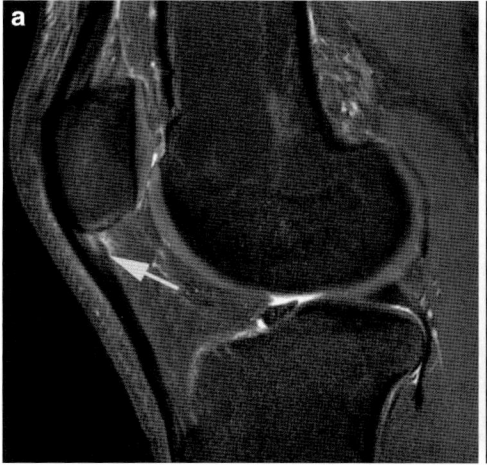
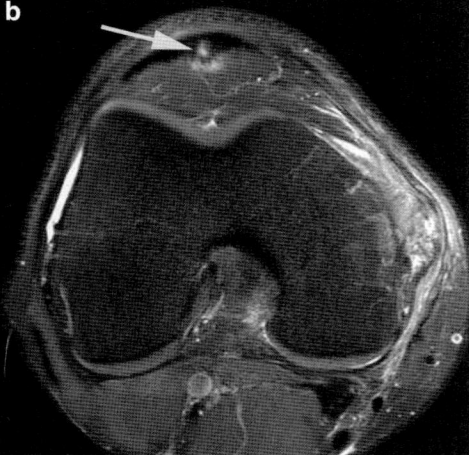

Fig. 1.33 Patellar tendinopathy (jumper's knee). Sagittal (**a**) and axial (**b**) proton density images with fat saturation. (**a**) The proximal patellar tendon is abnormally thickened with abnormal high signal within its deep fibres (*arrow*). Note also the signal change in the adjacent Hoffa's fat pad. The normal appearance to the more superficial fibres is typical. (**b**) The axial image demonstrates the very focal nature of the disease (*arrow*) and again shows the fat pad signal change. The location is very typical, slightly medial of the midline

extended which relaxes the tendon enabling vessels to demonstrate flow. With the tendon under tension these vessels tend to be occluded and the degree of neovascularisation underestimated. Examination with Doppler ensures vessels are not confused with fissure tears or cystic degeneration which may occur and will also appear as localised anechoic foci.

There are few comparison studies between ultrasound and MR imaging for patellar tendinopathy. One study showed a correlation between both MR imaging and ultrasound when compared with histopathology [34]. However, the technology of both MR imaging and ultrasound has advanced considerably since that paper was published.

Although the classic site for patellar tendinopathy as discussed above is in the proximal patellar tendon, tendinopathic change may be seen elsewhere within the tendon, particularly in association with the tibial insertion.

The patellar tendon is normally remarkably strong and able to transmit considerable force, the diseased tendon becomes weaker and may tear even with relatively minor trauma. Following patellar tendon rupture, imaging, including plain films, may show a high-riding patella due to retraction of the patella through the quadriceps mechanism. MR imaging and ultrasound readily show discontinuity in the tendon which may be palpable clinically.

Quadriceps Tendon Disease

The quadriceps tendon forms from tendon contributions from the four quadriceps muscles (vastus medialis, intermedius and lateralis and rectus femoris) and inserts into the proximal pole of the patella. A component of the tendon from rectus femoris continues over the superficial surface of the patella to become part of the patellar tendon. Additionally, components from the vastus medialis and lateralis, respectively, merge with the medial and lateral patellar retinaculae with attachments into the patella and the femoral condyles [35].

The quadriceps tendon has a complex appearance on both ultrasound and MR imaging, although classically a trilaminar appearance is described with the different tendon components from the four quadriceps muscles making up the layers [35]. Quadriceps tendinopathy is considerably less common than patellar tendinopathy but the symptoms of the two conditions may be very similar and imaging can play a useful role in distinguishing the two. As with the patellar tendon the findings are of thickening of the tendon and loss of definition of the individual layers of the tendon is usually noted.

Tendon Disease Involving Other Tendons About the Knee

Tendinopathy may be seen in other tendons about the knee although perhaps most frequently this is seen in the semimembranosus tendon when the pain is localised to the posteromedial region of the knee. This can be an exceptionally difficult area to examine with ultrasound due to its depth and due to the course the tendon takes to its insertion on the posteromedial aspect of the knee, but MR images may show thickening of the enthesis of the semimembranosus tendon with areas of increased signal intensity reflecting intra-substance change.

Tendinopathy may also be seen in the distal biceps tendon on the lateral aspect of the knee and also involving the pes anserinus tendons (semitendinosus, gracilis and sartorius). In cases involving the pes anserinus tendons there may also be an associated pes anserinus bursitis. Again, these changes can be demonstrated on MR imaging or ultrasound with the typical findings previously described.

Occasionally rupture of these tendons may be demonstrated using either MR imaging or ultrasound (Fig. 1.35).

Iliotibial Band Friction Syndrome

The iliotibial band (ITB) is a fascial band of tissue originating from the iliac crest and eventually inserting into the lateral tibia on Gerdy's tubercle.

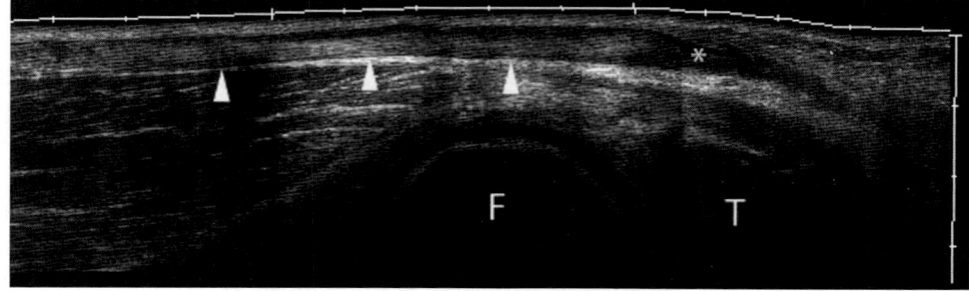

Fig. 1.35 Full thickness tear semitendinosus. Extended field of view longitudinal US along semitendinosus. More proximally the semitendinosus tendon is well visualised (*arrowheads*) but the more distal fibres become thickened and of low reflectivity. The tendon finally terminates suddenly (*) at its point of discontinuity. *F* medial femoral condyle; *T* medial tibial plateau

Iliotibial band friction syndrome is also known as "runner's knee" and there is considerable speculation as to its underlying cause. Originally thought to result from friction between the iliotibial band and the lateral femoral condyle during flexion and extension of the knee; it is now recognised that the story is rather more complicated and this conventional view has been challenged [36]. Whatever the aetiology, both MR imaging and ultrasound can demonstrate abnormalities associated with the distal ITB in patients presenting with the typical symptoms of tenderness and swelling of the lateral aspect of the knee. In patients with ITB friction syndrome, oedema or fluid is seen deep to the ITB as it passes over the lateral femoral condyle. Some studies have suggested a bursitis is seen and certainly discrete fluid collections can be seen deep to the ITB in this condition. However, there is disagreement as to whether a true bursa is actually present as often such fluid actually represents joint effusion within the lateral recess of the knee [36]. Studies have suggested that thickening of the ITB may develop, particularly in the more chronic stages of the disease but no abnormality in signal intensity is normally shown within the ITB itself on MR imaging.

Hoffa's Disease and Impingement

The infra-patellar fat pad also known as Hoffa's fat pad is the fat pad lying in the anterior aspect of the knee deep to the extensor mechanism. It is recognised that this structure may become inflamed following both acute trauma and chronic repetitive injury, a condition known as Hoffa's syndrome. This results in haemorrhage and fat necrosis of the fat pad and in the chronic situation fibrosis of the fat pad may be seen [37]. Acute inflammation within the fat pad is evident on MR scanning as diffuse or focal oedema within the fat pad. More chronic fibrotic change is seen as low signal change noted on all sequences but particularly evident on T1-weighted (T1w) imaging in contrast to the normal high signal fat.

In some patients, particularly those participating in sprinting and related sports, localised impingement (usually of the superolateral fat pad) may be seen as focal oedematous change within the fat pad between the femoral condyle and extensor mechanism (Fig. 1.36). This can be easy to miss and as has been noted by Saddik et al. is frequently under-reported [37].

Plica

Early in development the knee joint is divided into three compartments by synovial tissue which breaks down to create the single compartment knee joint most usually seen. Remnants of

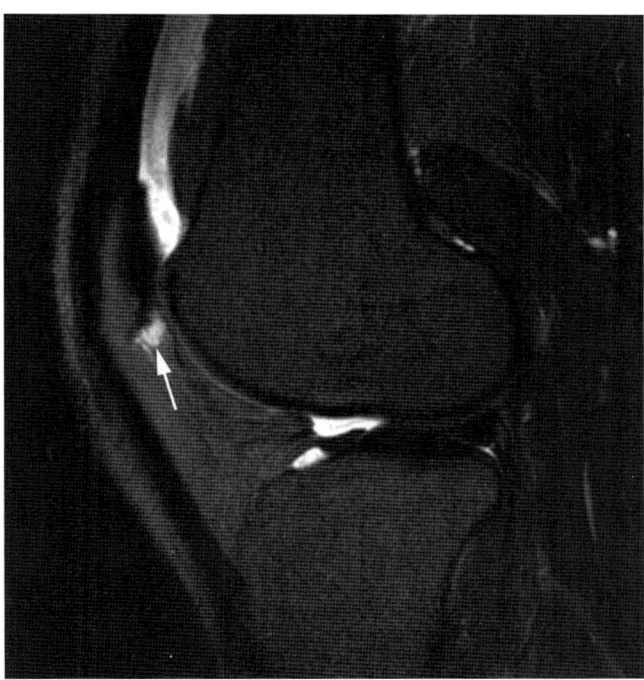

Fig. 1.36 Hoffa's impingement. Sagittal proton density image with fat saturation. Localised oedematous change is seen within the superolateral Hoffa's fat pad in this elite sprinter (*arrow*). The appearances represent impingement of the fat pad between the extensor mechanism and lateral femoral condyle, a cause of anterior knee pain in sprinters. Symptoms resolved following surgical resection

the synovial folds known as plica may be found in the normal adult knee and typically lie in one of three positions. The medial patellar plica arises from the medial wall of the knee joint and extends a variable distance into the knee joint. The supra-patellar plica embryologically divides the supra-patellar pouch from the remainder of the knee joint. The infra-patellar plica extends from the infra-patellar fat pad to the apex of the intercondylar notch. While a complete intact plica may persist completely dividing the knee joint into two or more cavities, more commonly a remnant of the plica persists as a synovial fold. The majority of synovial folds are entirely asymptomatic but occasionally as a result of trauma or impingement a plica may become thickened, fibrotic and inflamed. In the case of the medial patellar plica, this may be as a result of impingement between the extensor mechanism and medial femoral condyle. When this occurs there may be a secondary mechanical synovitis. Saddik et al. have commented on the overlap between symptomatic infra-patella plica and the Hoffa's fat pad syndrome described above. This exists because the plica itself may run through the fat pad [37].

The symptomatic plica will appear thickened and chronically shows low signal on all MR imaging sequences due to the formation of fibrous tissue. Plica are more easily identified in the presence of a joint effusion on MR imaging (Fig. 1.37).

Traction Enthesopathy in the Adolescent

Osgood–Schlatter disease occurs at the insertion of the patellar tendon into the tibial tubercle and is thought to result from chronic micro-trauma to the tendon insertion during growth. It characteristically occurs in adolescence and presents as pain and swelling in the region of the tibial tuberosity, particularly during activity. A similar but less frequently seen condition occurs at the insertion of the tendon into the lower pole of the patellar, known as Sindig–Larsen–Johanssen syndrome.

Radiographically there maybe bone irregularity and fragmentation at the site, but the soft tissue changes are best appreciated with MR imaging or ultrasound. In addition to bone fragmentation, thickening of the tendon with areas of increased signal seen on PD and T2 imaging is seen on MR imaging. Low reflective change and neovascularisation within the thickened tendon are appreciated on ultrasound. Adjacent to the abnormal tendon there may be oedematous change in Hoffa's fat pad and the surrounding soft tissues and in the case of Osgood–Schlatters disease, fluid may also be seen in the deep infrapatellar bursa (Fig. 1.38).

Bursae

Numerous bursae are present around the knee joint and may become inflamed as a result of sporting activity. Bursae are easily identified with either ultrasound or MR imaging as fluid-filled structures when inflamed. Examples include the popliteal (Baker's) cyst, semimembranosus bursa, pes anserine bursa and pre- and infrapatellar bursae (Fig. 1.38). These are amenable to ultrasound-guided injection, if necessary.

Patellofemoral Syndrome

Anterior knee pain is a frequent complaint amongst patients involved in sporting activity. It has a long differential diagnosis which includes many of the conditions already discussed (Table 1.6). However, the patellofemoral joint itself needs consideration as a primary cause of anterior knee pain. Osteoarthritis may occur at this joint and give rise to pain but other causes of pain from the joint include chondromalacia and chronic maltracking. These conditions are intimately associated but their relationship is poorly understood and more importantly the mechanism by which they generate pain remains obscure. The term patellofemoral syndrome has increasingly been used to refer to pain around the patella and has, in particular, largely replaced the term chondromalacia patellae. Three major contributing factors to the condition are recognised [38]:

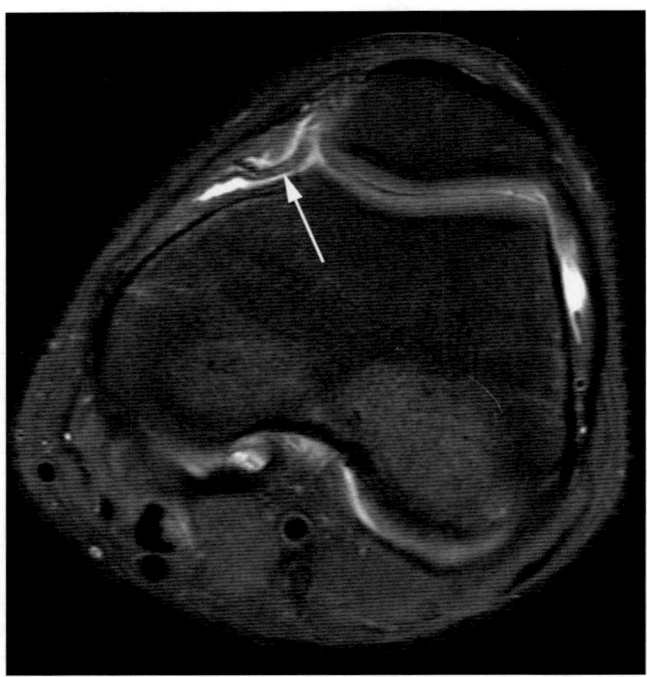

Fig. 1.37 Medial plica syndrome. Axial proton density image with fat saturation. A thickened oedematous medial plica is demonstrated (*arrow*). This was felt to be the cause of this athlete's anterior knee pain which resolved following resection

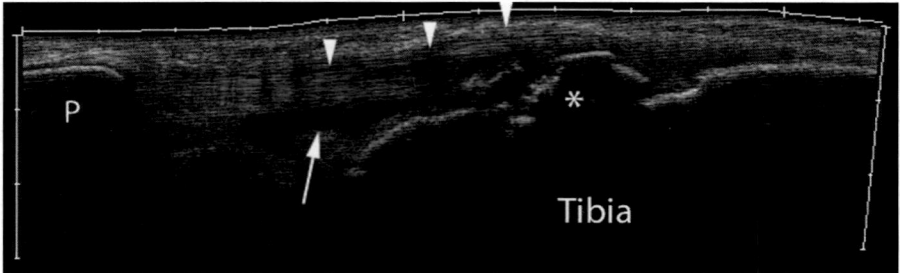

Fig. 1.38 Osgood–Schlatters disease. Extended field of view longitudinal US along the patellar tendon. There is bony fragmentation of the tibial tuberosity (*). The patellar tendon is demonstrated (*arrowheads*) and has lost its normal striated appearance close to its insertion. There is also fluid seen in the deep infra-patella bursa (*arrow*). *P* patella

Table 1.6 Causes of anterior knee pain in athletes

Tendon disease
- Patellar
- Quadriceps

Hoffas fat pad
- Trauma
- Impingement

Patellofemoral Joint
- Chronic maltracking
- Transient dislocation/recurrent subluxation
- Trauma/stress fracture
- Osteoarthritis
- Chondromalacia
- Synovitis

Other causes
- Bursitis
- Anterior meniscal injury
- Plica
- Referred hip pain

- Malalignment
- Muscular Imbalance
- Overactivity

Anatomy

The bony morphology of both the femoral trochlea and the articular surface of the patellar are vital in maintaining its stability. Nevertheless, the quadriceps muscle/tendon complex and patellar tendon do not act in a straight line through the patella, the angle created by the two structures is referred to as the Q angle. The patella is stabilised by medial and lateral retinacular structures. It is the medial retinacular structures which are responsible for resisting the tendency for the patella to move laterally which results from the Q angle geometry. These comprise the medial patellofemoral ligament (MPFL), the medial collateral ligament (MCL), the patellotibial ligament and the patellomeniscal ligament. Of these structures studies have shown it is the MPFL that provides the greatest restraint to lateral displacement of the patella [39]. The MPFL meshes with the fibres of vastus medius obliquus close to its patellar insertion suggesting that the MPFL acts as both a static and a dynamic restraint [39].

Transient Patellar Dislocation

Acute dislocation of the patellofemoral joint can occur and by the time the patient undergoes imaging, or even before the patient seeks medical attention the patella has usually relocated. Transient patellar dislocation can occur without the patient being aware of what has happened. While plain films may show an osteochondral loose body if there is an associated osteochondral injury, MR imaging is the imaging modality of choice. Often there will be evidence of a recent dislocation with a characteristic bone bruise pattern seen with increased T2 signal in the anterolateral aspect of the lateral femoral condyle and the medial aspect of the patella (Fig. 1.39). This occurs as a result of the impaction occurring between the patella and the lateral femoral condyle at the time of dislocation. In addition, MR imaging allows an assessment of the soft tissue damage to the medial retinacular structures. Medial retinacular damage is reported in a high number of these cases [40]. Multiple sites of medial retinacular damage may occur and Elias et al. noted 45% of patients showed signal change in keeping with oedema or haematoma in the inferior aspect of the vastus medialis obliquus [40].

There may be associated osteochondral injury to either the patella and/or the lateral femoral condyle which may be associated with loose body formation. Elias et al. found osteochondral injury to the patella was more common than to the lateral femoral condyle and most frequently involved the inferomedial patella [40] (Fig. 1.39). One study has shown that when osteochondral damage occurs to the lateral femoral condyle it may be more posterior than might be expected for the mechanism of injury and the site of any lateral femoral condyle bone bruise [41]. When a patient presents with MR imaging findings suggesting a transient patellar dislocation, patellofemoral alignment should be assessed. Malalignment may be contributing to the patellofemoral instability and is relatively common in this group of patients [40]. Such changes are discussed in the next section.

Chronic Patella Maltracking

As noted, the relationship between chronic maltracking of the patella and patellar chondromalacia is unclear, as is the mechanism by which these conditions result in pain. McNally has noted that two key anatomical relationships are important to allow normal tracking of the patella [42]. These are:

- The degree of lateralisation of the patellar tendon as it approaches its insertion into the tibia
- The congruency between the patella and femoral trochlea articular surfaces

The former of these is a reflection of the Q angle described above. This can be assessed clinically or with leg length plain radiographs by lines joining the anterior superior iliac spine and patellar and the tibial tubercle. A CT scanogram can also be used but the Q angle cannot be assessed from axial imaging. Instead, the trochlear-tubercle distance (TTD) can be obtained from superimposing axial images through the most superior part of the trochlear and through the tibial tuberosity. Lines perpendicular to the posterior bicondylar line are constructed through the deepest point of the trochlear groove and the middle of

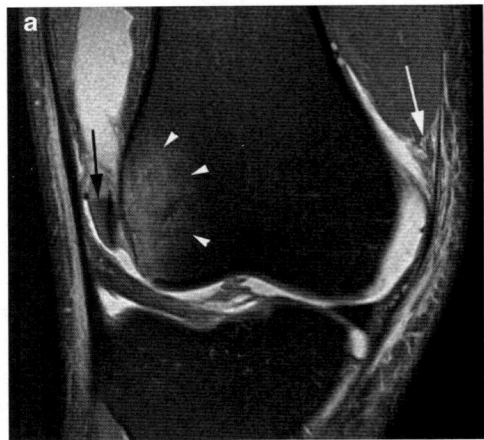 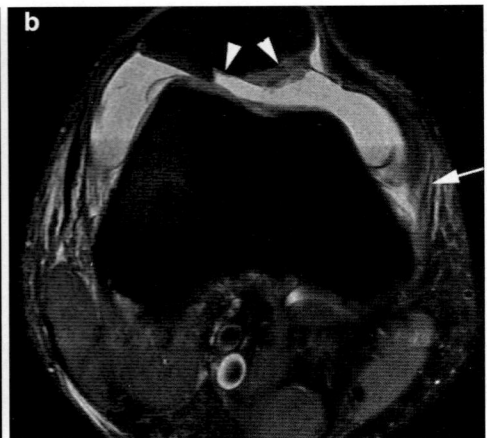

Fig. 1.39 Transient patellar dislocation. Coronal (**a**) and axial (**b**) proton density images with fat saturation. (**a**) There is characteristic bone bruising in the lateral aspect of the lateral femoral condyle (*arrowheads*). An intra-articular osteochondral body is identified in the lateral recess of the joint (*black arrow*). There is evidence of disruption of the inferior fibres of the vastus medius obliquus muscle (*white arrow*). (**b**) The axial image identifies the site of origin of the osteochondral body seen in **a** as from the patella (*arrowheads*). Note the sharp margin of the cartilage defect on the lateral side reflecting the traumatic nature of the injury. There is disruption of the medial patellofemoral ligament (*arrow*)

the tibial tuberosity and the distance between these two perpendiculars is measured to give the TTD [42].

Plain films provide limited information on the relationship of the patella to the trochlea and skyline views should be interpreted with caution. At best these only provide evidence of the relationship in a single position.

The lateral radiograph allows an assessment of patellar height. Patella alta is associated with anterior knee pain and patellofemoral instability. The patella height can be assessed by a variety of techniques but perhaps the most frequently used is the Insall–Salvati ratio which uses a ratio of the tendon length to the patella length defining patella alta as a ratio over 1.2 [43]. The Caton ratio is the ratio of the distance from the lower edge of the articular surface of the patella to the anterosuperior angle of the tibia, to the length of the articular surface of the patella [44]. Again, a ratio greater than 1.2 is said to represent patella alta. Although patella height can also be assessed on MR imaging, it is important to note that the same ratios may not apply. Shabshin et al. have suggested that on MR imaging the upper limit of normal for the patellar tendon to patellar length ratio is 1.5 [45].

Trochlea and dorsal patellar morphology can be assessed to some extent using plain films. However, evaluation is easier using cross-sectional imaging and a variety of angles and distances can be measured [42, 46]. While these measurements can be made on both CT and MR imaging the difference between measurements made to the articular cartilage and to the osseous surfaces of trochlea have been emphasised. Any bone dysplasia tends to be worsened by the overlying cartilage morphology which is poorly demonstrated on plain film and CT. Because of this MR imaging has advantages in assessing the trochlear morphology prior to surgical intervention [47]. Ultrasound has been found to be unreliable compared with CT and MR imaging for assessing the trochlear groove morphology [48].

Unfortunately, there is some disagreement within the literature over the normal ranges for measurements that can be made to assess patellofemoral alignment and dysplasia. McNally et al. found a TTD of greater than 2 cm to be highly specific but poorly sensitive for maltracking, while other specific but poorly sensitive measures include a femoral groove less than 5 mm deep and displacement of the lateral margin of the patella 5 mm or more beyond the lateral femoral condyle [42]. DeJour et al. suggest four factors are significant in knees with symptomatic patellar instability [46]:

- Trochlea dysplasia with a trochlea bump of >3 mm and a trochlear depth of <4 mm
- A patellar tilt >20°
- Patella alta (using the Caton index [44]) >1.2
- TTD >20 mm

Dynamic axial imaging techniques have been suggested for assessing the patellofemoral articulation. Some of these utilise CT or MR imaging in a series of static positions to generate a cine loop to evaluate the movement of the patella over the trochlea. However, abnormal motion is more likely to be demonstrated if there is active contraction of extensor mechanism against resistance. This has led a number of workers to develop techniques of dynamic MR imaging scanning while the knee is extended against resistance using a variety of kinematic devices of greater or lesser sophistication [49–51].

Bone and Articular Cartilage Injury

Acute bone injuries to the knee occur in athletes and may be clinically obvious or clearly demonstrated on conventional radiography. These may occur as a result of direct impaction or force applied to the bone. Alternatively they may arise through mechanisms of avulsion such as avulsion of a tibial spine (Fig. 1.18). A bone injury identified on conventional radiography may indicate a soft tissue injury which is much more dramatic and significant than the bone injury itself. Examples include the Segond fracture and its association with anterior cruciate ligament disruption (Figs. 1.18 and 1.22) and avulsion of the fibular styloid (the arcuate sign) and its association with posterolateral corner disruption and instability (Fig. 1.32). Some fractures are more subtle and associated with articular cartilage damage. While the ossific component of an osteochondral injury may be recognised on plain films it will often underestimate the actual damage done.

Cartilage and Osteochondral Injury

Articular cartilage injury may occur as a result of acute trauma, or due to more chronic insult, the latter resulting in a degenerative pattern of damage to the cartilage. Acute osteochondral injury in the knee is a relatively common sports injury and often occurs in association with soft tissue injuries such as cruciate or collateral ligament tears.

If cartilage damage is seen with clinically occult subchondral bone injury, loss of cartilage generally develops. Where no overt cartilage damage occurs, generally healing is seen. However, conflicting data exists in this area and it seems cartilage loss may occasionally be seen associated with a bone bruise in the absence of apparent initial cartilage damage [52–54].

Degenerative change in the cartilage involves both a change in the quality of the articular cartilage, as the composition of the cartilage changes, and, as the process progresses, loss of cartilage. Both these findings can be detected with MR imaging.

Although, it is possible to obtain exquisite imaging of the articular surfaces in the knee using CT arthrography and ultrasound, MR imaging remains the mainstay for articular cartilage imaging. CT arthrography is very sensitive to subtle cartilage lesions and may well be the imaging modality of choice for detecting such damage but it does not provide information about the intrinsic nature of the cartilage as can be assessed with MR imaging and gives little information relating to the subchondral bone changes.

MR imaging of articular cartilage is an area that has seen rapid development in recent years with the development of novel pulse sequences specifically designed to show cartilage morphology. Sophisticated techniques are available to aid detection of cartilage damage including T2 mapping techniques and measurement of magnetisation transfer coefficients. These techniques are predominantly research tools and conventional imaging techniques remain the basis of cartilage imaging in clinical practise.

Gradient echo sequences have been popular for assessing articular cartilage and are still used in many centres. Conventional spin echo T2w imaging has been shown to be relatively insensitive to articular cartilage defects [55, 56]. Proton density and T2 fat-suppressed FSE imaging provide excellent cartilage definition on modern machines and have been proven reliable in the assessment of articular cartilage damage [55, 56]. The use of FSE imaging gives the additional benefit of providing magnetisation transfer contrast in addition to the T2 contrast. These sequences have the advantage of being ubiquitous on modern systems and sensitive to other knee pathology which means they form the basis of most routine protocols.

Loss of articular cartilage may be seen as focal partial thickness thinning of the cartilage with an irregular surface or full thickness cartilage loss possibly with an associated underlying bone defect. In addition, traumatic injury may result in more subtle cartilage lesions such as fissures, clefts, flap tears and surface fibrillation. The Outerbridge scale for classifying cartilage lesions was originally developed for macroscopic assessment of the cartilage through arthroscopy but has been modified for use with MR imaging. This provides a useful tool for describing these lesions when reporting scan results (Table 1.7) [57].

It is difficult to distinguish cartilage damage that has occurred as a result of injury and more chronic cartilage loss occurring as a result of cartilage degeneration. An important clue is that cartilage defects resulting from injury are often sharply marginated and solitary (Figs. 1.39 and 1.40). They may have a flap-like configuration or show linear clefts or fissures. In contrast, cartilage damage resulting

Table 1.7 Modified outerbridge classification of cartilage damage [57]

Grade	Macroscopic	MRI
0	Normal	Normal
1	Swelling and softening	Intrachondral signal change but no surface damage
2	<50% cartilage loss	<50% cartilage loss
3	>50% cartilage loss but no exposure of subchondral bone	>50% cartilage loss but no exposure of subchondral bone
4	Full thickness cartilage loss exposing subchondral bone	Full thickness cartilage loss exposing subchondral bone

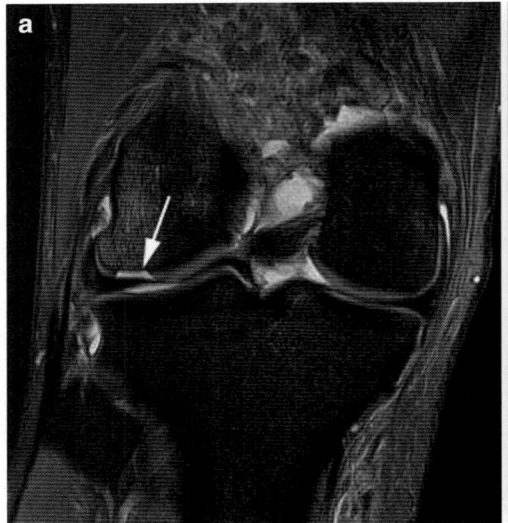 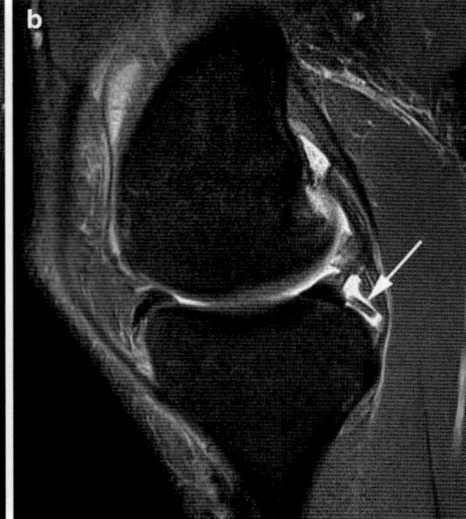

Fig. 1.40 Osteochondral fracture with loose body. Coronal (**a**) and axial (**b**) proton density images with fat saturation. (**a**) A focal articular cartilage defect is seen in the lateral femoral condyle with associated bone marrow oedema (*arrow*). Note the acute angle edges of the defect reflecting the traumatic nature of the injury. (**b**) On the sagittal image the osteochondral loose body that has arisen from the defect shown in **a** is identified posteriorly behind the posterior horn of the medial meniscus (*arrow*)

from chronic degeneration is usually more diffuse and there will often be multiple defects with variable size and depth. The margins of these defects are less well defined [55]. An important clue to cartilage damage is signal change in the subchondral bone and if this is seen a careful review of the overlying cartilage is necessary. While damaged cartilage may remain in situ or become partially detached, an unstable cartilage or osteochondral fragment will become loose and displaced into the joint space. If a cartilage defect is seen it is important to look for any displaced intra-articular chondral body (Fig. 1.40).

Cartilage Repair

In recent years, a variety of procedures have been developed for repairing articular cartilage in the knee joint. Broadly these fall into three groups:

1. Cartilage stimulation techniques such as abrasion and micro-fracture designed to stimulate the growth of fibro-cartilage within the cartilage defects.
2. Tissue-based cartilage repair such as mosaicplasty where osteochondral plugs are taken from normal weight-bearing areas of the joint and transplanted into the chondral defect. An alternative is allograft transplantation where cadaveric osteochondral material is used for transplantation.
3. Cell-based cartilage repair techniques. These involve autologous chondrocyte implantation which is undertaken after healthy chondrocytes been harvested and cultured in vitro. The reimplanted chondrocytes may be covered with a periosteal flap or more recently a collagen membrane or 3-D biological scaffold may be used.

The technical success of the procedure can be assessed with post-operative imaging [58–64]. The International Cartilage Repair Society recommends the use of the same sequences that would be used to evaluate normal articular cartilage [58, 65]. MR imaging allows an assessment of the degree of filling of the cartilage defect and how well the curvature of the joint surface has been restored. It also allows an assessment of complications of the procedure such as displacement of graft material.

References

1. Watanabe AT, Carter BC, Teitelbaum GP, Seeger LL, Bradley WG Jr (1989) Normal variations in MR imaging of the knee: appearance and frequency. AJR Am J Roentgenol 153(2):341–344
2. Sanders TG, Linares RC, Lawhorn KW, Tirman PF, Houser C (1999) Oblique meniscomeniscal ligament: another potential pitfall for a meniscal tear – anatomic description and appearance at MR imaging in three cases. Radiology 213(1):213–216
3. Warren LF, Marshall JL (1979) The supporting structures and layers on the medial side of the knee: an anatomical analysis. J Bone Joint Surg Am 61(1):56–62
4. Karachalios T, Hantes M, Zibis AH, Zachos V, Karantanas AH, Malizos KN (2005) Diagnostic accuracy of a new clinical test (the Thessaly test) for early detection of meniscal tears. J Bone Joint Surg Am 87(5):955–962

5. Helms CA (2002) The meniscus: recent advances in MR imaging of the knee. AJR Am J Roentgenol 179(5):1115–1122
6. Cheung LP, Li KC, Hollett MD, Bergman AG, Herfkens RJ (1997) Meniscal tears of the knee: accuracy of detection with fast spin-echo MR imaging and arthroscopic correlation in 293 patients. Radiology 203(2):508–512
7. Escobedo EM, Hunter JC, Zink-Brody GC, Wilson AJ, Harrison SD, Fisher DJ (1996) Usefulness of turbo spin-echo MR imaging in the evaluation of meniscal tears: comparison with a conventional spin-echo sequence. AJR Am J Roentgenol 167(5):1223–1227
8. Rubin DA, Kneeland JB, Listerud J, Underberg-Davis SJ, Dalinka MK (1994) MR diagnosis of meniscal tears of the knee: value of fast spin-echo vs conventional spin-echo pulse sequences. AJR Am J Roentgenol 162(5):1131–1135
9. Blackmon GB, Major NM, Helms CA (2005) Comparison of fast spin-echo versus conventional spin-echo MRI for evaluating meniscal tears. AJR Am J Roentgenol 184(6):1740–1743
10. Rohren EM, Kosarek FJ, Helms CA (2001) Discoid lateral meniscus and the frequency of meniscal tears. Skeletal Radiol 30(6):316–320
11. Stoller DW, Martin C, Crues JV 3rd, Kaplan L, Mink JH (1987) Meniscal tears: pathologic correlation with MR imaging. Radiology 163(3):731–735
12. Kornick J, Trefelner E, McCarthy S, Lange R, Lynch K, Jokl P (1990) Meniscal abnormalities in the asymptomatic population at MR imaging. Radiology 177(2):463–465
13. Helms CA, Laorr A, Cannon WD Jr (1998) The absent bow tie sign in bucket-handle tears of the menisci in the knee. AJR Am J Roentgenol 170(1):57–61
14. Wright DH, De Smet AA, Norris M (1995) Bucket-handle tears of the medial and lateral menisci of the knee: value of MR imaging in detecting displaced fragments. AJR Am J Roentgenol 165(3):621–625
15. Magee TH, Hinson GW (1998) MRI of meniscal bucket-handle tears. Skeletal Radiol 27(9):495–499
16. Harper KW, Helms CA, Lambert HS 3rd, Higgins LD (2005) Radial meniscal tears: significance, incidence, and MR appearance. AJR Am J Roentgenol 185(6):1429–1434
17. Rubin DA, Britton CA, Towers JD, Harner CD (1996) Are MR imaging signs of meniscocapsular separation valid? Radiology 201(3):829–836
18. McCauley TR (2005) MR imaging evaluation of the postoperative knee. Radiology 234(1):53–61
19. Deutsch AL, Mink JH, Fox JM, Arnoczky SP, Rothman BJ, Stoller DW et al (1990) Peripheral meniscal tears: MR findings after conservative treatment or arthroscopic repair. Radiology 176(2): 485–488
20. White LM, Kramer J, Recht MP (2005) MR imaging evaluation of the postoperative knee: ligaments, menisci, and articular cartilage. Skeletal Radiol 34(8):431–452
21. Applegate GR, Flannigan BD, Tolin BS, Fox JM, Del Pizzo W (1993) MR diagnosis of recurrent tears in the knee: value of intraarticular contrast material. AJR Am J Roentgenol 161(4):821–825
22. Mutschler C, Vande Berg BC, Lecouvet FE, Poilvache P, Dubuc JE, Maldague B et al (2003) Postoperative meniscus: assessment at dual-detector row spiral CT arthrography of the knee. Radiology 228(3):635–641
23. Gentili A, Seeger LL, Yao L, Do HM (1994) Anterior cruciate ligament tear: indirect signs at MR imaging. Radiology 193(3): 835–840
24. LaPrade RF, Resig S, Wentorf F, Lewis JL (1999) The effects of grade III posterolateral knee complex injuries on anterior cruciate ligament graft force. A biomechanical analysis. Am J Sports Med 27(4):469–475
25. Sonin AH, Fitzgerald SW, Hoff FL, Friedman H, Bresler ME (1995) MR imaging of the posterior cruciate ligament: normal, abnormal, and associated injury patterns. Radiographics 15(3):551–561
26. Schatz JA, Potter HG, Rodeo SA, Hannafin JA, Wickiewicz TL (1997) MR imaging of anterior cruciate ligament reconstruction. AJR Am J Roentgenol 169(1):223–228
27. Kobayashi M, Nakagawa Y, Suzuki T, Okudaira S, Nakamura T (2006) A retrospective review of bone tunnel enlargement after anterior cruciate ligament reconstruction with hamstring tendons fixed with a metal round cannulated interference screw in the femur. Arthroscopy 22(10):1093–1099
28. Bui-Mansfield LT, Youngberg RA (1997) Intraarticular ganglia of the knee: prevalence, presentation, etiology, and management. AJR Am J Roentgenol 168(1):123–127
29. Yu JS, Salonen DC, Hodler J, Haghighi P, Trudell D, Resnick D (1996) Posterolateral aspect of the knee: improved MR imaging with a coronal oblique technique. Radiology 198(1):199–204
30. Schweitzer ME, Tran D, Deely DM, Hume EL (1995) Medial collateral ligament injuries: evaluation of multiple signs, prevalence and location of associated bone bruises, and assessment with MR imaging. Radiology 194(3):825–829
31. Hughston JC, Jacobson KE (1985) Chronic posterolateral rotatory instability of the knee. J Bone Joint Surg Am 67(3):351–359
32. Dye SF, Campagna-Pinto D, Dye CC, Shifflett S, Eiman T (2003) Soft-tissue anatomy anterior to the human patella. J Bone Joint Surg Am 85-A(6):1012–1017
33. Yu JS, Popp JE, Kaeding CC, Lucas J (1995) Correlation of MR imaging and pathological findings in athletes undergoing surgery for chronic patellar tendinitis. AJR Am J Roentgenol 165(1):115–118
34. Khan KM, Bonar F, Desmond PM, Cook JL, Young DA, Visentini PJ et al (1996) Patellar tendinosis (jumper's knee): findings at histopathologic examination, US, and MR imaging. Victorian Institute of Sport Tendon Study Group. Radiology 200(3):821–827
35. Yu JS, Petersilge C, Sartoris DJ, Pathria MN, Resnick D (1994) MR imaging of injuries of the extensor mechanism of the knee. Radiographics 14(3):541–551
36. Fairclough J, Hayashi K, Toumi H, Lyons K, Bydder G, Phillips N et al (2007) Is iliotibial band syndrome really a friction syndrome? J Sci Med Sport 10(2):74–76, discussion 7–8
37. Saddik D, McNally EG, Richardson M (2004) MRI of Hoffa's fat pad. Skeletal Radiol 33(8):433–444
38. Thomee R, Augustsson J, Karlsson J (1999) Patellofemoral pain syndrome: a review of current issues. Sports Med 28(4):245–262
39. Panagiotopoulos E, Strzelczyk P, Herrmann M, Scuderi G (2006) Cadaveric study on static medial patellar stabilizers: the dynamizing role of the vastus medialis obliquus on medial patellofemoral ligament. Knee Surg Sports Traumatol Arthrosc 14(1):7–12
40. Elias DA, White LM, Fithian DC (2002) Acute lateral patellar dislocation at MR imaging: injury patterns of medial patellar soft-tissue restraints and osteochondral injuries of the inferomedial patella. Radiology 225(3):736–743
41. Sanders TG, Paruchuri NB, Zlatkin MB (2006) MRI of osteochondral defects of the lateral femoral condyle: incidence and pattern of injury after transient lateral dislocation of the patella. AJR Am J Roentgenol 187(5):1332–1337
42. McNally EG (2001) Imaging assessment of anterior knee pain and patellar maltracking. Skeletal Radiol 30(9):484–495
43. Insall J, Salvati E (1971) Patella position in the normal knee joint. Radiology 101(1):101–104
44. Caton J, Deschamps G, Chambat P, Lerat JL, Dejour H (1982) Patella infera. Apropos of 128 cases. Rev Chir Orthop Reparatrice Appar Mot 68(5):317–325
45. Shabshin N, Schweitzer ME, Morrison WB, Parker L (2004) MRI criteria for patella alta and baja. Skeletal Radiol 33(8):445–450
46. Dejour H, Walch G, Nove-Josserand L, Guier C (1994) Factors of patellar instability: an anatomic radiographic study. Knee Surg Sports Traumatol Arthrosc 2(1):19–26

47. van Huyssteen AL, Hendrix MR, Barnett AJ, Wakeley CJ, Eldridge JD (2006) Cartilage-bone mismatch in the dysplastic trochlea. An MRI study. J Bone Joint Surg Br 88(5):688–691
48. Toms AP, Cahir J, Swift L, Donell ST (2009) Imaging the femoral sulcus with ultrasound, CT, and MRI: reliability and generalizability in patients with patellar instability. Skeletal Radiol 38(4):329–338
49. Brossmann J, Muhle C, Schroder C, Melchert UH, Bull CC, Spielmann RP et al (1993) Patellar tracking patterns during active and passive knee extension: evaluation with motion-triggered cine MR imaging. Radiology 187(1):205–212
50. McNally EG, Ostlere SJ, Pal C, Phillips A, Reid H, Dodd C (2000) Assessment of patellar maltracking using combined static and dynamic MRI. European Radiol 10(7):1051–1055
51. Muhle C, Brossmann J, Heller M (1996) Kinematic MRI of the knee using a specially designed positioning device. J Comput Assist Tomogr 20(4):522–525
52. Boks SS, Vroegindeweij D, Koes BW, Hunink MG, Bierma-Zeinstra SM (2006) Follow-up of occult bone lesions detected at MR imaging: systematic review. Radiology 238(3):853–862
53. Costa-Paz M, Muscolo DL, Ayerza M, Makino A, Aponte-Tinao L (2001) Magnetic resonance imaging follow-up study of bone bruises associated with anterior cruciate ligament ruptures. Arthroscopy 17(5):445–449
54. Vellet AD, Marks PH, Fowler PJ, Munro TG (1991) Occult post-traumatic osteochondral lesions of the knee: prevalence, classification, and short-term sequelae evaluated with MR imaging. Radiology 178(1):271–276
55. Disler DG, Recht MP, McCauley TR (2000) MR imaging of articular cartilage. Skeletal Radiol 29(7):367–377
56. Yao L, Gentili A, Thomas A (1996) Incidental magnetization transfer contrast in fast spin-echo imaging of cartilage. J Magn Reson Imaging 6(1):180–184
57. Uhl M, Allmann KH, Tauer U, Laubenberger J, Adler CP, Ihling C et al (1998) Comparison of MR sequences in quantifying in vitro cartilage degeneration in osteoarthritis of the knee. Br J Radiol 71(843):291–296
58. Choi YS, Potter HG, Chun TJ (2008) MR imaging of cartilage repair in the knee and ankle. Radiographics 28(4):1043–1059
59. Chung CB, Frank LR, Resnick D (2001) Cartilage imaging techniques: current clinical applications and state of the art imaging. Clin Orthop Relat Res (391 Suppl):S370–S378
60. Link TM, Stahl R, Woertler K (2007) Cartilage imaging: motivation, techniques, current and future significance. Eur Radiol 17(5):1135–1146
61. Potter HG, Foo LF (2006) Magnetic resonance imaging of articular cartilage: trauma, degeneration, and repair. Am J Sports Med 34(4):661–677
62. Recht M, Bobic V, Burstein D, Disler D, Gold G, Gray M et al (2001) Magnetic resonance imaging of articular cartilage. Clin Orthop Relat Res (391 Suppl):S379–S396
63. Recht MP, Goodwin DW, Winalski CS, White LM (2005) MRI of articular cartilage: revisiting current status and future directions. AJR Am J Roentgenol 185(4):899–914
64. Trattnig S, Millington SA, Szomolanyi P, Marlovits S (2007) MR imaging of osteochondral grafts and autologous chondrocyte implantation. Eur Radiol 17(1):103–118
65. Bobic V (2000) ICRS articular cartilage imaging committee. ICRS MR imaging protocol for knee articular cartilage. International Cartilage Repair Society, Zollikon, Switzerland

Chapter 2
Hip, Pelvis and Groin Injuries

Philip Robinson

Introduction

The pelvis is the focus of marked biomechanical stresses during all athletic activity. It is an extremely complex anatomical area consisting of many powerful muscle groups as well as joints with varying degrees of mobility. Proximal thigh muscle strain is the most acute frequent injury in most running sports (from athletics to soccer). Overuse injuries affecting tendons, the symphyseal region (Pubalgia) and the hip joint are conditions that affect the majority of athletes across different sports.

This chapter will discuss and review the anatomy, biomechanics and injury processes that occur in the pelvis focussing on the hip joint, symphyseal region, surrounding muscles and tendons. Imaging features and strategies will be presented for all conditions outlining how these findings aid diagnosis, grade injury, affect prognosis and guide management (Table 2.1).

Pelvic Osseous Injury

Acute fractures or dislocations of the pelvis and femur are rare even in high energy sports but stress injuries are not infrequent. Femoral stress injuries are the third most frequent injury occurring in 10% of series [1]. Stress injury aetiology, risk factors and imaging strategies are discussed in detail in Chap. 4.

Femoral neck stress injury occurs either on the medial (compressive) or lateral (tensile) side (Fig. 2.1) [2]. It is important to detect early as the consequences for osteonecrosis or complete fracture are serious especially with lateral (tensile) stress injury. Other pelvic areas susceptible to stress injury include the pubic rami, sacrum and apophyses (Fig. 2.2).

Philip Robinson (✉)
Department of Radiology, Leeds Teaching Hospitals,
Leeds, LS7 4SA, UK
e-mail: p.robinson@leedsth.nhs.uk

In athletes stress injury normally relates to a sustained increase in training and more commonly presents in athletes who have suffered prior osseous injury, have concomitant lower limb injuries and are female. The increased incidence of femoral and pelvic stress injuries in women distance runners is thought to be due to the relatively lower bone mass and surrounding muscle bulk [3].

T2-weighted (fat-suppressed) magnetic resonance (MR) sequences are most sensitive for detecting the full spectrum of injury from periosteal, cortical and bone marrow oedema to the development of a low signal fracture line (Figs. 2.1 and 2.2). Although grading systems have been developed for stress injuries a more conservative approach is taken with femoral neck injuries because of the potential for displacement and osteonecrosis.

Internal Derangement of the Hip

Athletic injuries of the hip include femoroacetabular impingement (FAI), osteochondral lesions, ligamentous injuries and instability. All these processes can be insidious or acute.

Hip Joint Biomechanics and Anatomy

Biomechanically forces involving the hip joint act around the centre of the femoral head (its fulcrum) and are dependant on body weight [4, 5]. The body's centre of gravity acts through the centre of the pelvis and exerts a large moment of force on the hip joint. Subsequently the surrounding muscles must generate forces in excess of body weight to maintain equilibrium [4, 5]. These forces are two and a half times body weight while walking, five times while jogging and over eight times body weight during athletic activity or stumbling [4]. Forces are further increased in single stance which occurs when kicking, jumping or cutting-in (changing direction).

Table 2.1 Overview of athletic pelvic injuries and imaging choices (nb plain radiographs will be performed initially in the majority of cases)

	Primary modality	Why	Others	Why
Osseous	MR imaging	Stress injury	CR/CT	Acute injury
FAI	MR arthrography	1. Global joint assessment	CT	Osseous and cartilage detail
		2. Anaesthetic		
Muscle	MR imaging or US	See Chap. 6		
Paratenon	MR imaging	Very subtle oedema not seen on US	US	Guided injection
Snapping	US	Dynamic assessment and injection		
Pubalgia – parasymphyseal	MR imaging	Entheseal and subchondral oedema (not seen on US)	US	Injection
Pubalgia – inguinal	US	Exclude hernia (very rare)		

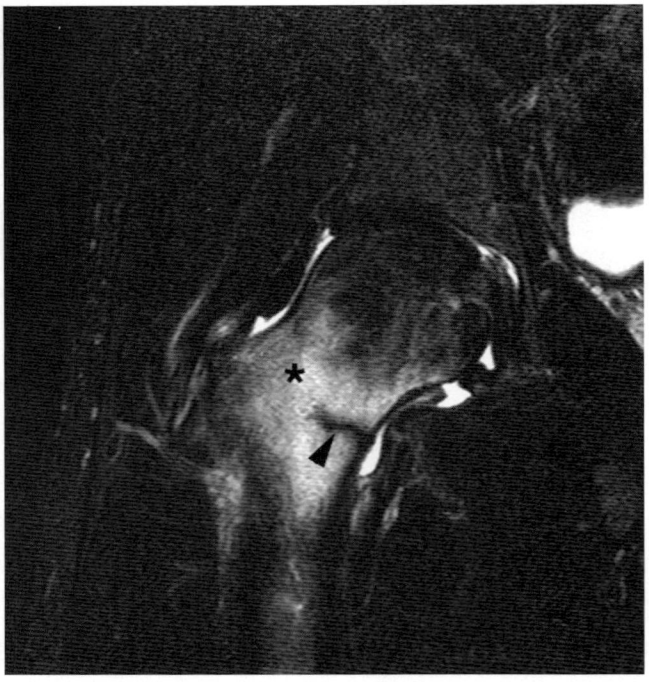

Fig. 2.1 Coronal T2w FS MR image shows basal femoral neck oedema (*) and low signal medial fracture (*arrowhead*)

The femoral head and acetabulum are also incongruent resulting in gliding as well as rotation of the femoral head as it reaches the limits of movement within the acetabulum. The fibrocartilagenous labrum is located along the outer margin of the articular cartilage increasing the acetabular volume by 20% [6]. In athletic activity the labrum undergoes compressive and shearing forces while limiting femoral head motion which can result in acute labral tears, capsular injury, impingement or chronic degeneration. Certainly in retired soccer players there is a high incidence of premature hip osteoarthritis and there is now an increasing recognition of osteochondral and labral injuries occurring during active playing careers.

Labral Abnormalities and Femoroacetabular Impingement

The labrum can undergo degenerative change or tear acutely but is more commonly involved in conjunction with femoroacetabular impingement [7].

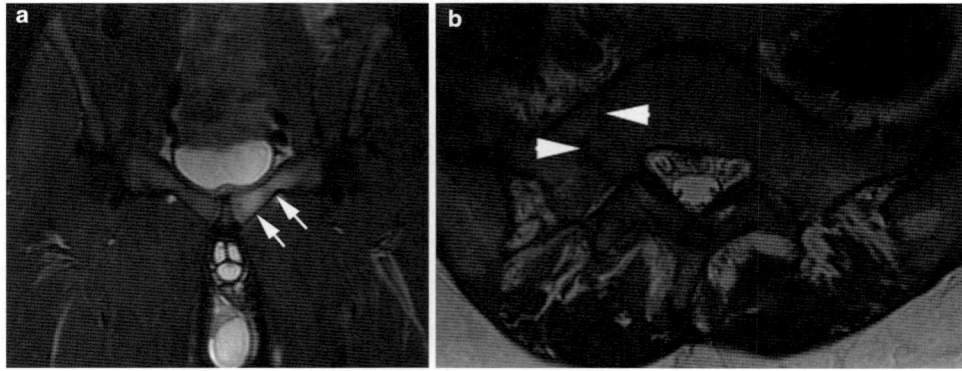

Fig. 2.2 (**a**) Coronal STIR MR image shows left pubic body and superior ramus oedema (*arrows*) with no fracture. (**b**) Axial T2w MR image shows low signal linear right sacral fracture (*arrowheads*)

Femoroacetabular Impingement

FAI develops because of abnormal femoral and acetabular impingement either due to a primary acetabular deformity (termed "pincer") or, more commonly in athletes, due to a prominence of the femoral head and proximal neck (termed "cam") [7]. There is a mixed pattern often present in the general population but there is usually cam dominance in athletes. Clinically there is deep groin discomfort with pain classically precipitated during passive hip flexion (to 90°) with forced internal rotation and adduction [7, 8].

In cam impingement the abnormal femoral head prominence leads to impaction on the anterosuperior labrum during hip flexion and internal rotation. The resultant shearing forces produce tears at the base of the labrum at its junction with the adjacent acetabular cartilage. It is not known whether this femoral head abnormality is congenital, secondary to previous epiphyseal injury or even part of the spectrum of mild dysplasia.

In pincer impingement the femoral head range of motion is limited by acetabular overcoverage or acetabular retroversion. The acetabular depth may be increased congenitally, by an elongated dysplastic labrum, or the presence of an os acetabuli. This limitation also results in impaction and anterosuperior joint damage but also contre-coup impaction with osteochondral damage posteriorly not typically seen in cam impingement.

Imaging

The role of imaging is not only to confirm the diagnosis but to assess the whole joint for cartilage damage. This extent will define suitability for surgical intervention and ultimately prognosis.

Magnetic Resonance Techniques

The primary imaging technique for FAI is MR arthrography although there are recognised limitations in the assessment of cartilage [7]. MR arthrography sequences performed are predominantly T1 weighted (with fat suppression) (Fig. 2.3) but protocols should include at least one T2-weighted fat-suppressed sequence to evaluate extra-articular and osseous pathology. Non-arthrographic MR studies rely predominantly on PD-weighted fat-suppressed sequences. Oblique axial sequences (parallel to the long axis of the femoral neck) should be performed to assess femoral morphology (Fig. 2.4) (see below).

Both techniques should utilise surface coils to allow a small field of view and slice thickness. An advantage of MR arthrography is that during arthrographic injection local anaesthetic can be added which can help clinicians diagnostically if examination findings are equivocal.

Normal Appearances and Pitfalls

The fibrocartilage labrum should normally have a low signal triangular shape. A normal cleft can occur inferiorly at its junction with the transverse ligament but pathology rarely occurs at this point (Fig. 2.3b). There is debate whether a cleft can normally exist between the anterosuperior labrum and adjacent acetabular cartilage with the current consensus favouring it to be pathological. Superior capsular recesses can allow contrast to bathe the superficial labral surface and should not be confused with a tear or cyst. A normal stellate cartilage region can occur in the mid-acetabular roof at the old physeal junction distal to where pathology normally

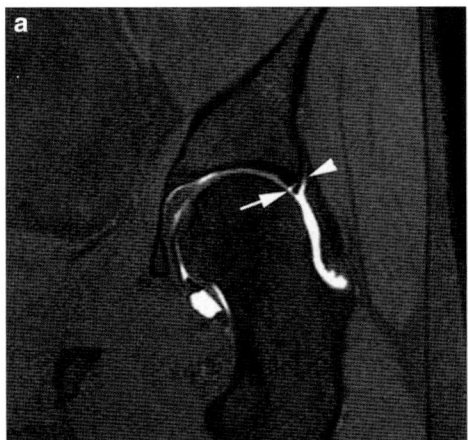 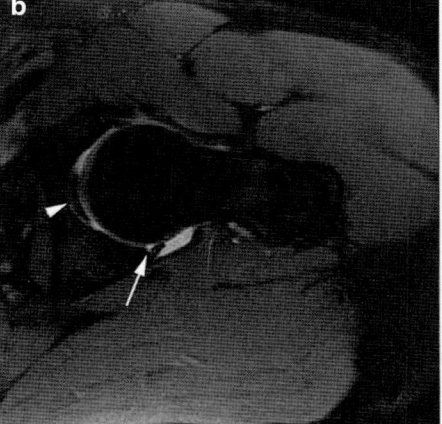 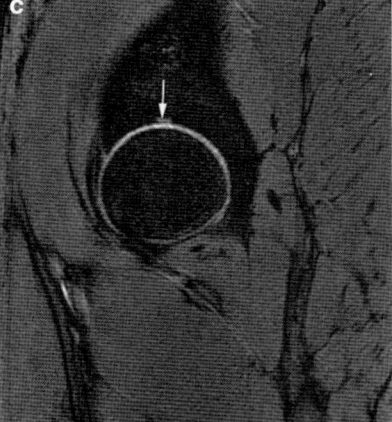

Fig. 2.3 (**a**) Coronal T1w FS MR arthrogram image shows normal superior recess (*arrowhead*) and partial labral tear (*arrow*). (**b**) Oblique axial T1w FS MR arthrogram image shows normal cleft (*arrow*) at the junction of inferior labrum and transverse ligament. Ligamentum teres (*arrowhead*). (**c**) Sagittal PDw MR image shows normal acetabular stellate cartilage (*arrow*)

occurs (Fig. 2.3c). Subcortical cystic change or herniation pits can occur anywhere throughout the femoral neck circumference and their presence in isolation is non-specific. However oedematous cystic change can be seen underlying the anterosuperior prominence in cam impingement (Fig. 2.5).

Appearances of FAI

Frequently in cam impingement there is a triad of femoral head deformity, labral and acetabular cartilage damage (Figs. 2.4–2.7). Labral tears occur at the base of labrum at its junction with the anterosuperior acetabular cartilage. This defect can be full or partial thickness but in early disease there is rarely any other labral deformity or cysts. However, similar to meniscal injury, chronic injury and subsequent degenerative change result in complex tears with associated labral deformity (Fig. 2.6). Paralabral cysts occur with full thickness tears and can extrude anteriorly and superiorly therefore it is important not to confuse this with iliopsoas tendon pathology radiologically or clinically (Fig. 2.8).

Femoral head deformity is assessed on oblique axial sequences by measuring the alpha angle which normally should not exceed 55° (Fig. 2.4). Other proposed measurements include radial measurements from the femoral head centre but to date these are not as widely utilised as the alpha angle.

Assessment of cartilage injury can be difficult given the relatively thin, closely apposed and highly curved articular surfaces. Even with MR arthrography there is little distensile pressure produced on the articular surfaces. Subchondral change (oedema or cysts) and reduced thickness are good indicators of cartilage damage (Fig. 2.7). Delaminating flap tears of the adjacent acetabulum or femoral head can be missed because thickness is maintained and there may be no superficial disruption to allow contrast within the flap (Fig. 2.6). Higher strength (3T) MR scanners may provide increased resolution for this area in the future.

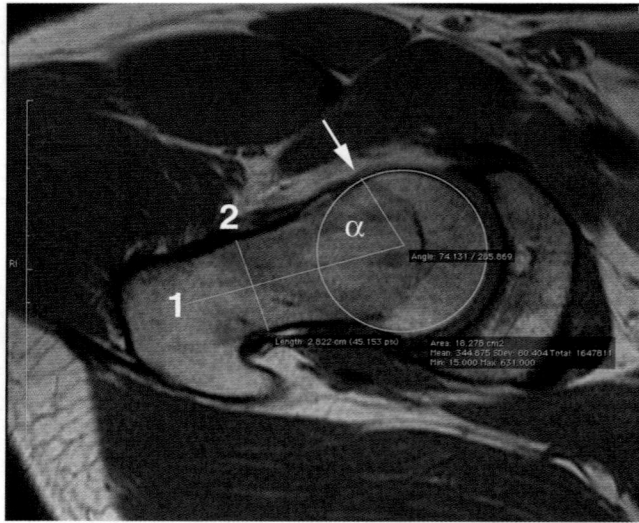

Fig. 2.4 Alpha angle of 74° (normal<55°). Oblique axial T1w MR arthrogram image through the neck with *circle* drawn to best fit femoral head. Line 1 from the *circle* centre and perpendicular to line 2 bisecting the neck. A line is drawn from the *circle centre* to where any prominence leaves the *circle* circumference (*arrow*) and the alpha angle measured

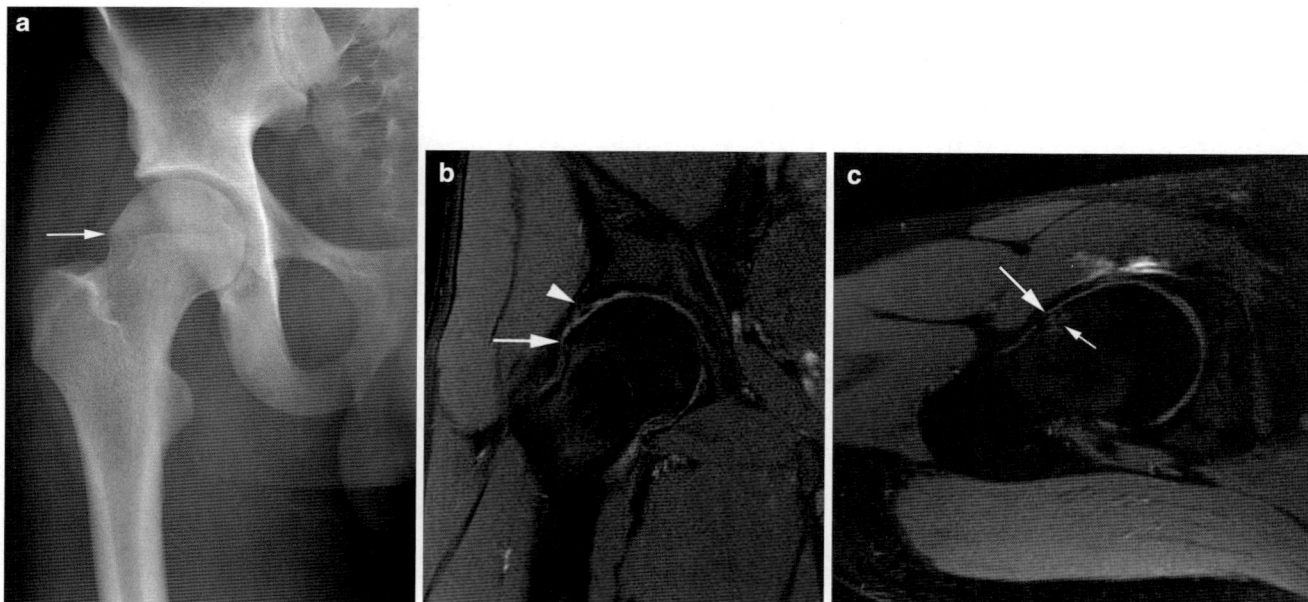

Fig. 2.5 Cam impingement. (**a**) Plain radiograph shows right "pistol grip" deformity with femoral prominence (*arrow*). (**b**) Coronal and (**c**) oblique axial T1w MR arthrogram images show femoral head prominence (*large arrows*) with underlying oedema (*small arrow*), basal labral tear (*arrowhead*) and cartilage thinning

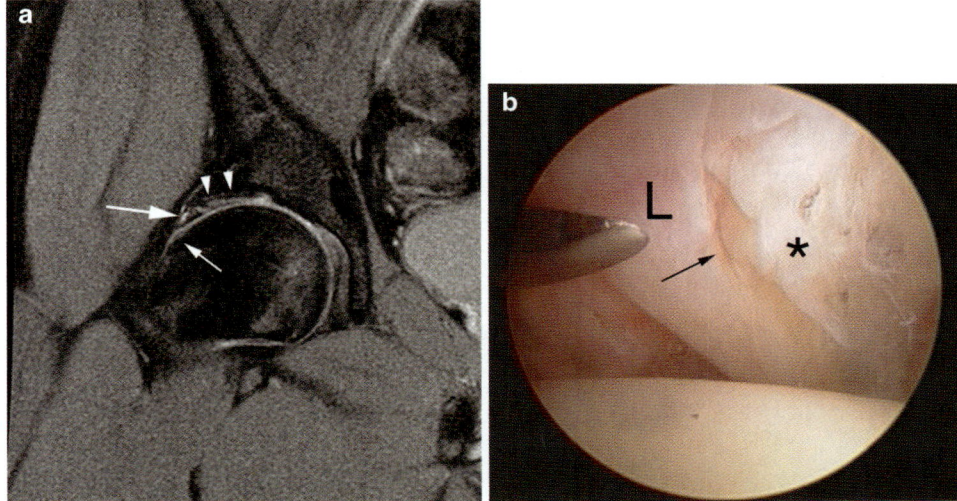

Fig. 2.6 Cam impingement. (**a**) Coronal T1w FS MR arthrogram images shows femoral head prominence (*small arrow*), basal tear extending into main labrum (*large arrow*) and delaminating acetabular cartilage tear (*arrowheads*). (**b**) Arthroscopic image shows labrum (L), basal tear (*arrow*) and delaminated acetabular cartilage (*) (courtesy of Mr. E. Schilders)

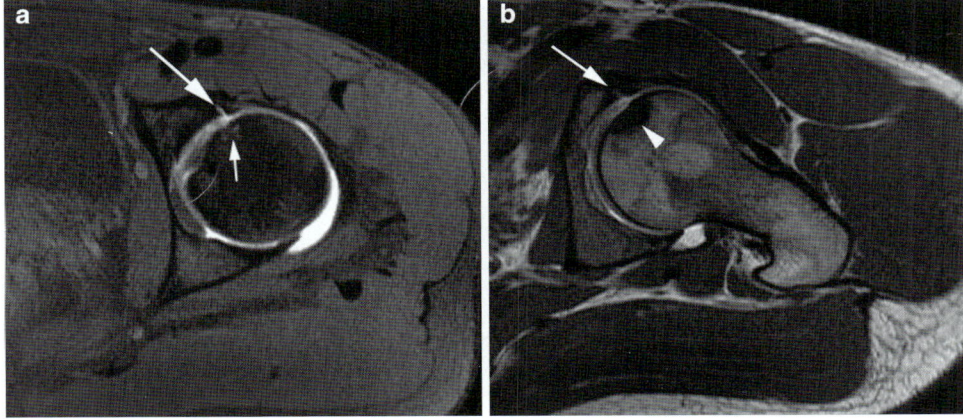

Fig. 2.7 Femoral osteochondral lesion. (**a**) Axial T1w FS MR arthrogram image shows basal labral tear (*arrow*) and apposing cartilage irregularity and feint subchondral high signal (*small arrow*). (**b**) Oblique axial T1w MR arthrogram image shows subchondral sclerosis (*arrowhead*) and irregularity more clearly

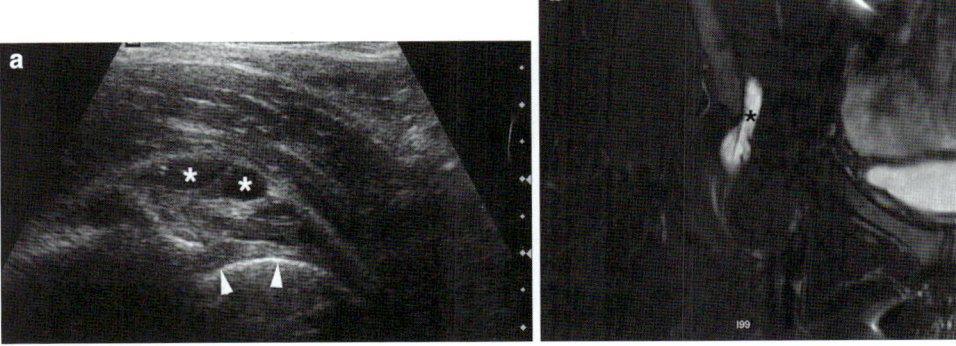

Fig. 2.8 Iliopsoas bursitis in athlete with hip pain sent for MRA. (**a**) Longitudinal sonogram prior to guided injection for MRA shows complex bursitis (*) and labrum (*arrowheads*). (**b**) Coronal T2w FS MRA image shows the bursa (*)

In pincer impingement the acetabular depth can be assessed as well as the usual labral and osteochondral abnormalities (especially posteriorly) (Figs. 2.9 and 2.10). Os acetabuli can be associated with this type of impingement and their presence should be noted (Fig. 2.10). The alpha angle is usually normal but should always be assessed in case a mixed picture is present that will need addressing at surgery.

Other Hip Abnormalities

Osteochondral lesions can also occur outside the setting of impingement secondary to shearing and compressive forces. During MR examination a non-fat-suppressed sequence is recommended to ensure chronic (non-oedematous) lowsignal sclerotic or fibrotic processes are not missed as well as highlighting bone marrow within intra-articular bodies (Figs. 2.7 and 2.11).

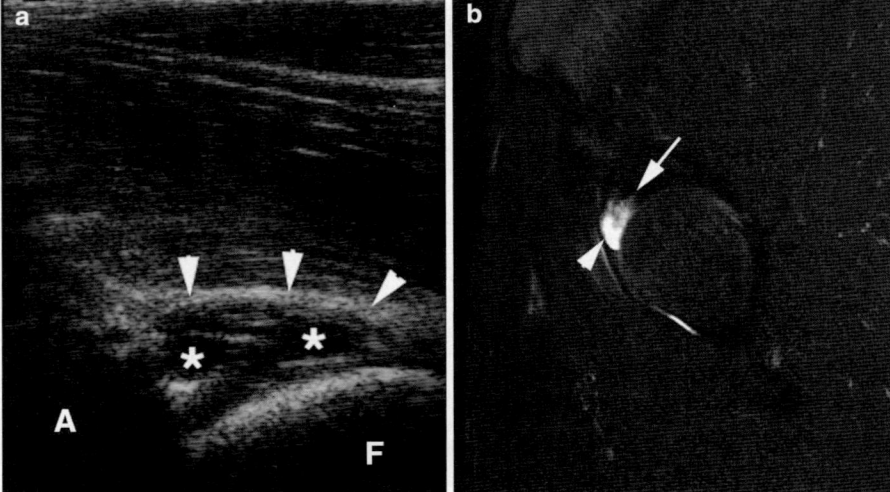

Fig. 2.9 Pincer impingement due to large intralabral cyst. (**a**) Longitudinal sonogram prior to injection shows enlarged cystic (*) labrum (*arrowheads*). *A* acetabulum; *F* femoral head. (**b**) Sagittal T2w FS MRA image shows cyst (*arrowhead*) with irregular labral margin (*arrow*)

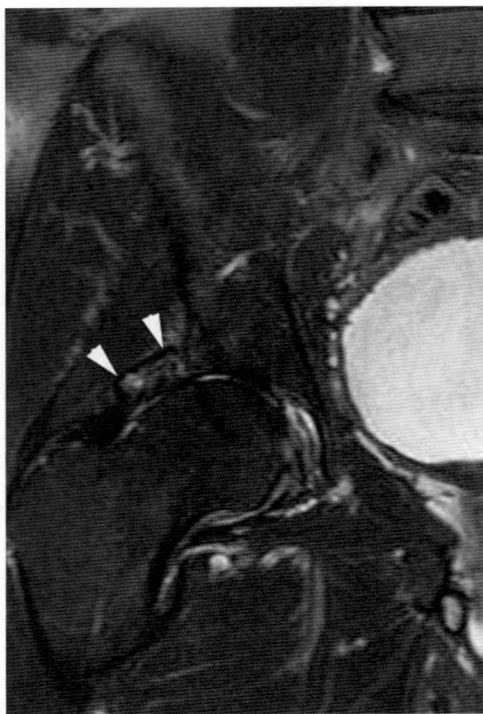

Fig. 2.10 Pincer impingement. Coronal T2w FS MR image shows large oedematous os acetabuli (*arrowheads*)

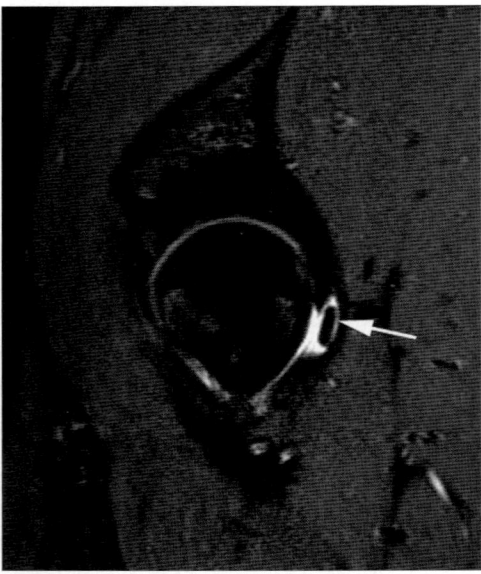

Fig. 2.11 Intermittent hip locking. Sagittal PDw FS MRA image shows posterior body (*arrow*)

Role of Other Modalities

Plain radiographs can define "pistol grip" femoral abnormality (cam) (Fig. 2.4a) and acetabular retroversion by the cross over sign (pincer). CT allows 3D reconstruction of femoral morphology but lacks soft tissue resolution and is therefore not routinely used.

Ultrasound only assesses the anterior and superior labrum (where most pathology occurs) but is still insensitive to undisplaced tears and cartilage abnormality. However ultrasound can aid diagnosis when the labrum is thickened or has an associated cyst (Fig. 2.9). Ultrasound also has an important role in intervention and detecting alternative diagnoses (Fig. 2.8) [9, 10].

Management in Athletes

Non-surgical management has not been fully evaluated in FAI with surgical osteotomy of the femoral prominence, labral repair/trimming and chondroplasty now commonly performed arthroscopically. The prognosis for elite athletes is excellent especially if intervention occurs before more extensive cartilage degeneration develops [8].

Injection of the hip joint or needling of associated paralabral cysts can provide temporary symptomatic relief allowing an athlete to complete a schedule prior to surgery. This strategy is not recommended in the medium or long-term as the anaesthetic and steroid can reduce pain but potentially allows the labral and articular cartilage damage to progress.

Post-operative Imaging of the HIP

If an athlete develops pain post-hip surgery or during rehabilitation, an open mind should be kept regarding the source of pain. This should include labral retear but also consider iliopsoas tendon irritation (or snapping) and referred adductor pain. Given this potential spectrum, conventional MR imaging best evaluates all these areas. The criteria for retear are the same as primary tear although it should be noted that the labrum may not look homogeneous due to granulation tissue and artefact may be present (Fig. 2.12).

Technique: Ultrasound-Guided Injection of the Hip and Soft Tissues

Direct needle visualisation is preferred for hip and soft tissue injection as it allows confirmation of needle and injectate position for diagnostic (local anaesthetic or gadolinium solution in MR arthrography) and therapeutic procedures (e.g. corticosteroid). It requires a needle skin entry site at the margin of the probe and can be performed in either the transverse or longitudinal plane of the femoral neck, although the transverse position is usually easier to perform. After skin preparation and local anaesthetic injection the main needle is advanced under direct guidance into the joint or soft tissue target (Fig. 2.13). Once the needle is on the femoral articular surface there should be little resistance to injection with injectate flowing away from the needle tip (if it does collect around the tip it indicates an extra-articular position).

Needle choice will vary with patient body habitus but is usually longer than 5 cm. An aseptic technique is essential to

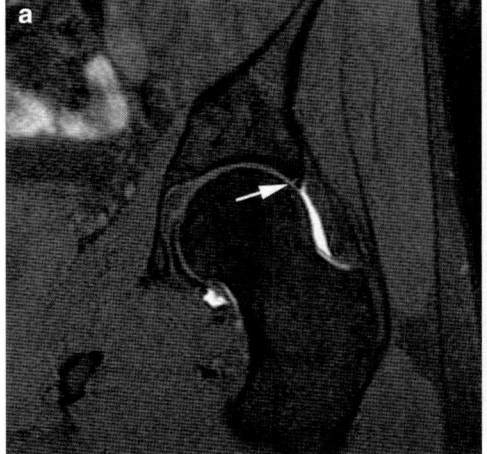
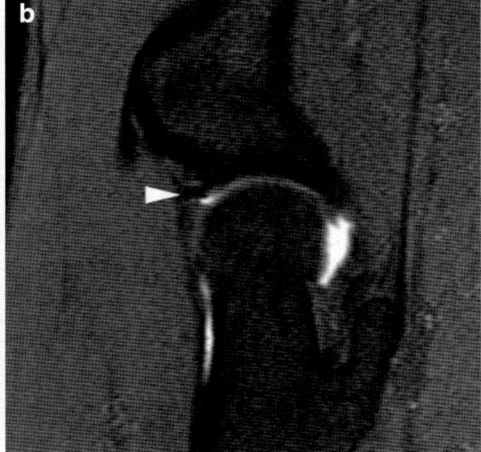

Fig. 2.12 Athlete with previously treated cam impingement (pre-op see Fig. 2.3a). (**a**) Post-op coronal and (**b**) sagittal T1w FS MRA images show granulation tissue (*arrow*) in the repaired labrum and surgical artefact (*arrowhead*)

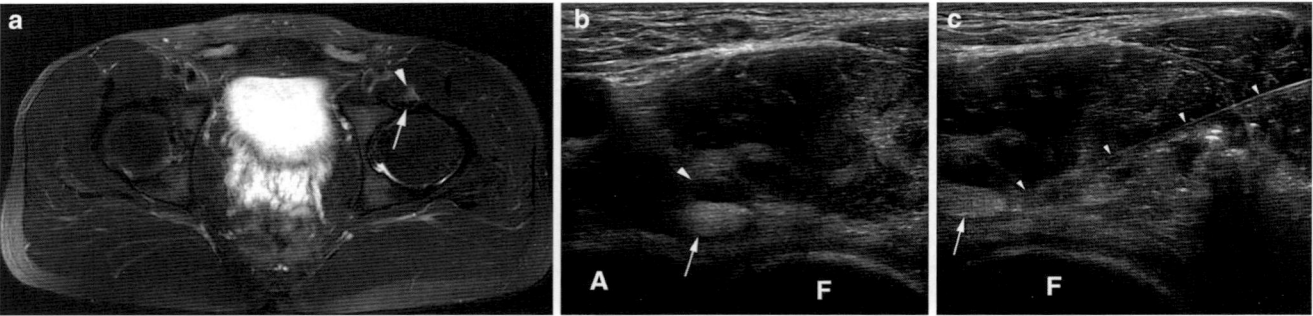

Fig. 2.13 Iliopsoas para tendinopathy. (**a**) Axial T2w FS MR image shows normal left iliopsoas tendon (*arrow*) with surrounding oedema (*arrowhead*). (**b**) and (**c**) Corresponding transverse sonograms show normal tendon (*arrow*), oedema (*large arrowhead*) and needle placement (*small arrowheads*) during injection. *A* acetabulum; *F* femoral head

reduce the risk of iatrogenic infection and this is the main risk explained during consent for the procedure although in reality the incidence is extremely low (<1/1,000) [11].

Pelvic Muscle and Tendon Injury

Acute pelvic muscle injuries are common but acute tears of normal tendons are rare with overuse injuries resulting in tendinopathy more frequent [12, 13]. Overuse (training errors), injury elsewhere in the kinetic chain, adjacent pathology (e.g. joint degeneration) or just increasing age can alter a tendon's matrix, collagen composition and subsequently its susceptibility to injury.

Imaging evaluation and findings for muscle injury are presented in Chap. 6 and the same principles apply when investigating the pelvic region. In this section the commoner muscle injuries seen in the pelvis will be briefly reviewed and the main focus will be on imaging and intervention for overuse tendon injuries.

Imaging Choice

Full pelvic muscle and tendon visualisation at ultrasound can be difficult due to frequent tendon obliquity and increased muscle bulk present when compared to the extremities. A careful technique is essential to eliminate anisotropy as a cause of hypoechoic change both from obliquity (e.g. iliopsoas) or crossing of multiple fibrils (e.g. adductor, hamstring and gluteal tendons). For these reasons, unless the clinical features are very focal, MR imaging is initially performed as it offers a larger and more consistent field of view. In addition, oedematous paratenon changes seen in athletes can be minor and more easily appreciated on MR imaging compared to ultrasound.

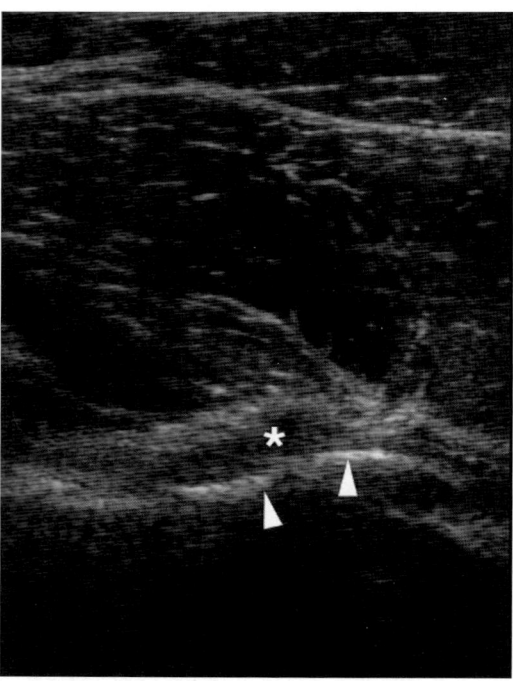

Fig. 2.14 Iliopsoas impingement due to acetabular osteophyte. Longitudinal sonogram shows the spur (*arrowheads*) displacing the hypoechoic tendon (*))

However ultrasound is still excellent for focussed and dynamic examination of muscle, tendon and adjacent bone abnormality, as well as targeted intervention (Figs. 2.13–2.15) [14].

Areas of mechanical friction are important for the development of chronic damage (and tendon snapping) and occur at the iliopectineal eminence (iliopsoas tendon), greater trochanter (gluteal tendons and tensor fascia lata (TFL)) or from overlap with adjacent tendons (gluteal and proximal hamstring tendons) [9, 15–17]. Adductor longus tendinopathy is common but can be asymptomatic while tenoperiosteal disease seems to be a more important source of chronic groin pain (see Pubalgia later).

Iliopsoas Tendinopathy and Snapping

This compound muscle has a primary function of hip flexion and lateral rotation originating from the spine and pelvis with its distal tendon attaching to the lesser trochanter [9, 16]. Overuse tendon or paratenon abnormality is increasing recognised in runners. This typically occurs at the iliopectineal eminence just medial to the anterior inferior iliac spine (Fig. 2.13). At this point, the tendon normally lies adjacent to the cortex and rotates smoothly as the hip flexes and extends. Secondary irritation can be due to adjacent hip disease or bony irregularity (osteophytes) (Fig. 2.14). Iliopsoas tendinopathy or bursitis can be difficult to clinically pinpoint and these abnormalities should always be evaluated as part of imaging for hip or groin pain (Fig. 2.8).

MR imaging typically shows a normal low signal tendon with a faint area of oedema in the adjacent muscle (Fig. 2.13a). Occasionally if there is marked impingement there may be a bursa and oedematous tendon change. Because of the high level of communication with the hip joint an effusion should always be evaluated in case tendon sheath fluid is due to this rather than a primary tenosynovitis (Fig. 2.8).

Ultrasound evaluation is made in the transverse plane at the level of the iliopectineal imminence and hip joint where it can assess tendinopathy, bursitis, snapping and any adjacent hip or iliopectineal abnormality [9, 17]. Minor but significant adjacent bony abnormality (spur or osteophyte) can often be better appreciated at ultrasound (Fig. 2.14).

Clinically iliopsoas snapping is felt as a sudden flick that can be reproduced on hip flexion and extension. The tendon may appear normal but there is usually some subtle paratenon oedema which may only be appreciated on MR imaging. However, ultrasound can confirm snapping on dynamic hip flexion with the tendon losing its normal smooth translation from lateral to medial being replaced by juddering and sudden displacement correlating with symptoms (Fig. 2.15) [17].

Ultrasound-guided injection of steroid and anaesthetic is an effective treatment to reduce inflammation and allow rehabilitation [9]. The injection is performed under direct guidance using a transverse position with the needle introduced from the lateral aspect thus avoiding the femoral vessels medially (Fig. 2.13c).

Quadriceps and Sartorius

The two rectus femoris tendons originate from the anterior inferior iliac spine (long head) and acetabulum (short or reflected head) adjacent to the hip capsular margin. Proximal tendon disease is rare but acute apophyseal avulsions can occur at the anterior inferior iliac spine in skeletally immature patients usually during kicking or tackling (Fig. 2.16). This injury mechanism also commonly affects sartorius and the superior iliac spine. If a large bone fragment is involved diagnosis can be confirmed on plain film but avulsions can sometime mainly involve the fibrocartilage at the tendon insertion with only a small flake of bone. Ultrasound can confirm the intact tendon continuous with fibrocartilage and any associated bone fragment. Accurate evaluation of displacement is relevant in dictating whether surgical reattachment is necessary (Fig. 2.17).

In skeletally mature athletes proximal myotendinous injuries occur at the merger of the two rectus femoris heads just distal to the level of the hip joint. This injury occurs particularly in kicking athletes when the leg is drawn back with hip

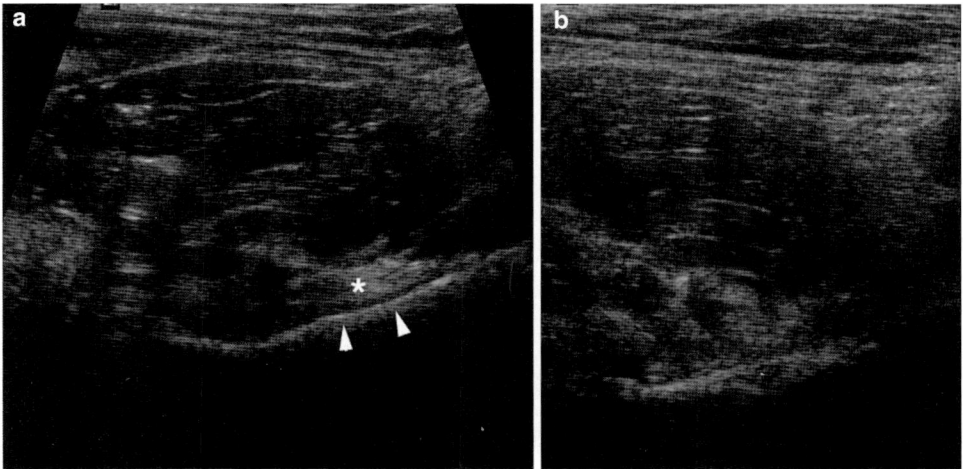

Fig. 2.15 Snapping iliopsoas. Transverse sonograms of iliopsoas tendon (*) at the iliopectineal eminence (*arrowheads*) (**a**) at rest and (**b**) in flexion show juddering rotation

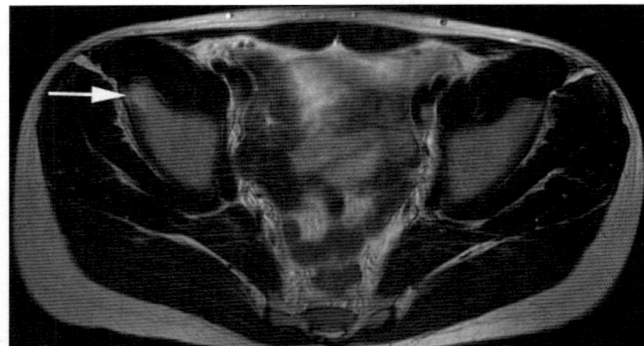

Fig. 2.16 Rectus femoris apophyseal injury. Transverse T2w MR image shows acute right anterior inferior iliac spine oedema (*arrow*) consistent with stress injury and no avulsion

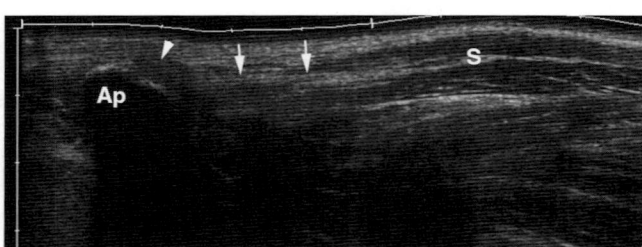

Fig. 2.17 Sartorius (S) apophyseal injury. Longitudinal eFOV sonogram shows acute anterior superior iliac spine (Ap) avulsion, intact cartilage (*arrowhead*) and tendon (*arrows*)

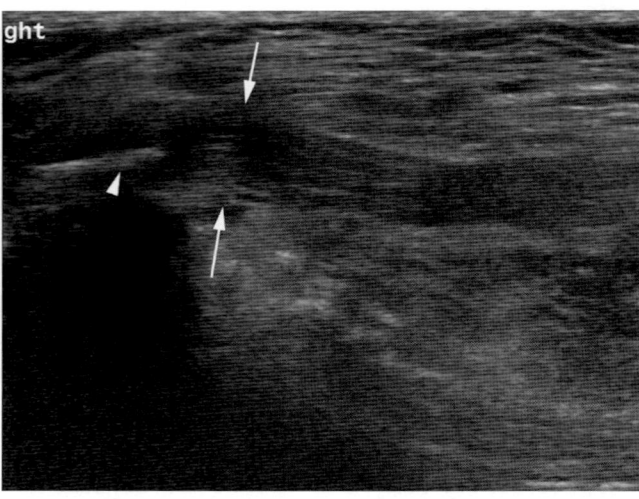

Fig. 2.18 Runner with lateral pain. Longitudinal sonogram shows chronically thickened hypoechoic tendon (*arrows*) arising from irregular iliac crest (*arrowhead*)

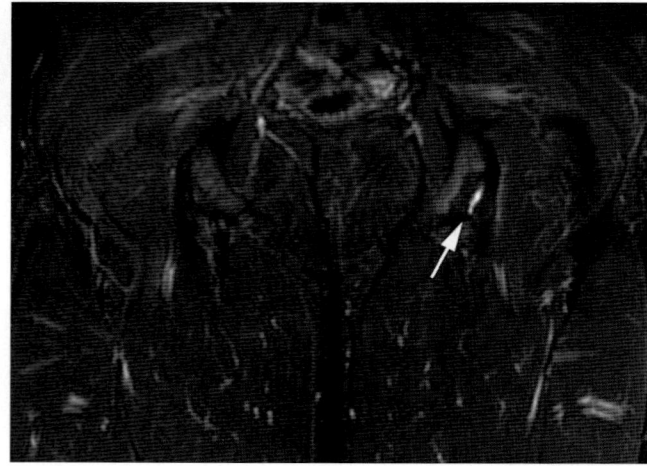

Fig. 2.19 Coronal STIR MR image shows partial left common hamstring avulsion with high signal oedema including small area of bone (*arrow*)

extension and knee flexion producing significant eccentric loading at this point. The quadriceps muscles are also a common area for scarring and myositis ossificans because of frequent athletic injury and contusion.

Tensor Fascia Lata

The TFL originates from the iliac crest with a broad short tendon and muscle which then forms the iliotibial band passing distally to the tibia. The muscle's main function is to stabilise the knee in flexion and extension during normal gait and athletic activity. The tendon can occasionally undergo a proximal partial tear or tendinopathy at the iliac crest and this feature is reported as a cause of groin pain in runners. At ultrasound the proximal tendon appears swollen, hypoechoic and has lost its normal fibrillar pattern (Fig. 2.18) [15].

Slightly more distally impingement of the iliotibial band over the greater trochanter and adjacent gluteal tendons can result in tendinopathy and snapping clinically. On MR imaging there may be oedema present, while on ultrasound the tendon may appear hypoechoic with abnormal movement on hip flexion [17].

A shearing injury can occur in contact sport athletes in relation to the TFL resulting in haematoma and fat necrosis at its junction with the overlying subcutaneous fat and fascia. The underlying TFL appears normal and this is easier to appreciate on ultrasound as the complex hypoechoic fluid and oedema overlying the fascia can obscure this detail on MR imaging.

Hamstring Group

Overuse hamstring tendinopathy and paratenon inflammation is most commonly seen in athletes particularly soccer players and distance runners and can result in quite debilitating symptoms due to sciatic nerve irritation (Figs. 2.19–2.21). The

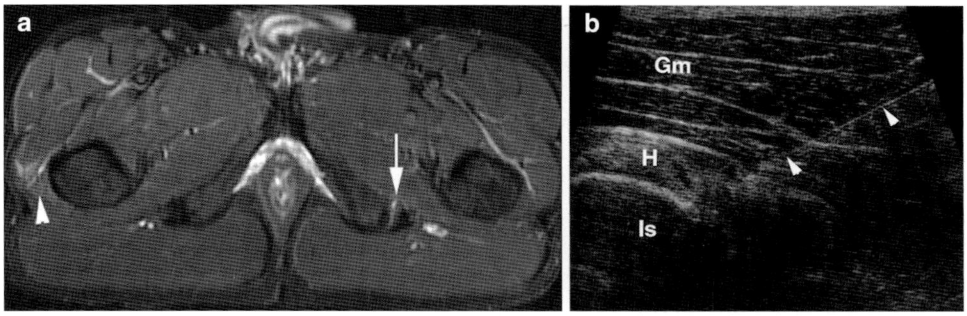

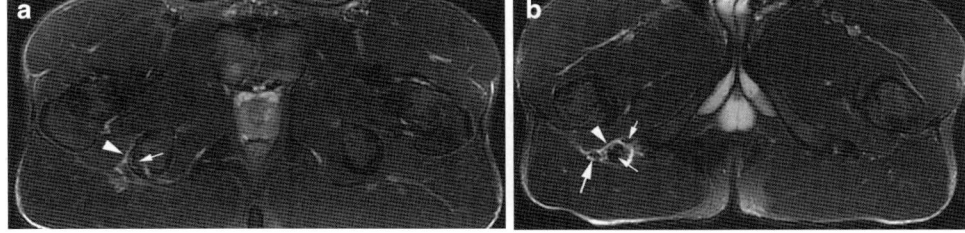

Fig. 2.20 Athlete with left posterior thigh pain. (**a**) Transverse T2w FS MR image shows left paratenon oedema (*arrow*), normal ischial tuberosity and low signal tendons. Note asymptomatic gluteal muscle oedema (*arrowhead*). (**b**) Transverse sonogram shows the ischial tuberosity (Is), hamstring tendons (H), overlying gluteus maximus (Gm), no discernable oedema and therapeutic injection (*arrowheads*)

Fig. 2.21 Athlete with right sciatic pain. Transverse T2w FS MR images show (**a**) right paratenon oedema (*arrowhead*) with normal ischial tuberosity and low signal thickened tendons (*small arrows*) and (**b**) more inferiorly oedema surrounding the sciatic nerve (*large arrow*)

tendons overlap as they originate from the ischial tuberosity which can also have a very variable surface contour normally. Although commonly described as bursitis, discrete fluid collections are rare with subtle paratenon oedematous change common and better seen at MR imaging than ultrasound (Fig. 2.20). The tendons often appear normal, however, they can be thickened if the process is longstanding, in an aged athlete or if there has been previous injury (Fig. 2.21).

Ultrasound can be used to guide injection of steroid and anaesthetic for treatment if resistant to conservative management. A transverse approach allows direct visualisation of the needle avoiding the sciatic nerve (Fig. 2.20b).

Gluteal Muscles

The gluteal muscles are important postural muscles acting on the hip and femur to produce abduction and external rotation during normal gait. Gluteal tendinopathy particularly of medius and minimus is a common symptomatic area where they attach to the greater trochanter and are crossed by gluteus maximus and TFL. Bursae are present between the individual tendons as well as between the tendons and the greater trochanter [18]. Bursitis or a fluid collection is rarely seen with tendinopathy and oedema more commonly found on imaging. Clinical correlation is always necessary as asymptomatic tendinopathy, tendon thickening and entheseal changes (greater trochanter irregularity) are commonly seen in mature athletes. Ultrasound can also be used to guide injection of steroid and anaesthetic for treatment. Acute athletic gluteal muscle and tendon tears are rare.

Adductor Group

The thigh adductor muscle group consists of adductors longus, brevis and magnus as well as gracilis. These muscles originate from the pubic body, symphyseal capsular tissues and inferior pubic ramus passing distally to the femur and tibia (see Pubalgia). Their main action is thigh adduction with some hip flexion and are functionally important in sports where frequent changes of direction are required [19]. Acute muscle injuries occur with forced abduction of the thigh and adductor longus is most commonly injured at the proximal or distal myotendinous junction. Pectineus lies superior to the adductor area originating from the superior pubic ramus. Injury to this muscle can be clinically confused with adductor longus injury; however, the prognosis for return to activity is much more rapid than adductor injury (Fig. 2.22).

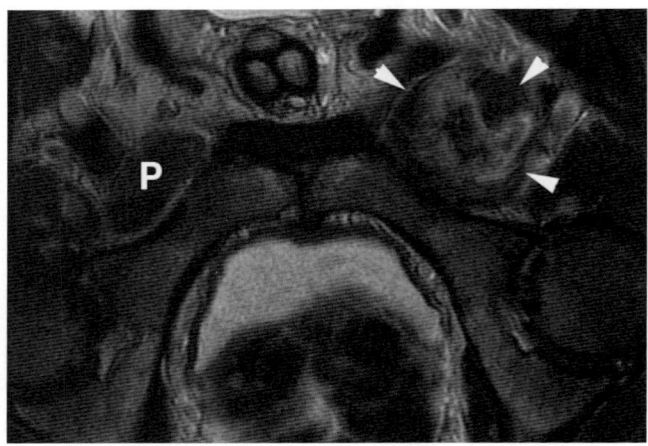

Fig. 2.22 Axial T2w MR image shows left pectineus muscle tear (*arrowheads*) with oedema and haemorrhage. Normal right muscle (P)

Proximal tendon avulsion is more common in mature athletes due to chronic tendinopathy (Fig. 2.23) [19]. On imaging, there is oedema and free fluid anterior to the pubis with a thickened and retracted tendon (Fig. 2.24). Although haemorrhage can pass along the aponeurosis, no muscle disruption is seen. However, because of the close relationship of the adductor origin, capsular tissues and inguinal soft tissues (see Pubalgia later) haemorrhage can extend into the inguinal canal and scrotum causing severe symptoms initially (Fig. 2.24).

Abdominal Muscles

The musculature of the lower abdominal wall has an important postural function. The rectus abdominis lies either side of the midline raphe running inferiorly to blend with the superior

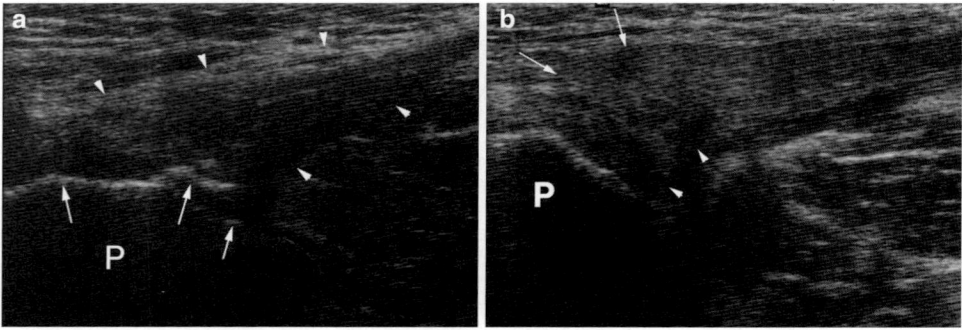

Fig. 2.23 Longitudinal sonograms show (**a**) normal adductor longus tendon (*arrowheads*) and insertion with asymptomatic hypoechoic tendinopathy and pubic irregularity (*arrows*). (**b**) Symptomatic thickened tendinopathic adductor longus origin (*arrows*) with hypoechoic deep partial tear (*arrowheads*). P Pubis

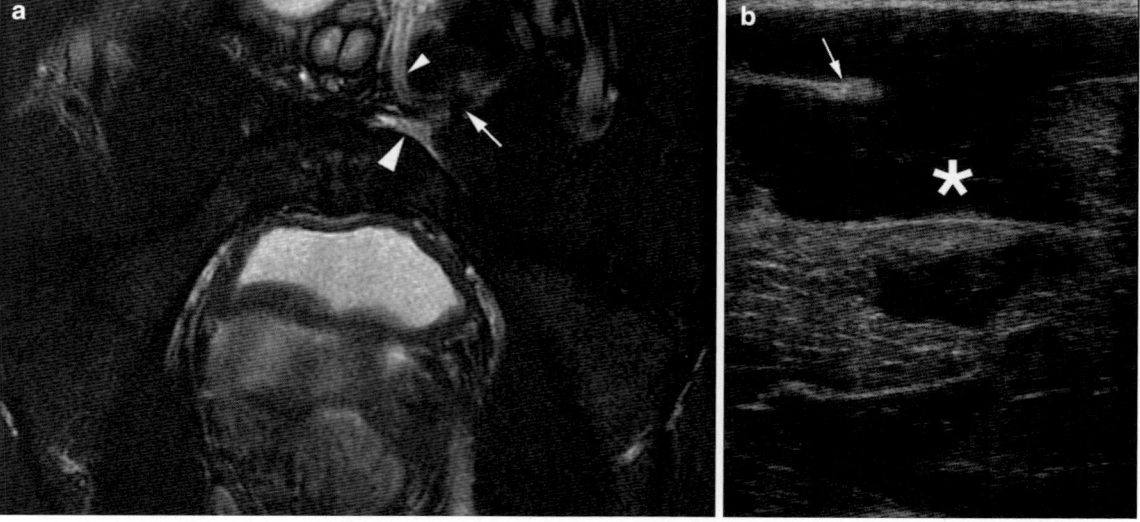

Fig. 2.24 Acute adductor longus tendon tear. (**a**) Axial T2w FS MR image shows retracted tendon (*arrow*), left-sided oedema and haemorrhage (*large arrowhead*) anterior to the pubis and extending into the scrotum and inguinal canal (*small arrowhead*). (**b**) Transverse sonogram shows pubic cortex, hypoechoic haematoma (*) and torn retracted tendon (*arrow*)

aspect of the symphysis pubis and the adductor musculature [20]. The other abdominal muscles form three layers at the lateral margin of the rectus abdominis with external oblique outermost, internal oblique and then transversus abdominis lying innermost [21]. Acute muscle injury is relatively rare except in athletes but rectus abdominis is most commonly affected (especially in weightlifters, tennis players and gymnasts). In athletes with "side on" activity (tennis and cricket) asymmetry of muscle bulk is commonly seen. The oblique muscles can undergo acute injury especially in cricketers where the bowling action requires violent torsion and side flexion which particularly affects the internal oblique and its attachment to the inferior 12th rib (see Chaps. 4 and 6).

23]. Considerable reactive forces (multiples of body weight) act through the anterior pelvis in particular the symphysis pubis, inguinofemoral aponeuroses and parasymphyseal muscles (abdominal and adductor groups). The pelvis is normally tilted anteriorly in relation to the hip and lower limb and this relationship must be maintained through complex athletic movements. This core stability is thought to be crucial for normal and repetitive athletic activity of the pelvis which in turns acts as the stabiliser for effective athletic function of the lower limb [24]. Pre-season weakness of the hip abductors and external rotators has been shown to predispose to lower limb injury while decreased adductor function predisposes to further ipsilateral adductor injury [24, 25].

Athletic Groin Pain (Pubalgia)

Pubalgia is defined as chronic athletic groin pain of insidious onset and over 6–12 weeks duration. Therefore, acute osseous, muscle or tendon injuries are not included and discussed elsewhere in this chapter.

Biomechanics and Core Stability

The pelvis contains the centre of gravity of the body with the symphysis pubis and rami functioning as an effective strut between the lower limbs and sacrum (and rest of spine) [22,

Anatomy

The symphysis pubis is a non-synovial diarthrodial joint with the pubic articular surfaces covered by hyaline cartilage and separated by an intervening fibrocartilagenous disc [20, 21, 26]. The joint is the confluence for the thigh adductors, rectus abdominis and the medial aspect of the inguinal ligament (Fig. 2.25) [20, 21]. Chronic degeneration and irregularity of the symphysis pubis is a common non-specific finding seen in professional athletes but can also occur secondary to chronic adductor enthesopathic change (Fig. 2.23). Importantly, the apophysis of the pubis covers its anteromedial articular surface and therefore this area can have an irregular contour normally before and after fusion (usually at 18–24 years of age) (Fig. 2.26) [20, 26].

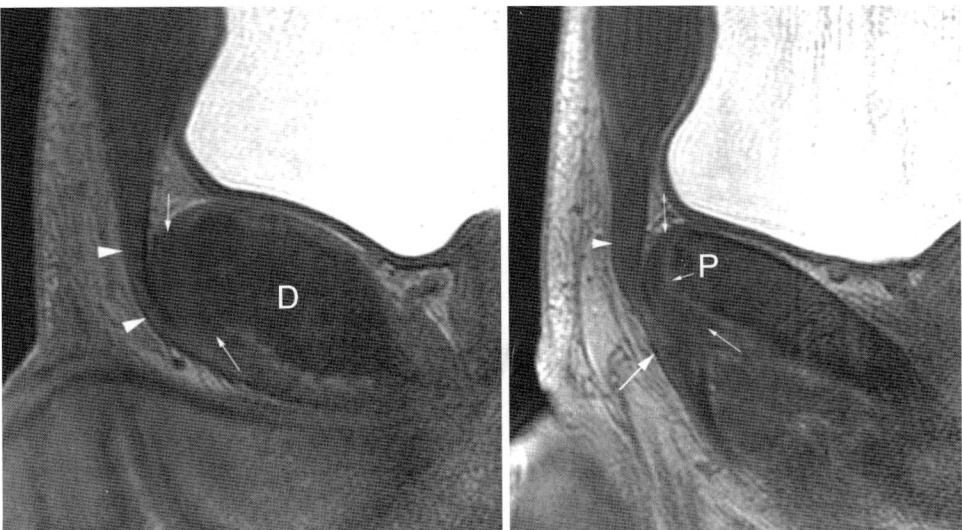

Fig. 2.25 Soft tissue anatomy. (**a**) Symphyseal and (**b**) parasymphyseal sagittal high resolution T2w MR volume images show the pubis (P), symphyseal disc (D) merging with the anterior capsular tissues (*small arrows*), rectus abdominis (*arrowheads*) and more laterally adductor longus (*large arrow*)

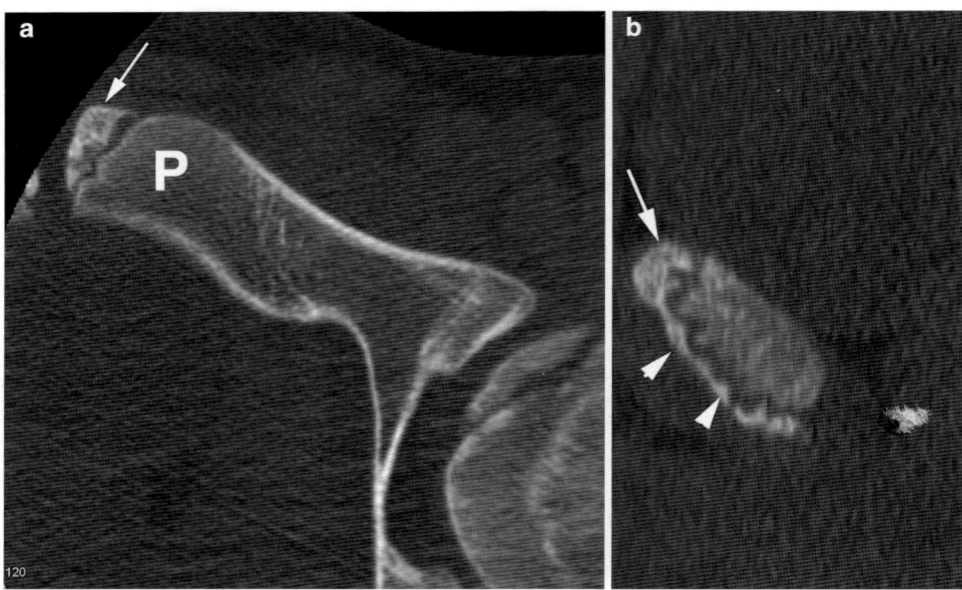

Fig. 2.26 Apophyseal anatomy (17-year old). (**a**) Axial and (**b**) sagittal reformatted CT images show extent of the anteromedial pubic apophysis (*arrow*) and its inferior extent (*arrowheads*). *P* main pubis

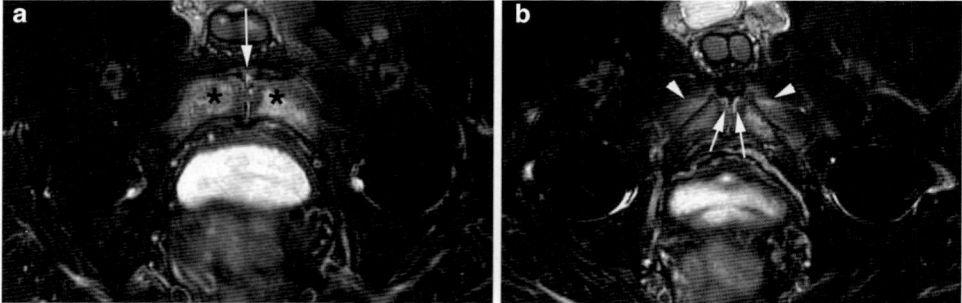

Fig. 2.27 Pubalgia – osteitis pubis clinically. (**a**) and (**b**) Axial oblique T2w FS MR images show marked bilateral pubic bone marrow oedema (***), capsular oedema (*arrow*), subchondral oedema (*arrows*) and surrounding soft tissue oedema (*arrowheads*)

The adductor longus, brevis and gracilis have attachments to the pubic bone, pubic symphysis capsular tissues (and disc) merging with rectus abdominis (Fig. 2.25) [21, 27]. This close anatomical relationship may explain why overuse injuries in this region can commonly produce diffuse symptoms radiating into the medial thigh and lower abdomen.

The junction of the pubic apophysis and soft tissues probably represents an area of biomechanical weakness which endures considerable forces during athletic single stance manoeuvres. This junctional area also represents the centre of abnormality detected in MR series of athletic pubalgia (Figs. 2.27–2.31). Attachments of the muscles to the capsule and therefore to the fibrocartilaginous disc mean changes to the cartilaginous structures, including cleft formation and adjacent bone marrow oedema may occur by transmission of repetitive stresses from the muscle groups directly to the soft tissues and joint.

Clinical Overview

Pubalgia is a significant clinical problem with potentially poor prognostic implications for athletes as it can be extremely difficult to diagnose and treat effectively [28]. Athletes describe slight discomfort at the end of a game which then gradually progresses to stiffness on waking in the mornings. Initially all these features ease with warming-up but soon symptoms begin to appear during playing and are exacerbated by cutting-in and kicking.

Fig. 2.28 Left publagia and cleft sign. (**a**) Coronal STIR and (**b**) oblique axial T2 FS MR images show left-sided defect (*arrow*) at junction of the capsular tissues and adductor longus continuous with joint (*arrowhead*)

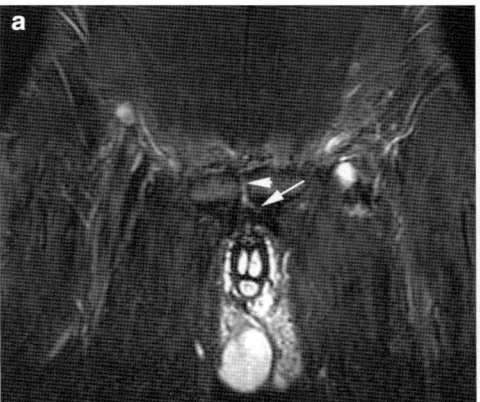
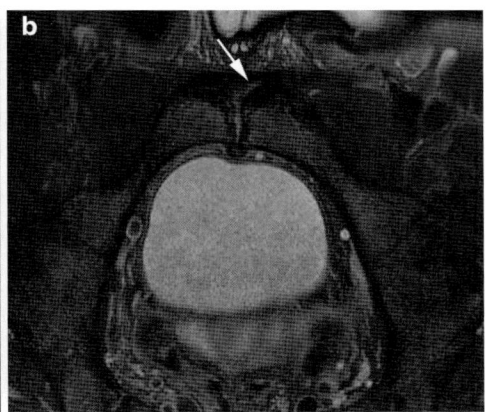

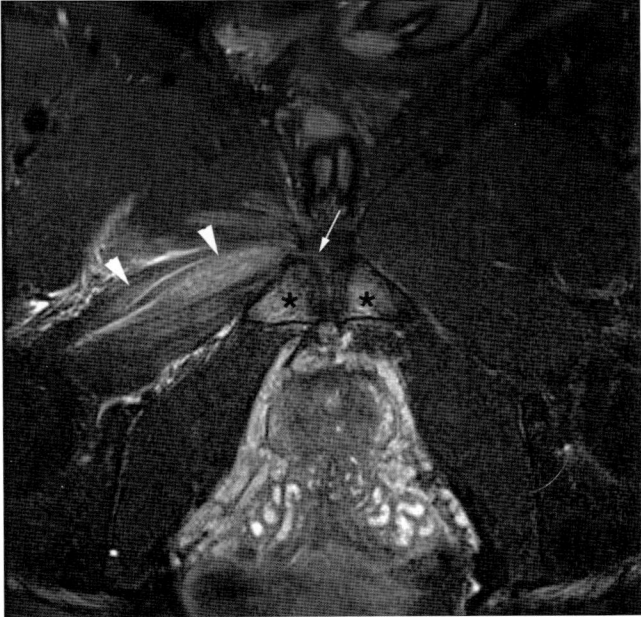

Fig. 2.29 Previous right pubalgia with sudden acute injury. Oblique axial T2 FS MR image shows bilateral pubic bone marrow oedema (*) and right capsular/adductor oedema (*arrow*) which had been present on previous MRI. However, there is now an acute right obturator externus tear (*arrowheads*) which because of the position and overlying muscle bulk would be difficult to define on ultrasound

The increased incidence in sports that require constant changing of direction and kicking, may relate to chronic shearing forces being further exacerbated if the player develops one dominant leg and is commonly in single stance [29]. Although not exclusive to soccer (e.g. ice hockey and Australian rules football) it is certainly described more frequently in soccer players and is estimated to comprise 10% of acute and 18% of chronic injuries [30–32].

There is no unifying theory how this complex process develops and further confusion over terminology with osteitis pubis and sportsman's hernia encompassing many different potential conditions to different clinicians [30, 33–36]. In an effort to decrease confusion the terms pubalgia and pubic bone stress injury are now being used in an effort to describe chronic exertional groin pain omitting references to specific anatomical regions or structures [30, 36].

Proposed Pathologies: Inguinal vs. Parasymphyseal (Table 2.2)

Clinical definition of these various pathologies can be difficult as symptoms and examination findings are similar or overlap markedly [19, 29, 33]. Referred pain should also be considered either from the spine or hip (FAI) [7].

Imaging

Radiological procedures utilised in the evaluation of athletic pubalgia include MR imaging, ultrasound and herniography [13, 30, 37, 38]. Although radiographs and scintigraphy have been previously described as integral investigations, these are often unhelpful in athletes. Pubic sclerosis, irregularity and increased isotope uptake are commonly seen in asymptomatic athletes presumably due to chronic shearing forces and remodelling. Resolution of bone scans is also poor for differentiating other causes of increased uptake or grading injury.

MR Imaging

MR imaging series have found a number of symphyseal and parasymphyseal changes that do correlate with clinical symptoms but minor changes can also be seen in asymptomatic athletes [13, 30, 32, 39]. In one series, diffuse pubic bone marrow oedema did correlate with symptoms but a recent series has shown this is not a prognostic marker for subsequent

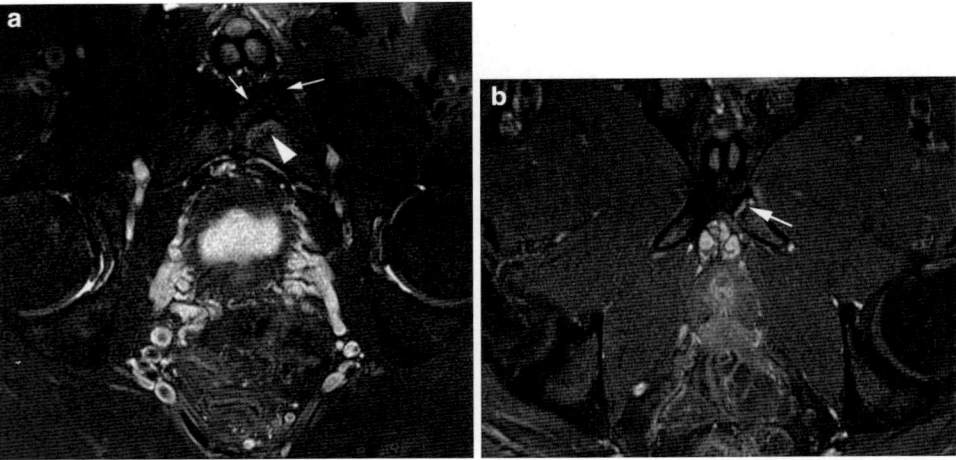

Fig. 2.30 Left pubalgia clinically. (**a**) oblique axial T2 FS and (**b**) T1 FS post-gadolinium MR images show subchondral oedema (*arrowhead*), left capsular/adductor oedema (*small arrows*) and marked inferior entheseal enhancement (*large arrow*)

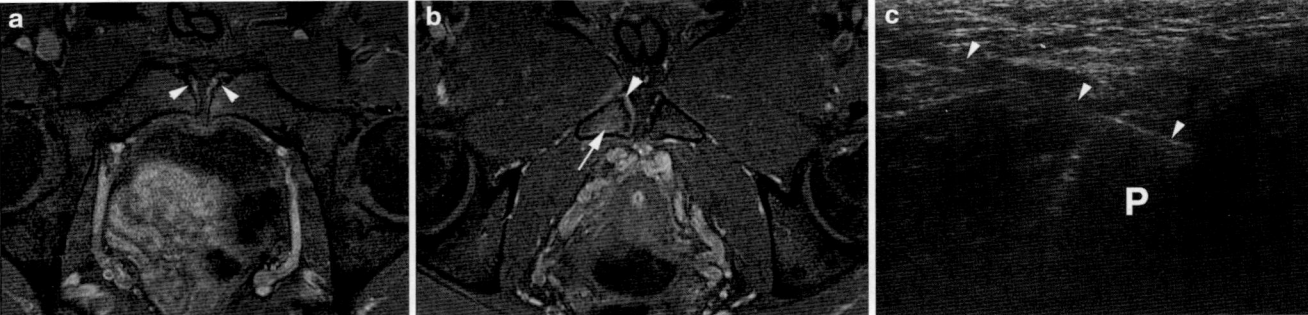

Fig. 2.31 Right pubalgia clinically. (**a**) and (**b**) oblique axial T1 FS post-gadolinium MR images show mild bilateral subchondral enhancement (*arrowheads*) in the old apophysis but marked right-sided inferior enhancement (*arrow* and *large arrowhead*). (**c**) Transverse sonogram shows needle placement (*arrowheads*) at right enthesis adjacent to inferior pubis (P) during injection

Table 2.2 Summary of proposed pathologies for pubalgia and optimal imaging modalities

Inguinal pathologies[a]	Imaging	Parasymphyseal pathologies[b]	Imaging
Inguinal canal ballooning/bulging	US (but ? significance)	Adductor/rectus enthesopathy	MR imaging
Microtears (e.g. External oblique, rectus abdominis)	Not detected	Pubic subchondral stress reaction[b]	MR imaging
Dehiscence (conjoint tendon, inguinal ligament)	Not detected	Symphyseal cleft[b]	MR imaging
Neuralgia (genitofemoral nerves)	Not detected	Osteitis pubis	MR imaging
Inguinal hernia	US (but rare in athletes)	Adductor tendinopathy	MR imaging and US but of questionable significance

[a]Sometimes loosely termed "Sportman's hernia" or "Gilmour's groin"
[b]Similar imaging features recorded with different emphasis placed by authors on primary injury process

development of pubalgia [32, 40, 41]. Severe symmetrical and diffuse bone and soft tissue oedema (Fig. 2.27) can be termed osteitis pubis but is not the predominant appearance in the majority of athletes.

A more reliable indicator is severity of localized subchondral oedema and enhancement of the anteromedial pubis and adjacent capsular tissues (Figs. 2.28–2.31) [13, 41]. This region encompasses the original pubic apophysis, capsular and aponeurotic tissues of the rectus abdominis and adductor muscle group. This appearance is the most common finding in athletes with pubalgia and although present bilaterally is often markedly asymmetrical. Severity of oedema/enhancement and extent (inferior extension to gracilis) correlates with side of symptoms and can allow targeting of soft tissue injection.

Other theories proposed for the primary origin of these MR imaging changes is symphyseal cleft extension or subchondral stress fractures (Table 2.2) [39, 41].

The Role of Ultrasound

Ultrasound is initially performed in parasymphyseal pain to rule out inguinal hernia or acute on chronic tendon or muscle strain (particularly of adductor longus). Features that suggest acute injury within chronic tendinopathy are superimposed acute changes within the tendon including haematoma or oedema causing convex swelling (Fig. 2.23b).

However, ultrasound is often "normal" and if the clinicians are confident of an inguinal soft tissue abnormality (e.g. external oblique or conjoint tendon tear) no other imaging is performed as ultrasound cannot detect the microtears described clinically or the subtle symphyseal changes detected by MR imaging [13, 29, 34].

Management

The majority of players will respond to active rehabilitation and core stabilisation but this can be of a relatively long duration taking many months to return to full activity [12]. A number of surgical procedures have developed in an effort to treat true non-responders but no controlled trials have been described (Table 2.1). These procedures include modified bassini inguinal repairs (with or without mesh), rectoplasty, neural division and adductor tenotomies either alone or often in combination [34–36].

Some studies report an earlier return to pain-free activity after symphyseal injection but no comparable control groups have been included [42–44]. Ultrasound-guided symphysis pubis injection can help refine the clinical diagnosis or provide long-term symptom relief [43]. When unilateral symptoms predominate infiltration around the adductor tendon origin (enthesis) may be sufficient.

Injection Technique

For both types of injection a freehand technique can be used visualising the relevant anatomy (symphyseal joint or adductor tendons). A 22-gauge spinal or long 20-gauge needle is introduced using a transverse oblique or sagittal approach as a pure transverse position may lead to piercing of the medial inguinal contents (Fig. 2.32). When infiltrating around the adductor tendon origins a 20-gauge needle usually suffices, as the adductor muscle is relatively superficial when the thigh is abducted and externally rotated (Fig. 2.31c).

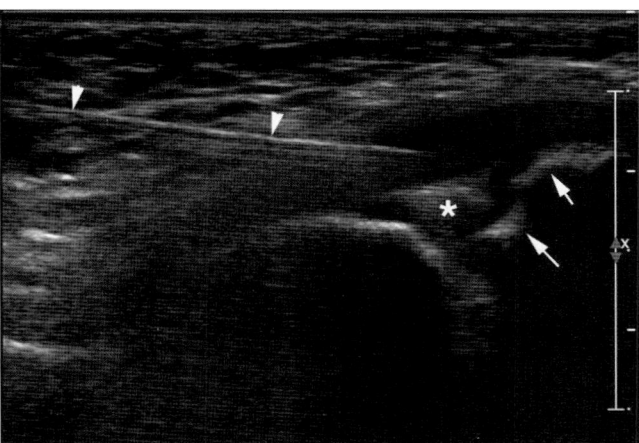

Fig. 2.32 Transverse sonogram shows needle placement (*arrowheads*) during symphyseal injection. Note normal bony irregularity at old apophysis (*arrows*) and disc (*)

Hernias

Hernias are a rare cause of athletic pubalgia and a detailed review of aetiology and imaging evaluation will not be presented but a fuller description is available from the listed references [10, 11, 37].

Overview and Differing Imaging Modalities

Herniography has been evaluated in athletes and is a very sensitive but potentially non-specific technique with demonstration of asymptomatic hernias in 6–18% of athletes. Herniography has a low complication rate but the procedure is still relatively invasive and requires ionising radiation [38]. False-negative herniography findings can occur with small hernias or hernias predominantly consisting of fat [10]. MR imaging and CT have not been evaluated in athletes with clinical hernias.

Ultrasound has been shown to be an accurate technique for confirming and classifying hernias (sensitivity 86–100% and specificity 82–97%) [10, 45]. Ultrasound can also detect fat-filled hernias not seen at herniography, but false-positive findings have been attributed to over-reporting of bulging as direct hernias [45].

Inguinal Canal Evaluation by Ultrasound

A longitudinal image of the inguinal canal is obtained with the linear fibrillar echogenic inguinal ligament seen deep to the subcutaneous fat with multiple hyperechoic and hypoechoic

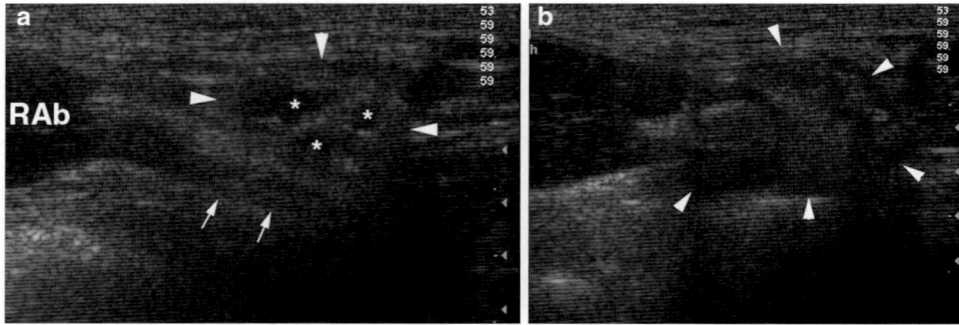

Fig. 2.33 Asymptomatic soccer player. Sagittal sonograms (**a**) at rest show short axis oval inguinal canal (*arrowheads*), contents (*), inferior epigastric vessels (*arrows*) and rectus abdominis (RAb). (**b**) Straining shows expansion (*arrowheads*) by entry of an indirect hernia

linear structures (representing vessels, nerves and cords) within the canal. The inferior epigastric vessels are an important landmark, because after their origin from the external iliac vessels they lie immediately medial to the deep inguinal ring. Deep to the canal are the psoas muscle, echogenic peritoneum, hypoechoic bowel and pre-peritoneal fat [10].

The canal should also be assessed in its short axis which is the anatomical sagittal plane where it appears oval in shape with peritoneum and bowel postero-superiorly (Fig. 2.33).

Normally on performing a slow Valsalva manoeuvre there can be mild bulging of the posterior wall, slight vessel dilatation and sliding of contents but bowel should only move towards the canal and not completely enter or efface it [10].

In the transverse plane an indirect hernia arises lateral to the epigastric vessels and extends through the long axis of the canal. When scanning sagittally (short axis of the canal) the indirect hernia can be seen distending the canal and effacing its contents (Fig. 2.33). Direct inguinal hernias protrude through a posterior wall defect medial to the epigastric vessels rarely continuing distally along the inguinal canal and are more localised in comparison to indirect hernias. In the sagittal plane the direct hernia will push into the canal from the posterior aspect and efface its contents.

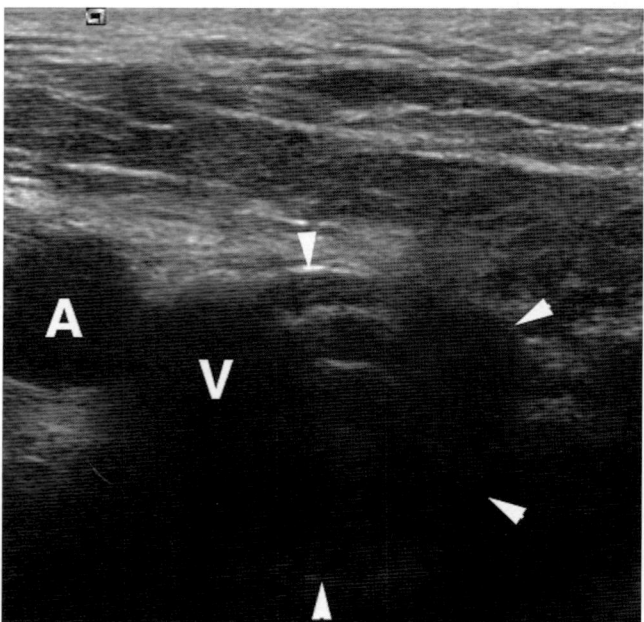

Fig. 2.34 Right publagia in player with previous inguinal repair. Transverse sonogram during straining shows right femoral artery (A), vein (V) and expanding femoral hernia (*arrowheads*)

"Bulging" and "Pre-hernia Complex"

Bulging of the transversalis fascia, where the posterior inguinal wall almost occludes the canal on straining but with no actual herniation has been proposed as a source of pain or "pre-hernia" condition. To date, ultrasound [10, 37, 46] and herniography [38] studies do not confirm that this feature correlates with pain or is part of the spectrum of direct hernia. This finding should be cautiously interpreted as a positive feature, but useful comment may be made when wall bulging occurs on the symptomatic side and is markedly asymmetrical with the asymptomatic side.

Other Hernias

Although uncommon, femoral hernias can occur in male athletes after previous inguinal surgery where bowel preferentially heads deep and inferior to the inguinal canal presumably because of scar tissue. On ultrasound the femoral canal is located just below the inguinal canal and lies medial to the femoral vein [10]. On Valsalva a femoral hernia expands the canal compressing or preventing the normal expansion of the femoral vein (Fig. 2.34).

Spigelian hernias occur through a weakness of the lateral rectus abdominis sheath at its margin with the oblique muscles (linea semilunaris).

Conclusion

The pelvis is a complex anatomical area and a common site for acute and overuse injuries in athletes. Muscle bulk and subtle oedema associated with overuse soft tissue injuries makes MR imaging an excellent tool for diagnosis and grading in pelvic sports injury. Femoroacetabular impingement and pubalgia are complex injury processes which are not yet fully understood but have significant abnormalities on MR imaging.

Ultrasound has a definite role to play in dynamic and focussed evaluation of acute and overuse tendon abnormalities. Increasingly ultrasound-guided injection is playing an important role in athlete management reducing the need for surgical intervention and accelerating recovery.

References

1. Kaufman KR, Brodine S, Shaffer R (2000) Military training-related injuries: surveillance, research, and prevention. Am J Prev Med 18:54–63
2. Nordin M, Frankel VH (2001) Biomechanics of bone. In: Nordin M, Frankel VH (eds) Basic biomechanics of the musculoskeletal system, 3rd edn. Lippincott Williams & Wilkins, Philadelphia, pp 26–58
3. Jones BH, Bovee MW, Harris JM 3rd, Cowan DN (1993) Intrinsic risk factors for exercise-related injuries among male and female army trainees. Am J Sports Med 21:705–710
4. Bergmann G, Graichen F, Rohlmann A (1993) Hip joint loading during walking and running, measured in two patients. J Biomech 26:969–990
5. Davy DT, Kotzar GM, Brown RH et al (1988) Telemetric force measurements across the hip after total arthroplasty. J Bone Joint Surg Am 70:45–50
6. Robertson DD, Britton CA, Latona CR, Armfield DR, Walker PS, Maloney WJ (2003) Hip biomechanics: importance to functional imaging. Semin Musculoskelet Radiol 7:27–41
7. Pfirrmann CW, Mengiardi B, Dora C, Kalberer F, Zanetti M, Hodler J (2006) Cam and pincer femoroacetabular impingement: characteristic MR arthrographic findings in 50 patients. Radiology 240:778–785
8. Espinosa N, Rothenfluh DA, Beck M, Ganz R, Leunig M (2006) Treatment of femoro-acetabular impingement: preliminary results of labral refixation. J Bone Joint Surg Am 88:925–935
9. Adler RS, Buly R, Ambrose R, Sculco T (2005) Diagnostic and therapeutic use of sonography-guided iliopsoas peritendinous injections. AJR Am J Roentgenol 185:940–943
10. Robinson P, Hensor E, Lansdown MJ, Ambrose NS, Chapman AH (2006) Inguinofemoral hernia: accuracy of sonography in patients with indeterminate clinical features. AJR Am J Roentgenol 187:1168–1178
11. McNally E (2004) Ultrasound of the hip. In: McNally E (ed) Practical musculoskeletal ultrasound. Churchill Livingston, London
12. Holmich P, Uhrskou P, Ulnits L et al (1999) Effectiveness of active physical training as treatment for long-standing adductor-related groin pain in athletes: randomised trial. Lancet 353: 439–443
13. Robinson P, Barron DA, Parsons W, Grainger AJ, Schilders EM, O'Connor PJ (2004) Adductor-related groin pain in athletes: correlation of MR imaging with clinical findings. Skeletal Radiol 33:451–457
14. Van Holsbeeck M, Introcasco J (2001) Musculoskeletal ultrasound. Mosby, St. Louis, MO
15. Bass CJ, Connell DA (2002) Sonographic findings of tensor fascia lata tendinopathy: another cause of anterior groin pain. Skeletal Radiol 31:143–148
16. Blankenbaker DG, Tuite MJ (2008) Iliopsoas musculotendinous unit. Semin Musculoskelet Radiol 12:13–27
17. Pelsser V, Cardinal E, Hobden R, Aubin B, Lafortune M (2001) Extraarticular snapping hip: sonographic findings. AJR Am J Roentgenol 176:67–73
18. Pfirrmann CW, Chung CB, Theumann NH, Trudell DJ, Resnick D (2001) Greater trochanter of the hip: attachment of the abductor mechanism and a complex of three bursae – MR imaging and MR bursography in cadavers and MR imaging in asymptomatic volunteers. Radiology 221:469–477
19. Anderson K, Strickland SM, Warren R (2001) Hip and groin injuries in athletes. Am J Sports Med 29:521–533
20. Robinson P, Salehi F, Grainger A et al (2007) Cadaveric and MRI study of the musculotendinous contributions to the capsule of the symphysis pubis. AJR Am J Roentgenol 188:W440–W445
21. Agur A (1991) Grant's atlas of anatomy. Williams and Wilkins, Baltimore, MD
22. Lavignolle B, Vital JM, Senegas J et al (1983) An approach to the functional anatomy of the sacroiliac joints in vivo. Anat Clin 5:169–176
23. Meissner A, Fell M, Wilk R, Boenick U, Rahmanzadeh R (1996) [Biomechanics of the pubic symphysis. Which forces lead to mobility of the symphysis in physiological conditions?]. Unfallchirurg 99:415–421
24. Leetun DT, Ireland ML, Willson JD, Ballantyne BT, Davis IM (2004) Core stability measures as risk factors for lower extremity injury in athletes. Med Sci Sports Exerc 36:926–934
25. Tyler TF, Nicholas SJ, Campbell RJ, McHugh MP (2001) The association of hip strength and flexibility with the incidence of adductor muscle strains in professional ice hockey players. Am J Sports Med 29:124–128
26. Gamble JG, Simmons SC, Freedman M (1986) The symphysis pubis. Anatomic and pathologic considerations. Clin Orthop Relat Res 261–272
27. Tuite DJ, Finegan PJ, Saliaris AP, Renstrom PA, Donne B, O'Brien M (1998) Anatomy of the proximal musculotendinous junction of the adductor longus muscle. Knee Surg Sports Traumatol Arthrosc 6:134–137
28. Lynch SA, Renstrom PA (1999) Groin injuries in sport: treatment strategies. Sports Med 28:137–144
29. Fricker PA (1997) Management of groin pain in athletes. Br J Sports Med 31:97–101
30. Verrall GM, Slavotinek JP, Fon GT (2001) Incidence of pubic bone marrow oedema in Australian rules football players: relation to groin pain. Br J Sports Med 35:28–33
31. Hawkins RD, Hulse MA, Wilkinson C, Hodson A, Gibson M (2001) The association football medical research programme: an audit of injuries in professional football. Br J Sports Med 35:43–47
32. Lovell G (1995) The diagnosis of chronic groin pain in athletes: a review of 189 cases. Aust J Sci Med Sport 27:76–79
33. Fredberg U, Kissmeyer-Nielsen P (1996) The sportsman's hernia – fact or fiction? Scand J Med Sci Sports 6:201–204
34. Ziprin P, Williams P, Foster ME (1999) External oblique aponeurosis nerve entrapment as a cause of groin pain in the athlete. Br J Surg 86:566–568
35. Irshad K, Feldman LS, Lavoie C, Lacroix VJ, Mulder DS, Brown RA (2001) Operative management of "hockey groin syndrome": 12 years of experience in National Hockey League players. Surgery 130:759–764, discussion 764–756

36. Meyers WC, Foley DP, Garrett WE, Lohnes JH, Mandlebaum BR (2000) Management of severe lower abdominal or inguinal pain in high-performance athletes. PAIN (Performing Athletes with Abdominal or Inguinal Neuromuscular Pain Study Group). Am J Sports Med 28:2–8
37. Orchard JW, Read JW, Neophyton J, Garlick D (1998) Groin pain associated with ultrasound finding of inguinal canal posterior wall deficiency in Australian Rules footballers. Br J Sports Med 32:134–139
38. Smedberg SG, Broome AE, Gullmo A, Roos H (1985) Herniography in athletes with groin pain. Am J Surg 149:378–382
39. Brennan D, O'Connell MJ, Ryan M et al (2005) Secondary cleft sign as a marker of injury in athletes with groin pain: MR image appearance and interpretation. Radiology 235:162–167
40. Lovell G, Galloway H, Hopkins W, Harvey A (2006) Osteitis pubis and assessment of bone marrow edema at the pubic symphysis with MRI in an elite junior male soccer squad. Clin J Sport Med 16:117–122
41. Slavotinek JP, Verrall GM, Fon GT, Sage MR (2005) Groin pain in footballers: the association between preseason clinical and pubic bone magnetic resonance imaging findings and athlete outcome. Am J Sports Med 33:894–899
42. Holt MA, Keene JS, Graf BK, Helwig DC (1995) Treatment of osteitis pubis in athletes. Results of corticosteroid injections. Am J Sports Med 23:601–606
43. Schilders E, Bismil Q, Robinson P, O'Connor PJ, Gibbon WW, Talbot JC (2007) Adductor-related groin pain in competitive athletes. Role of adductor enthesis, magnetic resonance imaging, and entheseal pubic cleft injections. J Bone Joint Surg Am 89:2173–2178
44. O'Connell MJ, Powell T, McCaffrey NM, O'Connell D, Eustace SJ (2002) Symphyseal cleft injection in the diagnosis and treatment of osteitis pubis in athletes. AJR Am J Roentgenol 179:955–959
45. Kraft BM, Kolb H, Kuckuk B et al (2003) Diagnosis and classification of inguinal hernias. Surg Endosc 17(12):2021–2024
46. Steele P, Annear P, Grove JR (2004) Surgery for posterior inguinal wall deficiency in athletes. J Sci Med Sport 7:415–421, discussion 422–413

Chapter 3
Ankle and Foot Injuries

Ne Siang Chew, Justin Lee, Mark Davies, and Jeremiah Healy

Introduction

The ankle and foot is a common site of injury amongst sportsmen [1]. According to the International Olympic Committee, 55% of injuries sustained during the 2008 XXIX Beijing Olympic Games affected the lower extremity while five out of the top ten injuries sustained during the XXVIII Athens Olympic Games in 2004 related to the ankle and foot (Table 3.1) [2].

This chapter aims to provide an illustrative guide to normal anatomy, biomechanics of injury and common imaging appearances of foot and ankle injuries in elite athletes.

Osseous Pathology

There is a spectrum of osseous pathology affecting the elite athlete, ranging from fractures to osteochondral injuries. The aetiology may be traumatic but is frequently the consequence of overuse. For each injury the associated biomechanical cause, clinical presentation, and imaging findings are described.

Fractures

Fracture in the athlete can be secondary to a mechanical injury or due to increased physiological stress on normal bone as a consequence of overuse or overload leading to a stress fracture.

Jeremiah Healy (✉)
Chelsea and Westminster Hospital,
369 Fulham Road, London, SW10 9NH, UK
and
London Foot and Ankle Centre, Hospital of St John and St Elizabeth, Grove End Road, London, NW8, UK
e-mail: j.healy@ic.ac.uk

Mechanical (Non-stress) Fractures

Ankle Fractures

Up to 55% of ankle fractures sustained are sports or leisure activity related [3]. Displaced and unstable fractures require open reduction and internal fixation.

- Biomechanics of injury

Ankle fractures usually result from excessive rotational forces applied to the ankle. The position of the foot and the direction and severity of the forces involved, determines the pattern of injury.

- Imaging

Plain Radiographs

The Weber classification system was developed to guide surgical treatment of ankle fractures. It describes fractures by the level of the fibula fracture with type A distal to the tibio-talar joint, type B at the syndesmosis and type C proximal to the syndesmosis but involving the syndesmotic ligaments (Fig. 3.1). Whilst this system is easy to apply, it does not apply to injuries of the medial malleolus or deltoid ligament.

Pilon Fractures

The ankle joint resembles a mortar and pestle, the tibial plafond being the mortar and the talus being the pestle or pilon. In a pilon fracture, the talus impacts upon the tibial plafond, resulting in an intra-articular fracture of the tibial plafond. Pilon fractures were first reported in skiers.

- Clinical

Pilon fractures are more serious injuries than standard ankle fractures and are associated with a poorer prognosis. Low-energy pilon fractures as a result of skiing are more

Table 3.1 Injuries sustained during the World Olympics of 2004

Type of injury sustained during the Olympics, 2004 (not in order of frequency)
Fractures, stress fractures and stress reactions
Achilles tendinosis
Plantar fasciitis
Tears of the plantar fascia and plantar plate
Lateral ligamentous complex injuries of the ankle
Muscles strains
Rotator cuff tendinosis/tears
Shoulder labral tears
Disc herniation and spondylolysis of the lumbar spine
Ligamentous and meniscal injuries to the knee

Plain Radiographs

Radiographic criteria for diagnosis include:

1. Extensive comminution of the distal tibia with circumferential distribution of fracture fragments (Fig. 3.2).
2. Presence of an intra-articular fracture involving the tibial plafond.
3. Presence of a talar fracture in some pilon fractures.
4. Anatomical relationship of between the talus and lateral malleolus is maintained.

CT Imaging

CT is more sensitive in providing information regarding fracture fragment size, degree of communition and impaction which can alter surgical management [4].

Anterior Process Fracture of Calcaneus

- Clinical

Patients present with a history of an ankle sprain complicated by persistent lateral foot pain long after the injury. An un-united fragment may need surgical excision.

- Biomechanics of injury

This injury usually occurs due to forced inversion/adduction with plantar flexion of the foot [5]. The injury is a result of an avulsion injury of the bifurcate ligament, which connects the anterior process to the cuboid and navicular bone.

- Imaging

Plain Radiographs

This is usually radiographically occult as the fracture line is almost always vertical and the fracture fragments are not commonly displaced [5].

CT/MR Imaging

CT or MR imaging will clearly delineate the fracture (Fig. 3.3).

Lateral Talar Process Fractures/Snowboarder's Fracture

Fractures of the lateral process of the talus are seen typically in snowboarders and account for 2.3% of snowboarding injuries [6]. Prior to development of this sport, these fractures were uncommon and related to falls from a height, road-traffic accidents and inversion injuries [7].

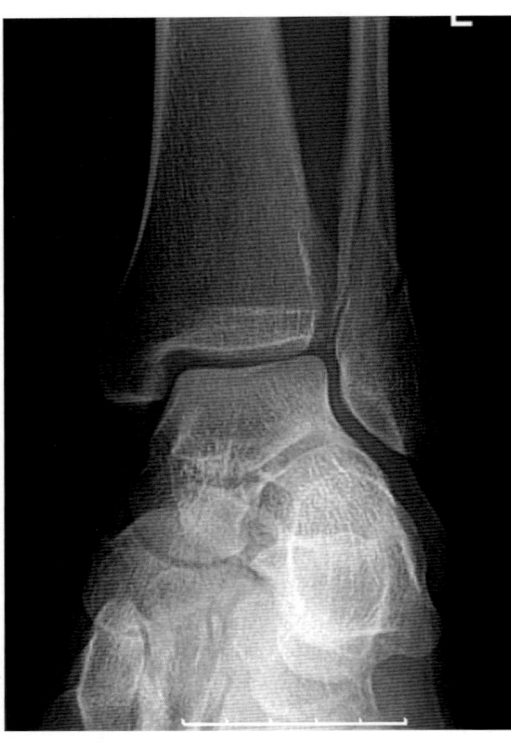

Fig. 3.1 AP X-ray of the ankle demonstrating a fracture of the distal fibula at the level of the lower end of the syndesmosis (Weber Type B). Fractures distal to this level are classified as Weber Type A whilst fractures above this level are classified as Weber Type C

benign than high-energy pilon fractures seen for example in Motor Vehicle Accidents (MVAs). Soft tissue problems early on and later stiffness and post-traumatic arthritis make this a particularly unpleasant injury.

- Biomechanics of injury

The fracture arises from axial compression due to a fall from a height.

- Imaging

Fig. 3.2 (a) AP X-ray of the ankle in a 24-year-old female with a pilon fracture of the distal tibia following a fall. There is a comminuted fracture of the distal tibia due to impaction of the talar dome into the tibial plafond. (b) Surface-shaded 3D reconstruction CT of pilon fracture

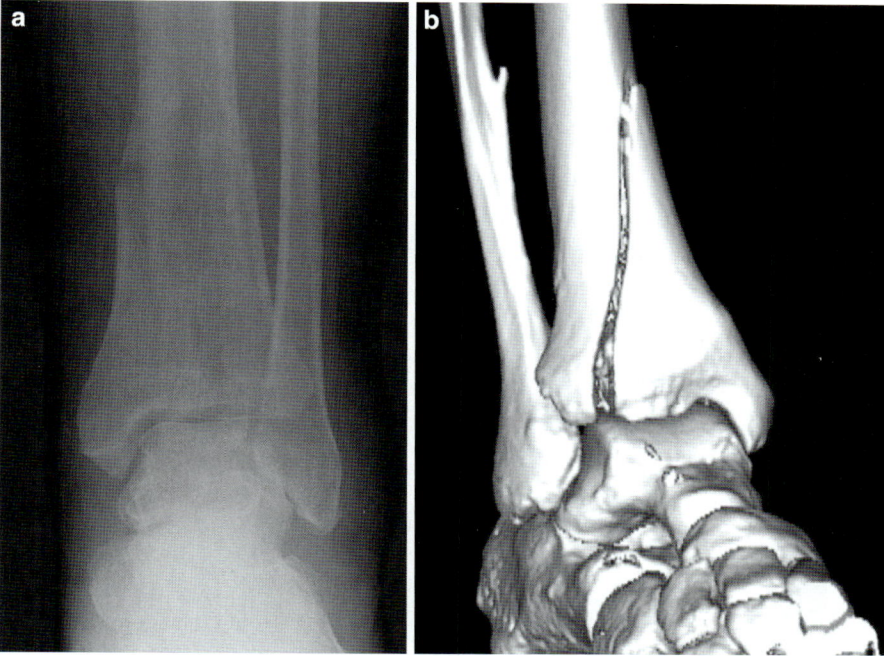

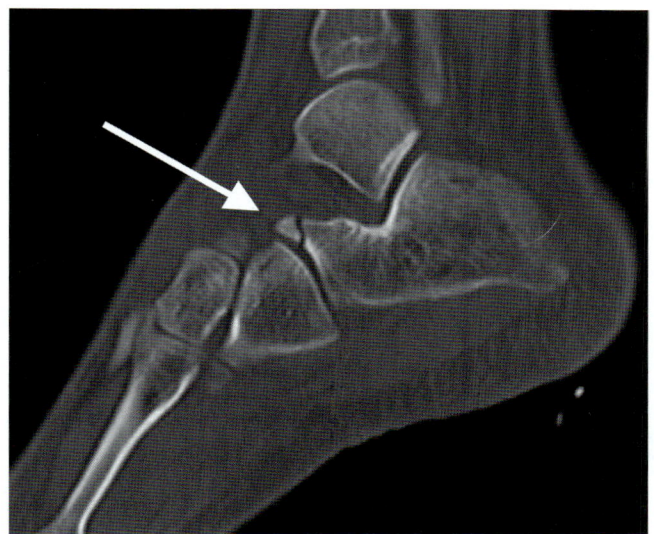

Fig. 3.3 Sagittal CT planar reformat of the hindfoot demonstrating a minimally displaced anterior process of os calcis fracture

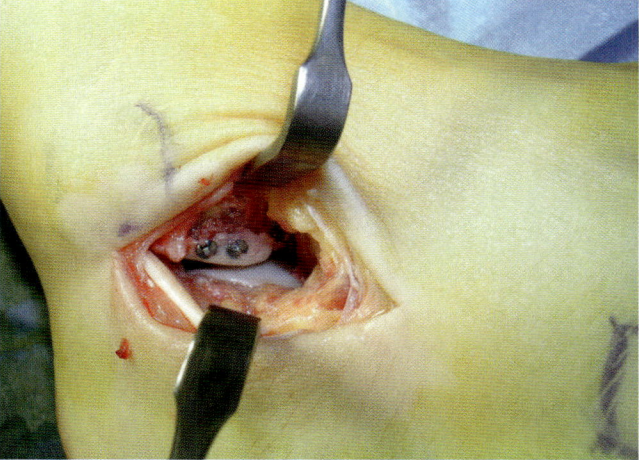

Fig. 3.4 Operative photograph illustrating internal fixation of a lateral talar process fracture

Anatomically, the lateral process of the talus is a broad-based triangular bony projection which lies between the lateral malleolus and the calcaneus. This bony projection articulates dorsolaterally with the fibula and inferomedially with the calcaneum. The lateral talar process as such forms the lateral part of the subtalar joint.

- Clinical

Patients present with lateral ankle pain and stiffness of the subtalar joint. This fracture is often misdiagnosed as lateral ankle sprain [6]. Acute displaced fractures need fixation of the fragment (Fig. 3.4) or excision if the fragment if it is displaced and small. Delayed diagnosis may result in persistent pain, instability, premature osteoarthritis subsequently requiring subtalar fusion.

- Biomechanics of injury

The injury is due to inversion with the ankle dorsiflexed. Shearing forces are transmitted across the subtalar joint from the calcaneus to the lateral talar process.

- Imaging

Both CT and MR imaging can clearly demonstrate the fracture. The fracture is best viewed in the coronal and sagittal planes (Fig. 3.5).

Stress Fractures

Stress fractures account for 10% of patients in a typical sports medical practise. Sporting activities implicated in foot stress fractures include, dancing (43%), athletics (21%), long-distance running (12%), aerobics (7%), basketball and racquet games (2%) and others (12%) [8]. Most frequent anatomical sites of stress fractures include: the talar bones (57.5%), the metatarsal bones (35.7%), the upper part of the talocrural joint (3.4%), sesamoids and accessory ossicles (2.6%) and digits (0.6%) [9].

- Clinical

Clinically, stress fractures are associated with intense pain and swelling but as there is often no history of "injury," they are frequently overlooked.

- Biomechanics of injury

Normally, there is homeostasis between bone tissue breakdown and repair in response to physical activity. In physical overuse, tissue breakdown exceeds repair, resulting in a stress response within bone. Female athletes are more predisposed to stress injury due to impaired repair mechanisms which are a consequence of menstrual irregularity and eating disorders (female athlete triad) [10].

The formation of a stress fracture is considered the end point in the spectrum of bone response to overuse injury. Initially there is bone marrow oedema, then periostitis, which represents activation of the acute repair process. Repeated microtrauma within the bone cortex and medulla lead to the end-stage stress fracture [11].

- Imaging

The physician should investigate the patient further if the initial plain radiograph is normal as pathology is frequently not demonstrated early in the context of a stress/overuse injury. MR imaging is preferred over scintigraphy as it is more specific [12]. Periostitis is recognised on the MR image as areas of increased STIR/T2 signal intensity (Fig. 3.6).

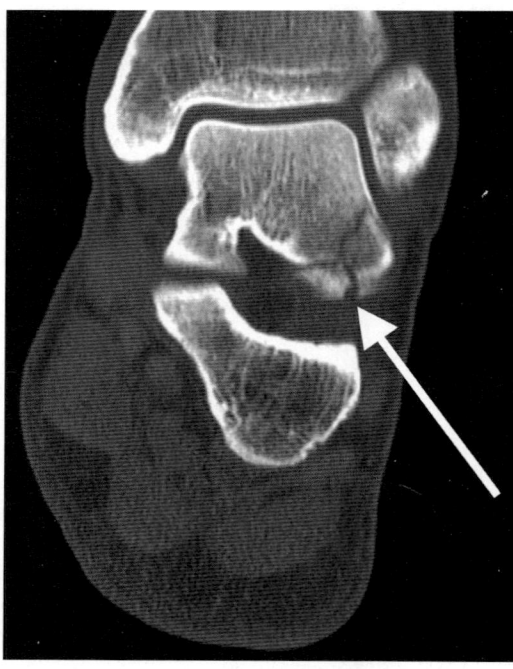

Fig. 3.5 Coronal CT reformatted image of the ankle. There is a multipart fracture of the lateral process of the talus (*arrow*)

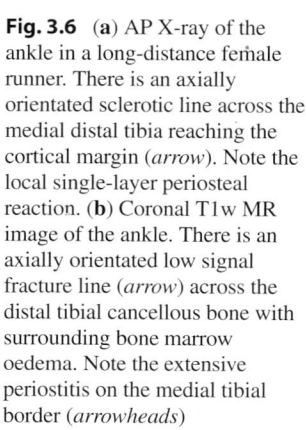
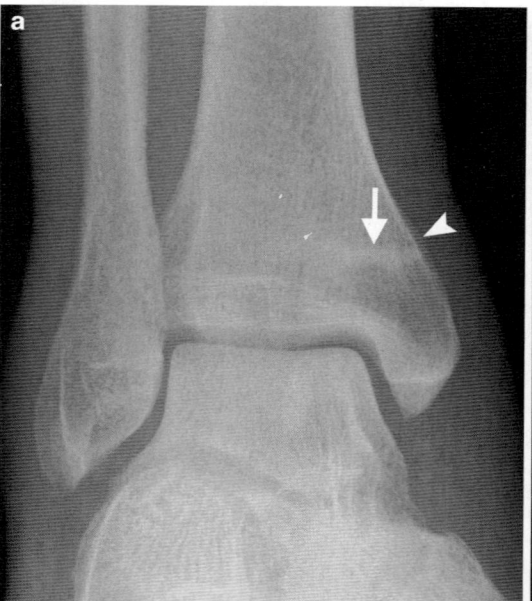
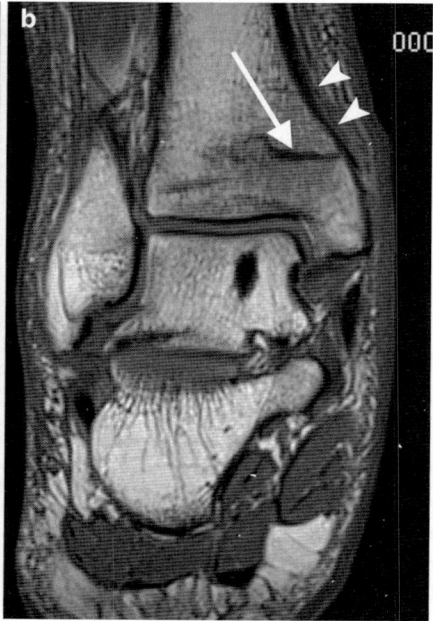

Fig. 3.6 (**a**) AP X-ray of the ankle in a long-distance female runner. There is an axially orientated sclerotic line across the medial distal tibia reaching the cortical margin (*arrow*). Note the local single-layer periosteal reaction. (**b**) Coronal T1w MR image of the ankle. There is an axially orientated low signal fracture line (*arrow*) across the distal tibial cancellous bone with surrounding bone marrow oedema. Note the extensive periostitis on the medial tibial border (*arrowheads*)

MR Appearances

Characteristic MR findings of stress fractures include [13]:

1. Low signal linear areas within the medulla on T1/T2/STIR imaging, extending towards the cortex
2. Marked bone marrow oedema and haemorrhage which is low SI on T1 and high signal on T2 and STIR
3. Periostitis

Calcaneal Stress Fractures

Calcaneal fractures are a common site of a stress fracture in the hind foot.

- Clinical

Patients present with diffuse heel pain and tenderness.

- Biomechanics of injury

Overuse injury typically occurring in running and jumping athletes.

- Imaging

These fractures are vertically oriented, usually involving the posterior calcaneum, particularly posterior–superiorly. Detection of stress fractures on plain radiography at presentation is poor, and only detected in up to 50% at follow-up [13].

Navicular Stress Fractures

Navicular stress fractures predominantly occur in sprinting and jumping athletes and are common in football and rugby.

- Clinical

The patient complains of pain in the "ankle" but will point to the navicular bone as the site of pain. These injuries can be devastating and often require surgical fixation but even this is no guarantee of return to sport.

- Biomechanics of injury

Navicular stress fractures typically occur in the sagittal plane in the central and lateral thirds of the navicular bone. This is the site of maximum shear stress on the navicular from the surrounding bones. The fracture commences at the proximal dorsal articular surface and spreads plantar and distally.

- Imaging

Plain radiographs often miss the fracture as the fracture lies in an oblique direction.

On MR imaging and CT the fracture usually extends inferiorly in the sagittal plane from a prominent superior navicular osteophyte (Fig. 3.7). The fracture may pass on either side of a osteophyte giving an "inverted mercedes benz" sign on coronal imaging.

Metatarsal Stress Fractures

Metatarsal stress fractures are common in runners, ballet dancers and gymnasts [14]. Stress fractures have a predilection for the mid-shaft or neck of the second, third or fourth metatarsal bones. In ballet dancers, however, the proximal metatarsal bases are frequently affected.

- Biomechanics of injury

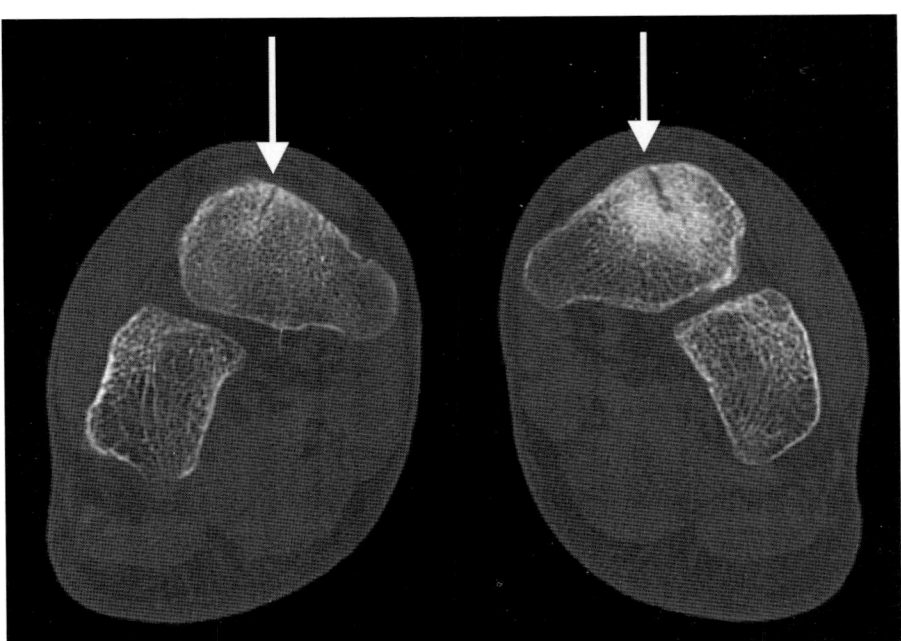

Fig. 3.7 Coronal CT of the ankle in a 22-year-old soccer player demonstrating bilateral stress fractures of the navicular

Overuse injury.

- Imaging appearances.

MR imaging will demonstrate the characteristic appearances of a stress fracture (Fig. 3.8). Trabecular bony detail is shown well on CT imaging which can also be used to assess healing by demonstrating bony bridging, sclerosis and periosteal bony deposition.

Proximal Fifth Metatarsal Stress Fractures

Proximal fifth metatarsal stress fractures have a high incidence in footballers and basketball players [15].

- Clinical

The patient presents with lateral foot pain and point tenderness over the site of fracture. In the athlete, these fractures are best treated with percutaneous screw fixation (Fig. 3.9).

- Biomechanics of injury

The injury is due to overuse [16].

- Imaging

Proximal diaphyseal fifth metatarsal stress fractures are in the zone immediately distal to the Jones fracture anatomic area. True Jones fractures are located at the junction between the diaphysis and metaphysis of the fifth metatarsal without distal extension beyond the fourth to fifth intermetatarsal articulations. This fracture should be distinguished from an avulsion fracture at the peroneus brevis insertion.

Sesamoid Stress Fractures

The great toe sesamoids act to diminish pressure on the first metatarsal head. They elevate the first metatarsals so that they are at level with or higher than the other metatarsal heads. In addition, they protect the flexor hallucis longus (FHL) tendon, which lies between them. Dancers are particularly susceptible to stress fractures of the sesamoids [17]. Stress fractures of the sesamoids are also recognised in rhythmic sports such as gymnastics and long/triple jump [18].

- Clinical

The patient exhibits tenderness directly over the affected sesamoid bone on the plantar aspect of the first metatarsophalangeal joint. Treatment is generally conservative.

- Biomechanics of injury

Overuse injury. Repeated trauma is the mechanism of injury. In ballerinas, stress fractures occur due to repeated trauma when the foot is in the demi-pointe position.

The medial sesamoid is slightly more susceptible to a stress fracture as it lies directly under the first metatarsal head [15].

- Imaging

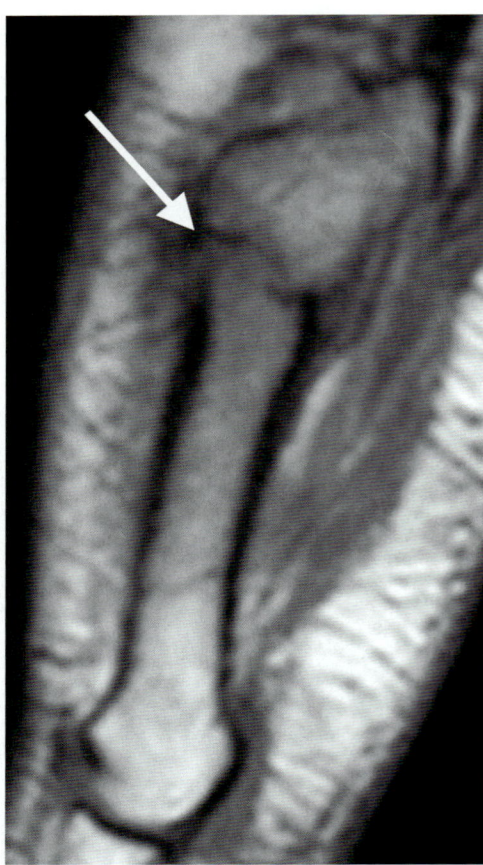

Fig. 3.8 Sagittal T1 MR image of the fifth metatarsal in a 25-year-old male soccer player. Note the low signal line traversing the cortex and medullary bone with surrounding bone marrow oedema and periosteal thickening (*arrow*) consistent with a stress fracture

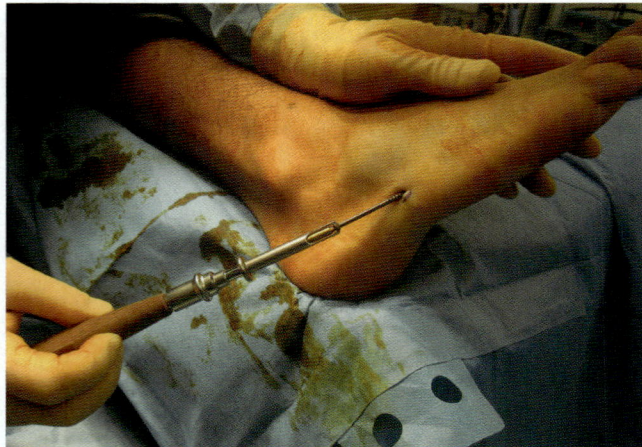

Fig. 3.9 Operative photograph demonstrating technique of inserting screw fixation of a proximal fifth metatarsal base fracture

Differentiation of a stress fracture from a bipartite sesamoid can be difficult.

MR imaging may demonstrate the fracture line within a markedly oedematous sesamoid bone. Secondary synovitis in the metatarsophalangeal joint and reactive changes in the undersurface of the first metatarsal head is not uncommon (Fig. 3.10). CT may be useful as bipartite sesamoids have more rounded margins at the cleft whereas stress fractures have congruous margins and may show signs of healing such as bony bridging.

Osteochondral Injuries

Osteochondral injuries (OCI) are defined as the separation of articular cartilage, with or without separation of subchondral bone. This may be a result of a single or multiple traumatic events [19]. They occur most commonly in the second to third decades of life in active sportsmen. OCI of the talus can be bilateral in 10% of cases. This is reported to be associated with ankle sprains, where the incidence of OCI following ankle sprains has been reported to be as high as 6.5% [20, 21]. OCI occur in both medial and lateral talus in equal frequency, specifically at the posterior third of the medial border and the middle third of the lateral border.

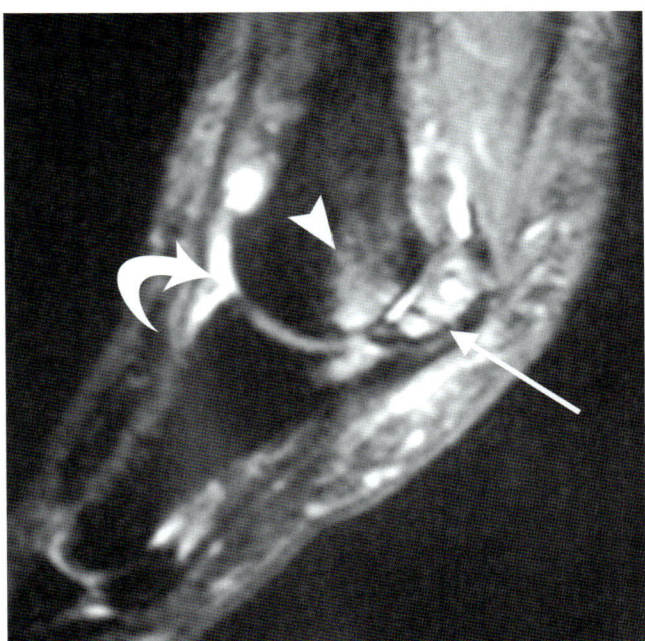

Fig. 3.10 Sagittal STIR MR image of the forefoot in a 27-year-old female runner. There is marked inflammation within the medial sesamoid surrounding a low signal stress fracture line (*arrow*). Note the reactive bone marrow oedema in the adjacent undersurface of first metatarsal head (*arrowhead*) and the marked synovitis in the first metatarsophalangeal joint (*curved arrow*)

- Biomechanics

The mechanisms of osteochondral injury were elegantly described by Berndt and Harty in 1959. The medial talar injury is explained by inversion, plantarflexion and external rotation, which result in the posterior medial talus being impacted upon the tibial ceiling. The anterolateral OCI occurs due to inversion combined with dorsiflexion, whereby the anterolateral talus impacts against the fibula.

- Clinical

Patients present with exercise-related pain which is poorly localised, mild swelling and infrequently, sensations of clicking and catching. Arthroscopic debridement or microfracture is sometimes necessary (Fig. 3.11).

- Imaging

Plain Radiographs

Plain radiographs may demonstrate cortical defects on the talar dome.

MR/CT Imaging

Whilst a plain radiograph may demonstrate a small cortical defect, these lesions may be subtle and radiologically occult. MR imaging can evaluate and demonstrate abnormality within the cartilage as well as the underlying bone (Fig. 3.12). A rim of high signal fluid partially or completely surrounding the osteochondral fragment on T2/STIR imaging indicates the presence of an unstable injury in the skeletally mature patient (Fig. 3.13). In the skeletally immature child,

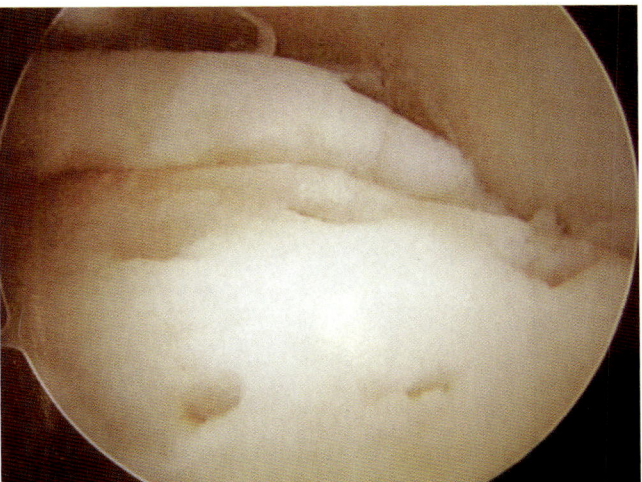

Fig. 3.11 Arthroscopic image of the ankle joint following microfracture of the talar dome. Note the typical "Swiss-cheese" appearance of the cartilage surface following the procedure

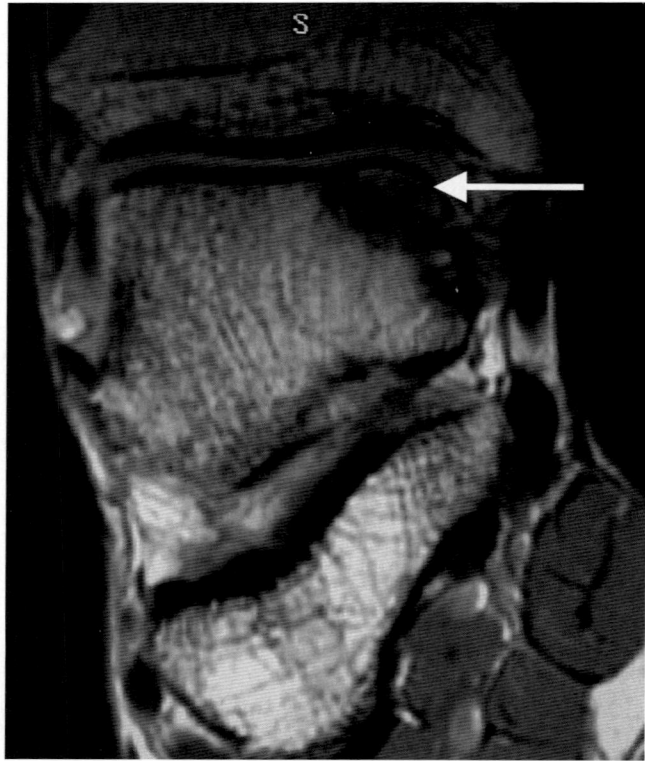

Fig. 3.12 Coronal T1 MR image of the ankle demonstrating a mature osteochondral fragment which has corticated margins. The overlying talar dome cartilage appears to be intact

Table 3.2 Osteochondral injury grading system

Grade	Description	Treatment
I	Subchondral compression fracture. Overlying cartilage intact	Conservative
II	Partially detached osteochondral fragment	Conservative
III	Osteochondral fragment completely detached from talus but not displaced	Surgical, conservative if lesion is medial
IV	Osteochondral fragment detached and displaced	Surgical

the presence of a high signal intensity rim or cysts surrounding the osteochondral fragment is not an unequivocal sign of instability; these OCI have been described to heal with conservative treatment [22]. Unstable OCI left untreated in the skeletally mature adult can result in a detached loose body and may give rise to symptoms of joint locking. The lack of a T2/STIR high signal intensity interface between the osteochondral fragment and the parent bone indicates a stable or healed osteochondral fragment.

CT may be useful in identifying any loose bodies within the joint complicating OCI [23]. MR or CT arthrography may identify cartilage flap tears and communication between the joint and the base of an OCI confirming instability [24]. The grading system of osteochondral injuries according to Berndt and Harty and their surgical implications are described in the Table 3.2.

Ligamentous Injuries

Whilst bony deformities secondary to athletic trauma may be easily detected on radiographs, the radiologist should not ignore accompanying soft tissue ligamentous and tendinous injuries.

Lateral Ligamentous Injuries

The lateral collateral ligamentous complex comprises three components: the anterior talofibular ligament (ATFL), posterior talofibular ligament (PTFL) and the calcaneofibular ligament (CFL). On MR imaging, the anterior talofibular ligament is a thin flat or triangular band which connects the anterior tip of the distal fibula to the lateral talar process (Fig. 3.14). The posterior talofibular ligament (PTFL) which is seen at the same level is broader and has a fan-shaped origin from the fibular fossa of the distal fibula. It attaches to the posterior aspect of the distal talus and has internal striations due to interspersed fat. This should not be misinterpreted as a tear.

Both ATFL and PTFL are best viewed axially at the level of the malleolar fossa. The malleolar fossa is recognised just

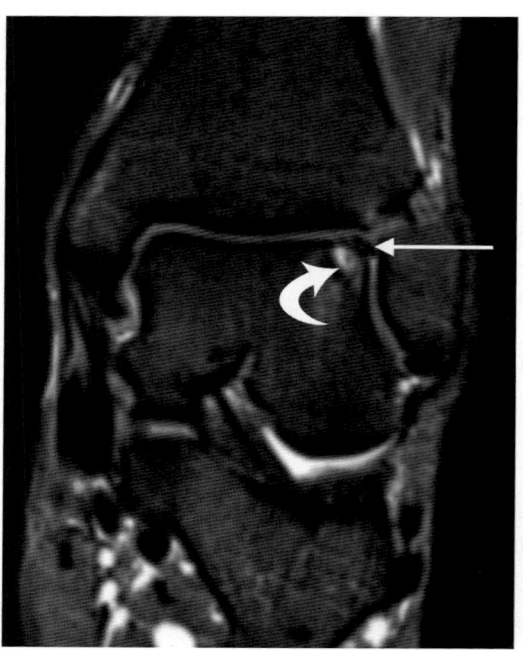

Fig. 3.13 Coronal STIR MR image of the ankle in a 32-year-old male rugby player 12 months after an inversion injury. Note the unstable displaced osteochondral fragment (*arrow*) which is separated from the underlying talar dome by focal cystic change (*curved arrow*)

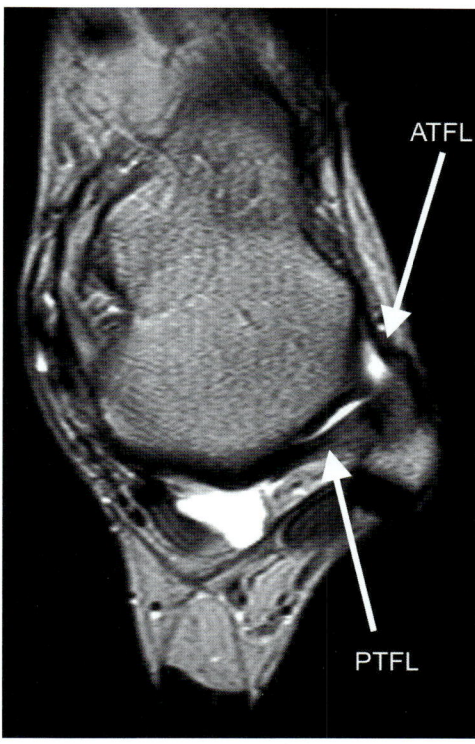

Fig. 3.14 Axial T2w MR image of the ankle in a healthy volunteer. The anterior talofibular ligament (ATFL) is a well-defined low signal band between the anterior margin of the distal fibula and the anterior margin of the lateral process of the talus. The posterior talofibular ligament (PTFL) is identified at the same level extending from the lateral tubercle of the posterior process of the talus to the medial margin of the malleolar fossa of the fibula

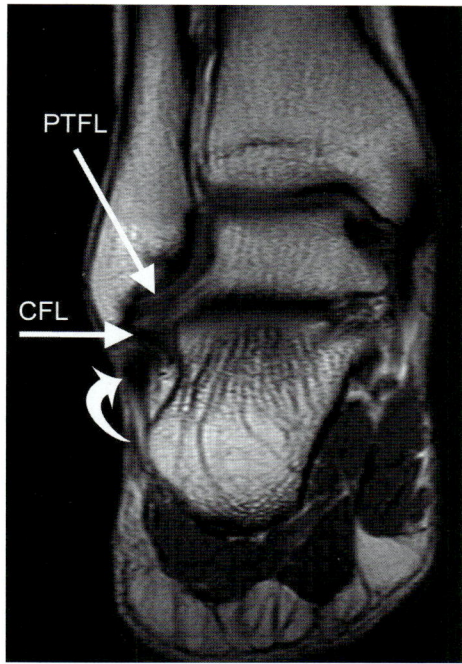

Fig. 3.15 Coronal T1w MR image of the ankle. The calcaneofibular ligament (CFL) lies deep to the peroneal tendons (*curved arrow*) and attaches to the fibula malleolus alongside the posterior talofibular ligament (PTFL)

below the tibio-talar joint where the medial aspect of the lateral malleolus assumes a "c" shape.

The calcaneofibular originates from the inferior tip of the distal fibula and inserts onto the lateral cortex of the calcaneum. It is seen deep to the peroneal tendons. The ligament can be appreciated in both the coronal and axial planes (Figs. 3.14 and 3.15).

The lateral ankle ligaments are most commonly injured accounting for 85% of ankle sprains. Lateral ligamentous sprains represent 16–21% of all sports-related ankle injuries [19]. As the ATFL is the weakest ligament, it is the first torn, followed by the CFL and subsequently the PTFL.

ATFL Injury

- Clinical.

Most lateral ligament sprains are treated with rest, ice, compression and elevation (RICE). If instability persists, surgical reconstruction may be required (Fig. 3.16).

- Biomechanics of injury

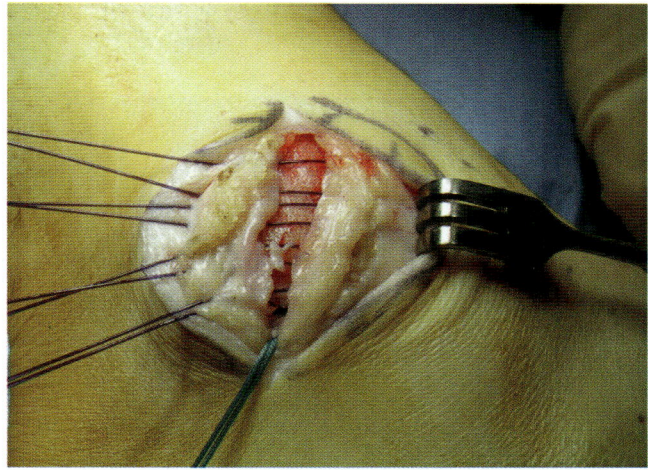

Fig. 3.16 Operative photograph demonstrating the plication of the ATFL remnant and anterolateral joint capsule during a Brostrum repair of a full-thickness ATFL tear

The function of the ATFL is to resist ankle inversion in plantarflexion. Two accessory functions of the ATFL are to resist anterior talar displacement from the mortise (can be elicited clinically through the anterior drawer test) and resist internal rotation within the mortise. Injuries to the ATFL occur when the foot is forced into internal rotation during plantarflexion and inversion.

- Imaging

MR/US Imaging

An acute ATFL tear demonstrates discontinuity and detachment of the ligament from its talar or fibula attachment. On MR imaging, there is high signal fluid surrounding the thickened disrupted ligament (Fig. 3.17) [25]. The ATFL is part of the joint capsule and when torn allows leakage of joint fluid into the surrounding soft tissues. On US the ligament is markedly thickened and hypoechoic, if completely ruptured it will appear as a hypoechoic mass in the anterolateral gutter (Fig. 3.18).

Acute injuries may be associated with avulsion fractures from either side of the ligament attachments. This will produce underlying bone marrow oedema on MR imaging in the talus or fibula. US is sensitive in identifying avulsion fractures as linear echogenic flakes of bone attached to a thickened, hypoechoic, injured ligament (Fig. 3.19) [26].

MR imaging with intravenous gadolinium will identify post-traumatic synovitis, which frequently complicates inversion injury which increases the length of rehabilitation. This sometimes necessitates US-guided steroid injection for effective management.

Chronic tears of the ATFL may demonstrate discontinuity of the ligament without the soft tissue or bone marrow oedema changes. The ATFL can appear intact in cases of chronic injury but will be irregular in outline and attenuated or thickened as a consequence of healing with variable amount of scarring (Fig. 3.20) [25].

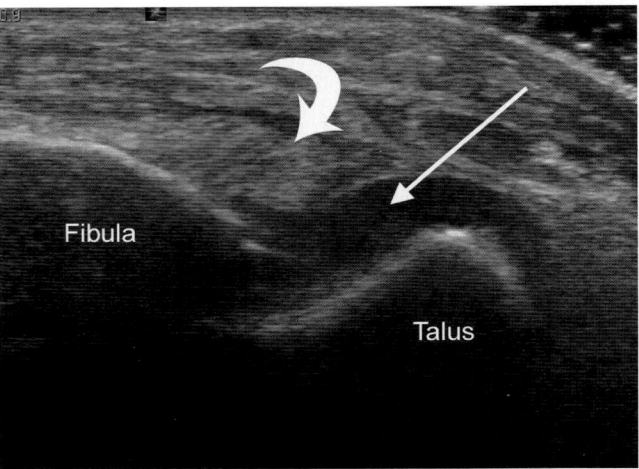

Fig. 3.18 Sonogram of the anteolateral ankle with the transducer aligned to the anterior talofibular ligament (*curved arrow*). Note the disruption of the talar attachment of the ATFL allowing fluid to escape freely from the joint (*arrow*)

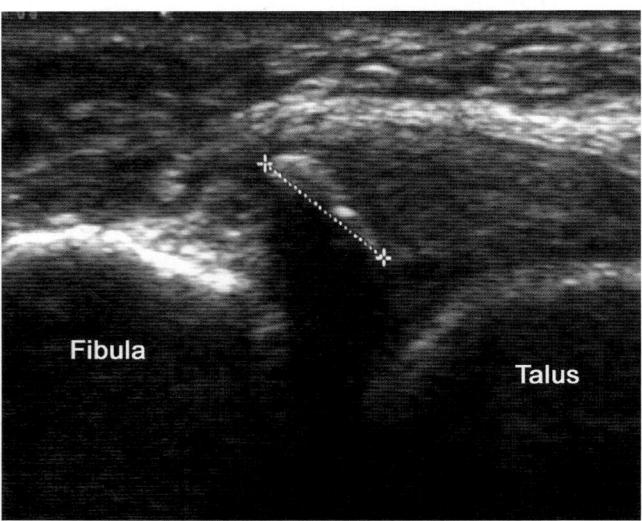

Fig. 3.19 Sonogram of the anteolateral ankle with the transducer aligned to the anterior talofibular ligament. There is an avulsed fragment within the proximal part of the ligament arising from the fibular attachment

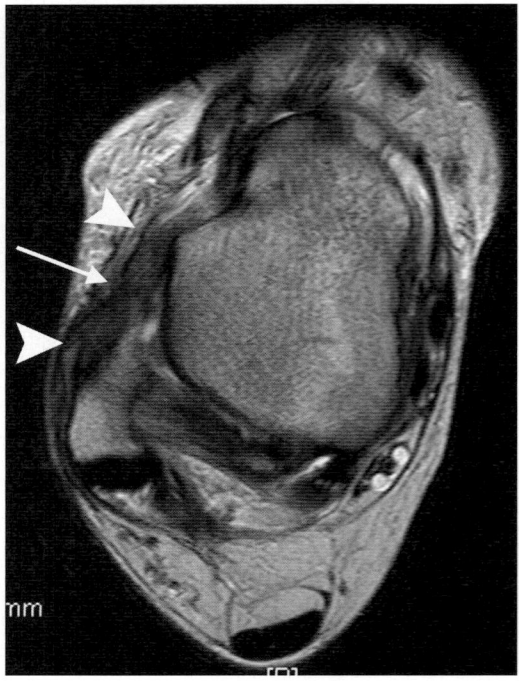

Fig. 3.17 Axial T2w MR image of the ankle. The anterior talofibular ligament is markedly thickened (*arrowheads*) and there is a focal defect centrally within the ligament (*arrow*)

Classification of lateral ankle sprains is described in the Table 3.3.

Medial Ligamentous Injuries

The medial collateral ligament complex or deltoid ligament forms part of the ankle joint capsule (Fig. 3.21). These ligaments function to resist eversion and external rotation.

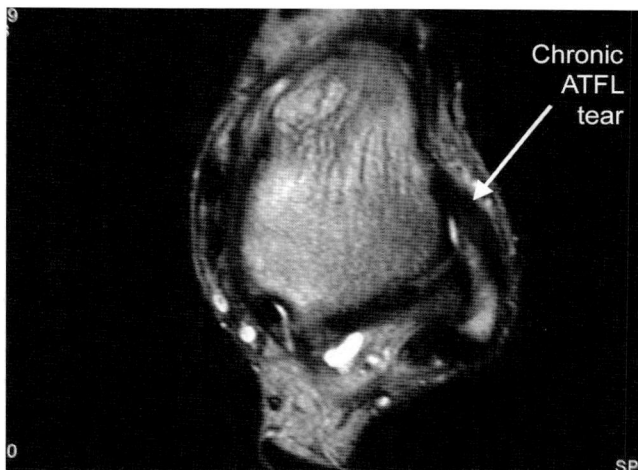

Fig. 3.20 Axial T2w MR image demonstrating a thickened anterior talofibular ligament consistent with a chronic tear with over-exuberant healing by fibrous tissue

Table 3.3 Lateral ankle sprain classification

Degree of sprain	Description
First	Partial/completed tear of ATFL
Second	Partial/completed tear of ATFL + CFL
Third	Partial/completed tear of ATFL + CFL + PTFL

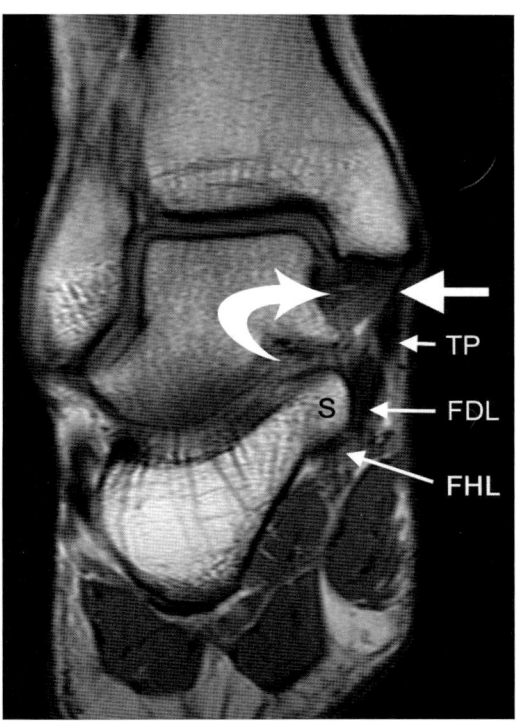

Fig. 3.21 Coronal T1w MR image of the ankle joint in a healthy volunteer. The deep tibio-talar component of the deltoid ligament has a typical striated appearance on T1w MR images due to the presence of fat interspersed between the ligament fibres (*curved arrow*). The thinner tibiocalcaneal component (*large block arrow*) extends from the medial malleolus to the sustentaculum tali of the os calcis. Tibialis posterior (TP), flexor digitorum longus (FDL) and flexor hallucis longus (FHL) S, Sustentaculum tali

It consists of five components:

(a) Three superficial components, all of which arises from the distal tip of the medial malleolus:

   (i) Tibiocalcaneal ligament attaches to the sustentaculum tali of the calcaneus.

   (ii) The tibiocalcaneal ligament runs deep to the flexor retinaculum and is superficial to the tibio-talar ligament.

   (iii) Tibionavicular ligament attaches anterior to the calcaneus onto the navicular.

   (iv) Tibiospring ligament attaches to the spring ligament.

(b) The two deeper components are:

   (i) Anterior tibio-talar ligament which runs from the distal tip of the medial malleolus to the talar neck, and

   (ii) Posterior tibio-talar ligament which runs from the distal tip of he medial malleolus to the medial talar surface

Deltoid Ligament Injury

- Clinical

The deltoid ligament is rarely injured in isolation and when injured alone is usually associated with an ankle fracture. The ligament rarely needs surgical repair.

- Biomechanics of injury

Deltoid ligamentous injuries may occur secondarily to forced eversion and inversion. Generally, it is more common to identify an avulsion fracture of the medial malleolus than a tear of the deltoid ligament in an eversion injury. Isolated deltoid injuries are uncommon and account for 5% of all ankle sprains. They may follow forced eversion and lateral rotation. When the deltoid ligament is completely or partially disrupted, there is usually high signal fluid outlining the defect on MR imaging.

Inversion injuries can also lead to partial tears of the posterior tibio-talar ligament. This is secondary to the compression between the medial talar wall and the medial malleolus.

- Imaging

MR Imaging

When the ligament is sprained, MR findings include loss of normal striations within the deltoid ligament and increased signal intensity within the ligament on both T1w and T2w images (Fig. 3.22). An effusion within the posterior tibialis tendon may also be present. Partial tears of the deep surface are best seen in the coronal plane on T2/STIR sequences.

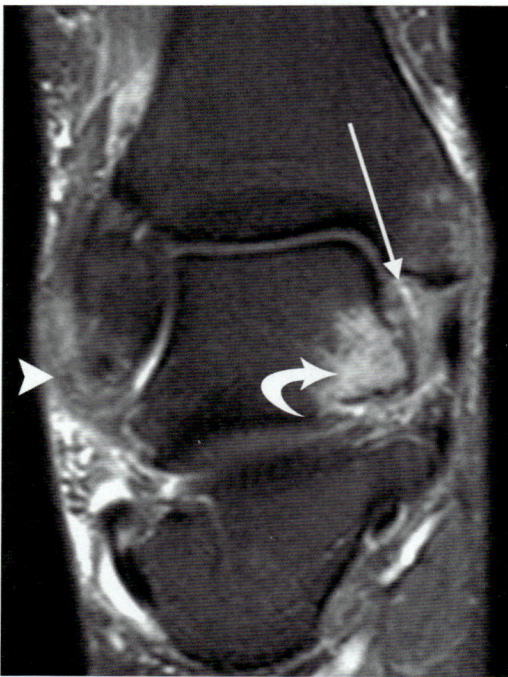

Fig. 3.22 Coronal STIR MR image of the ankle following an inversion injury. Note the torn lateral collateral ankle ligament (*arrowhead*) and bone bruise in the medial talar process (*curved arrow*). There is diffuse high signal throughout the deltoid ligament with a focal partial thickness vertical tear centrally within the ligament substance (*arrow*)

Lisfranc Ligamentous Injury

The tarso-metatarsal joints, also known as the Lisfranc joints are important in stabilisation of the mid-foot and longitudinal arch. Architecturally shaped as a Roman arch, the Lisfranc joint is stable. Two keystones in this Roman arch formation are the second metatarsal and the middle cuneiform (C2) bones. Disruption to the keystones will lead to arch failure.

The first to third tarso-metatarsal joints are formed by opposing articular facets of the three metatarsals with their respective cuneiforms. The base of the second metatarsal (M2) is unique in that it is recessed proximally compared to other metatarsal bases. This adds stability to the joint.

The Lisfranc ligament primarily attaches the medial cuneiform (C1) to the base of the second metatarsal. There are two components to the Lisfranc ligament; the dorsal component arises from the lateral surface of the C1 and courses distally to insert onto the medial aspect of M2. The plantar component which is stronger arises from the lateral base of C1 and inserts onto the plantar aspect of M2. It is of note that there is no intermetatarsal ligament between the base of the first and second metatarsal bones.

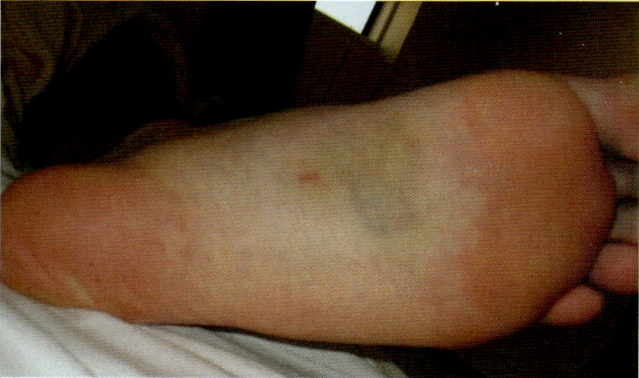

Fig. 3.23 Clinical photograph of the plantar aspect of the foot in a soccer player with an acute Lisfranc ligament injury. Note the ecchymosis in the medial mid-foot as well as the bruising in the bases of the second and third toes

Whilst the function of the Lisfranc joint is to stabilise the foot, the main function of the Lisfranc ligament is to keep the mid-foot congruent.

- Biomechanics of Injury to the Lisfranc ligament

True dislocation of the tarso-metatarsal joints occurs predominantly as a result of severe non-athletic trauma including fall from a height and road-traffic accidents. The mechanism of injury involved is plantarflexion with forced pronation or supination; this causes fractures of the metatarsal bases and/or injures to the ligaments. In sports and recreation, cases of Lisfranc ligament injuries are not uncommon in football players, ballet dancers and windsurfers as a consequence of trauma following a jump or as a consequence of a direct blow to the plantar aspect of the mid-foot in football [27].

Injuries to this area are classically divided into homolateral or divergent types. In homolateral fractures, all five metatarsal bases are displaced in the same direction in the coronal plane. In divergent fractures, there is separation of the first and second metatarsal bases.

- Clinical

Patients complain of immediate pain and swelling and will often describe a popping sensation. Clinical examination reveals swelling and plantar bruising (Fig. 3.23) and as the swelling subsides the foot shape will often be "flatter".

- Imaging

Plain Radiography

In Lisfranc ligamentous injuries, plain radiographs may demonstrate:

1. Loss of the in-line arrangement of the lateral margin of the first metatarsal base with the lateral edge of the medial cuneiform (C1).

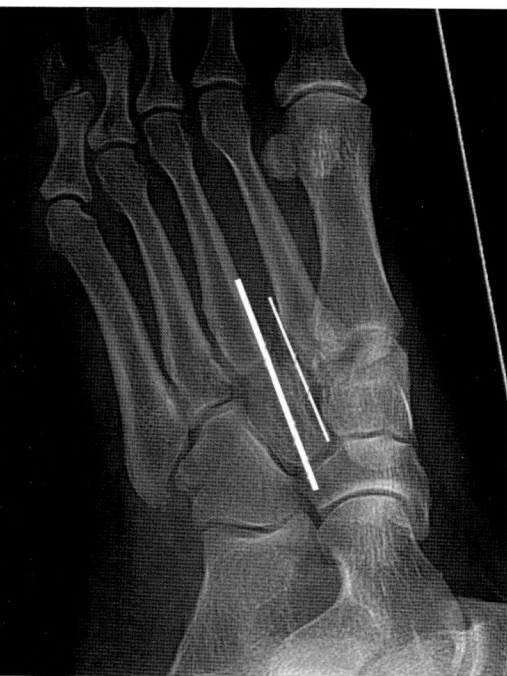

Fig. 3.24 DP X-ray of the foot demonstrating misalignment of the medial border of the third metatarsal (*thick line*) and the medial border of the lateral cuneiform (*thin line*)

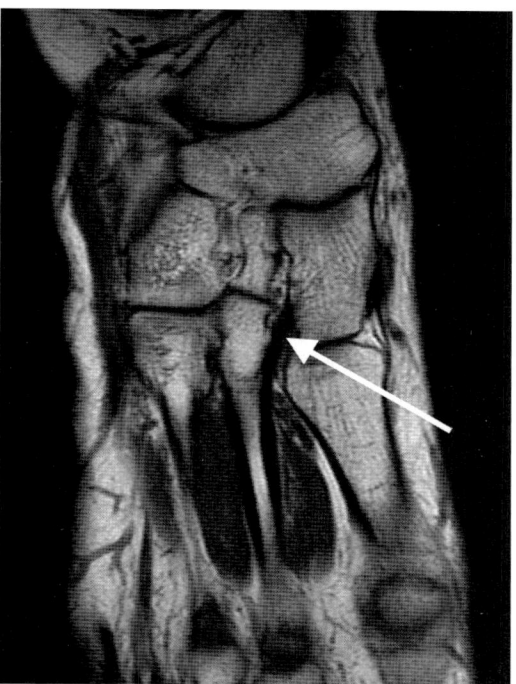

Fig. 3.25 T1w axial MR image of the mid-foot demonstrating an intact normal Lisfranc ligament passing from the medial cuneiform to the base of the second metatarsal (*arrow*)

2. Loss of the in-line arrangement of the medial margin of the second metatarsal base with the medial edge of the intermediate cuneiform (C2) in the anterior–posterior weightbearing view (Fig. 3.24). Note however, in a study by Nunley et al., 50% of patients with diastasis of the first and second metatarsals appeared normal on non-weight-bearing radiographs [28].
3. Presence of avulsed fragments (fleck sign) between the base of the second metatarsal and medial cuneiform may be identified. The fleck represents either a proximal or distal avulsion of the Lisfranc ligament.

Lisfranc ligamentous injuries may be missed in up to 50% of cases on plain radiographs [28]. MR and CT imaging are more reliable techniques for this injury.

MR Imaging

The Lisfranc ligament is clearly seen in the long axis/coronal plane on MR imaging (Fig. 3.25). When torn, the Lisfranc ligament demonstrates discontinuity and is associated with soft tissue oedema. Secondary signs of bone marrow oedema within the inferior aspect of the middle cuneiform or M2 should also make the radiologist suspect a Lisfranc injury. Fractures of the metatarsal bases and tarsal bones should be sought along with tears of the intermetarsal ligaments. Long axis/coronal imaging will demonstrate loss of the Roman arch with loss of alignment between the medial cortex of M2 and the C2.

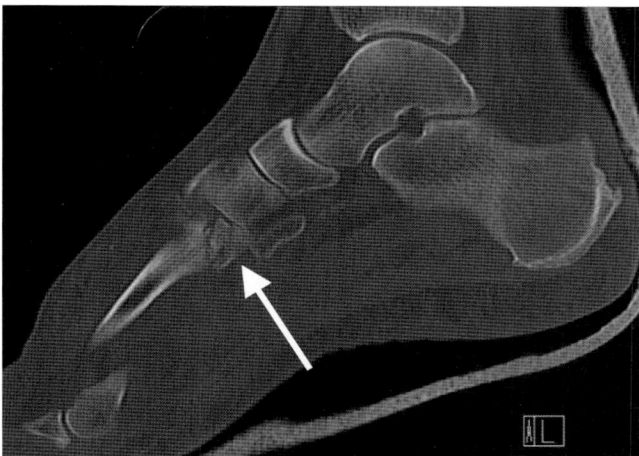

Fig. 3.26 Sagittal CT planar reformat of the mid-foot demonstrating a comminuted fracture subluxation of the base of the second metatarsal consistent with a bony Lisfranc injury

CT Imaging

CT imaging gives better fracture delineation and aids pre-operative planning (Fig. 3.26). CT allows recognition and evaluation of all tarso-metatarsal bony injuries, provides imaging in a multiple planes not available from the plain radiographs, and may help detect fractures not identified on plain radiographs or MR images [29].

Syndesmotic Ligamentous Injury/High Ankle Sprain

Syndesmotic injuries or *high ankle sprains* are more common than lateral ankle sprains in sports which necessitate rigid immobilisation of the ankle and in collision sports [30]. In the late 1970s, when ski boots became more rigid, Fritschy identified a change from a pattern of injury of lateral ankle sprain to syndesmotic injuries in skiers. Syndesmotic injuries are prevalent in collision sports such as hockey, football, rugby, wrestling and lacrosse [30].

Stability of the syndesmosis is secondary to the unique architecture of the distal tibia and fibula and the syndesmotic ligaments. The fibula is located within a groove deepened by the anterior and posterior tibial processes, giving bony stability to the syndesmosis. In addition, the four syndesmotic ligaments, namely the anterior inferior tibiofibular, posterior inferior tibiofibular, transverse tibiofibular and interosseous ligaments also contribute to stability. Although not a syndesmotic ligament per se, the deep component of the deltoid ligament also provides stability to the syndesmosis and should therefore be evaluated in the context of acute or chronic injury.

- Clinical

Syndesmotic ligament injuries can occur in isolation. They are frequently missed and usually take twice as long to recover from than lateral ankle ligament injuries. Whether isolated or part of an ankle fracture, all but the syndesmotic sprains without displacement require surgical stabilisation.

- Biomechanics of injury

The most common mechanism of syndesmotic injury is external rotation of the foot and forced ankle dorsiflexion with axial loading [31]. When the foot is plantar fixed in this position and externally rotated, the fibula separates from the tibia, disrupting the anterior inferior tibiofibular ligament. The external rotation of the talus with respect to the tibia may also cause injury to the deep deltoid ligament. Other mechanisms of injury including eversion, inversion, plantarflexion, pronation and internal rotation have also been reported [31].

- Imaging

Plain Radiographs

Plain radiographs may demonstrate a fracture and presence of diastasis of the syndesmosis. Diastasis is defined as an increase in the tibiofibular clear space on an anteroposterior radiograph of 6 mm or greater. However, diagnosis on plain radiographs may be difficult due to the inability to consistently position patients [32].

MR/CT Imaging

The main modality for diagnosis is MR, where the sensitivity and specificity for detection of an AITFL tear was 100 and 93%, respectively, using arthroscopy as gold standard. The sensitivity and specificity of the diagnosis of a PITFL tear was 100%, respectively. On MR, features of syndesmotic injury include:

1. Sprain injury – AITFL intact but thickened, with fluid seen around the ligament.
2. Tear of the anterior inferior tibiofibular and posterior inferior tibiofibular ligaments manifested as [33]:

    1. Ligament discontinuity
    2. Wavy of curved ligament contour (Fig. 3.27)
    3. Non-visualisation of ligament
    3. Oedema or partial tear seen in the lower end of the interosseous ligament
    4. Bone marrow oedema or fracture through the posterior malleolus of the tibia

CT identifies bony injuries within the posterior malleolus and will also identify flake fractures at the tibial insertions of both the AITFL and PITFL. These flake fractures especially posteriorly may contribute to persistent symptoms as a consequence of local synovitis.

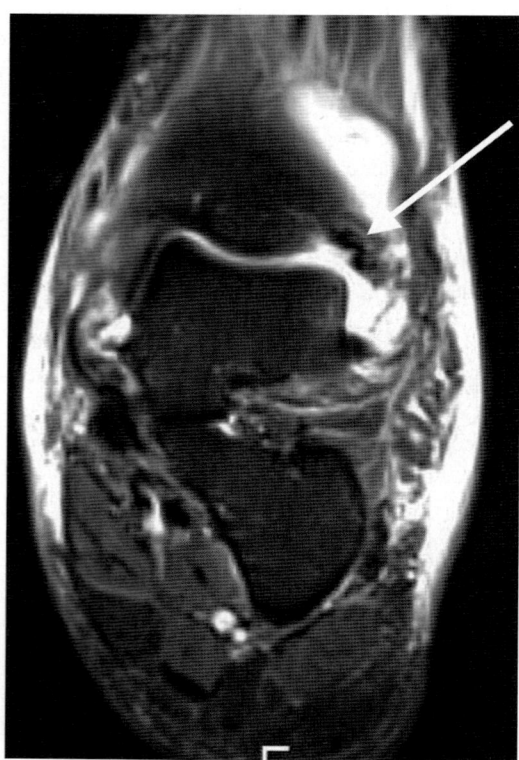

Fig. 3.27 Coronal STIR MR image of the ankle. Note the wavy contour of the anterior inferior tibiofibular ligament consistent with a full-thickness tear

Ultrasound

The anterior and posterior inferior tibiofibular ligaments can be readily visualised on ultrasound. In cases of acute injury, the ligament loses its normal fibrillar pattern and becomes diffusely hypoechoic (Fig. 3.28).

Impingement Syndromes

Ankle impingement is a painful condition of the ankle resulting from pinching of joint tissues secondary to altered ankle joint anatomy, e.g. osteophytes, synovial hypertrophy, calcific fragments and loose bodies.

Ankle impingement syndromes can be divided anatomically into anterior and posterior subtypes. Subtypes of the anterior impingement syndromes include anterolateral, anterior and anteromedial syndromes. Mimics of ankle impingement should be considered before the diagnosis is made (see Table 3.4).

Anterolateral Impingement

Anterolateral impingement (ALI) is the most common type of ankle impingement related to ankle inversion. The main pathology is secondary to presence of synovial scarring, inflammation and hypertrophy within the anterolateral recess.

The anterolateral recess (Fig. 3.29) is a potential space bounded superiorly by the anterior inferior tibiofibular, and inferiorly by the anterior talofibular and calcaneofibular ligaments. Its lateral border is the fibula whereas its medial border is the talus. The recess extends superiorly to the level of the tibial plafond and distal tibiofibular syndesmosis and inferiorly to the level of the calcaneofibular ligament.

- Clinical

The typical patient presents with sharp anterolateral ankle pain with dorsiflexion. In addition, there is often a degree of instability as consequence of previous inversion injury.

- Biomechanics of Injury

ALI is thought to occur following minor trauma involving forced ankle plantar flexion and supination. The initial trauma resulting in the tearing of the anterolateral ligaments and soft tissues may not cause mechanical instability. However, subsequent instability is caused by synovial scarring, inflammation and hypertrophy within the anterolateral recess from repeated microtrauma and soft tissue haemorrhage [34–36].

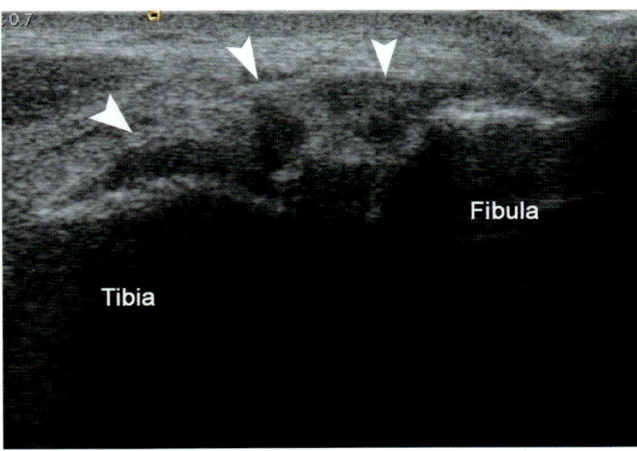

Fig. 3.28 Axial sonogram of a markedly thickened anterior inferior tibiofibular ligament (*arrowheads*) consistent with a significant ligament sprain

Table 3.4 Mimics of ankle impingement

Mimics of ankle impingement that should be considered include
- Osteochondral fractures
- Calcaneal talar stress fractures
- Mechanical instability from ligament tears
- Peroneal tendon pathology including rupture, tenosynovitis and subluxation
- Sinus tarsi syndrome

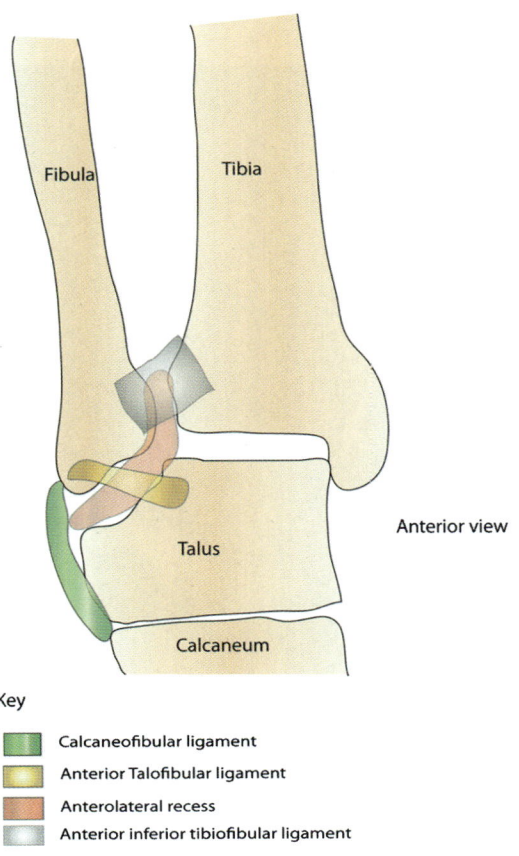

Fig. 3.29 Schematic diagram of the anterolateral gutter of the ankle joint

In advanced cases, a hyalinised meniscoid lesion may be present within the anterolateral gutter.

- Imaging

MR Imaging

MR demonstrates soft tissue thickening or a fibrous band, separate from the ATFL within the anterolateral recess [34, 35]. This band is low signal on T1 and intermediate or low signal on T2 imaging (Fig. 3.30). Additionally, on MR arthrography, there is absence of a recess, secondary to presence of adhesions preventing contrast from entering the normal recess [34, 35].

Anterior Ankle Impingement/"Footballer's Ankle"

Anterior impingement is a relatively common cause for anterior ankle pain, particularly in patients who perform repeated ankle dorsiflexion movements. This type of impingement is typically seen in footballers.

Anatomically, this type of impingement affects soft tissues between the anterior part of the tibial plafond and the dorsum of the talus, within the joint capsule.

- Clinical

Anterior ankle pain in a footballer may be provoked by certain movements which is sometimes a result of large osteophytes. These can be removed arthroscopically or via an open approach (Fig. 3.31).

- Biomechanics of injury

Anterior ankle impingement is characterised by presence of anterior tibio-talar spurs, at the anterior rim of the tibial plafond and the opposing face of the talus. Previously, the bony spurs were suspected to be secondary to chronic traction on the anterior joint capsule [37]. Nonetheless, cadaveric studies by Tol et al. demonstrated that the anterior tibio-talar spurs are formed within the anterior joint capsule instead of at the site of the capsular insertion [38]. In these anatomical specimens, the antero-superior joint capsule attaches onto the tibia on average 6 mm proximal to

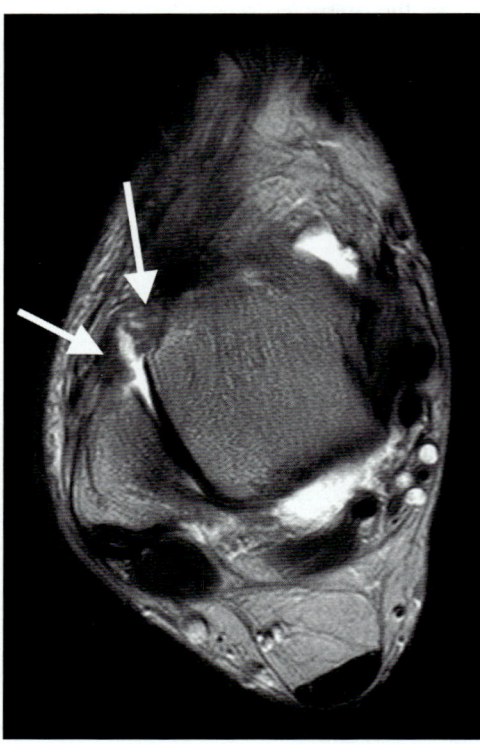

Fig. 3.30 Axial T2w MR image demonstrating fibrous proliferation (*arrows*) in the anterolateral recess associated with clinical anterolateral impingement syndrome

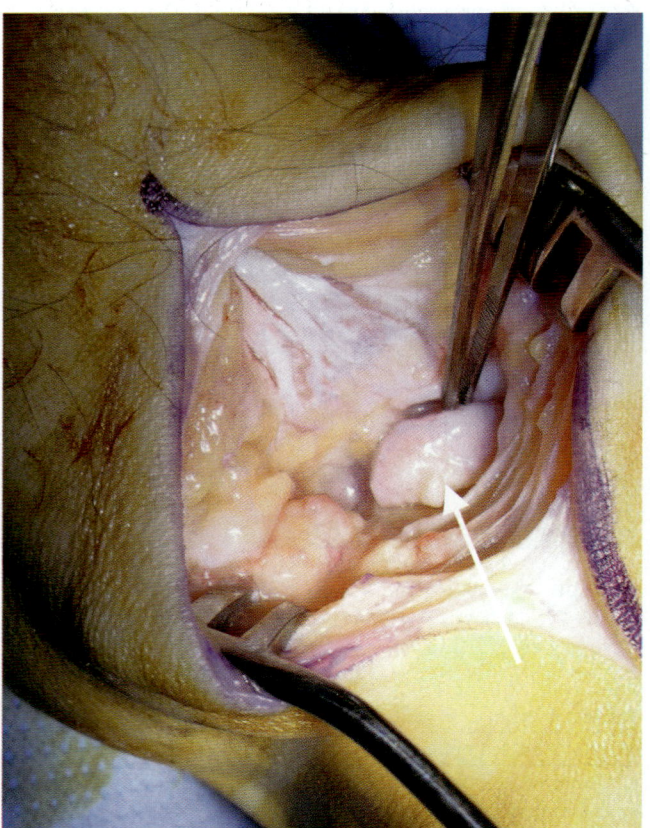

Fig. 3.31 Operative photograph demonstrating a large anterior tibial plafond osteophyte at the tip of the surgical instrument (*arrow*) in footballer with anterior impingement syndrome

the cartilage rim. Antero-inferiorly, the capsule attaches approximately 33 mm from the distal cartilage border [38]. This evidence makes the hypothesis of chronic repetitive capsular traction to be an unlikely cause of anterior impingement [38].

Causative theories in the pathogenesis and formation of bony spurs include:

1. Bony spurs arise due to repetitive trauma to the anterior articular cartilage rim secondarily either to
   (a) Repeated dorsiflexion (causing impaction between the anterior tibia and talus) [38] or
   (b) Direct trauma to the anterior ankle joint including articular cartilage rim during ball strike in football players. The average kicking velocity is 96 km/h and in a match, there are 60–120 ball contacts per player.
2. Trabecular microfractures with periosteal haemorrhage from repetitive microtrauma that heals to form new bone [39].
   - Imaging

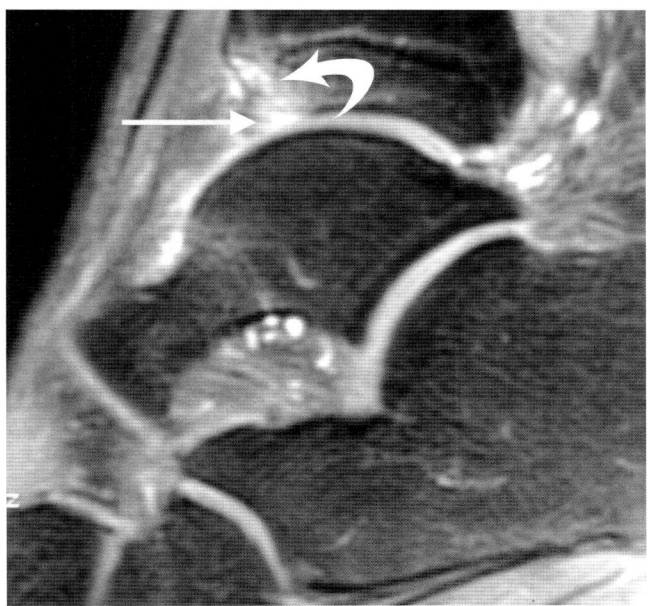

Fig. 3.32 Sagittal T1 STIR MR image of the ankle in a soccer player with anterior ankle impingement syndrome. Note the prominent anterior tibial plafond marginal osteophyte (*straight arrow*) with surrounding bone marrow oedema (*curved arrow*)

Plain Radiography/CT

Plain radiographs are often the only imaging study necessary; they allow evaluation of osseous spurs, which are present in anterior impingement and their effect on the anterior tibio-talar joint space [34]. CT is sometimes necessary as it accurately locates the osteophytes and identifies loose bodies within the tibio-talar joint, which helps plan the surgical approach for osteophyte excision.

MR Imaging

MR demonstrates the position of the tibio-talar spurs within the capsular margin (Fig. 3.32). Bone marrow oedema within the spurs can occur but is uncommon. Synovial thickening, evidenced by low signal intensity changes on T1 and low to intermediate signal intensity on T2 imaging with irregular contours can also be identified [34].

Anteromedial Ankle Impingement Syndrome

Anteromedial ankle impingement syndrome is an uncommon cause of chronic ankle pain. This condition is rarely an isolated injury. It is most commonly associated with an inversion injury with medial and lateral ligamentous complex injuries [34, 40].

- Biomechanics of injury

There are two theories of causation. The first theory is that it results from the impingement upon a meniscoid lesion located anterior to the tibio-talar ligament [34, 40]. The second theory is that impingement is secondary to a thickened anterior tibio-talar ligament, with impingement of the anteromedial soft tissues upon dorsiflexion [34, 40].

On dorsiflexion, both lesions impinge upon the anteromedial corner of the talus. Chondral damage and osteophyte formation may ensue [34, 40], worsening the impingement (Fig. 3.33).

- Imaging

MR Imaging

Conventional MR imaging may miss the meniscoid lesion unless a joint effusion is present. MR arthography may demonstrate a medial meniscoid lesion, a thickened anterior tibio-talar ligament and any chondral or osteochondral lesion [34, 40].

Posterior Ankle Impingement Syndromes

Posterior ankle impingement syndromes can be further subdivided into:

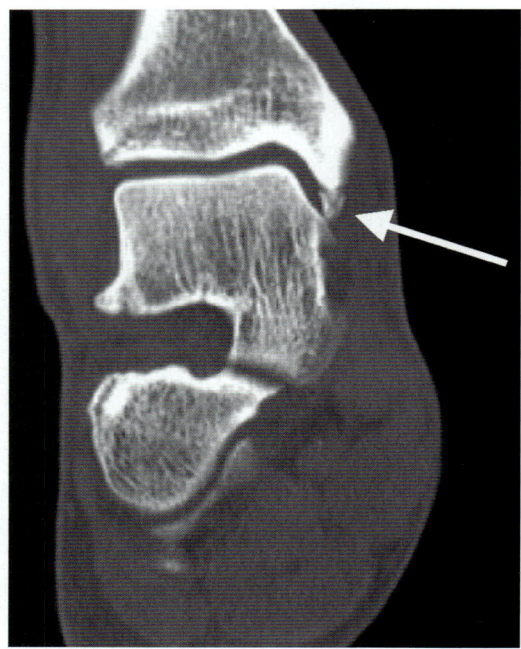

Fig. 3.33 Coronal CT planar reformat demonstrating an ossicle in the anteromedial recess of the ankle joint causing clinical anteromedial impingement

1. True posterior ankle impingement syndrome
2. Posteromedial ankle impingement (PoMI)
3. Haglund's phenomenon

Posterior Ankle Impingement

Posterior ankle impingement (PAI) is rare in the general population but an important cause of chronic ankle pain in footballers and ballet dancers [34, 41–43].

- Biomechanics of injury

This painful condition is caused by compression of the soft tissues in the region of the postero-lateral aspect of the talus, between the posterior margin of the tibia and the calcaneus by posterior ankle osseous anatomical variants.

The key players in the pathogenesis of PAI can be divided into osseous and soft tissue components. Osseous components which predispose or exacerbate PAI include presence of [43, 44]:

(i) A downsloping posterior tibial plafond
(ii) An os trigonum, an unfused lateral tubercle of the posterior process of the talar body (Fig. 3.34)
(iii) "Stieda process," an unusually long lateral posterior process of the talar body
(iv) Haglund's deformity, an enlarged posterosuperior calcaneal tuberosity, which is also classically associated with insertional Achilles tendinopathy and retrocalcaneal bursitis.

The soft tissue components which are involved in PAI include [43, 44]:

(i) Posterior ankle ligaments; including the posterior inferior tibiofibular ligament, a thickened transverse tibiofibular ligament, the "tibial slip" (connecting the PTFL to the medial malleolus), and the posterior talofibular ligament
(ii) Joint capsule and synovium
(iii) The flexor hallucis longus

PAI syndrome may be secondary to an acute injury such as a posterior talofibular ligament avulsion, an acute disruption of the os trigonum or fracture of the lateral talar process. PAI syndrome is not secondary to the presence of an os trigonum per se but secondary to a traumatic event causing inflammation [44]. The three initiating factors described above lead to thickening of posterior capsule and adjacent soft tissues,

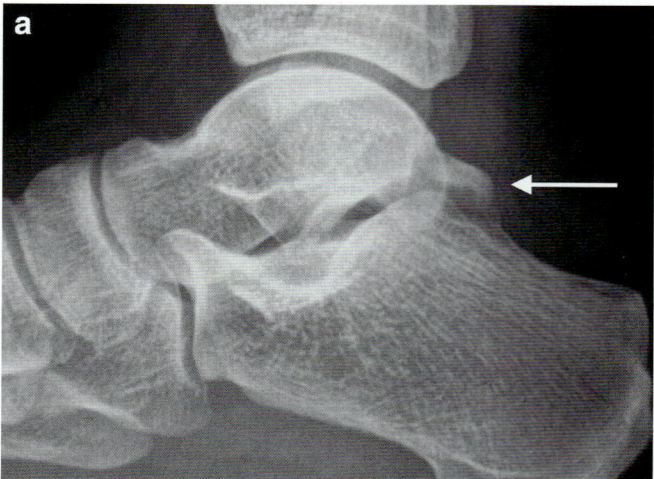 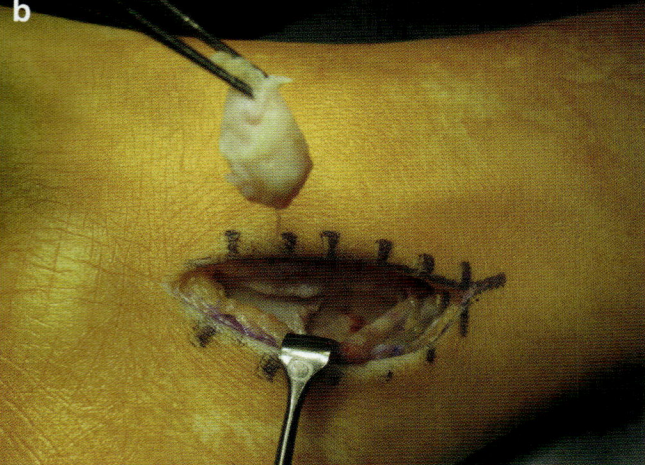

Fig. 3.34 (a) Lateral X-ray of the ankle demonstrating an os trigonum (*arrow*). (b) Operative photograph demonstrating removal of the os via a medial approach

which results in PAI syndrome. Additionally, loose bodies collecting within the posterior recess may also contribute to symptoms.

- Clinical

Symptoms of PAI syndrome are reproduced on repeated forced plantar flexion and repeated full-weight bearing in the extreme plantar-flexed position. When the ankle is forced into plantar flexion, the posterior talar process or os trigonum is compressed between the posterior rim of the tibia and calcaneus, reproducing the symptoms. If conservative measures such as rest and anti-inflammatory medication fail to alleviate symptoms, surgery which may be open or arthroscopic is indicated (Fig. 3.34).

- Imaging

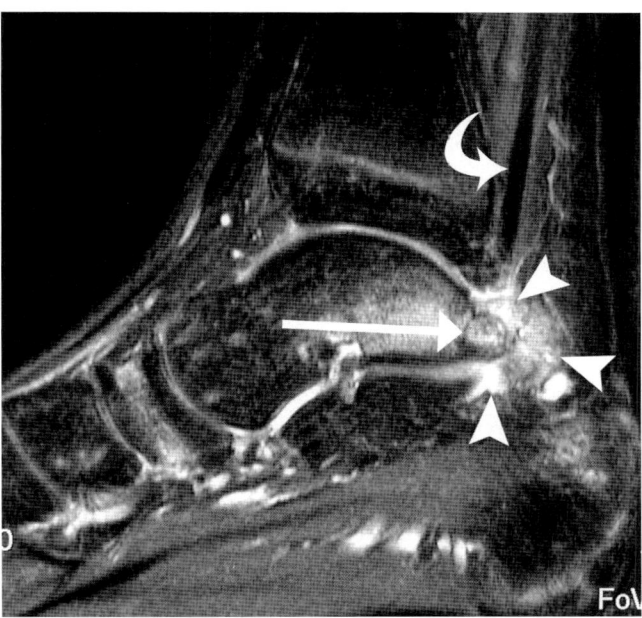

Fig. 3.35 Sagittal MR image of the ankle joint in a 17-year-old ballet dancer. There is an inflamed os trigonum (*long arrow*) with surrounding synovitis (*arrowheads*). The flexor hallucis longus tendon (*curved arrow*) runs into the inflamed tissues

MR/US Imaging

MR findings can be divided into osseous and soft tissue abnormalities:

1. Osseous abnormalities

Bone marrow oedema within and surrounding the os trigonum is demonstrated. In addition, there may be fragmentation of *os trigonum*, lateral tubercle and talar lateral process with loose body formation [43, 44]. There may also be bone marrow oedema in the posterior tibia, posterior talus and calcaneus (Fig. 3.35).

2. Soft tissue abnormalities

Oedema surrounding the os trigonum or postero-lateral tubercle of the talus is seen (Fig. 3.35). Flexor hallucis longus tenosynovitis and posterior capsular synovitis, evidenced by enhancement following Gadolinium intravenous injection is also present [43, 44]. Furthermore, thickening and tears of the PTFL, PITF, intermalleolar ligament may be demonstrated [44].

Posterior impingement may be demonstrated on MR imaging with the foot plantar-flexed using rapid sequences. US can also demonstrate impingement and synovitis dynamically and can guide injection as a diagnostic/therapeutic test.

Haglund's Syndrome

Originally described by Patrick Haglund in 1928, Haglund's deformity is the presence of a prominent physical "pump bump" and radiographically abnormal prominence of the posterior superior tubercle of the os calcis.

- Clinical

Haglund's syndrome (HS) is the presence of pain and a Haglund's deformity (Fig. 3.36). Surgical excision of the bony deformity along with the overlying bursa may be required for symptomatic relief.

- Biomechanics of injury

HS is due to friction of the prominent posterior superior tubercle of the os calcis with:

1. Anterior structures including Kager's fat pad and the retrocalcaneal bursa
2. Posterior structures including the Achilles tendon

following repeated contractions of the gastrocnemius–soleus complex [44].

- Imaging

MR Imaging

Radiologically, Haglund's syndrome is manifested as insertional Achilles tendonitis and retrocalcaneal bursitis. MR demonstrates presence of Haglund's deformity of posterior calcaneus, and an expanded Achilles tendon insertion with intra-tendinous mucinous degeneration shown as high signal on T2/STIR images (Fig. 3.37) [44]. The retrocalcaneal bursa is enlarged and demonstrates inflammation on images following IV gadolinium. There may also be marked oedema on T2/STIR images within the posterior superior calcaneus.

Posteromedial Ankle Impingement Syndrome

Posteromedial ankle impingement syndrome is an uncommon cause of chronic posteromedial ankle pain and is the least described ankle impingement syndrome.

- Clinical

Chronic posteromedial ankle pain.

- Biomechanics of injury

PoMI syndrome typically occurs following a supination/inversion injury of the ankle. During forced inversion of the ankle, the anterior talofibular ligament which resists oversupination of the tibio-talar joint may be disrupted. Medially, there is compression of the posteromedial structures, which can lead to PoMI. The soft tissues involved include the [44]:

1. Posterior tibio-talar ligament
2. Posteromedial tibio-talar joint capsule
3. Posteromedial long flexor tendons
4. Posterior tibialis tendon
5. Flexor digitorum longus
6. Less frequently, flexor hallucis longus.

- Imaging

MR Imaging

ATFL injury may be demonstrated with possible signs of anterolateral impingement and or presence of an osteochondral injury of the talar dome (Fig. 3.38) [44].

Posteromedially, loss of normal fat striation within the PTTL is demonstrated [45]. Posteromedial synovitis and synovial hypertrophy may be present. Additionally, posterior and postero-lateral synovitis may be evident (Fig. 3.38) [46].

Tendinous Pathology

In athletes, the most common tendon pathologies occur in the Achilles and peroneal tendons. Less commonly, tendinous pathology may also be seen in the flexor and extensor tendon groups around the ankle.

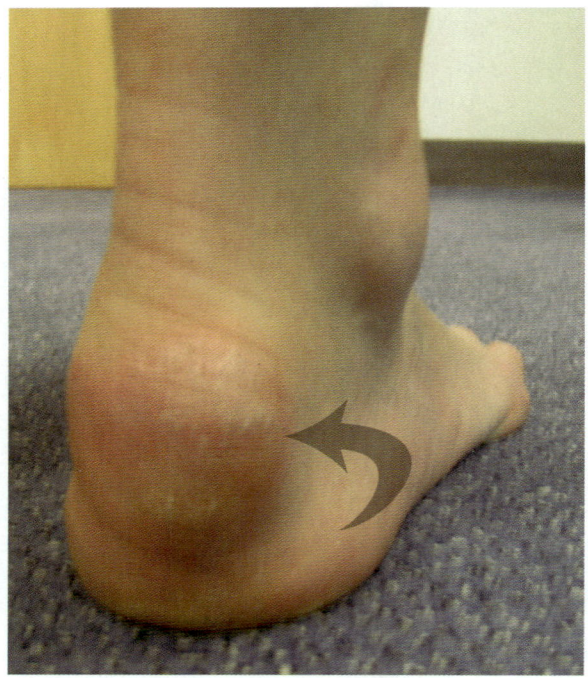

Fig. 3.36 Clinical photograph showing the prominent "pump bump" of a Haglund's deformity of the posterosuperior os calcis

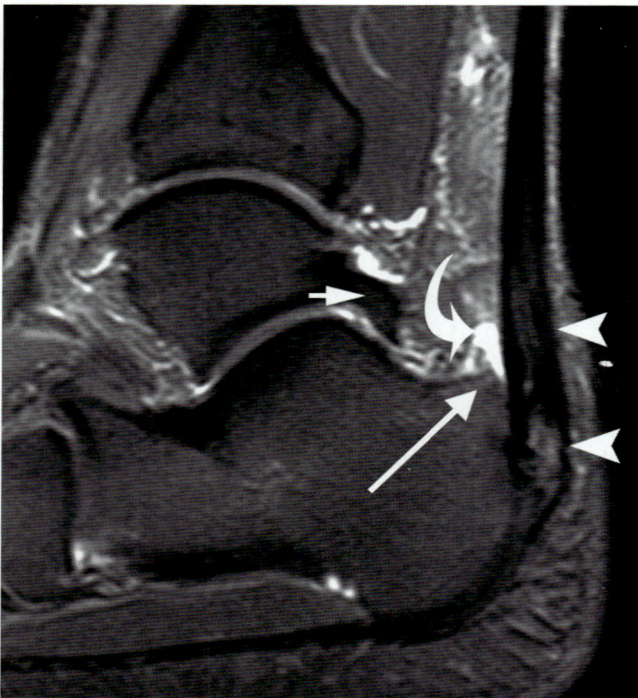

Fig. 3.37 Sagittal STIR MR image of a 39-year-old marathon runner with Haglund's syndrome. Note the enlarged posterosuperior tubercle of the os calcis (*long arrow*) associated with retrocalcaneal bursitis (*curved arrow*) and insertional Achilles tendonitis (*arrowheads*). Note the enlarged Stieda process of the posterior talus (*short arrow*), which may be associated with Haglund's syndrome

The Achilles Tendon

The Achilles tendon (AT) is the thickest, longest and strongest tendon in the body.

Measuring 12–15 cm, it is formed by the confluence of the aponeuroses of the medial and lateral heads of gastrocnemius and soleus tendon. These insert into the posterior os calcis. On descending inferiorly, the shape of the tendon changes from being flat to a crescent shape with a flat or concave deep surface. Note however, its shape changes again just superior to its insertion, where it assumes a convex deep margin and may appear bulbous. It is important to appreciate these changes in the interpretation of ultrasound and MR imaging.

The AT does not have a tendon sheath but instead is enveloped dorsally, medially and laterally by a thin membrane which has network of blood vessels, known as a paratenon. The paratenon facilitates tendon gliding.

The spectrum of pathology involving the Achilles tendon includes tears/partial tears, tendinopathy (insertional and non-insertional), paratendinitis and bursitis.

Tendinopathy

Achilles tendinopathy can be insertional or non-insertional. Non-insertional injuries occur 4–6 cm above the distal insertion of the Achilles tendon, a watershed area, which is relatively hypovascular.

- Clinical

Patients present with a fusiform swelling of the Achilles tendon, which can range from being asymptomatic to extremely painful.

- Biomechanics of injury

This is multifactorial but is predominantly due to overuse injury leading to collagen and tenocyte necrosis [47, 48].

- Imaging

Ultrasound

US demonstrates tendon swelling, most commonly fusiform and less commonly focal or nodular, affecting the hypovascular middle third territory of the Achilles tendon (Fig. 3.39). There is loss of the normal echogenic fibrillar pattern within the tendon, which becomes hypoechoic and granular in its sonographic appearance.

Neovascularity and intra-tendinous cysts may also be evident (Fig. 3.40). The significance of tendon neovascularity is unknown but they do correlate with pain and these vessels may be accompanied by small nerves [49–51].

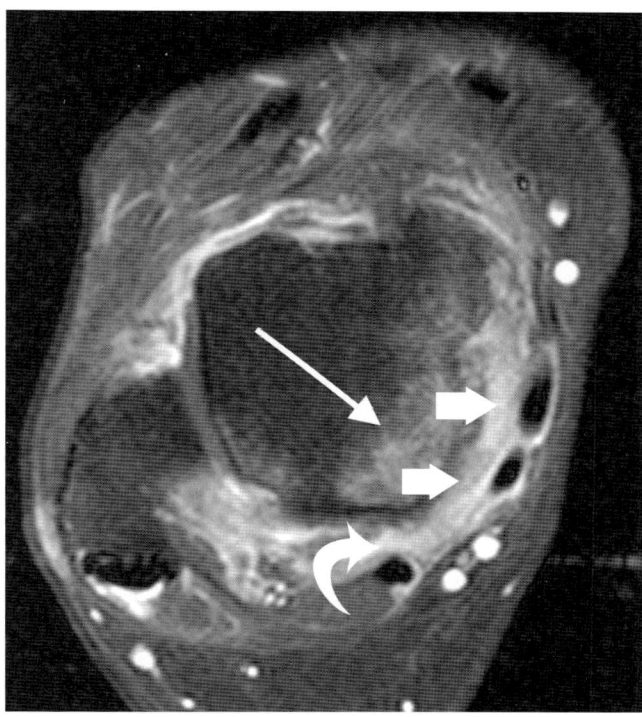

Fig. 3.38 Twenty-seven-year-old hockey player 6 weeks following an inversion injury. There is marked inflammation within the tibio-talar ligament (*block arrows*) deep to the flexor tendons. Posterior synovitis is also present around the flexor hallucis longus tendon (*curved arrow*). Bone marrow oedema is seen in the posteromedial talar dome (*long arrow*)

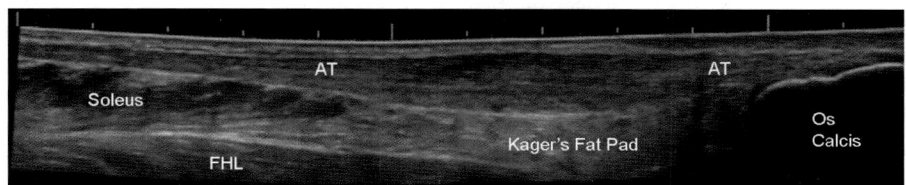

Fig. 3.39 Longitudinal extended-field-of-view sonogram of a 34-year-old female middle-distance runner. There is fusiform expansion of the Achilles tendon (AT) consistent with non-insertional Achilles tendinopathy. Note the flexor hallucis (FHL) muscle belly deep to the Achilles tendon and Kager's fat pad

Various therapies including sclerotherapy of the neovessels have been reported to improve patient symptoms [52].

MR Imaging

MR imaging shows diffuse intra-tendinous swelling producing fusiform expansion. This occurs with or without a focal or diffuse increase in signal. Insertional tendinopathy can be identified on MR imaging as increased signal intensity and swelling at the site of its insertion. This may be associated with retrocalcaneal bursitis. Calcaneal reactive bone marrow oedema may also be present. Haglunds deformity may also be associated with insertional tendinopathy [44] (see also section "Haglund's Syndrome").

Paratendinitis

In paratendinitis, the Achilles tendon is intact. However, there is peritendinous inflammation, effusions, adhesions and scarring of the paratenon (Fig. 3.41).

- Clinical

This condition can be extremely painful and even light palpation of the area can be excruciatingly painful. Sometimes stripping of the paratenon by injecting saline and local anaesthetic or surgical debridement of the paratenon may be required.

- Imaging

Ultrasound

Paratendinitis is manifested by hypoechoic thickening around the Achilles tendon (Fig. 3.42). This may demonstrate increased vascularity on Doppler imaging. There may be impingement with the adjacent retrocalcaneal fat identified on dynamic imaging secondary to adhesion formation.

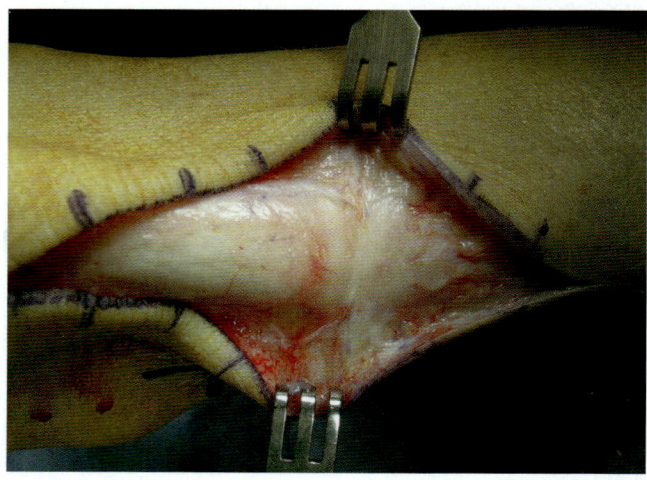

Fig. 3.41 Operative photograph demonstrating scar tissue and hyperaemia draping over the posterior surface of the Achilles tendon

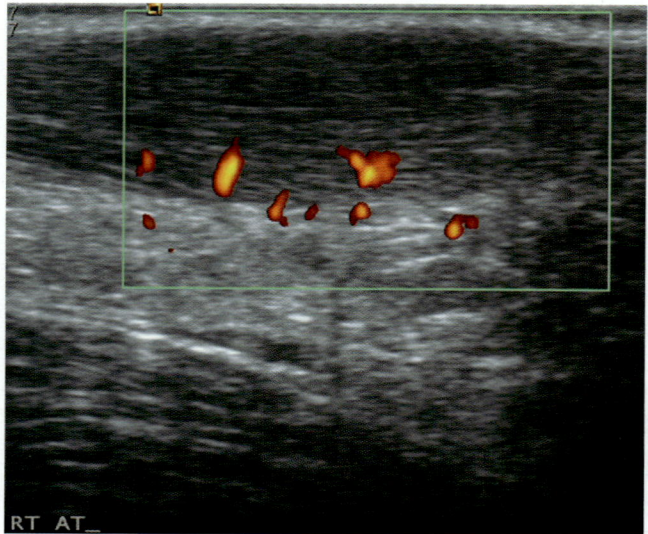

Fig. 3.40 Power Doppler longitudinal sonogram of the Achilles tendon. The tendon demonstrates fusiform expansion consistent with chronic tendinopathy. The colour represents flow within areas of neovascularisation of the tendon. Note the typical location of the vascularity arising from the deep surface and branching into the tendon

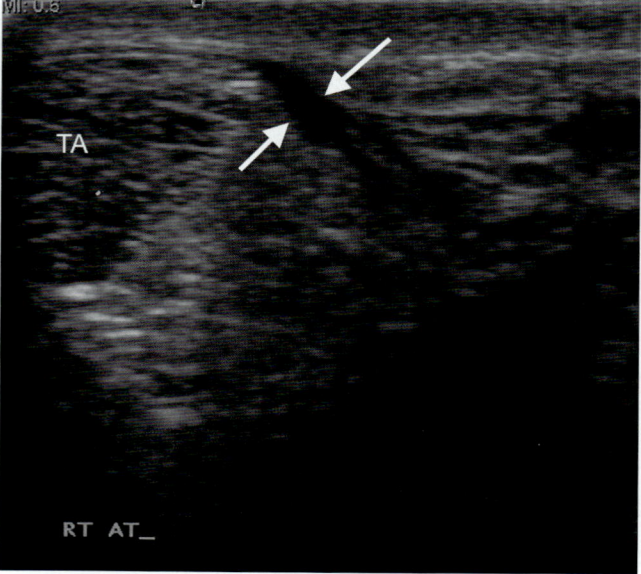

Fig. 3.42 Transverse sonogram of a 22-year-old runner with posterior ankle pain. Note the fluid (*arrows*) around the medial surface of the Achilles tendon consistent with paratendinitis

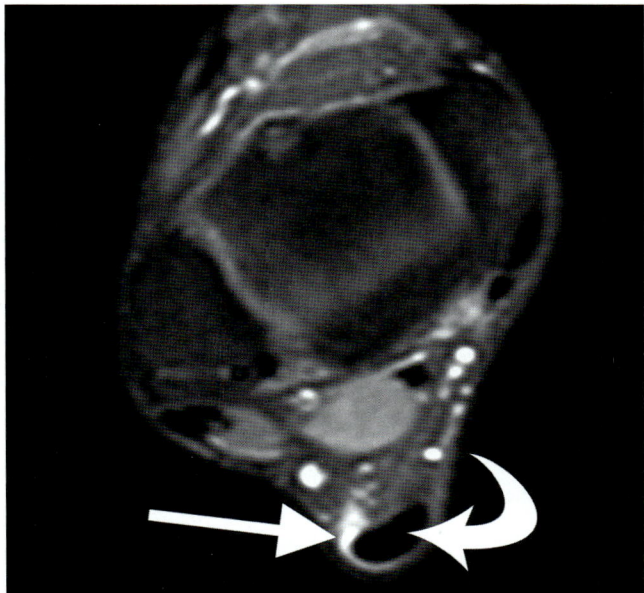

Fig. 3.43 Axial fat-saturated T1w MR image of the ankle following IV gadolinium. Note the marked enhancement (*arrow*) around the medial and posterior border of the Achilles tendon consistent with paratendinitis

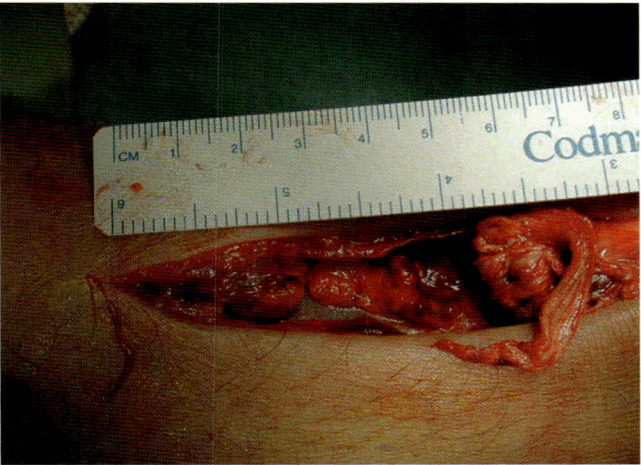

Fig. 3.44 Operative photograph exposing a full-thickness rupture of the Achilles tendon. Note the macerated distal end of the tendon

MR Imaging

On MR imaging, there is high signal fluid on T2/STIR imaging surrounding a normal Achilles tendon, which may show enhancement on post-contrast images following IV gadolinium (Fig. 3.43). In addition, there may be linear or irregular signal intensity changes in the pre-Achilles fat pad indicating adhesion formation [53].

Achilles Tendon Tears

The Achilles tendon commonly ruptures 2–6 cm above the calcaneal insertion; this critical area is relatively hypovascular.

- Clinical

This injury is caused by a violent push-off and is associated with racquet sports but can also occur as a result of a "missed" step. There is always bruising and swelling but due to the fact that patients can still walk and plantar flex the ankle, the diagnosis is often missed. Most surgeons treat rupture of the Achilles tendon surgically. (Fig. 3.44).

- Imaging

Ultrasound

On US, a complete rupture of the Achilles tendon can be seen as a focal defect between the torn tendon edges (Fig. 3.45). The free ends of the acutely torn tendon can be easily appreciated. An intervening tendon gap with acute haematoma can be identified; this can be anechoic or hypoechoic in its appearance. The tendon gap should be measured with the foot in the plantar-flexed position as this is the casting position.

In addition, there may be fat herniation into the tendon defect with improved visualisation of the plantaris tendon (Fig. 3.46) [54]. Posterior acoustic shadowing at the site of tendon end relates to US beam refraction at the frayed tendon ends can also be detected and is useful for determining the tendon gap, thus differentiating a partial from a full-thickness tear [54].

If there is still doubt as to whether a tear/rupture is present, gentle dynamic passive dorsiflexion will make separation of tendon ends more apparent and confirm apposition of the tendon ends in plantar flexion.

A partial thickness tear is identified on US as a hypoechoic interstitial defect usually in the longitudinal plane, paralleling the tendon fibres. There is disruption of the normal fibrillar pattern at this site.

MR Imaging

On MR imaging, complete tendon tears are evidenced by complete tendon discontinuity with fraying and retraction of tendon ends (Fig. 3.47). In acute tendon ruptures, the tendon gap is filled with haematoma (intermediate signal on T1) and oedema (high signal on T2/STIR) [19].

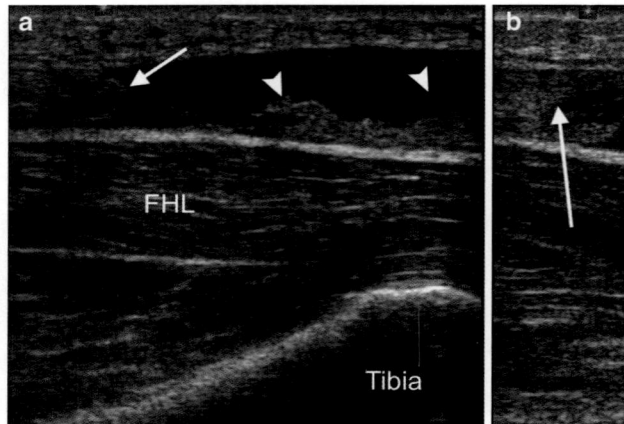

Fig. 3.45 Longitudinal sonogram of the Achilles tendon taken from patient in Fig. 3.44. (**a**) There is a full-thickness tear of the tendon with the rounded proximal end (*arrow*) separated from the macerated distal end by a fluid filled gap. In plantar flexion (**b**), the tendon edges appose but the patient was treated surgically due to the macerated distal end

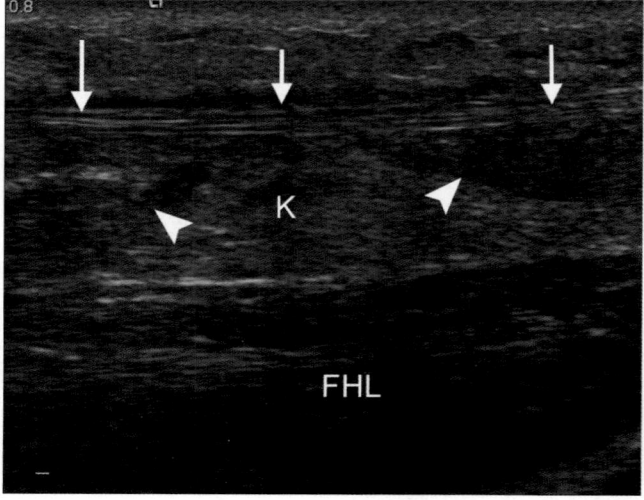

Fig. 3.46 Longitudinal sonogram of a 34-year-old male squash player with acute onset posterior ankle pain. Kager's fat pad (K) has herniated into the defect between the torn ends of the Achilles tendon (*arrowheads*) enhancing the visualisation of the plantaris tendon (*arrows*)

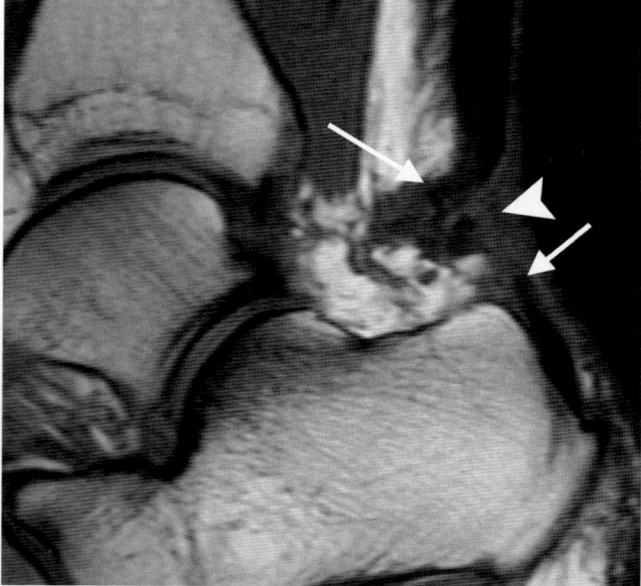

Fig. 3.47 Sagittal T1w MR image of the hindfoot in a 35-year-old female netball player. There is a complete tear of the Achilles tendon (*arrows*) with an intervening haematoma (*arrowhead*)

Partial thickness tears on MR imaging can be identified as intra-tendinous high T2/STIR signal intensity (Fig. 3.48) [55]. There is no complete disruption of the tendon [19]. Subcutaneous oedema and haemorrhage within Kager's fat pad may be present [19].

In describing AT tears, it is important to remark upon the integrity of the plantaris tendon. When a complete AT tear occurs, the plantaris tendon may move posteriorly to mimic intact fibres of the AT. Clinically, it may give a false-negative test.

Peroneal Tendons

There are two main peroneal tendons, the peroneus longus and brevis which plantar flex and evert the ankle and foot. Peroneus longus arises from the posterior lateral condyle of the tibia, the interosseous membrane and proximal fibula whereas peroneus brevis arises from the distal fibula and interosseous membrane, deep to the peroneus longus.

3 Ankle and Foot Injuries

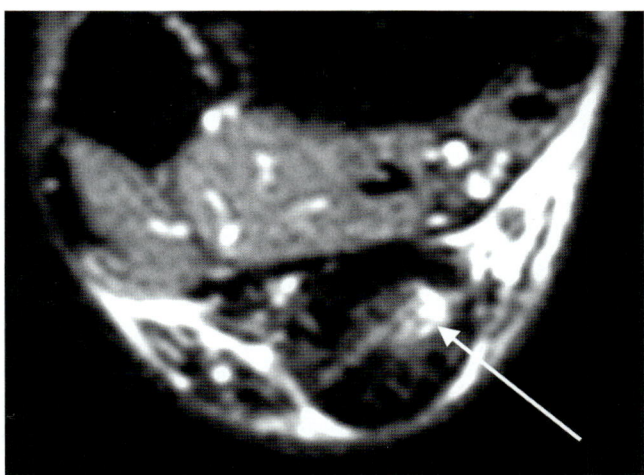

Fig. 3.48 Axial STIR MR image of the Achilles tendon. There is linear high signal within the central/medial side of the Achilles tendon consistent with an intrasubstance partial thickness tear

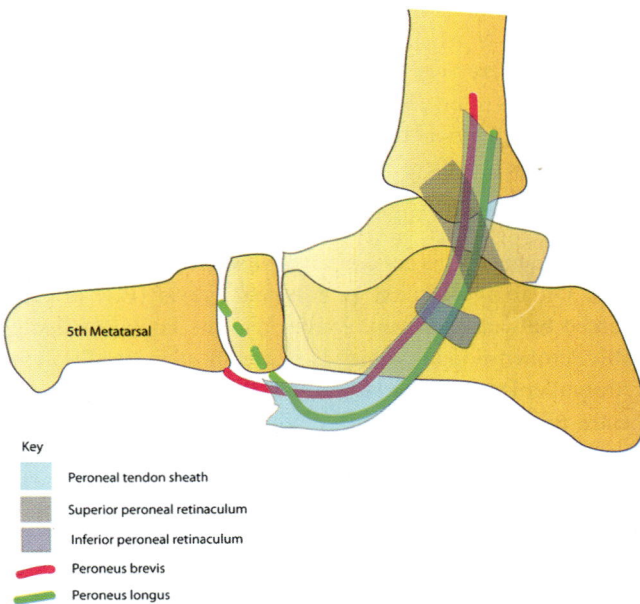

Fig. 3.49 Schematic drawing of the peroneal tendons and retinacula

At the ankle, both tendons run within a fibro-osseous tunnel located posterior to the lateral malleolus, known as the *retromalleolar groove*. The roof of the groove is formed by the superior peroneal retinaculum (SPR). The SPR is a fibrous band which arises from the posterior ridge of the distal fibula and inserts into the lateral wall of the calcaneus, or rarely merges with the Achilles tendon.

At the level of the retromalleolar groove, the peroneus longus is located posterolaterally and is oval. By comparison, the peroneus brevis tendon is anteromedial and is flat or mildly crescentic and is rarely bifurcated. When crescentic, it should not be thinner in the middle than at its periphery [56].

Both peroneal longus (PL) and brevis share a common tendon sheath that originates approximately 4 cm above the lateral malleolus proximally to the level of the calcaneocuboid joint distally [57].

More distally at the level of the calcaneum, both peroneal tendons are stabilised by an inferior peroneal retinaculum and located superficial to the calcaneofibular ligament (Fig. 3.49).

The peroneus longus subsequently changes its course medially, running within the cuboid tunnel deep to the cuboid bone and inserts into the plantar surface of the lateral cuneiform and base of the first metatarsal. The peroneus brevis continues anteriorly to insert into the base of the fifth metatarsal.

A spectrum of injuries to the peroneal tendons, ranging from tenosynovitis, tendinopathy, rupture and dislocation can occur.

Peroneal Tenosynovitis

Acute peroneal tenosynovitis is encountered typically in athletes who resume their activities after a layoff period and ballet dancers who spend considerable time standing in the *demi-pointe* position [58].

- Clinical

Patients complain of pain and slight swelling behind the fibula, extending down towards the fifth metatarsal base.

- Biomechanics of injury

Tenosynovitis may be secondary to increased stress around fixed pulleys, which include the retromalleolar groove, peroneal tubercle and undersurface of cuboid bone. It is noteworthy that fluid in the common peroneal tendon sheath may also be caused by a tear of the calcaneofibular ligament due to the close relationship between the ligament and the sheath [58].

- Imaging

MR/US Imaging

Peroneal tenosynovitis is defined as fluid within the common peroneal tendon sheath and/or thickening and inflammation of the tendon sheath in association with a normal peroneal tendon appearance. A small amount of fluid around the common peroneal tendon sheath on MR imaging is considered physiological. However calcaneofibular ligament (CFL) injury can give rise to fluid accumulation in the common peroneal tendon sheath and thus may be a marker of CFL injury [58].

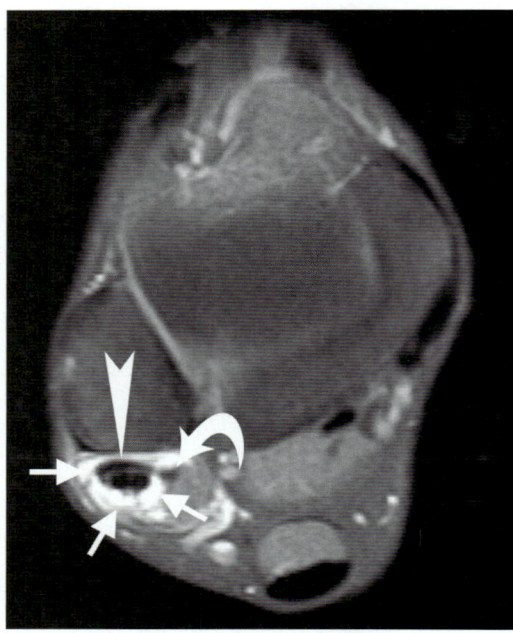

Fig. 3.50 Axial T1w FS MR image of the ankle following IV gadolinium. There is avid enhancement of the peroneal tenosynovium (*short arrows*). Note the marked flattening of the peroneus brevis tendon (*arrowhead*) with early development of a split in the medial margin of the tendon (*curved arrow*)

On MR, a pathological effusion is diagnosed if the radius of the fluid is greater than 2 mm or 25% of the width of the tendon or if the tendon is completely surrounded by fluid [55]. There may be marked tendon sheath enhancement following IV gadolinium (Fig. 3.50). Whilst there is no current literature on the US characteristics of peroneal tenosynovitis, we use imaging characteristics similar to MR imaging for this diagnosis in our institution. If the sheath is thickened, increased vascularity may be seen on colour Doppler imaging.

Stenosing tenosynovitis may occur following synovial proliferation and fibrosis surrounding the tendons, preventing their free movement. MR imaging demonstrates thickening of the tenosynovium with low signal adhesion formation within the sheath [58]. Enhancement post-Gadolinium is also seen [58]. Tendinopathy may also occur; this results in enlargement and/or increased T2 signal within the tendons [55].

Peroneal Brevis Tendon Tear/Rupture

Peroneal splits or longitudinal tears of the peroneus brevis tendon is frequently seen in young athletes [58].

- Clinical

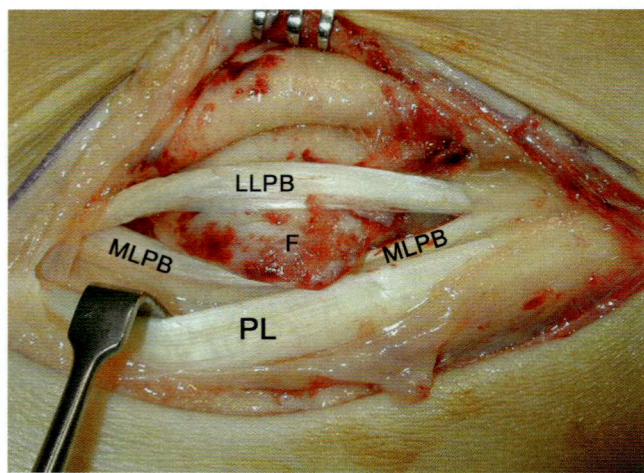

Fig. 3.51 Peroperative photograph demonstrating a split peroneus brevis tendon. The lateral limb of the peroneus brevis tendon (LLPB) has dislocated over the posterior margin of the fibula malleolus (F). The peroneus longus (PL) and medial limb of peroneus brevis (MLPB) remain behind the fibula malleolus

The findings are very similar to those of peroneal tenosynovitis. There is often a history of trauma but not always. Many tears require surgical repair (Fig. 3.51) and neglecting them can lead to a complete rupture.

- Biomechanics of injury

The peroneus brevis tendon is predisposed to degenerative tears. On foot dorsiflexion, peroneal brevis (PB) is compressed between peroneus longus and the lateral malleolus [58]. Peroneus longus, which is located posterior to PB in the retromalleolar groove acts as a bowstring which cuts into the centre to the PB tendon [55]. When the PB tears, the peroneus longus tendon migrates anteriorly into the PB defect.

- Imaging

On axial MR imaging, the PB assumes a *boomerang* or *c-shaped* configuration [55], enveloping the peroneus longus tendon. The central portion of the PB anterior to the peroneus longus becomes markedly attenuated and is not well visualised [58]. The signal intensity of PB is increased on T1w and T2/STIR-weighted images [58]. Clefts, fragmentation and irregularity of tendon contour may also be evident (Fig. 3.52) [58]. This cleft or splitting in the PB tendon is often better evaluated on US because of the superior spatial resolution (Fig. 3.53).

Secondary signs associated with PB tears should also be sought:

1. Shallow or convex retromalleolar groove – this is present in 95% of patients with a PB tear [55]
2. Subluxation of the peroneal tendons; tears are more common with subluxed peroneal tendons, secondary to a

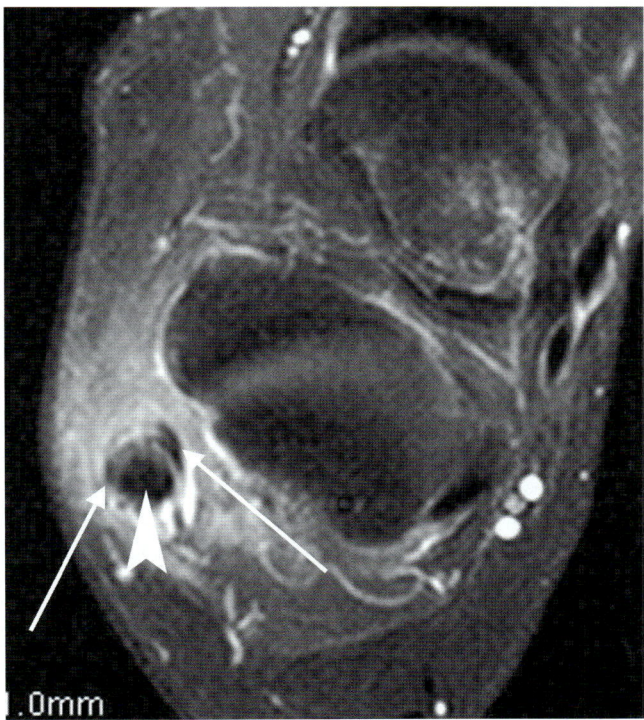

Fig. 3.52 Axial gadolinium enhanced fat-suppressed T1w MR image of the ankle. There is a split of the peroneal tendon into medial and lateral limbs (*arrows*) with the peroneus longus interposed between the two (*arrowhead*)

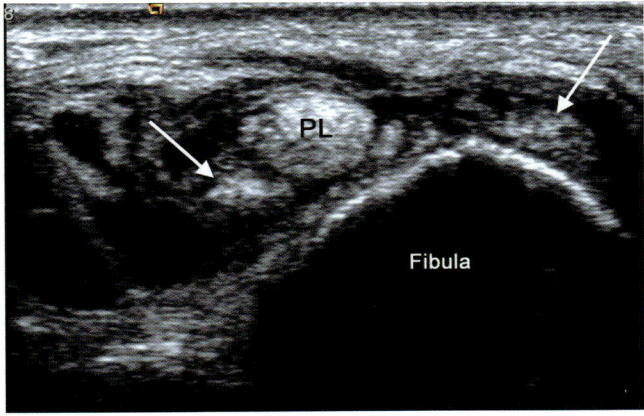

Fig. 3.53 Axial sonogram of same patient subsequently operated on in Fig. 3.57. The peroneus brevis tendon has split in two (*arrows*) with the peroneus longus tendon (PL) interposed between the two

shallow retromalleolar groove and/or a lax superior retinaculum [55]
3. Presence of a spur at the lateral aspect of the lateral malleolus, secondary to repeated traction of the superior retinaculum on the fibula [55]
4. Crowding within the retromalleolar groove from presence of a peroneus quartus tendon [55]
5. Presence of bone marrow oedema in the lateral malleolus [55]
6. Peroneus longus pathology; this may be peroneus longus thickening or a partial tear [55]

Imaging pitfalls include a normal bifurcated peroneus brevis may simulating a tear; this mistake can be avoided by examining the muscle-tendon unit proximal to the ankle [58]. A mildly crescentic PB tendon at the retromalleolar groove is a normal finding [58].

Peroneal longus Tendon Tear/Rupture

Tears of the PL tendon occur commonly in association with a PB tendon tear at the level of the retromalleolar groove [56]. Isolated PL tendon tears occur more distally, at the level of the peroneal tubercle or within the cuboid tunnel.

- Clinical

Tears of the peroneus longus tendon are rarer than those of peroneus brevis. Treatment strategies are however similar. In rare instances, the sesamoid bone within the peroneus longus tendon can fracture at the level of the cuboid tunnel.

- Biomechanics of injury

These may be sports related or associated with trauma, e.g. calcaneal fracture or calcaneocuboid joint direct crush injury.

Friction of the PL against either a hypertrophic peroneal tubercle or cuboid bone as the tendon curves underneath may predispose to a PL tear [58].

- Imaging

MR Imaging

MR imaging demonstrates abnormal signal intensity within the PL with morphological abnormalities including longitudinal splits and disruption [58]. Secondary signs including presence of increased marrow T2/STIR signal within the peroneal tubercle, lateral calcaneal wall or cuboid may be evident [58]. The two common sites of peroneus longus pathology are demonstrated in the Fig. 3.54.

Peroneal Retinaculum Injuries and Peroneal Dislocation

Superior retinacular injuries are more common although inferior retinacular injuries are described in footballers. Superior retinacular injuries have been reported amongst

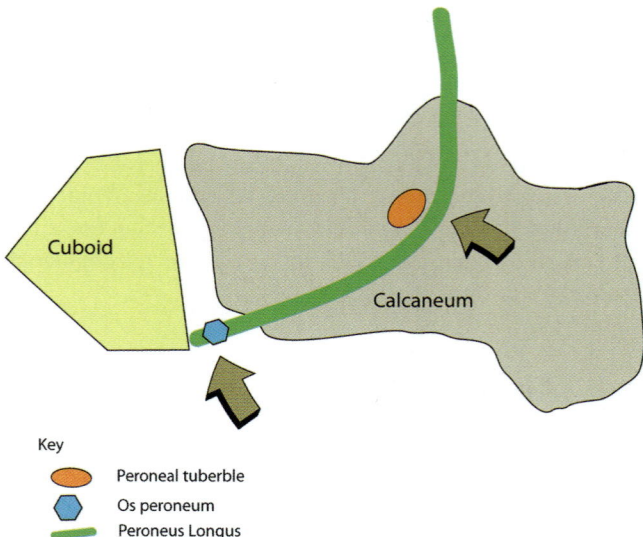

Fig. 3.54 Schematic drawing of the potential sites of inflammation within the peroneus longus tendon

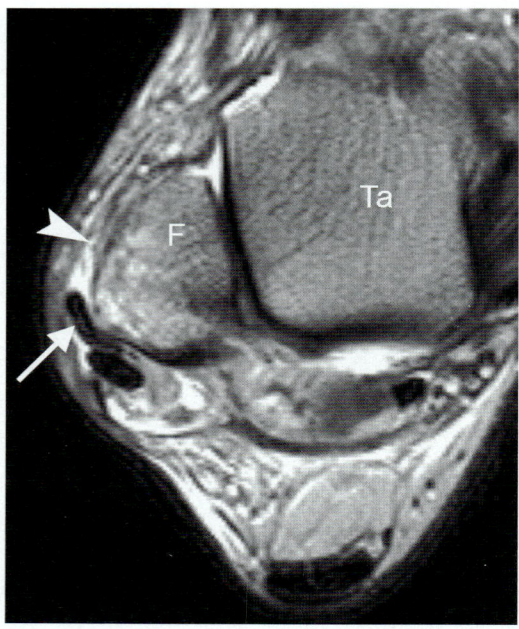

Fig. 3.55 Axial T2w MR image of the ankle in a ballet dancer. The peroneus brevis tendon (*arrow*) has dislocated over the lateral margin of the fibula (F). The fibula attachment of the superior peroneal retinaculum (*arrowhead*) is deficient. *Ta* talus

skiers when both tips of their skis catch in the snow, causing the skier to be thrown forward suddenly. In this process, the skier experiences sudden acute ankle dorsiflexion.

- Clinical

Superior retinacular injury is difficult to distinguish in the early stages from lateral ligament sprain. However the patient will often complain of a snapping sensation as the tendons subluxate over the fibula. Treatment involves relocating and securing the peroneii behind the fibula.

- Biomechanics of injury

Peroneal tendon dislocation occurs as a result of sudden foot dorsiflexion with violent contraction of the peroneal muscles; this causes stripping of the superior peroneal retinaculum from its distal fibular attachment. This allows the peroneal tendons to sublux anterolaterally from the retromalleolar groove [58].

- Imaging

Plain Radiographs

A flake-like fracture of the distal fibular metaphysis may be evident; this is indicative of an avulsed or stripped peroneal retinaculum [19].

MR Imaging

The axial plane is best for demonstrating dislocation of the tendons anterior and lateral to the distal fibula (Fig. 3.55). They are often seen within a "pouch" formed by a stripped-off superior peroneal retinaculum [19].

Other secondary/associated findings include [19], tenosynovitis and tears of the peroneal tendons, a convex fibular groove, avulsion fracture of the distal fibula with underlying bone marrow oedema and tears of the lateral ankle ligaments.

Ultrasound

US demonstrates the position of the subluxed, peroneal tendons lateral to the distal lateral malleolus, instead of posterior (Fig. 3.53) [59]. In addition, a small, echogenic, flake fracture paralleling the distal fibular metaphysic can be identified.

Dynamic US during dorsiflexion and eversion can help improve detection of intermittent subluxation [59].

Painful Os Peroneum Syndrome (POPS)

The os peroneum (OP) is a sesamoid bone within the peroneus longus tendon. It is normally located at the calcaneocuboid articulation, proximal to the peroneal groove on the underside of the cuboid (Fig. 3.56). Occasionally it can be seen at the plantar aspect of the cuboid and articulate with it [60]. It is present in everyone in a cartilaginous or fibrocartilaginous

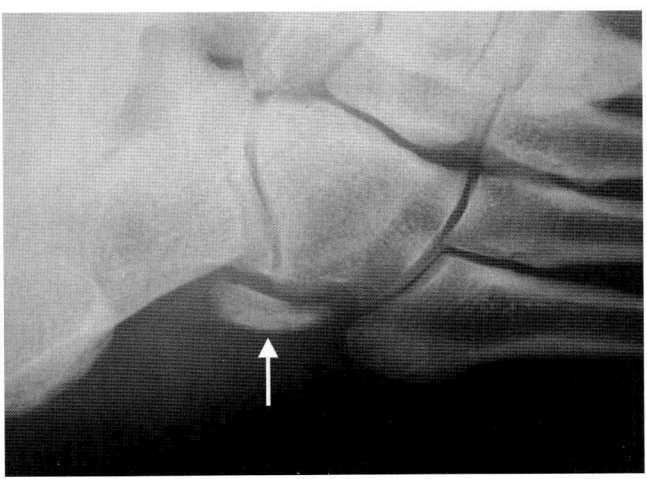

Fig. 3.56 Oblique X-ray of the foot in a tennis player with lateral foot pain. A large os peroneum was present. Subsequent MR imaging showed inflammation around the os consistent with painful os peroneum syndrome (POPS)

form but ossified (and radiologically evident) in 3–26% of the population and is bipartite or multipartite in 25–30% of these cases [60]. Painful os peroneum syndrome (POPS) can be secondary to acute and chronic injuries. Rarely the os peroneum needs to be excised.

- Biomechanics of injury

Acute injuries include OP fractures, diastasis of a multipartite OP or peroneal tendon ruptures. An acute OP fracture may either be secondary to a direct blow or forced contraction of the peroneus longus tendon. The latter may occur due to forced supination or dorsiflexion of the foot with eccentric contraction [60].

Chronic injuries leading to POPS include stenosing tenosynovitis of the peroneus longus tendon secondary to a healing fracture of the OP with callus or chronic diastasis of an OP fracture. Attritional thinning of the tendon and an enlarged lateral peroneal tubercle causing entrapment of the tendon and OP may also lead to chronic POPS [60].

- Clinical

In POPS, patients present with lateral foot pain, between the lateral malleolus and cuboid. Pain is reproduced on resisted plantar flexion of the foot and heel rise and the sensation of "stepping on a pebble" [60].

- Imaging

Plain Radiographs

On plain radiography, differentiation between a fractured os peroneum and a multipartite OP can be made; in the acute setting, the fracture margins are relatively non-sclerotic and the fracture fragments fit like "pieces of a puzzle" [61]. On the contrary a smooth, rounded sclerotic margin makes the lesion more likely to be a multipartite OP (Fig. 3.56) [61].

Additional radiographic signs which may help differentiation are [61]

1. OP fragments of 6 mm or more suggest os peroneus fracture and an associated full-thickness peroneus longus tendon tear.
2. However, separation of 2 mm or less may be seen in nondisplaced OP fractures and bipartite OP. MR imaging/CT may be useful if there is still clinical doubt.

MR Imaging

On MR imaging, the OP may demonstrate normal marrow signal or low cartilaginous signal. This should not be confused with an intrasubstance tear of the peroneus longus. MR imaging appearances of an acute fracture include bone marrow oedema within the fracture fragments.

Tibialis Posterior Tendon Pathology

The posterior tibialis muscle originates from the interosseous membrane, and the proximal tibia and fibula. The tibialis posterior tendon (TPT) forms within the distal one-third of the lower limb close to the posteriormedial tibia. Just above the ankle joint, TPT lies within the retrotibial groove, posterior to the medial malleolus. The flexor retinaculum holds TPT within the retrotibial groove. At this site, TPT should be twice the size of its more lateral flexor digitorum longus (FDL) counterpart. Further inferiorly, medial to the talar head, TPT lies superficial to the deltoid and the superomedial calcaneonavicular (spring) ligaments.

TPT then inserts into:

1. The navicular tuberosity or into an accessory navicular bone (seen in 4% of the population [62])
2. Extensive plantar insertions include small slips to the cuneiforms, cuboid and bases of the second to fourth metatarsals

The tibialis posterior tendon serves to plantarflex and inverts the foot. It is the main supporting structure for the medial longitudinal arch. A rupture of the tendon results in pes planus or flatfoot.

Whilst the posterior tibialis tendon is the second most common injured tendon after the Achilles tendon, this injury is uncommon in amongst the younger athletic population [63]. Acute PTT rupture has been described in runners, tennis players and basketball players. When it occurs, it usually occurs at its insertion to the navicular bone [64].

- Clinical

This condition usually affects overweight individuals who already have a flat foot. It rarely affects the athlete but when it occurs there is difficulty in running and performing any sports requiring a powerful push-off action [65]. Initially there is pain and swelling but with time the foot becomes flatter and eventually but uncommonly the tendon actually ruptures. The treatment of acute PTT rupture in the athlete is early surgical intervention (Fig. 3.57). Long-term effects of PTT rupture include degenerative mid-foot arthritis requiring triple arthrodesis for pain relief and stabilisation.

- Biomechanics of injury

Acute tenosynovitis of the PTT may be seen in young athletes secondary to tendon overuse injuries [19]. This is the first stage of PTT dysfunction.

Tendinopathy most commonly occurs in the midportion of the tendon, at the level of and just distal to the medial malleolus. This area is commonly affected as it is a relative zone of tendon hypovascularity and subjected to friction.

When tibialis posterior dysfunction/rupture occurs in athletes, the effects can be debilitating due to loss of function: in PTT partial or complete rupture, there is increased stress placed on static hindfoot constraints, such as the superomedial calcaneonavicular (spring) ligaments and interosseous ligaments. Additionally, there will be progressive collapse of the medial longitudinal arch, resulting in pes planus.

- Imaging

MR Imaging

Pathology involving the PTT includes tenosynovitis, tendinopathy, tendon dislocation and tears (Fig. 3.58). Collectively, these pathologies are named *posterior tibial tendon dysfunction*.

Acute tenosynovitis is demonstrated by presence of a high signal effusion measuring >2 mm but with normal tendon morphology. The PTT is of normal size and of normal dark signal.

In chronic tenosynovitis, there is nodular or diffuse thickening of the tendon with scarring of the paratenon [19].

Tendinopathy manifests as mild to severe heterogeneous increase in signal and tendon thickening on T2/STIR-weighted sequences [19] associated with the development of a fusiform shape [66]. Acute partial or complete rupture of the posterior tibial tendon is usually seen at the insertion of the tendon on the navicular bone [19]. Partial tears are identified as increased tendon thickness with linear and/or heterogeneous increased signal on all sequences [66]. When a complete tear occurs, the tendon gap is fluid filled [66].

A simple classification of PTT tendinopathy/tears have been described by Rosenberg [67] and these have been correlated with treatment options in the Table 3.5.

Three pitfalls in the MR interpretation of the TPT include:

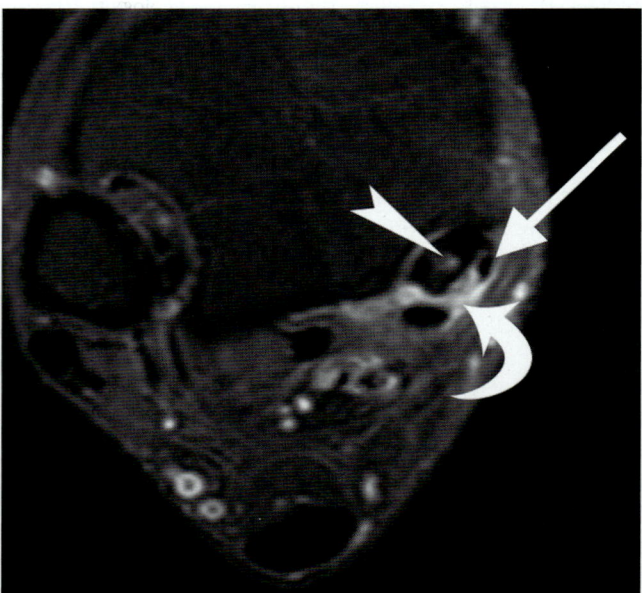

Fig. 3.58 Axial T1w FS MR image of the ankle from patient illustrated in Fig. 3.57. There is intra-tendinous enhancement within tibialis posterior (*arrowhead*) consistent with tendonitis. The separated limb from the longitudinal split is also visualised (*arrow*) and there is marked inflammation in the tenosynovium (*curved arrow*)

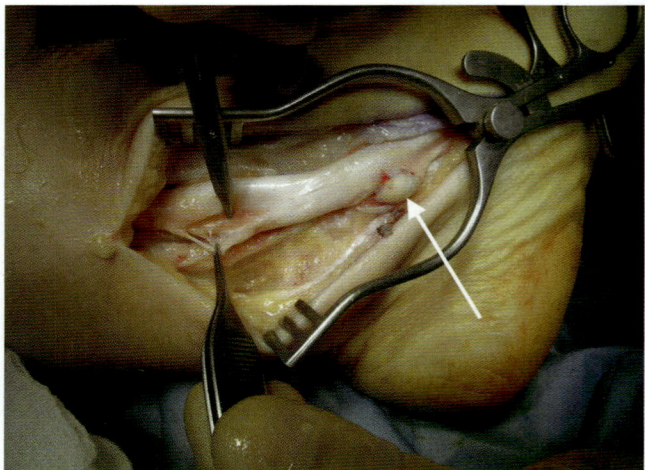

Fig. 3.57 Peroperative photograph of a patient with a longitudinal split in the tibialis posterior tendon. Note the presence of an accessory navicula at the insertion (*arrow*)

1. The tendon is typically low signal on all MR pulses. However, when imaged using short echo time sequences (<37 ms), it may exhibit increased signal due to the *magic angle effect*, especially if the foot is imaged at 90° to the lower leg.
2. There is enlargement and heterogeneity of the tendon as its inserts into the navicular tuberosity on T1 imaging due to a combination of:
    (a) Interposition of connective tissue
    (b) Partial volume averaging of the adjacent spring ligament and the tibionavicular and tibio-talar components of the deltoid ligament.
3. A small amount of fluid can normally be seen within the tendon sheath, this should be no more than 2 mm and should not be circumferential [68]. The tendon sheath ends at the mid-talar level. Fluid around the distal 1–2 cm should be considered abnormal as there is no tendon sheath at this level [68]. The criteria of the normal posterior tibialis tendon is summarised in Table 3.6.

Ultrasound

US can be used to evaluate pathology in the TPT including tenosynovitis, tendinopathy and tears with signs described already for the similar pathology in the peroneal tendons.

Table 3.5 Correlation between MR imaging morphology and surgical treatment in TPT dysfunction

Type	MRI description of tendon tear	Type of treatment
I	Hypertrophy with thickening of tendon	Conservative
II	Atrophy with attenuation of tendon	Surgery
III	Complete tear	Surgery

However, it is worth noting that TPT dysfunction can be present clinically despite normal US findings.

Painful Os Naviculare Syndrome (PONS)

The accessory navicular is located adjacent to the posteromedial margin of the navicular bone. Three types of accessory navicular bones exist.

The type 1 variant is not typically associated with pain. It is a small sesamoid bone located within the distal aspect of the posterior tibial tendon.

The type 2 variant is an accessory centre of ossification.

The type 3 variant is an enlarged medial horn of the navicular, also known as cornuate navicular.

Both type 2 and 3 variants are accessory navicular bones associated with pain [60].

- Clinical

Medial foot pain is the presenting symptom. The type 2 variant is more frequently seen in females in their 20s and is usually bilateral.

- Biomechanics of injury

The type 2 accessory bones may become symptomatic secondary to stress across the syndrondrosis or on the accessory bone, causing osteonecrosis.

The type 3 variant rarely becomes symptomatic when overlying soft tissue is irritated.

- Imaging

The symptomatic accessory navicular appears unremarkable on plain radiographs (Fig. 3.59). MR imaging demonstrates bone marrow oedema within the accessory bone and occasionally within the adjacent navicular (Fig. 3.60) [60].

Table 3.6 The normal posterior tibialis tendon

What is the *normal* posterior tibialis tendon?		
Parameter	Normal criteria for PTT	Knowledge application in interpretation
Size	2 × size of adjacent flexor digitorum longus (FDL)	If PTT is 5–10× larger than FDL, appearances are in keeping with a type I tear
	PTT should be slightly smaller than the anterior tibialis tendon	
	PTT should be slightly smaller than summated measurements of peroneus brevis and longus	If < 2 × size of adjacent FDL, suspect atrophy or type II tear of PTT
Location	Appears adjacent to FDL at the level of retromalleolar groove	If only one tendon present at retromalleolar groove, PTT may have ruptured. The intact FDL may shift forward in the retromalleolar groove mimicking an intact PTT
Tendon signal	Normally low signal	Intrasubstance high signal signifies an interstitial tear
Distal 2 cm of PTT	No fluid is seen surrounding the distal 2 cm of PTT as there is no tendon sheath at this site	Presence of high T2 signal fluid is abnormal and signifies metaplastic synovium

Anterior Tibialis Tendon Pathology

Three tendons are within the anterior ankle compartment. From medial to lateral, these are the anterior tibialis, extensor hallucis longus and extensor digitorum longus tendons.

The main function of these tendons is to dorsiflex the ankle. The anterior tendons are rarely affected in ankle pathology in athletes.

Anterior Tibialis Tendon Pathology

The anterior tibialis tendon (ATT) is the strongest dorsiflexor of the foot. It is the medial-most tendon and is stabilised and retained at the ankle by two retinaculae, namely the superior extensor retinaculum and inferior extensor retinaculum. The ATT inserts into the anteromedial aspect of the medial cuneiform and inferomedial aspect of the base of the first metatarsal. The presence of a short longitudinal split proximal to its insertion is normal.

Tendon tears are rare due to its relatively straight course and the lack of significant mechanical stress but can be caused by direct trauma. The most common pathology is tenosynovitis seen in athletes who actively run downhill and in footballers (Fig. 3.61).

- Imaging

MR/US Imaging

The tendons exhibits low signal on all MR pulse sequences and has fibrillar echogenicity on US. The ATT is oval at the level of the ankle and assumes a flat appearance more distally [66]. Tenosynovitis produces fluid in the tendon sheath, tendon sheath thickening, and inflammation following IV gadolinium on MR imaging, or increased vascularity on colour Doppler imaging (Fig. 3.62).

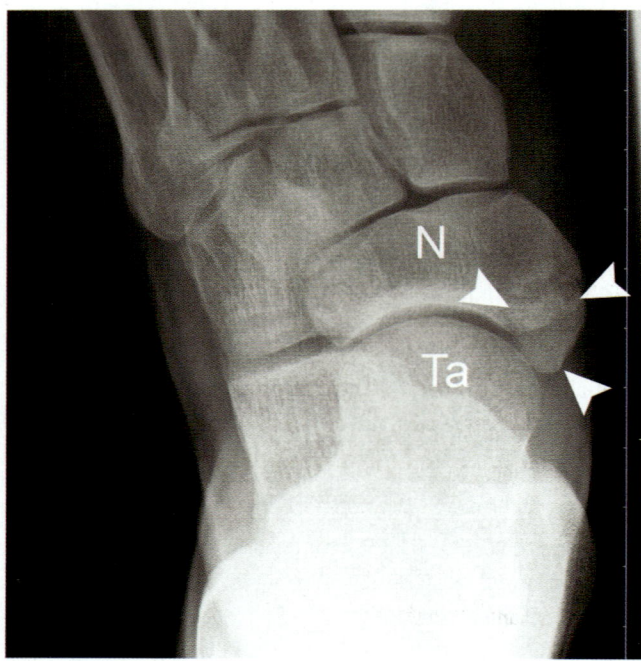

Fig. 3.59 DP X-ray of the foot. There is a large accessory navicular (os tibiale externum) (*arrowheads*) adjacent to the navicula (N) and head of the talus (Ta)

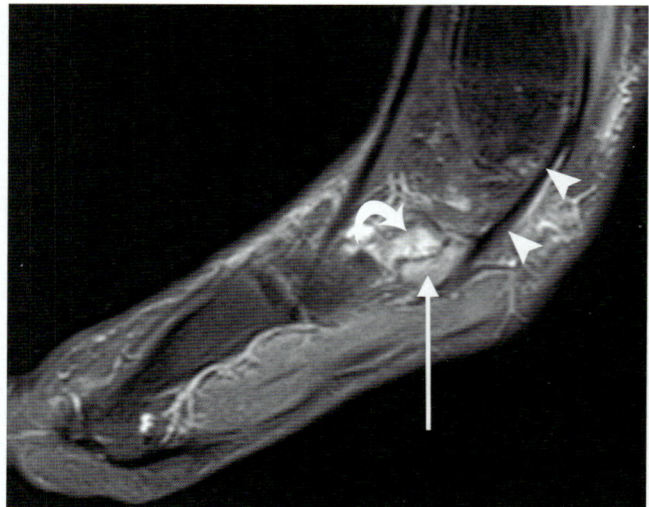

Fig. 3.60 Sagittal T1w FS MR image following IV gadolinium. There is marked inflammation at the synchondrosis (*arrow*) between the accessory and main navicula (*curved arrow*). The tibialis posterior tendon (*arrowheads*) is intimately related to the accessory navicula

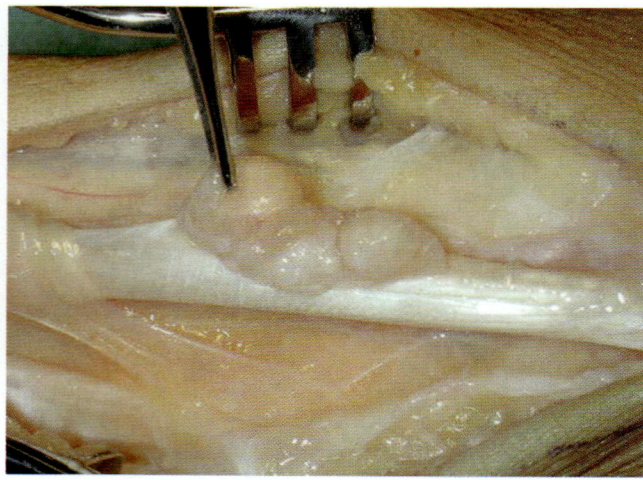

Fig. 3.61 Operative photograph demonstrating florid thickening of the tibialis anterior tenosynovium (held by the surgeon's forceps)

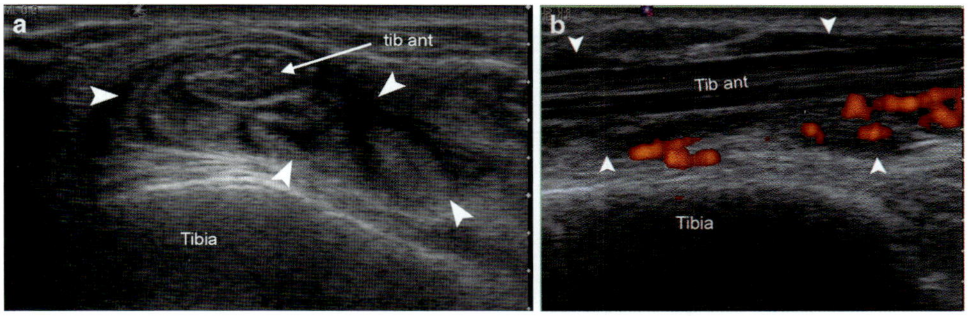

Fig. 3.62 Sonography of the tibialis anterior tendon in an amateur skier. The axial image (**a**) demonstrates marked thickening of the tibialis anterior (TA) tenosynovium (*arrowheads*). (**b**) The longitudinal power Doppler sonogram illustrates avid blood flow within the thickened tenosynovium

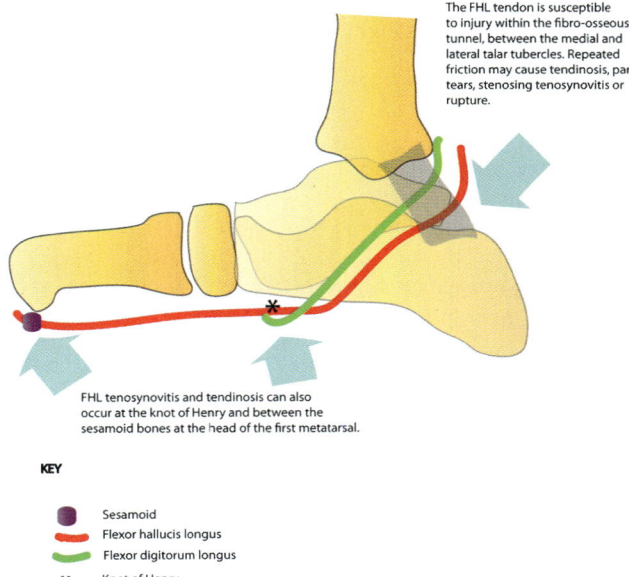

Fig. 3.63 Schematic drawing to show sites of flexor hallucis longus tendon pathology

Flexor Hallucis Longus Tendon

The FHL tendon begins just above the medial malleolus. More distally, it lies between the medial and lateral talar tubercles, within a synovial sheath lined fibro-osseous tunnel, deep to the flexor retinaculum. At the sustentaculum tali it crosses the flexor digitorum longus at the Knot of Henry, then inserts into plantar aspect of the base of the distal phalanx of the great toe via the inter-sesamoid groove (Fig. 3.63).

FHL Tenosynovitis

FHL tenosynovitis is not uncommon; typically seen in athletes and ballet dancers [55].

Table 3.7 Is fluid within the FHL tendon sheath abnormal?

If there is a large ankle effusion, fluid within the FHL tendon sheath is normal. It signifies communication between the tendon sheath and the joint
If there is only a little fluid in the ankle joint and synovial fluid surrounding an intact tendon, this appearance is characteristic of *chronic tenosynovitis* of the FHL

- Clinical

Patients present with pain in the posteromedial with signs of posterior impingement.

- Biomechanics of injury

Due to repeated forceful push-off from their forefoot [55].

- Imaging

US and MR Imaging

Tenosynovitis commonly occurs within the fibro-osseous tunnel, between the medial and lateral talar tubercles (Fig. 3.63). It can also occur at the knot of Henry [55].

US and MR imaging demonstrate large amounts of fluid within the tendon sheath in the absence of an ankle joint effusion (Table 3.7) [55]. The FHL sheath communicates with the ankle joint in 20% of individuals; hence fluid within the FHL tendon sheath common with large ankle joint effusions [19]. Left undiagnosed and untreated, FHL tenosynovitis may progress to stenosing tenosynovitis. The FHL tendon sheath appears thickened with decreased signal on T1 and T2 imaging with associated fluid within the tendon sheath [55]. This occurs at the trigonal groove and is common in ballet dancers as consequence of grand-plie, and in javelin-throwers due to hyper dorsiflexion of the lead foot (Fig. 3.64).

MR/US imaging demonstrates thickening of the synovium, abrupt change in the volume of synovial fluid at the level of the origin to the trigonal groove, and oedema in the

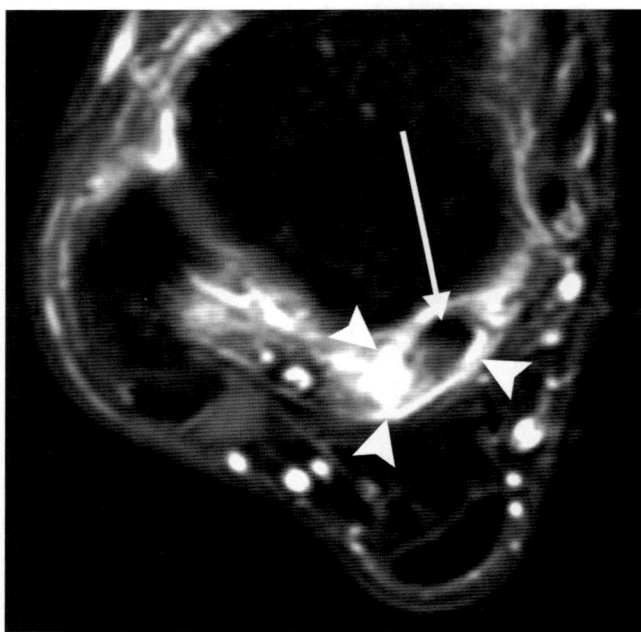

Fig. 3.64 Axial T1w FS MR image following IV gadolinium. There is avid enhancement of the FHL tendon sheath (*arrowheads*) around an intermediate signal inflamed FHL tendon

distal flexor hallucis muscle belly, which may become impinged within the trigonal groove. This can be demonstrated dynamically on US during provocative movements.

Plantar Fascial Pathology

The plantar fascia is a multilayered fibrous aponeurosis, which originates along the plantar aspect of the calcaneus. It has central, medial and lateral components which support the longitudinal arch of the foot. Typically, the term plantar fascia refers to the large central component, which originates from the medial calcaneal tuberosity and extends anteriorly, fanning out and splitting into five bands at the mid-metatarsal level. Each band in turn, attaches onto the base of the proximal phalanges of each toe. The structure deep to the large central band is the flexor digitorum brevis.

The medial and lateral components merely act as fascia overlying the intrinsic muscles, namely the abductor hallucis and abductor digiti minimi.

In the normal population, the plantar fascia has uniform thickness from the calcaneal tuberosity to its midpoint. Thereafter, it thins out to insert into the phalanges. This can be assessed on MR or US imaging. The normal fascia is 2–4 mm thick and is uniformly low signal on all MR pulse sequences [69–71] and has an echogenic fibrillar pattern on US.

Plantar Fasciitis

Plantar fasciitis is a low-grade inflammation of the plantar fascia and peri-fascial tissues [72]. It is the most common cause of inferior heel pain and commonly seen in running athletes [72].

- Clinical

The pain typically occurs when weight bearing after a period of rest and improves with ordinary walking. Excessive walking exacerbates the condition. This condition settles spontaneously in 95% of individuals within 18 months of symptom onset.

- Biomechanics of Injury

Plantar fasciitis is thought to be secondary to repetitive microtears.

- Imaging

Plain Radiographs

Plain radiography may reveal presence of a calcaneal spur but this not thought to be a causative factor.

Ultrasound

On ultrasound (Fig. 3.65), the main findings are increased plantar fascial thickness (>4 mm) and hypoechoic echotexture with loss of normal fibrillar pattern [73, 74]

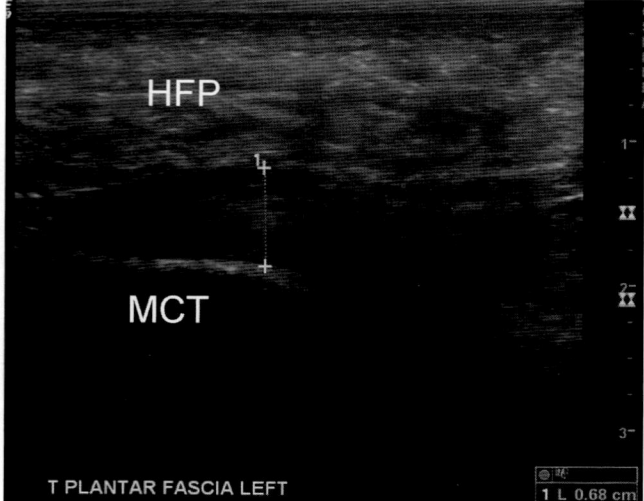

Fig. 3.65 Longitudinal sonogram of the plantar fascia. The fascia is attached to the medial calcaneal tubercle (MCT) and is covered by the heel fat pad (HFP). Note the measurement of the fascia exceeds 4 mm consistent with plantar fasciitis

In acute plantar fasciitis, Doppler imaging may demonstrate hyperaemia within the fascia and surrounding soft tissues [75]. However, frequently the only sonographic finding is thickening of the medial cord of the plantar fascia.

MR Imaging

The main MR findings (Fig. 3.66) are:
1. Fusiform fascial thickening (>4 mm), involving the proximal portion and calcaneal insertion.
2. High signal on T2/STIR imaging.
3. Enhancement within and around the plantar fascia following IV gadolinium.
4. There may be additional peri-fascial oedema within the fat pad and underlying soft tissues, and oedema in the medial calcaneal tuberosity.
5. A calcaneal spur may also be present [69–71].

Plantar Fascial Tear/Rupture

Plantar fascial tears or ruptures are typically sports related and seen in athletes who run and jump, including long-distance runners, basketball, football and tennis players [76]. Plantar fascial ruptures usually affect the proximal portion of the fascia close to its calcaneal insertion [76].

- Clinical

The patient experiences sudden plantar heel pain associated with bruising. It is rare unless a cortisone injection has been administered beforehand.

- Biomechanics of injury

Thought to be secondary to repetitive minor trauma [76]
- Imaging

MR Imaging

In an acute tear, there is partial or complete disruption of the normal low signal intensity fascia which is replaced by areas of increased T2/STIR signal (Fig. 3.67) and enhancement following intravenous contrast. Peri-fascial fluid collections and an underlying tear of the flexor digitorum brevis may also be evident [76]. Acute and subacute muscle tears are seen as high signal intensity changes with a feathery appearance on T2/STIR imaging [76].

It can be difficult to identify a tear within the plantar fascia on US as this is often obscured by haematoma formation which can be misinterpreted as plantar fasciitis.

Great Toe

Turf Toe

Turf toe or disruption of the plantar capsule, is a common pathology seen in athletes who run and rapidly change speed, especially in football players. This injury is common when playing on hard artificial surfaces which do not absorb shock whilst wearing soft flexible shoes which do not limit hyperextension at the metatarsophalangeal (MTP) joint [77]. Older sportsmen and ones with a longer professional sporting history are more likely to be affected [78].

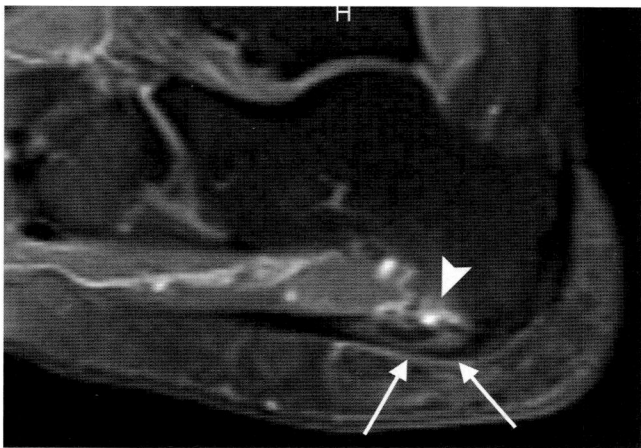

Fig. 3.66 Sagittal T1w FS MR image following IV gadolinium. There is marked inflammation within the medial plantar fascia at the insertion (*arrows*) associated with bone marrow oedema in the medial calcaneal tubercle (*arrowhead*)

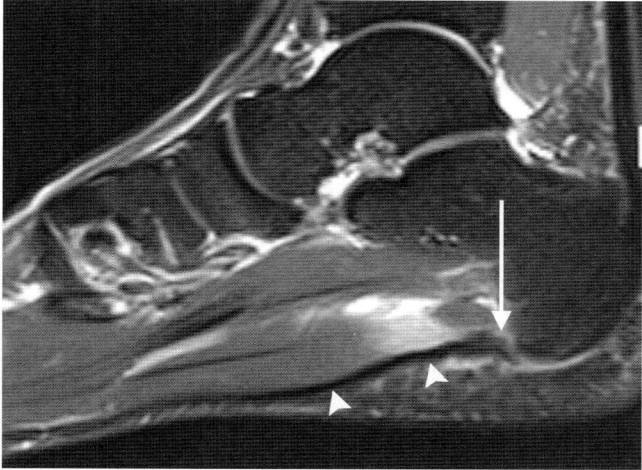

Fig. 3.67 Sagittal T1w FS MR image following IV gadolinium of the hindfoot in a professional footballer. There is a tear of the plantar fascia at the medial calcaneal tubercle (*arrow*) the plantar fascia distal to the tear has lost its normal taut appearance (*arrowheads*)

- Biomechanics of injury

This injury is due to violent hyperextension at the first MTP joint, resulting in partial or complete tear of the fibrocartilaginous plantar plate [77]. This plate extends from the volar aspect of the metatarsal neck to the proximal phalanx of the toe. The plantar plate serves to reinforce the MTP joint capsule.

- Clinical

Patients present with pain swelling and bruising in the region of the big toe following a hyperextension injury to the MTP joint of the great toe. These injuries can be quite debilitating and need to be taken seriously. A rupture of the medial ligament or disruption of the sesamoid complex may require surgery.

- Imaging

Radiographs and CT may be normal.

MR Imaging

The primary finding of turf toe is disruption to the plantar plate (Fig. 3.68). Other findings include:
1. High signal changes on T2 and STIR within the soft tissues plantar to the sesamoid bones [77].
2. Concomitant injury to the articular cartilage and subchondral bone demonstrated by subchondral high signal change on STIR [77].
3. Disruption/laxity of the medial collateral ligament (Fig. 3.69).
4. Disruption of the sesa2moid complex/fracture of the sesamoids.

Hallux Rigidus

The main function of the hallux is to allow dorsiflexion of the first metatarsal during the propulsive phase of the human gait. With normal locomotion, the amount of hallux dorsiflexion during this phase is must approximate 65–75°. This function of the hallux can be limited due to osteoarthritis of the first MTP joint, a common degenerative condition secondary to repetitive loading injury. This results in restricted movement due to pain, and is termed *hallux rigidus*.

- Biomechanics of injury

Repetitive loading.

- Clinical

Patients present with pain at the first MTP joint associated with palpable osteophytes and a reduction in movement. Sometimes, in severe cases, there is virtually no movement at the joint. Surgical treatment usually involves a debridement (Fig. 3.70) (cheilectomy) or fusion. Joint replacement has been tried but is not the treatment of choice for the majority of cases of hallux rigidus.

- Imaging

Both plain radiographs and MR imaging demonstrated loss of joint space, dorsal and lateral osteophytes, sesamoid proliferation and geodes. MR imaging is more sensitive for sesamoid proliferation and osteophytes compared to conventional radiographs [79].

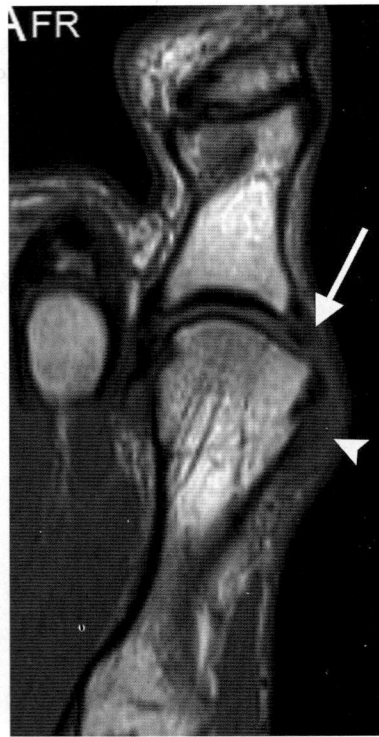

Fig. 3.69 Coronal T1 MR image of the big toe in a rugby union footballer. There is a tear of the medial collateral ligament (*arrow*) of the big toe metatarsophalangeal joint with adjacent haematoma (*arrowhead*)

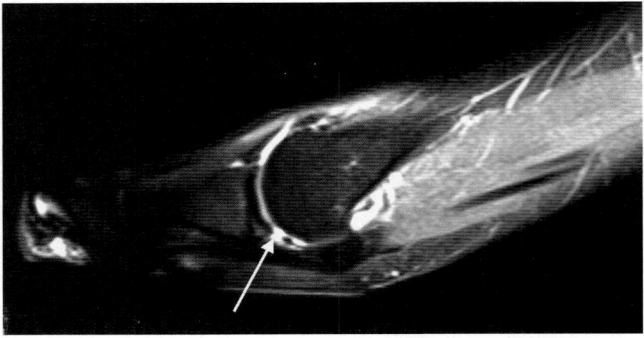

Fig. 3.68 Sagittal STIR MR image of the big toe. There is a tear of the plantar plate (*arrow*) consistent with "turf toe"

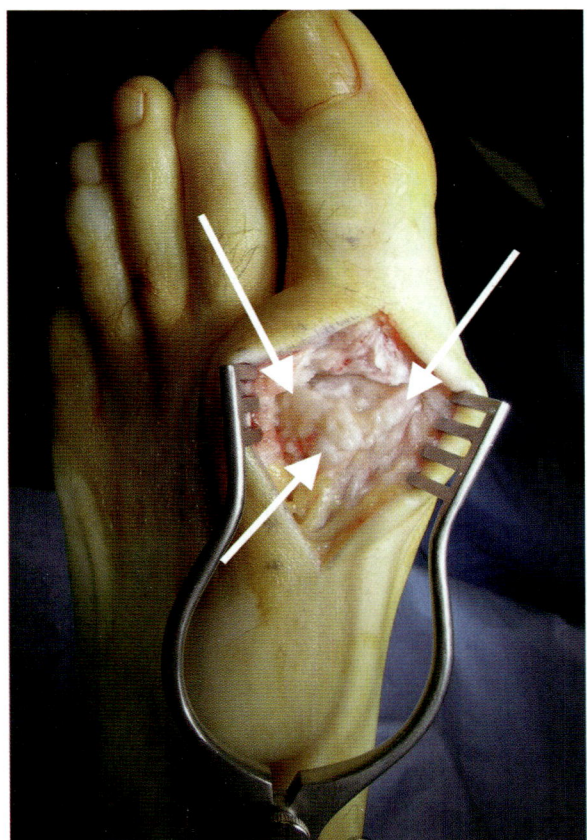

Fig. 3.70 Operative photograph of the big toe metatarsophalangeal joint. There are several large osteophytes on the dorsal surface of the metatarsal head that were soon to be removed by cheilectomy

Conclusion

This chapter highlights the imaging manifestations of important and common ankle and foot pathology in the athlete. Plain films are always useful as a starting point for the evaluation of symptoms and essential when examining trauma. CT is essential when delineating trauma to influence and advise on management.

MR imaging and US both have a place to play in refining our diagnosis of occult foot and ankle pain. The strengths of MR imaging include its wide field of view and with the administration of IV gadolinium the ability to identify mild inflammation which may be enough to produce symptoms and affect performance, especially in the elite athlete.

The strengths of US relate to its superior spatial resolution allowing interrogation of the internal anatomy of soft tissues especially tendons, the ability to evaluate structures dynamically, and finally to administer injections as diagnostic and therapeutic agents.

References

1. Fong DT, Hong Y, Chan LK, Yung PS, Chan KM (2007) A systematic review on ankle injury and ankle sprain in sports. Sports Med 37:73–94
2. Papakonstantinou O, Kelekis AD, Kelekis NL, Kelekis DA (2007) Sports-specific injuries, 1st ed. Springer. Imaging of Orthopaedic Sports Injuries. ed Vanhoenacker F
3. Jensen SL, Andresen BK, Mencke S, Nielsen PT (1998) Epidemiology of ankle fractures. A prospective population-based study of 212 cases in Aalborg, Denmark. Acta Orthop Scand 69:48–50
4. Tornetta P 3rd, Gorup J (1996) Axial computed tomography of pilon fractures. Clin Orthop Relat Res 273–276
5. Ouellette H, Salamipour H, Thomas BJ, Kassarjian A, Torriani M (2006) Incidence and MR imaging features of fractures of the anterior process of calcaneus in a consecutive patient population with ankle and foot symptoms. Skeletal Radiol 35:833–837
6. Kirkpatrick DP, Hunter RE, Janes PC, Mastrangelo J, Nicholas RA (1998) The snowboarder's foot and ankle. Am J Sports Med 26:271–277
7. Mukherjee SK, Pringle RM, Baxter AD (1974) Fracture of the lateral process of the talus. A report of thirteen cases. J Bone Joint Surg Br 56:263–273
8. Bennell KL, Brukner PD (1997) Epidemiology and site specificity of stress fractures. Clin Sports Med 16:179–196
9. Niva MH, Sormaala MJ, Kiuru MJ, Haataja R, Ahovuo JA, Pihlajamaki HK (2007) Bone stress injuries of the ankle and foot: an 86-month magnetic resonance imaging-based study of physically active young adults. Am J Sports Med 35:643–649
10. Barrow GW, Saha S (1988) Menstrual irregularity and stress fractures in collegiate female distance runners. Am J Sports Med 16:209–216
11. Bennell KL, Malcolm SA, Brukner PD et al (1998) A 12-month prospective study of the relationship between stress fractures and bone turnover in athletes. Calcif Tissue Int 63:80–85
12. Ishibashi Y, Okamura Y, Otsuka H, Nishizawa K, Sasaki T, Toh S (2002) Comparison of scintigraphy and magnetic resonance imaging for stress injuries of bone. Clin J Sport Med 12:79–84
13. Anderson MW, Greenspan A (1996) Stress fractures. Radiology 199:1–12
14. Weinfeld SB, Haddad SL, Myerson MS (1997) Metatarsal stress fractures. Clin Sports Med 16:319–338
15. Boden BP, Osbahr DC (2000) High-risk stress fractures: evaluation and treatment. J Am Acad Orthop Surg 8:344–353
16. Chuckpaiwong B, Queen RM, Easley ME, Nunley JA (2008) Distinguishing Jones and proximal diaphyseal fractures of the fifth metatarsal. Clin Orthop Relat Res 466:1966–1970
17. Burton EM, Amaker BH (1994) Stress fracture of the great toe sesamoid in a ballerina: MRI appearance. Pediatr Radiol 24:37–38
18. Biedert R, Hintermann B (2003) Stress fractures of the medial great toe sesamoids in athletes. Foot Ankle Int 24:137–141
19. Rosenberg ZS, Beltran J, Bencardino JT (2000) From the RSNA Refresher Courses. Radiological Society of North America. MR imaging of the ankle and foot. Radiographics 20 Spec No:S153–S179
20. Flick AB, Gould N (1985) Osteochondritis dissecans of the talus (transchondral fractures of the talus): review of the literature and new surgical approach for medial dome lesions. Foot Ankle 5:165–185
21. Elias I, Jung JW, Raikin SM, Schweitzer MW, Carrino JA, Morrison WB (2006) Osteochondral lesions of the talus: change in MRI findings over time in talar lesions without operative intervention and implications for staging systems. Foot Ankle Int 27:157–166
22. Kijowski R, Blankenbaker DG, Shinki K, Fine JP, Graf BK, De Smet AA (2008) Juvenile versus adult osteochondritis dissecans of the knee: appropriate MR imaging criteria for instability. Radiology 248:571–578

23. Bohndorf K (1999) Imaging of acute injuries of the articular surfaces (chondral, osteochondral and subchondral fractures). Skeletal Radiol 28:545–560
24. Schmid MR, Pfirrmann CW, Hodler J, Vienne P, Zanetti M (2003) Cartilage lesions in the ankle joint: comparison of MR arthrography and CT arthrography. Skeletal Radiol 32:259–265
25. Schneck CD, Mesgarzadeh M, Bonakdarpour A (1992) MR imaging of the most commonly injured ankle ligaments. Part II. Ligament injuries. Radiology 184:507–512
26. Martinoli C, Bianchi S (2007) Ankle. In: Ultrasound of the musculoskeletal system. Springer, Berlin, pp 773–834
27. Meyer SA, Callaghan JJ, Albright JP, Crowley ET, Powell JW (1994) Midfoot sprains in collegiate football players. Am J Sports Med 22:392–401
28. Nunley JA, Vertullo CJ (2002) Classification, investigation, and management of midfoot sprains: Lisfranc injuries in the athlete. Am J Sports Med 30:871–878
29. Goiney RC, Connell DG, Nichols DM (1985) CT evaluation of tarsometatarsal fracture-dislocation injuries. AJR Am J Roentgenol 144:985–990
30. Williams GN, Jones MH, Amendola A (2007) Syndesmotic ankle sprains in athletes. Am J Sports Med 35:1197–1207
31. Dattani R, Patnaik S, Kantak A, Srikanth B, Selvan TP (2008) Injuries to the tibiofibular syndesmosis. J Bone Joint Surg Br 90:405–410
32. Beumer A, van Hemert WL, Niesing R et al (2004) Radiographic measurement of the distal tibiofibular syndesmosis has limited use. Clin Orthop Relat Res 227–234
33. Oae K, Takao M, Naito K et al (2003) Injury of the tibiofibular syndesmosis: value of MR imaging for diagnosis. Radiology 227:155–161
34. Robinson P, White LM (2002) Soft-tissue and osseous impingement syndromes of the ankle: role of imaging in diagnosis and management. Radiographics 22:1457–1469, discussion 70–71
35. Robinson P, White LM, Salonen DC, Daniels TR, Ogilvie-Harris D (2001) Anterolateral ankle impingement: mr arthrographic assessment of the anterolateral recess. Radiology 221:186–190
36. Rubin DA, Tishkoff NW, Britton CA, Conti SF, Towers JD (1997) Anterolateral soft-tissue impingement in the ankle: diagnosis using MR imaging. AJR Am J Roentgenol 169:829–835
37. McMurray T (1950) Footballer's Ankle. J Bone Joint Surg 32:68–69
38. Tol JL, van Dijk CN (2004) Etiology of the anterior ankle impingement syndrome: a descriptive anatomical study. Foot Ankle Int 25:382–386
39. Cerezal L, Abascal F, Canga A et al (2003) MR imaging of ankle impingement syndromes. AJR Am J Roentgenol 181:551–559
40. Robinson P, White LM, Salonen D, Ogilvie-Harris D (2002) Anteromedial impingement of the ankle: using MR arthrography to assess the anteromedial recess. AJR Am J Roentgenol 178:601–604
41. Bureau NJ, Cardinal E, Hobden R, Aubin B (2000) Posterior ankle impingement syndrome: MR imaging findings in seven patients. Radiology 215:497–503
42. Robinson P, Bollen SR (2006) Posterior ankle impingement in professional soccer players: effectiveness of sonographically guided therapy. AJR Am J Roentgenol 187:W53–W58
43. Peace KA, Hillier JC, Hulme A, Healy JC (2004) MRI features of posterior ankle impingement syndrome in ballet dancers: a review of 25 cases. Clin Radiol 59:1025–1033
44. Lee JC, Calder JD, Healy JC (2008) Posterior impingement syndromes of the ankle. Semin Musculoskelet Radiol 12:154–169
45. Koulouris G, Connell D, Schneider T, Edwards W (2003) Posterior tibiotalar ligament injury resulting in posteromedial impingement. Foot Ankle Int 24:575–583
46. Messiou C, Robinson P, O'Connor PJ, Grainger A (2006) Subacute posteromedial impingement of the ankle in athletes: MR imaging evaluation and ultrasound guided therapy. Skeletal Radiol 35:88–94
47. Riley G (2008) Tendinopathy – from basic science to treatment. Nat Clin Pract Rheumatol 4:82–89
48. Khan KM, Cook JL, Bonar F, Harcourt P, Astrom M (1999) Histopathology of common tendinopathies. Update and implications for clinical management. Sports Med 27:393–408
49. Alfredson H (2003) Chronic midportion Achilles tendinopathy: an update on research and treatment. Clin Sports Med 22:727–741
50. Richards PJ, Win T, Jones PW (2005) The distribution of microvascular response in Achilles tendinopathy assessed by colour and power Doppler. Skeletal Radiol 34:336–342
51. Zanetti M, Metzdorf A, Kundert HP et al (2003) Achilles tendons: clinical relevance of neovascularization diagnosed with power Doppler US. Radiology 227:556–560
52. Ohberg L, Alfredson H (2002) Ultrasound guided sclerosis of neovessels in painful chronic Achilles tendinosis: pilot study of a new treatment. Br J Sports Med 36:173–175, discussion 6–7
53. Karjalainen PT, Soila K, Aronen HJ et al (2000) MR imaging of overuse injuries of the Achilles tendon. AJR Am J Roentgenol 175:251–260
54. Hartgerink P, Fessell DP, Jacobson JA, van Holsbeeck MT (2001) Full- versus partial-thickness Achilles tendon tears: sonographic accuracy and characterization in 26 cases with surgical correlation. Radiology 220:406–412
55. Tuite MJ (2002) MR imaging of the tendons of the foot and ankle. Semin Musculoskelet Radiol 6:119–131
56. Rosenberg ZS, Beltran J, Cheung YY, Colon E, Herraiz F (1997) MR features of longitudinal tears of the peroneus brevis tendon. AJR Am J Roentgenol 168:141–147
57. Tjin ATER, Schweitzer ME, Karasick D (1997) MR imaging of peroneal tendon disorders. AJR Am J Roentgenol 168:135–140
58. Wang XT, Rosenberg ZS, Mechlin MB, Schweitzer ME (2005) Normal variants and diseases of the peroneal tendons and superior peroneal retinaculum: MR imaging features. Radiographics 25:587–602
59. Magnano GM, Occhi M, Di Stadio M, Toma P, Derchi LE (1998) High-resolution US of non-traumatic recurrent dislocation of the peroneal tendons: a case report. Pediatr Radiol 28:476–477
60. Miller TT (2002) Painful accessory bones of the foot. Semin Musculoskelet Radiol 6:153–161
61. Brigido MK, Fessell DP, Jacobson JA et al (2005) Radiography and US of os peroneum fractures and associated peroneal tendon injuries: initial experience. Radiology 237:235–241
62. Lim PS, Schweitzer ME, Deely DM et al (1997) Posterior tibial tendon dysfunction: secondary MR signs. Foot Ankle Int 18:658–663
63. Lysholm J, Wiklander J (1987) Injuries in runners. Am J Sports Med 15:168–171
64. Conti SF (1994) Posterior tibial tendon problems in athletes. Orthop Clin North Am 25:109–121
65. Woods L, Leach RE (1991) Posterior tibial tendon rupture in athletic people. Am J Sports Med 19:495–498
66. Mengiardi B, Pfirrmann CW, Zanetti M (2005) MR imaging of tendons and ligaments of the midfoot. Semin Musculoskelet Radiol 9:187–198
67. Rosenberg ZS, Cheung Y, Jahss MH, Noto AM, Norman A, Leeds NE (1988) Rupture of posterior tibial tendon: CT and MR imaging with surgical correlation. Radiology 169:229–235
68. Nazarian LN, Rawool NM, Martin CE, Schweitzer ME (1995) Synovial fluid in the hindfoot and ankle: detection of amount and distribution with US. Radiology 197:275–278
69. Berkowitz JF, Kier R, Rudicel S (1991) Plantar fasciitis: MR imaging. Radiology 179:665–667
70. Kier R (1994) Magnetic resonance imaging of plantar fasciitis and other causes of heel pain. Magn Reson Imaging Clin N Am 2:97–107

71. Roger B, Grenier P (1997) MRI of plantar fasciitis. Eur Radiol 7:1430–1435
72. Kwong PK, Kay D, Voner RT, White MW (1988) Plantar fasciitis. Mechanics and pathomechanics of treatment. Clin Sports Med 7:119–126
73. Cardinal E, Chhem RK, Beauregard CG, Aubin B, Pelletier M (1996) Plantar fasciitis: sonographic evaluation. Radiology 201:257–259
74. Gibbon WW, Long G (1999) Ultrasound of the plantar aponeurosis (fascia). Skeletal Radiol 28:21–26
75. Walther M, Radke S, Kirschner S, Ettl V, Gohlke F (2004) Power Doppler findings in plantar fasciitis. Ultrasound Med Biol 30:435–440
76. Narvaez JA, Narvaez J, Ortega R, Aguilera C, Sanchez A, Andia E (2000) Painful heel: MR imaging findings. Radiographics 20:333–352
77. Ashman CJ, Klecker RJ, Yu JS (2001) Forefoot pain involving the metatarsal region: differential diagnosis with MR imaging. Radiographics 21:1425–1440
78. Rodeo SA, O'Brien S, Warren RF, Barnes R, Wickiewicz TL, Dillingham MF (1990) Turf-toe: an analysis of metatarsophalangeal joint sprains in professional football players. Am J Sports Med 18:280–285
79. Schweitzer ME, Maheshwari S, Shabshin N (1999) Hallux valgus and hallux rigidus: MRI findings. Clin Imaging 23:397–402

Chapter 4
Osseous Stress Injury in Athletes

Melanie A. Hopper and Philip Robinson

Introduction

Stress fractures can be classified into two main groups, those occurring due to normal forces placed upon weakened bone are termed insufficiency fractures, and the second group are fatigue fractures where bone failure is due to abnormal stresses placed upon physiologically normal bone. Sports training necessitates high volume, repetitive activity and so it is unsurprising that overuse injuries are common, constituting up to 10% of all injuries [1]. Particularly in athletes, the early diagnosis of stress injury is essential to prevent the development of more serious injury, to facilitate rehabilitation and to enable early return to training and competition. Imaging plays a central role in prompt diagnosis as clinical evaluation alone may not be able to differentiate stress injury from other common causes of musculoskeletal trauma.

Lower extremity injuries are more commonly encountered, particularly in runners and military recruits. Overall the tibia is most affected by stress injury, followed by the bones of the mid and forefoot [2]. Specific osseous stress injuries are associated with different sporting activities and reflect the particular stresses placed upon a bone during training.

Bone Anatomy

Bone is a dynamic, specialised and highly adaptive connective tissue composed of cells and a surrounding extracellular matrix. Approximately 90% of the extracellular matrix is organic, containing the type I collagen fibres that give bone its flexibility. Unlike other connective tissues, bone has a high inorganic content, predominantly crystalline mineral salts and calcium in the form of hydroxyapatite that combines with the organic matrix to give bone its rigidity.

The hard dense outer compact or cortical bone is highly organised and due to the longitudinal orientation of its constituents is adapted to resist compressive stress. The central cancellous bone forms a thin irregular network that resists forces according to the alignment of its fibre matrix. Cortical bone is covered, except at articular surfaces, by periosteum, a vascular, dense connective tissue containing fibroblasts in its outer layer. The inner layer of periosteum, or cambium, holds progenitor cells responsible for new bone formation during growth and repair. Interstices between the cancellous bone mesh are filled with red marrow providing the bone with nutrients via the blood vessels that pass through it.

Bone Biomechanics

The complexities of the mechanical properties of bone are beyond the remit of this text, however, there are several important factors to consider in the understanding of the osseous response to stress.

Bone is a biphasic material, the combination of mineral and collagen matrix is more able to withstand force than each component independently. As increasing load is applied to bone there is a phased response that can be represented by a load deformation curve (Fig. 4.1).

Due to its composition, bone is anisotropic, exhibiting different mechanical properties in response to different types of loading. Bone experiences complex stresses during activity and most acute and fatigue fractures occur in response to a combination of loading patterns. Compact (cortical) bone is better able to withstand compressive loading than other stresses due to the orientation of its constituents.

Aetiology of Fatigue Fractures

Acute fractures and apophyseal avulsions occur due to a single direct insult and are frequently seen in the athletic population, these are not detailed in this chapter as they

Philip Robinson (✉)
Department of Radiology, Leeds Teaching Hospitals,
Leeds LS7 4SA, UK
e-mail: p.robinson@leedsth.nhs.uk

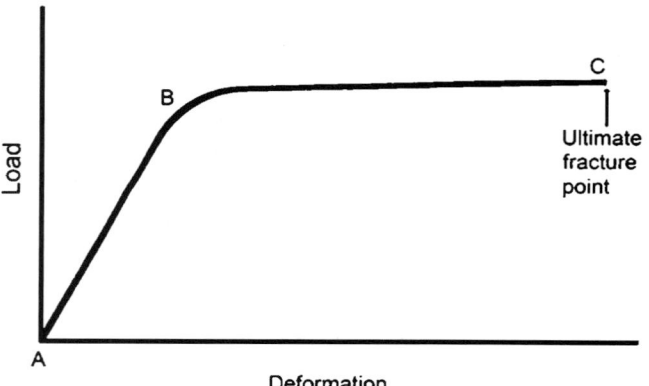

Fig. 4.1 Load deformation curve. Load applied within the elastic range (A–B) causes no persisting deformation. Beyond the yield point (B) loading within the plastic range (B–C) causes permanent deformity, further increases in load cause bone to fracture at its failure point (C)

Table 4.1 Common sites for acute traumatic (non-stress) fractures

Upper limb	Clavicle
	Scaphoid
	Metacarpals and phalanges
Lower limb	Tibia and medial malleolus
	Fibula and lateral malleolus
	Fifth Metatarsal

Table 4.2 Risk factors for stress injury

Intrinsic	Extrinsic
Female gender	Improper equipment
Poor diet	Poor technique
Hormone levels	Rapid changes in training regimen
Low bone mineral density	High impact training
Low muscle:bone ratio	Repetitive activity
Recent injury	Muscle fatigue
Anatomical variants/abnormalities	

rarely represent an imaging problem (Table 4.1). Stress fractures occur due to the cumulative effect of forces to a localised area of bone over time and are dependent upon the load exerted, repetition of loading and the capacity of bone to remodel and repair in response to injury [3].

During activity, muscle acts to decrease the load exerted on bone by dissipating forces and absorbing shock [4]. Contracting muscle allows more uniform distribution of tensile stress, a process known as stress shielding, particularly important in preventing fracture. This redistribution decreases the tensile stress and increases the compressive forces that bone is intrinsically more able to withstand [5]. Fatigued or injured muscles are less able to store energy and provide support, increasing tensile forces and the risk of stress injury.

When introducing a new stress, such as changing a training regimen, muscle tone increase occurs more rapidly than bone strength. This mechanical imbalance causes excessive loads to be experienced by bone and is thought to contribute towards fatigue fracture development [4–6].

Bone requires stress for normal development; changes in environmental forces cause a dynamic response via remodelling and repair enabling bone to function and adapt. This is summarised by Wolff's Law (Wolff 1892) that states that the remodelling of bone is influenced and modulated by mechanical stress. Stress fractures develop when repetitive mechanical loading exceeds the capacity of bone to remodel and compensate.

During the initial phase of remodelling, bone is resorbed by osteoclasts, a process that takes approximately 30 days. This is followed by the generation of new matrix by osteoblasts and finally by replacement of the weak woven bone by stronger fully mineralised osteonal bone. Consequently, there is a vulnerable period during which bone has a reduced capacity to resist stress. In normal physiological remodelling this is not of concern, however, when remodelling is accelerated due to increased stress as in overuse injury, bone is at increased risk of fracture if abnormal loading persists. From the initiation of osteoclast activity to the formation of fully mineralised bone, remodelling occurs over a period of approximately 90 days and ultimately results in bone that is better adapted to resist the forces placed upon it.

Risk Factors

Several intrinsic and extrinsic risk factors for athletic stress injury have been identified (Table 4.2). Training has a major role to play in the prevention of overuse injuries as athletes with better technique are less likely to incur injury. Developing a new technique or rapid increases in training intensity and duration are associated with increased risk of stress fracture [1]. Use of incorrect equipment is also implicated; this ranges from inadequate footwear to the wrong tennis racquet grip. Anatomical considerations such as leg length inequality and concomitant injury are particularly important in lower limb injury and are discussed below.

Stress injuries are more common in female military recruits and athletes. This may not be due to innate gender differences but instead is likely to represent sex-related factors, sometimes termed the "female athletic triad" of amenorrhoea, anorexia and low bone mineral density [4, 7, 8].

Disuse has a profound effect on bone quality with resorption of periosteal and endosteal bone and a subsequent decrease in the ability of bone to withstand mechanical stress. Although this may not be of consideration in the fit athlete, it is important in the return of an athlete to full training following injury and may also in part explain why these athletes are more prone to developing stress injuries.

Table 4.3 Imaging modality advantages and disadvantages for diagnosing stress injury

	Advantages	Disadvantages
Plain radiography	Readily available	Low sensitivity
	Inexpensive, fast	Ionising radiation
Ultrasound	Readily available	Operator dependent
	Inexpensive, fast	Low sensitivity
	No ionising radiation	Useful for superficial bones only
Nuclear medicine	Sensitive	Lengthy examination, ionising radiation
		Non-specific
CT	Readily available, fast	Insensitive
	Allows fracture evaluation	Ionising radiation
MR imaging	Sensitive, specific	Lengthy examination
	No ionising radiation	Contraindicated in some patients

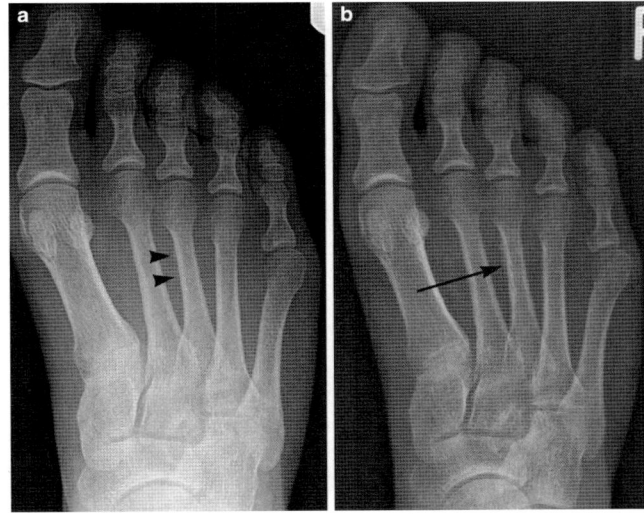

Fig. 4.2 Serial radiographs in runner with forefoot pain, initial image was normal. (**a**) Radiograph at 2 weeks shows subtle periosteal reaction at medial aspect of third metatarsal diaphysis (*arrowheads*). (**b**) Radiograph at 6 weeks shows stress fracture, mature periosteal reaction (*arrow*) but no visible fracture line

Imaging

Osseous stress response has been identified as a continuum ranging from bone oedema to full thickness cortical fracture and this is mirrored by changes in imaging findings. Early diagnosis of stress injuries is essential to allow evaluation of injury extent, to prevent deterioration and to guide training and rehabilitation. The advantages and disadvantages of each imaging modality are summarised in Table 4.3.

Radiography

Although plain radiographs continue to play an important role in preliminary evaluation, stress fractures are initially radiographically occult in up to 85% with up to 50% of follow-up radiographs remaining normal (Fig. 4.2) [1, 9, 10]. Positive findings on radiography have been shown to be strongly associated with higher-grade injury on MR imaging [11, 12].

Long bone diaphyses have a high proportion of cortical bone on cross-section. Radiographs show a range of features such as endosteal cortical thickening and periosteal reaction. Later a linear cortical radiolucency develops representing the fracture line that may be preceded by subcortical infraction. Long bone epiphyses, metaphysis and bones such as the talus have a high proportion of cancellous bone and radiographic findings reflect this. Characteristically, stress fractures in cancellous bone cause condensation of trabeculae represented by focal sclerosis on plain radiography, periosteal reaction is not a prominent finding (Fig. 4.3). In even later stages of healing, callus formation may mimic more aggressive lesions such as infection or tumour and it is therefore important to correlate imaging findings with clinical history to guide further investigation.

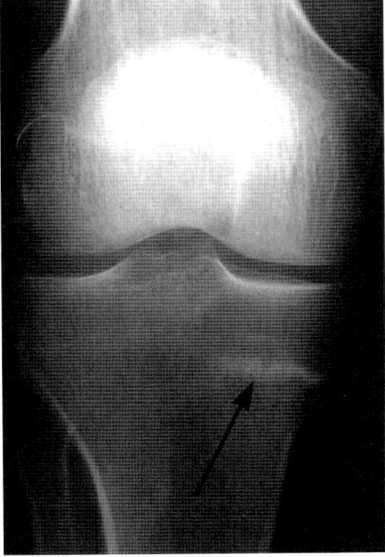

Fig. 4.3 Radiograph in athlete with proximal tibia stress fracture shows sclerotic fracture line (*arrows*) due to predominantly trabecular bone within metaphysis

Ultrasound

Ultrasound has the advantage of being widely available, fast and accessible. Little literature has been published detailing the use of ultrasound in the detection and evaluation of stress injuries; however, abnormalities may be detected in superficial bones such as the metatarsals and anterior tibia. Periosteal reaction may be seen as an area of cortical elevation still

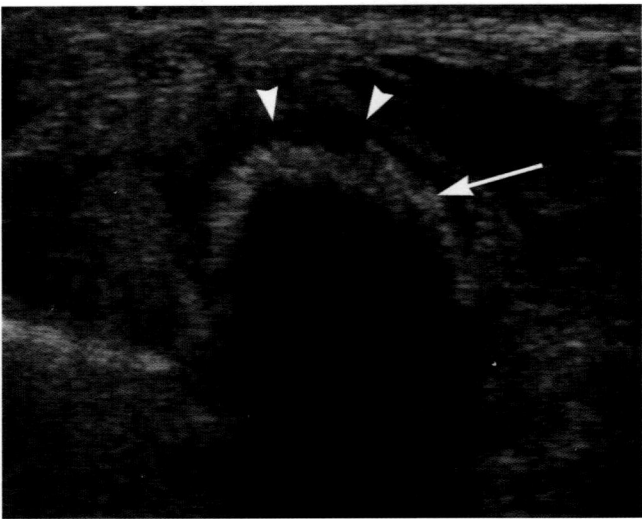

Fig. 4.4 Second metatarsal stress fracture in runner with normal radiographs. Transverse sonogram shows periosteal thickening and irregularity (*arrow*), note rim of hypoechogenicity representing periosteal oedema (*arrowheads*)

occult on radiography (Fig. 4.4). Thickened hypoechoic periosteum can amplify posterior acoustic shadowing due to increased sonographic reflection. Despite this, ultrasound is not the imaging modality of choice because of its low sensitivity in early stress injury.

Bone Scintigraphy

Bone scintigraphy is highly sensitive for osseous injury although false-negative imaging has been reported [13, 14]. Bone scintigraphy detects increased osteoblastic activity and can be used to evaluate the entire range of stress response (Fig. 4.5). Triple phase bone scintigraphy (TPBS) is advocated with angiographic, blood pool and delayed skeletal imaging to allow differentiation between bone and soft tissue injury. Previously TPBS represented the gold standard for evaluation of stress injury however, several studies have shown MR imaging to have similar sensitivity but increased

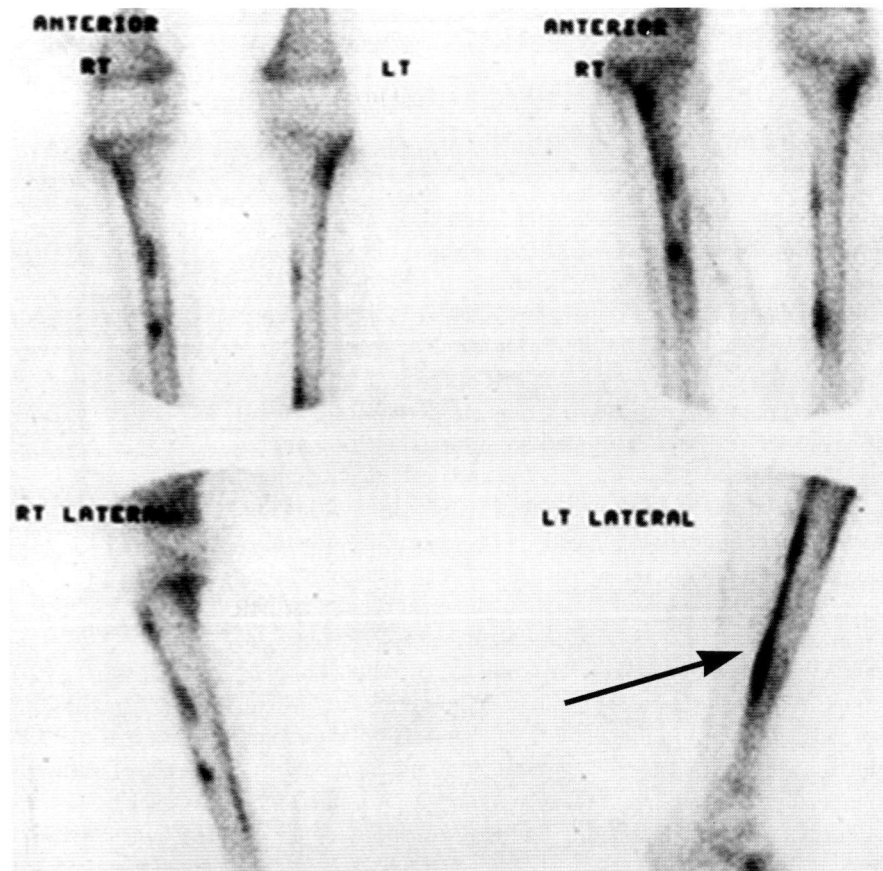

Fig. 4.5 Bone scintigraphy in athlete with left lower leg pain. Longitudinal increased uptake within left posterior tibia (*arrow*) corresponding to medial tibial stress syndrome

specificity with the additional benefit of not involving ionising radiation.

Abnormal increase in radiotracer uptake can be seen between 6 and 72 h following the onset of symptoms [15]. With time and worsening severity of symptoms, uptake becomes more intense and focal. Soft tissue injury causes increased uptake only in the angiographic and blood pool phase whereas acute stress fractures demonstrate increased radionuclide uptake in all three phases of the scan.

While being highly sensitive, TBPS is non-specific with abnormal increase in radiotracer uptake seen in degeneration, tumour and infection making clinical correlation essential. TPBS has also been reported to show non-symptomatic stress injuries [16] while abnormalities can persist for many months after the resolution of symptoms limiting its role in follow-up [4].

Computed Tomography

Although not as sensitive as MR imaging or bone scintigraphy, computed tomography (CT) is of particular use when cortical detail is required and is particularly sensitive in the detection of osteopaenia, one of the first features of impending stress fracture. Later appearances of resorption cavities, cortical striations and the presence of a fracture line can aid in differentiating stress response from alternative pathology (e.g. osteoid osteoma) when other imaging modalities are equivocal [4].

Multiplanar reconstruction allows easier diagnosis of fractures in the axial plane (Fig. 4.6). CT is specifically of use in certain areas such as the hook of hamate, talus, pars interarticularis and sacrum where other modalities may not provide sufficient fracture line delineation. CT also has a significant role, and may be marginally more sensitive than MR imaging, in the evaluation of longitudinal stress fractures of the tibia.

MR Imaging

MR imaging has the advantage of similar sensitivity compared to bone scintigraphy but with increased specificity and no ionising radiation. The high spatial resolution of MR imaging provides precise anatomical definition and when used appropriately is cost effective.

The sensitivity of MR imaging to water allows diagnosis of the entire injury spectrum from early stress response to complete fracture. STIR and T2 fat-suppressed images are particularly useful showing periosteal, bone marrow and muscle oedema as markers of early stress injury (Fig. 4.7) [4, 9, 13]. Even in cancellous bone, trabecular microfractures

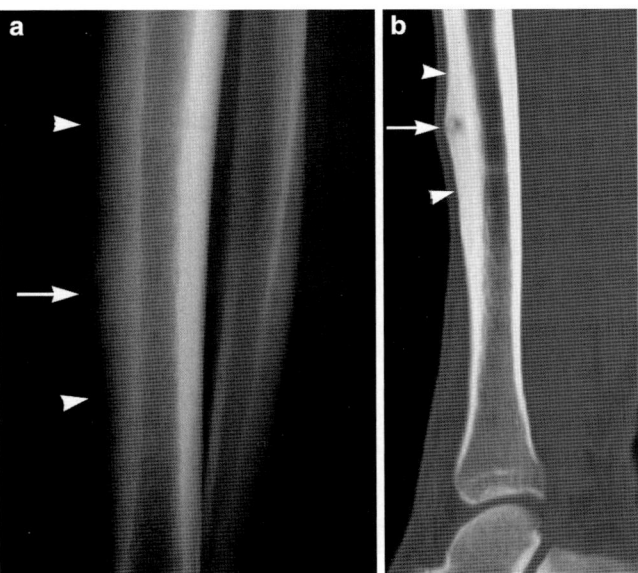

Fig. 4.6 (a) Anterior tibial stress fracture in soccer player. Lateral radiograph shows cortical expansion (*arrowheads*) and radiolucent fracture line (*white arrow*). (b) Sagittal CT reconstruction of anterior tibial stress fracture in an elite cricket fast bowler shows periosteal thickening (*arrowheads*) and resorption cavity (*arrow*)

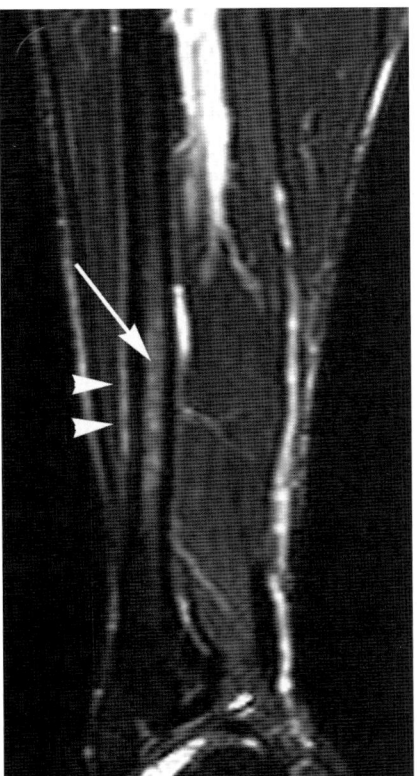

Fig. 4.7 Stress response in the distal fibula of an elite rugby player. Sagittal STIR MR image shows high bone marrow signal (*arrow*) without fracture line and periosteal oedema (*arrowheads*)

Table 4.4 MR classification system for tibial stress injury

Injury grade	MR imaging finding
0	No abnormality
1	Periosteal oedema with no bone marrow abnormality
2	Periosteal and bone marrow oedema only evident on T2w images
3	Periosteal oedema and bone marrow abnormality evident on T1 and T2w images
4	Intracortical signal abnormality and bone marrow oedema evident on T1 and T2w images

can be assessed. As stress response evolves, MR imaging usually demonstrates a focal low signal fracture line, typically surrounded by more diffuse bone marrow oedema. With florid bone marrow oedema the fracture band can be obscured and longitudinal fractures may also be difficult to appreciate and, in these circumstances, CT may provide additional information.

MR imaging abnormalities correlate well with bone scintigraphy changes and are thought to more accurately mirror the clinical findings. A grading system of MR abnormalities proposed by Fredericson et al. in the evaluation of tibial stress injuries is now widely used and has been shown to correlate well with clinical findings (Table 4.4) [1]. As with bone scintigraphy, changes can be seen in asymptomatic individuals [16, 17] and so imaging findings need to be correlated with symptoms. Disadvantages of MR imaging include the lack of cortical definition compared to CT, exam duration and the potential for patient claustrophobia. Some findings are non-specific, however, for most authors MR imaging has replaced bone scintigraphy as the gold standard in the investigation and diagnosis of osseous stress injury [1, 18].

Site-Specific Stress Injuries

Upper Extremity Stress Fractures

Significantly less common than lower extremity stress injuries, upper extremity fatigue fractures are predominantly seen in upper limb dominant sports such as baseball, tennis and golf.

Shoulder Girdle

The overwhelming majority of shoulder girdle injuries in athletes are soft tissue rather than osseous. Specific fatigue fractures include the coracoid process in trapshooters, the acromion in golfers and the inferior edge of the glenoid in baseball pitchers.

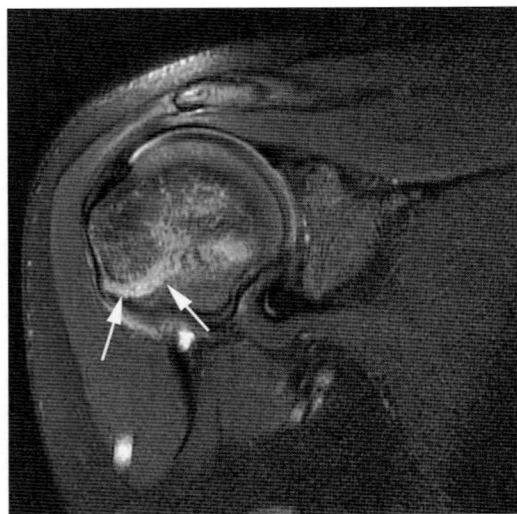

Fig. 4.8 Little leaguer's shoulder (*right*). Coronal oblique T2w FS MR image shows epiphyseal plate widening and oedema (*arrows*) (Courtesy of Dr. PF. Tirman)

Humerus

Mid and distal humeral fractures have been described in tennis players attributed to repetitive overarm serving with good clinical outcome from conservative therapy. Symptomatic bone marrow oedema of the humerus, is also reported in elite tennis players, and presumably represents an early stress response.

Skeletally immature throwing athletes are at risk of stress injury to the proximal humeral epiphyseal plate, termed "Little Leaguers Shoulder." Characterised by proximal humeral epiphyseolysis the exact aetiology is uncertain but most authors propose repetitive rotational stress as a cause of growth plate fracture or inflammation. Although typically seen in young male baseball players similar features have been described in adult pitchers and in athletes participating in other overhand sports (cricket and volleyball). Radiographs show subtle widening and irregularity of the epiphysis with adjacent demineralisation, sclerosis and fragmentation. MR imaging when required shows asymmetric growth plate widening, adjacent bone marrow and periosteal oedema (Fig. 4.8). Conservative management with rest and gradual reintroduction to throwing is required.

Forearm

Fatigue injuries to the ulna, although still uncommon, represent the majority of reported upper extremity stress fractures with the bone particularly vulnerable to stress injury at two sites, the olecranon and the mid-diaphysis.

As in acute olecranon fractures, the pull of triceps is implicated in the development of chronic stress injury and avulsion-type stress fractures have been described in throwing athletes such as baseball pitchers (Fig. 4.9). Javelin throwers, however, develop fatigue injury at the tip of the olecranon due to repetitive impaction with the olecranon fossa in hyperextension.

Mid-diaphyseal fatigue fractures of the ulna occur in sports such as badminton where alternating supination/pronation with wrist flexion and extension exerts torsional stress upon the mid-shaft where the small cross-section makes the bone vulnerable to fatigue injury.

Radius stress fractures are rare, the majority being described at the wrist in skeletally immature gymnasts. Gymnastic elements such as floor work, the beam and vault require support of body weight through the wrists combined with rotation and this has been suggested as the mechanism of injury. The relative inability of the growth plate to withstand torsional and compressive forces puts it at risk in young athletes (Fig. 4.10) [19].

Hand

Although a common site for acute injury, the hand is relatively unaffected by stress fracture.

Scaphoid

There are few cases in the literature of scaphoid stress fractures, all except one report repetitive forced wrist dorsiflexion as the underlying aetiology causing transverse fractures at the scaphoid waist.

Lunate

Acute fracture of the lunate is rare but avascular necrosis secondary to repetitive trauma (Keinbocks disease) is well described. Stress fractures of the lunate are of particular concern in racquet sports with one review of injuries in elite tennis players reporting 11% of stress injuries occurring in the lunate (Fig. 4.11) [20]. This may be related to repetitive wrist hyperextension causing compromise of blood supply in those players already at risk due to anatomical vascular variation. Symptoms can be non-specific; insidious pain and tenderness with reduced range of movement and grip strength.

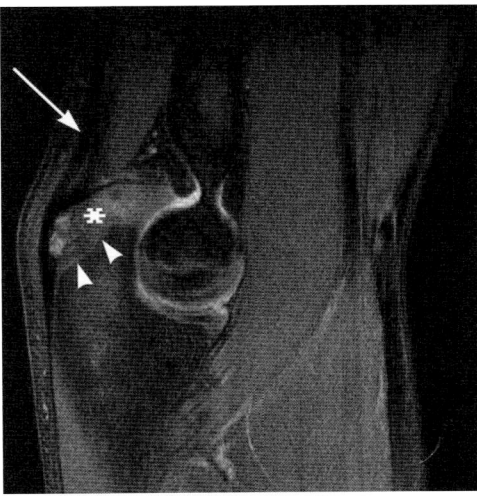

Fig. 4.9 Olecranon stress response. MR images shows triceps tendon (*arrow*), epiphyseal line (*arrowheads*) and olecranon apophyseal oedema (*)

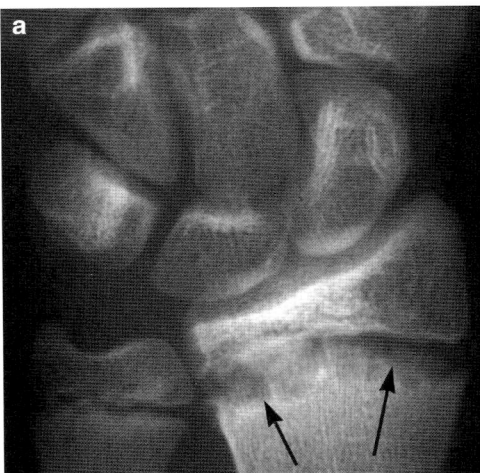
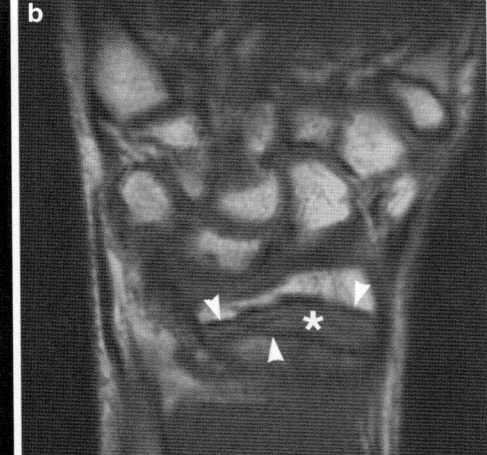

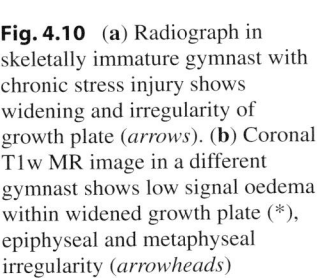

Fig. 4.10 (**a**) Radiograph in skeletally immature gymnast with chronic stress injury shows widening and irregularity of growth plate (*arrows*). (**b**) Coronal T1w MR image in a different gymnast shows low signal oedema within widened growth plate (*), epiphyseal and metaphyseal irregularity (*arrowheads*)

Early diagnosis is crucial as joint levelling procedures performed in minimal lunate collapse allow the majority of athletes to return to sporting activity whereas surgical intervention in later cases often leaves significant limitations in wrist movement.

Hamate

Fatigue fractures of the hook of the hamate occur due to recurrent abutment or shearing force from gripping and so are seen in sports such as golf, baseball and tennis. These are discussed more fully in Chap. 7.

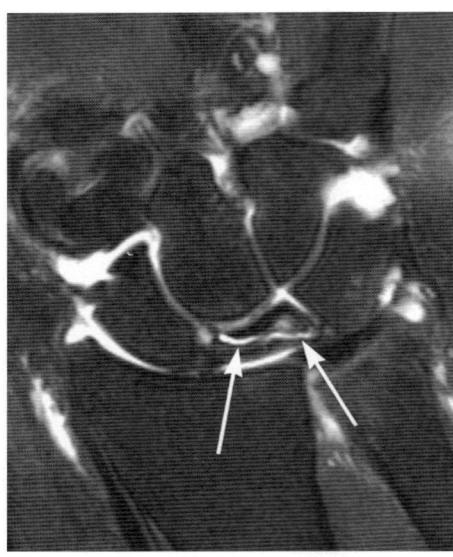

Fig. 4.11 Coronal T2w FS MR image shows lunate stress fracture with fluid between the fragments (*arrows*), adjacent bone marrow oedema and collapse

In general, plain radiography is unhelpful and TPBS lacks the required spatial resolution to fully assess stress injuries of the wrist. Carpal tunnel or supinated oblique views may demonstrate fractures of the hook of the hamate but in the main they have been superseded by CT. Both CT and MR have been shown to be of use in scaphoid, lunate and hamate injuries. MR has the advantage of allowing early evaluation of possible avascular complication and assessment of associated soft tissue injury. CT is particularly recommended in fractures of the hook of the hamate where a fracture line may be obscured by bone marrow oedema on MR imaging.

Metacarpals and Phalanges

Stress fractures of the metacarpals and phalanges are rare. Reported cases principally affect the dominant hand of young athletes, the index finger metacarpal being most often involved. Unlike other areas, case reports describe a high incidence of positive findings on plain radiography (periosteal reaction) at presentation.

Chest Wall

Fatigue fractures of the bony thorax are unusual injuries. There are case reports of lower rib stress injuries in golfers and rowers associated with changes in sporting technique and training. Imaging the chest with MR is generally more challenging than the extremities due to respiratory artefact and the obliquity of the chest wall but even early stress reaction is evident with fluid sensitive sequences (Fig. 4.12).

Spine – injuries of the spine are covered in Chap. 10.

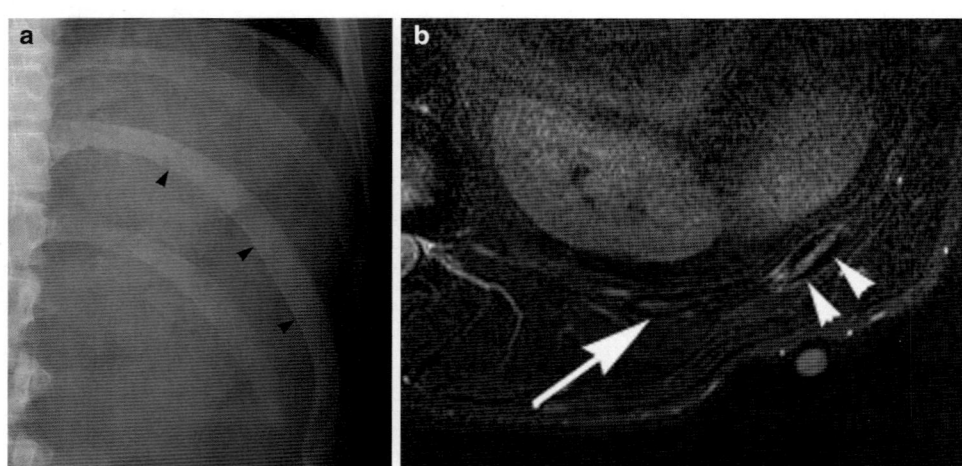

Fig. 4.12 Stress injury of the 11th rib in an elite cricket player. (**a**) Radiograph shows sclerosis (*black arrowheads*) and rib expansion. (**b**) Axial STIR MR image shows bone marrow oedema and cortical thickening (*arrowheads*) when compared to normal adjacent rib (*arrow*)

Lower Extremity Stress Injuries

Factors implicated in the development of lower extremity stress injury include leg length inequality, abnormalities of foot anatomy, Achilles tendon contracture and first ray hypermobility. Stress injuries of the lower limb are common, with the tibia most affected (50%) followed by the foot (40%) and femur (10%) [2]. Early diagnosis of stress fracture is particularly important in weight-bearing bones such as the femoral neck to prevent displacement and further serious complication.

Pelvis

Stress injuries of the pelvis are relatively uncommon accounting for an estimated 1–2% of all fatigue fractures.

Sacral stress fractures are seen in runners and athletes participating in similar high impact sports with females more commonly affected. Stress injuries to the sacrum are associated with other fractures especially parasymphyseal fractures, due to associated pelvic ring forces. Sacral fatigue fractures may be bilateral or unilateral with unilateral fractures linked to limb length discrepancy (see Chap. 2).

Stress injury to the sacrum presents typically with vague sacroiliac joint pain, gluteal pain and tenderness. The fracture line usually runs parallel to the sacral ala. Having a high ratio of cancellous to cortical bone, plain radiographs, when positive, usually show linear sclerosis along the fracture line.

Pubic Rami and Symphysis

Unlike insufficiency fractures which typically involve the superior ramus, fatigue fractures in athletes are much more common in the inferior pubic ramus. They are particularly seen in runners and female athletes who experience greater forces through the rami due to pelvic geometry and decreased muscle-to-bone ratio.

Osteitis pubis is a self-limiting non-infective inflammatory condition of the symphysis pubis originally described in fencers. More frequently it is seen in runners where it is caused by repetitive shearing forces across the symphysis or in soccer players where it is due to excessive pivoting in single leg stance. Acetabular stress fractures are rare and affect the acetabular roof or anterior column and have a strong association with other fatigue fractures, particularly of the inferior pubic ramus, femoral neck and shaft [21].

Imaging

Plain radiography is rarely helpful in assessment of pelvic stress injuries. Pelvic outlet views may be more sensitive than a direct AP radiograph but positive findings such as cortical thickening, periosteal reaction and fracture line sclerosis tend to occur late.

TPBS and MR imaging are highly sensitive with the additional benefit of demonstrating associated pelvic ring injury. Within the sacrum MR imaging will demonstrate bone marrow oedema and the fracture may be evident, particularly on T1 weighted or PD sequences. CT can be useful in confirmation and accurate delineation of the fracture line. The pathognomonic Honda sign is described in bone scintigraphy of sacral insufficiency fractures but the same features may be evident in bilateral sacral fatigue fractures. A study of MR imaging of insufficiency fractures of the hip region showed that sagittal sequences have increased sensitivity compared to other planes in demonstration of fracture lines [22].

Femur

Femoral stress fractures account for up to 10% of all stress fractures, the vast majority involving the femoral neck. They cause particular problems in long distance runners with improper footwear, coxa vara and uneven running surfaces all implicated.

Most frequently femoral neck stress fractures involve the inferomedial aspect of the neck (Fig. 4.13) and are compression type injuries. These are stable injuries with a generally benign clinical course, once diagnosed, and respond well to non-operative management with 6–8 weeks of full or partial non-weight-bearing. Tensile femoral neck fractures involve the superior aspect of the femoral neck and in comparison, are unstable with an increased risk of displacement and long-term complication such as avascular necrosis and osteoarthritis.

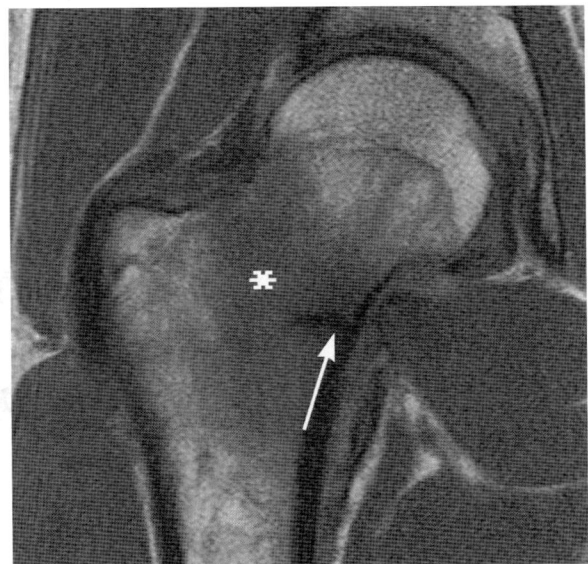

Fig. 4.13 Coronal T1w MR image in runner shows low signal bone marrow oedema (*) and low signal fracture line at inferior femoral neck (*arrow*)

Groin pain, as discussed in Chap. 2, is a common complaint in athletes and femoral neck stress injuries may be difficult to clinically differentiate from other causes of groin injury.

Plain radiographs are typically normal in undisplaced fractures as the trabecular pattern is unaffected. As the clinical course progresses compression fractures show callus formation and tensile fractures may reveal radiolucency of the superior femoral neck and fracture displacement. As with acute femoral neck fractures it is important to consider the tenuous vascular supply to the femoral head in displaced fractures. MR imaging allows assessment of the full range of stress response and can also diagnose avascular necrosis of the femoral head.

Stress fractures of the femoral diaphysis are uncommon with abrupt changes in training regimen and running surface identified as precipitating factors. Unlike military recruits where femoral shaft injuries occur distally in greater than 50% of cases, in athletes the majority of fractures occur within the proximal femur (Fig. 4.14).

Shaft injuries often lack localising symptoms, which makes them more difficult to diagnose clinically. Specific clinical tests such as the hop test and the fulcrum test have been suggested as useful in initial diagnosis and for follow-up [15, 23].

Tibia and Fibula

The tibia is the most common location for stress fracture particularly affecting runners in whom they represent up to 50% of all stress fractures [2] but other causes of exertional leg pain are also frequently encountered. Medial tibial syndrome, chronic compartment syndrome and popliteal entrapment syndrome may all present with similar symptoms, imaging allows accurate diagnosis and correct treatment implementation. The site of stress injury within the tibia is sport dependent, but all generally affect the diaphysis where the tibia has the smallest cross-sectional area and has little surrounding muscle to dissipate forces and absorb shock. Fractures of the proximal third of the tibia occur in jumping athletes, of the middle third in dancers and the mid to distal thirds in runners [9]. Tibial stress fractures occur in runners due to compression and typically involve the posteromedial cortex. Stress fractures of the anterior tibial cortex are seen in jumping athletes, caused by tensile forces and are particularly prone to non-union. Longitudinal fractures of the tibia are significantly less common than transversely orientated injuries; however, these also have an increased risk of non-union and so require more aggressive treatment or follow-up (Figs. 4.6 and 4.15) [1, 24].

Tibial stress fractures cause progressive exertional pain, localised tenderness and pain elicited on percussion [9, 25] this has been shown to be an indicator of the severity of injury [1].

The aetiology of medial tibial stress syndrome (also termed posterior shin splints) has been a controversial subject. Symptoms have been attributed to muscular traction of periosteum causing localised inflammation [9, 25]. However, imaging has revealed positive findings distal to the origin of the main muscle groups making traction an unlikely aetiology. Current thinking is that medial tibial stress syndrome represents early bony stress response as part of the spectrum of fatigue injuries seen in the lower leg. As in tibial stress fractures, the majority of patients experience symptoms in the distal tibia. There is an increased incidence in female

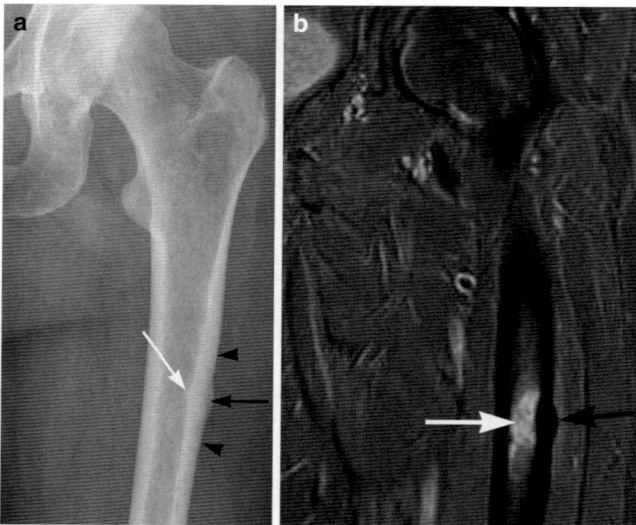

Fig. 4.14 Proximal femoral stress response in long distance runner. (**a**) Radiograph shows subcortical infraction (*black arrow*), endosteal thickening (*white arrow*) and periosteal cortical thickening (*black arrowheads*). (**b**) Coronal STIR MR image shows bone marrow oedema (*white arrow*) and cortical thickening (*black arrow*)

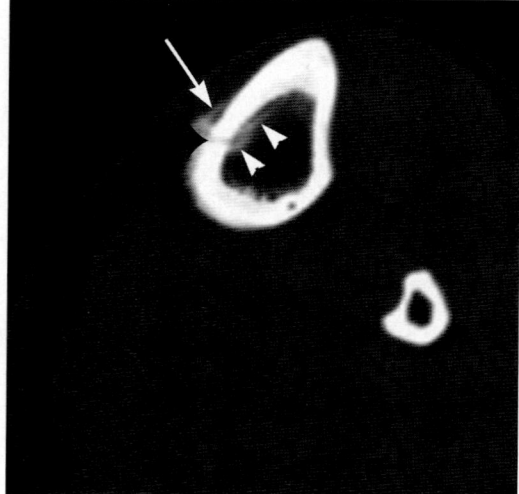

Fig. 4.15 Longitudinal tibial stress fracture. Axial CT image shows fracture line (*curved black arrow*), periosteal reaction (*white arrow*) and endosteal cortical reaction (*arrowheads*)

Fig. 4.16 Fibular stress injury. (**a**) Axial CT image shows eccentric cortical thickening (*black arrow*) and subcortical infraction (*white arrow*). (**b**) Corresponding axial STIR MR image shows cortical oedema (*white arrow*)

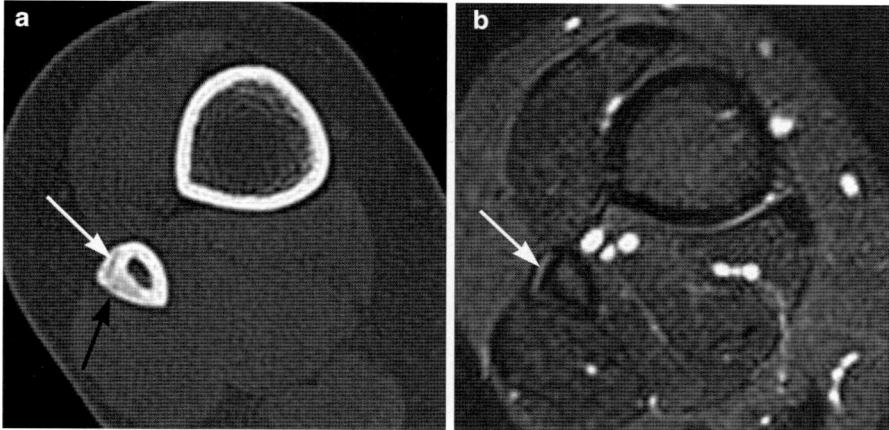

athletes and a strong association with foot pronation and a history of current or recent lower limb injury [9, 25].

Fibular stress injuries are relatively uncommon. Approximately 75% involve the distal lateral cortex and are seen predominantly in runners (Figs. 4.7 and 4.16). The second most common location is the posterior aspect of the proximal fibular cortex [12]. Several studies describe an association between fibular stress fractures and jumping activity [26].

The imaging of tibial stress injuries has been well described. Radiography is insensitive, periosteal reaction is the most commonly seen abnormality but occurs late [1, 11]. Bone scintigraphy is sensitive, medial tibial stress syndrome classically causes longitudinally orientated increase in radiotracer uptake whereas in tibial stress fracture the radionuclide accumulation is more focal (Fig. 4.5). MR is the single most useful imaging modality but is not 100% sensitive.

Foot

Calcaneus and Tarsals

Fatigue fractures of the calcaneus are mostly seen in military recruits. They are related to the action of the achilles and plantar tendons and typically affect the posterior calcaneal margin. The fracture line lies perpendicular to the trabecular pattern and as with other cancellous bones, positive radiographs reveal trabecular malalignment and sclerosis.

Talar stress fractures are uncommon affecting athletes such as gymnasts who experience repetitive axial loading during training. The talar neck is most often involved and persistent activity-related pain that increases on dorsiflexion should raise clinical suspicion [27]. MR is the imaging modality of choice but if marrow oedema obscures the fracture line this is generally better delineated using axial CT (Fig. 4.17).

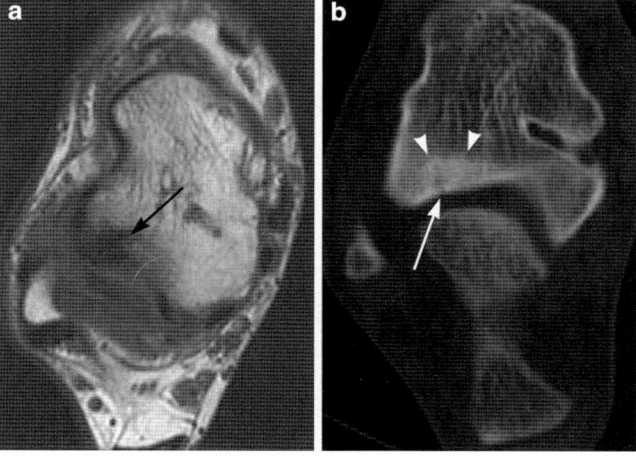

Fig. 4.17 Talar stress fracture in rugby player. (**a**) Axial T1 MR image shows bone marrow oedema of talus (*black arrow*) without a fracture line. (**b**) Axial CT image shows lucent fracture line (*white arrow*) and adjacent sclerosis (*arrowheads*)

Navicular stress fractures present particular diagnostic and treatment challenges. Seen predominantly in sports such as running and basketball the fractures are typically sagittally orientated and affect the central third and dorsal aspect of the navicular. The relative avascularity of the navicular places it at high risk of complication (Fig. 4.18).

Metatarsals

Stress fractures of the metatarsals are common, second in incidence only to the tibia. Eighty per cent develop within the second and third metatarsals although any can be affected (Figs. 4.4 and 4.19). They are particularly associated with distance runners, dancers and military recruits ("March" fracture).

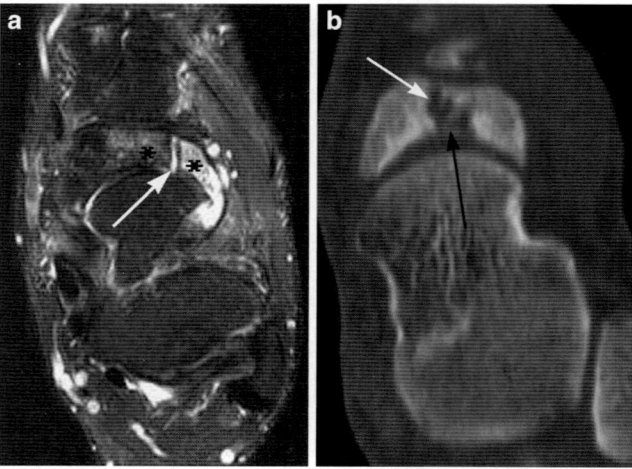

Fig. 4.18 Navicular stress fracture in soccer player. (**a**) Axial STIR MR image shows bone marrow oedema (*) and sclerotic edges to fracture line (*white arrow*) consistent with non-union. (**b**) Axial CT image shows sagittally orientated fracture line (*black arrow*) and confirms sclerotic fracture edges (*white arrow*)

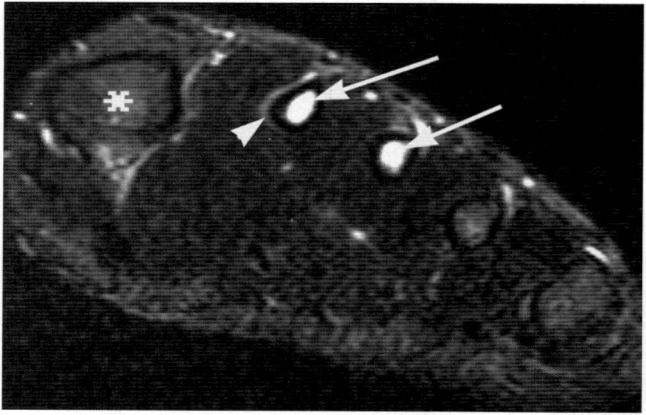

Fig. 4.19 Athlete with forefoot pain and normal radiographs. Short axis STIR MR image shows bone marrow oedema within the second and third metatarsal diaphyses (*arrow*), compare to normal bone marrow signal (*). Eccentric cortical thickening and periosteal oedema of the second metatarsal (*arrowhead*)

Ninety-five per cent of fractures of the second metatarsal occur within the mid-diaphysis with the remainder affecting the proximal aspect. Despite gait analysis and evaluation of biomechanics the reason for this is unclear but the distinction is important as proximal diaphyseal fractures have an increased incidence of non-union and may require surgical fixation [28]. There are several theories as to the contributing anatomical factors behind second metatarsal fractures. Relative achilles tendon shortening increases plantar pressure which is thought to alter forces experienced by the metatarsals. Fractures develop perpendicular to the long axis of the metatarsal and like other stress fractures, they are initially radiographically occult although they may develop exuberant callus during the healing process.

CT, MR imaging and TPBS can all be of use in initial diagnosis, MR imaging demonstrates marrow oedema that persists after clinical resolution and so is not of use in imaging follow-up. CT is more useful in further evaluation of suspected non-union.

Lisfranc injuries – injuries of the foot are further covered in Chap. 3.

High-Risk Stress Fractures

The majority of stress injuries are uncomplicated and heal satisfactorily with reduction or cessation of injury provoking activity. High-risk fractures occur due to tensile forces and relative avascularity putting them at increased risk of complete fracture or delayed/non-union. Sites for concern include the superior aspect of the femoral neck, anterior tibia, patella, talus, navicular, proximal fifth metatarsal and sesamoids (Figs. 4.18 and 4.20) (Table 4.5). Due to the heightened possibility of complication, these fractures often require more aggressive management and follow-up.

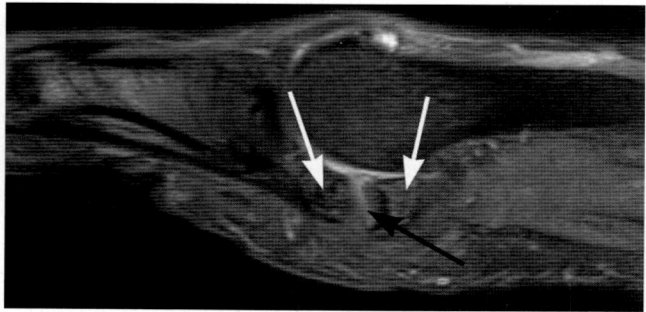

Fig. 4.20 Stress fracture of first toe medial sesamoid in rugby player. Sagittal STIR MR images show fracture (*black arrow*), separation of fragments and oedema within the sesamoid (*white arrows*)

Table 4.5 High-risk stress fractures

Tensile femoral neck
Patella
Anterior tibia
Medial malleolus
Talus
Navicular
Proximal fifth metatarsal
Sesamoids

Differential Diagnosis

A clinical history of pain that is worse at night or at rest is suggestive of an underlying osteoid osteoma. Stress injury pain is typically activity related but as symptoms progress pain becomes more persistent and the clinical picture can become more confusing. Pain caused by either process may be relieved by non-steroidal anti-inflammatory drugs and so imaging may be required to differentiate between the two. Radiography is not a reliable differentiator between stress reaction and osteoid osteoma as both may demonstrate cortical thickening with associated lucency. MR imaging shows highly variable appearances in osteoid osteoma, the nidus may not be evident or it may be seen as a focus of low-to-intermediate T1-weighted signal with higher signal on T2-weighted sequences [29]. CT is the preferred modality for the exclusion or confirmation of an osteoid osteoma.

In general, imaging of osteogenic sarcoma is diagnostic and with the clinical history, allows differentiation from stress injury. Although both occur in the young population and cause periosteal reaction, marrow signal and juxtacortical signal changes, stress fractures unlike sarcomas, do not show bone destruction or large associated soft tissue masses.

Conclusion

Bony fatigue injuries encompass a wide spectrum of abnormalities from early marrow oedema to displaced fractures. Low-grade injuries have been shown to require a significantly shorter time for return to full activity when compared to higher-grade injuries. MR imaging, in particular, plays a central role in evaluation of the symptomatic athlete as clinical evaluation alone may not be sufficient to discriminate between stress injury and other common causes of musculoskeletal injury. Prompt diagnosis is crucial to guide treatment and rehabilitation, to enable a timely return to training and to help prevent further injuries.

References

1. Fredericson M, Bergman AG, Hoffman KL, Dillingham MS (1995) Tibial stress reaction in runners. Correlation of clinical symptoms and scintigraphy with a new magnetic resonance imaging grading system. Am J Sports Med 23(4):472–481
2. Kaufman KR, Brodine S, Shaffer R (2000) Military training-related injuries: surveillance, research, and prevention. Am J Prev Med 18(3 Suppl):54–63
3. Anderson MW, Ugalde V, Batt M, Gacayan J (1997) Shin splints: MR appearance in a preliminary study. Radiology 204(1):177–180
4. Anderson MW, Greenspan A (1996) Stress fractures. Radiology 199(1):1–12
5. Spitz DJ, Newberg AH (2002) Imaging of stress fractures in the athlete. Radiol Clin North Am 40(2):313–331
6. Ross J (1993) A review of lower limb overuse injuries during basic military training. Part 1: types of overuse injuries. Mil Med 158(6): 410–415
7. Boden BP, Osbahr DC (2000) High-risk stress fractures: evaluation and treatment. J Am Acad Orthop Surg 8(6):344–353
8. Bennell KL, Malcolm SA, Thomas SA et al (1996) Risk factors for stress fractures in track and field athletes. A twelve-month prospective study. Am J Sports Med 24(6):810–818
9. Batt ME, Ugalde V, Anderson MW, Shelton DK (1998) A prospective controlled study of diagnostic imaging for acute shin splints. Med Sci Sports Exerc 30(11):1564–1571
10. Stafford SA, Rosenthal DI, Gebhardt MC, Brady TJ, Scott JA (1986) MRI in stress fracture. AJR Am J Roentgenol 147(3):553–556
11. Kijowski R, Choi J, Mukharjee R, de Smet A (2007) Significance of radiographic abnormalities in patients with tibial stress injuries: correlation with magnetic resonance imaging. Skeletal Radiol 36(7):633–640
12. Woods M, Kijowski R, Sanford M, Choi J, De Smet A (2008) Magnetic resonance imaging findings in patients with fibular stress injuries. Skeletal Radiol 37(9):835–841
13. Gaeta M, Minutoli F, Scribano E et al (2005) CT and MR imaging findings in athletes with early tibial stress injuries: comparison with bone scintigraphy findings and emphasis on cortical abnormalities. Radiology 235(2):553–561
14. Milgrom C, Chisin R, Giladi M et al (1984) Negative bone scans in impending tibial stress fractures. A report of three cases. Am J Sports Med 12(6):488–491
15. Matheson GO, Clement DB, McKenzie DC, Taunton JE, Lloyd-Smith DR, MacIntyre JG (1987) Stress fractures in athletes. A study of 320 cases. Am J Sports Med 15(1):46–58
16. Zwas ST, Elkanovitch R, Frank G (1987) Interpretation and classification of bone scintigraphic findings in stress fractures. J Nucl Med 28(4):452–457
17. Bergman AG, Fredericson M, Ho C, Matheson GO (2004) Asymptomatic tibial stress reactions: MRI detection and clinical follow-up in distance runners. AJR Am J Roentgenol 183(3): 635–638
18. Arendt EA, Griffiths HJ (1997) The use of MR imaging in the assessment and clinical management of stress reactions of bone in high-performance athletes. Clin Sports Med 16(2):291–306
19. Liebling M, Berdon W, Ruzal-Shapiro C, Levin T, Roye D Jr, Wilkinson R (1995) Gymnast's wrist (pseudorickets growth plate abnormality) in adolescent athletes: findings on plain films and MR imaging. Am J Roentgenol 164(1):157–159
20. Maquirriain J, Ghisi JP (2006) The incidence and distribution of stress fractures in elite tennis players. Br J Sports Med 40(5):454–459, discussion 9
21. Williams TR, Puckett ML, Denison G, Shin AY, Gorman JD (2002) Acetabular stress fractures in military endurance athletes and recruits: incidence and MRI and scintigraphic findings. Skeletal Radiol 31(5):277–281
22. Grangier C, Garcia J, Howarth NR, May M, Rossier P (1997) Role of MRI in the diagnosis of insufficiency fractures of the sacrum and acetabular roof. Skeletal Radiol 26(9):517–524
23. Johnson AW, Weiss CB Jr, Wheeler DL (1994) Stress fractures of the femoral shaft in athletes – more common than expected. A new clinical test. Am J Sports Med 22(2):248–256
24. Edwards PH Jr, Wright ML, Hartman JF (2005) A practical approach for the differential diagnosis of chronic leg pain in the athlete. Am J Sports Med 33(8):1241–1249

25. Yates B, White S (2004) The incidence and risk factors in the development of medial tibial stress syndrome among naval recruits. Am J Sports Med 32(3):772–780
26. Symeonides PP (1980) High stress fractures of the fibula. J Bone Joint Surg Br 62-B(2):192–193
27. Rossi F, Dragoni S (2005) Talar body fatigue stress fractures: three cases observed in elite female gymnasts. Skeletal Radiol 34(7):389–394
28. Chuckpaiwong B, Cook C, Pietrobon R, Nunley JA (2007) Second metatarsal stress fracture in sport: comparative risk factors between proximal and non-proximal locations. Br J Sports Med 41(8):510–514
29. Davies M, Cassar-Pullicino VN, Davies AM, McCall IW, Tyrrell PN (2002) The diagnostic accuracy of MR imaging in osteoid osteoma. Skeletal Radiol 31(10):559–569

Chapter 5
Shoulder Injuries

Andrew J. Grainger and Phillip F.J. Tirman

Introduction

The shoulder has the greatest range of movement of any joint in the body and is used in a wide variety of sporting activities, particularly those involving overhead activities such as throwing or serving in racket sports. The shallow glenoid cup in part allows the large range of movement but also contributes anatomically to an inherently unstable joint which is particularly vulnerable to injury through direct trauma such as may be sustained in contact sports and when falling. The humeral head balanced on the relatively small glenoid is analogous to a golf ball sitting on a tee, additionally requiring the soft tissue stabilising labrum, which increases the surface area of the glenoid, and the rotator cuff which stabilises the shoulder through the wide range of motion. Besides acute traumatic sports injuries, the shoulder is also prone to a range of chronic injuries resulting from recurrent and repetitive movements.

With modern imaging techniques, and in particular since the advent of ultrasound and magnetic resonance (MR) imaging, the radiologist is able to demonstrate a wide range of bone and soft tissue injuries and in many cases can assist in treatment through guided intervention. Currently the principal imaging techniques available for assessing the shoulder are conventional radiographs, CT, ultrasound, MR imaging, and MR and CT arthrography. Conventional radiographs supplemented by CT are particularly useful for assessing bone injury. However many of the important injuries of the shoulder joint involve soft tissues such as the rotator cuff, glenoid labrum and biceps tendon. MR imaging is readily able to identify abnormalities associated with these structures and is also useful for evaluating osteochondral injuries. Supplementing MR imaging or CT with arthrographic techniques can increase sensitivity to injuries to the structures. While ultrasound has not yet proved useful for the assessment of the static stabilisers of the shoulder (glenohumeral ligaments and glenoid labrum) it is able to provide a high-resolution assessment of the dynamic stabilisers (rotator cuff) and biceps tendon and has particular advantages in being able to assess the structures dynamically, in real time and also guide intervention.

Anatomy

The shallow glenoid cup articulates with the humeral head and is deepened by a circumferential fibrocartilage labrum. This potentially unstable arrangement requires soft tissue structures to help maintain the stability of the joint. The stabilisers of the joint are generally divided into two groups:

1. The dynamic stabilisers. These are the rotator cuff tendons which function throughout the large range of motion keeping the humeral head centred on the glenoid by competent neuromuscular function
2. The static stabilisers. These comprise the glenoid labrum and glenohumeral ligaments which function at the end range of motion keeping the humeral head from subluxing or dislocating by acting as a check rein

The Rotator Cuff

The rotator cuff muscles act to control the position of the humeral head on the glenoid drawing it towards the glenoid and maintaining it in a central position while the more powerful muscles of the shoulder girdle such as the deltoid, pectoralis major and latissimus dorsi act on the arm. For instance, during adduction of the arm by pectoralis major and latissimus dorsi, the muscles of the rotator cuff resist the tendency of the powerful adductors to translate the humeral head inferiorly on the glenoid.

The rotator cuff is made up of four muscles and tendons:

- Supraspinatus
- Infraspinatus
- Subscapularis
- Teres minor

Andrew J. Grainger (✉)
Department of Radiology, Leeds Teaching Hospitals,
Leeds LS7 4SA, UK
e-mail: andrew.grainger@leedsth.nhs.uk

All four muscles arise from the scapula and insert into the tubercles of the humeral head. The subscapularis arises from the anterior aspect of the scapula and inserts into the lesser tubercle of the humerus. Supraspinatus arises from the supraspinatus fossa of the scapula, while infraspinatus and teres minor arise from the posterior aspect of the scapula, inferior to the spinous process. These latter three muscles insert via their tendons into the greater tuberosity of the humerus. The tendons of supraspinatus, infraspinatus and teres minor blend together at their insertion to form a continuous cuff, but are separated from the subscapularis tendon by a small gap known as the rotator interval. The long head of biceps tendon passes through the rotator interval as it tracks from its origin on the superior glenoid to the upper arm. As it transits the rotator interval it emerges from the joint capsule and is surrounded by a synovial sheath that is continuous with the joint cavity. It is now generally accepted that the long head of biceps tendon is important in maintaining shoulder stability.

The majority of fibres in the rotator cuff tendons are arranged longitudinally but a focal, deep portion of the supraspinatus and infraspinatus tendons contains fibres running transversely. These perpendicularly arranged tendon fibres on the articular side of the cuff extend in an arc from the anterior insertion of supraspinatus to the posterior insertion of infraspinatus and are known as the rotator cable. The longitudinal tendon fibres lateral to the cable are thinner and are known as the rotator crescent [1]. The crescent zone is particularly vulnerable to tears.

The Static Stabilisers

The glenoid labrum and the glenohumeral ligaments make up the labroligamentous complex The coracohumeral ligament which anatomically forms the roof of the rotator interval between the subscapularis and supraspinatus and also stabilises the biceps tendon will also be discussed.

The glenoid labrum is fibrous in nature and forms a ring of tissue around the bony glenoid. While it plays a role in deepening the cup of the glenoid, thereby increasing the contact area to the humerus and contributing to joint stability; it also provides a fibrous attachment for the glenohumeral ligaments and the longhead of biceps which insert onto the labrum and glenoid. This second feature is important when mechanisms of injury to the static stabilisers are considered.

It is well recognised that there are many variations in normal labral morphology. While the labrum can be firmly attached to the glenoid along its outer and central edge throughout its attachment (which occurs via a transitional zone made of fibrocartilage); a well-recognised variant is that the central edge is mobile with a meniscoid appearance. This occurs as a feature of the superior labrum above the

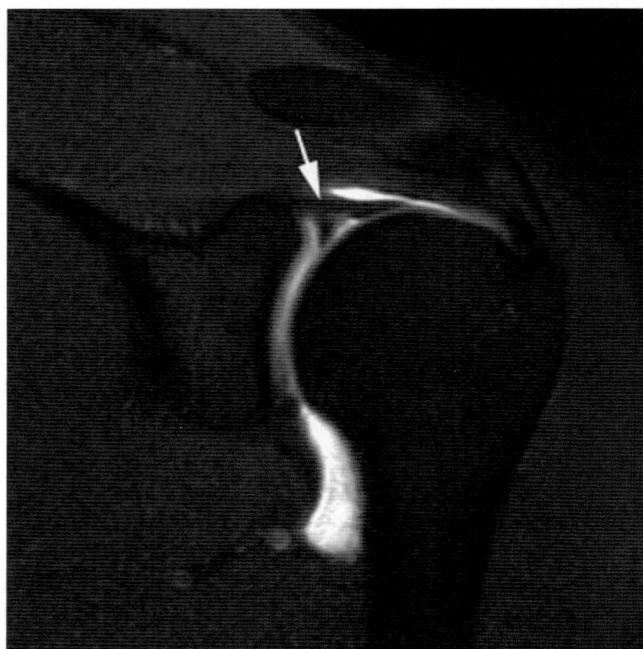

Fig. 5.1 Coronal oblique T1w FS MR arthrogram. There is a sublabral sulcus (filled with contrast) between the bicipital/labral complex (*arrow*) and the superior glenoid

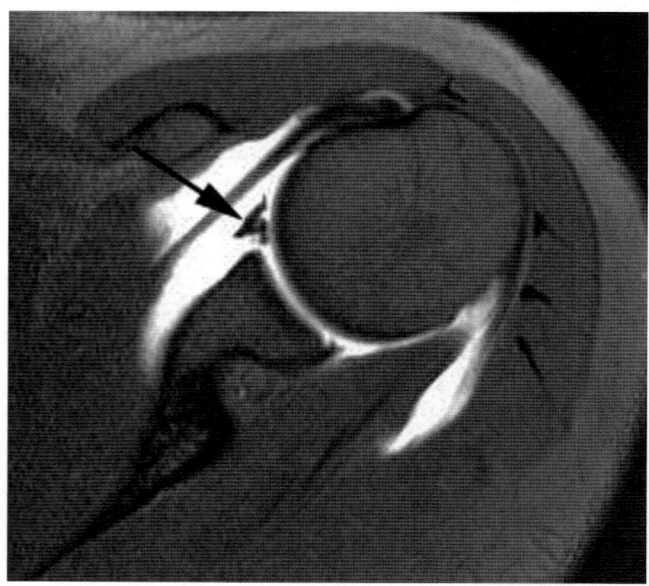

Fig. 5.2 Axial T1w FS MR arthrogram. There is a sublabral foramen separating the labrum (here shown adjacent to the middle glenohumeral ligament – *arrow*)

equator of the glenoid. When seen the space between labrum and glenoid is known as a sublabral recess or sulcus (Fig. 5.1). In some normal cases there is a complete detachment of the labrum superiorly. This generally occurs in the anterosuperior quadrant and the sublabral recess becomes known as a sublabral foramen (Fig. 5.2).

The glenohumeral ligaments represent thickened bands within the joint capsule and attach to both the margin of the glenoid (through the labrum) and to the proximal humerus. Although they are normally lax they become taut at the extremes of movement. It is at this point that they become vulnerable to disruption should movement continue beyond the endpoint reached. Three glenohumeral ligaments are recognised:

1. The Inferior glenohumeral ligament (IGHL). This is the most important of the glenohumeral ligaments and comprises an anterior and posterior band. Between the two bands lies the axillary pouch which forms a "hammock" between the two components of the IGHL. The bands of the IGHL, along with the axillary pouch, are flaccid in the adducted neutral position. However as the arm is abducted they become taut and the inferior aspect of the articular surface of the humeral head becomes cradled between the two components of the ligament in the "hammock" of the axillary pouch. The two bands of the IGHL have fairly wide attachments to the glenoid via the glenoid labrum in the region of the 3–5 o'clock and 7–9 o'clock positions.
2. The middle glenohumeral ligament arises from the anterosuperior glenoid rim, attaching via the labrum. It passes inferiorly across the anterior aspect of joint capsule to its insertion into the anatomical neck of the humerus close to the less tuberosity. It resists extreme external rotation in the lower ranges of abduction. The middle glenohumeral ligament is extremely variable. Studies have found that it is absent in around about 30% of cases. On the other hand it may be extremely prominent and cord like. In this latter situation it may be associated with an absence of the anterosuperior labrum, a normal variant known as the Buford Complex (Fig. 5.3).
3. The superior glenohumeral ligament is a smaller structure arising from the interval between the middle glenohumeral ligament and the biceps tendon. It inserts in the region of the bicipital groove and has an important function in stabilising the biceps tendon by contributing to the biceps pulley of the rotator interval (see later discussion).

Between the middle and superior glenohumeral ligaments is an opening into a synovial recess which has a saddlebag configuration over the subscapularis tendon – the subscapularis recess (Fig. 5.4) [2].

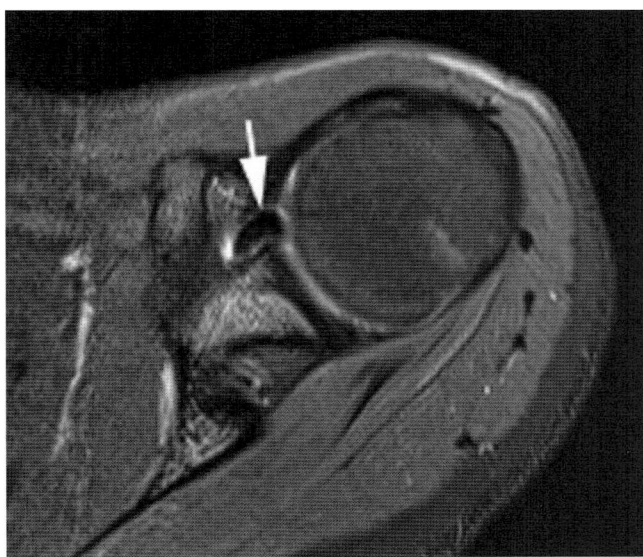

Fig. 5.3 Axial T1w FS MR arthrogram. An enlarged middle glenohumeral ligament is seen (*arrow*) in the absence of a labrum. The appearances are of a Buford complex

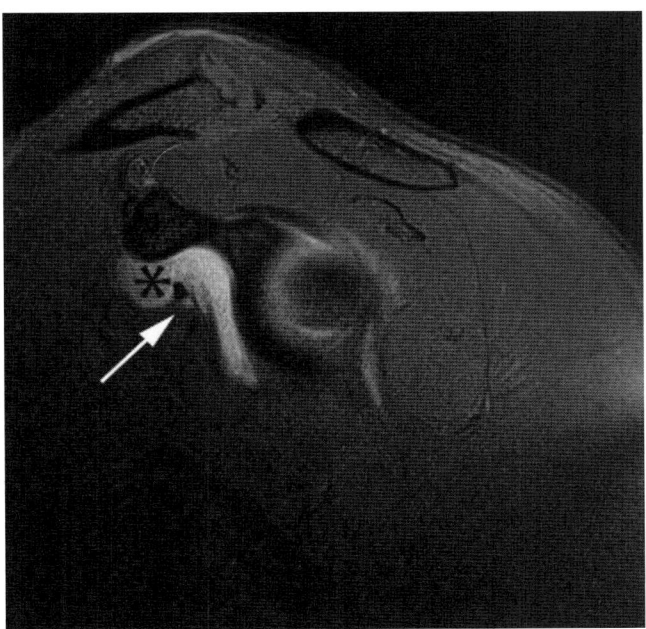

Fig. 5.4 Sagittal T1w FS MR arthrogram. There is a subscapular recess (*) seen "saddlebagged" over the subscapularis muscle and tendon (*arrow*)

The Longhead of Biceps and Rotator Interval

The long head of biceps arises from the superior glenoid with a variable attachment from the bony glenoid (superior glenoid tubercle) and the labrum. Due to the continuity with the labrum the unit is best referred to as the biceps labral complex. There are well-recognised variations in the way the biceps labral complex attaches to the glenoid. The attachment ranges from a firmly adherent attachment with no sublabral sulcus or foramen, through to an attachment with a very deep sulcus giving the labrum a meniscoid configuration.

The biceps origin is closely associated with the origins of the middle and superior glenohumeral ligaments which arise immediately anterior to the biceps.

The biceps tendon initially runs within the capsule of the shoulder joint passing between the supraspinatus and subscapularis tendons in the rotator interval. Here it passes into the intertubercular groove which in the normal anatomical position necessitates a significant change in direction. At this point the biceps tendon is stabilised by the biceps pulley mechanism. The tendon then passes out of the joint capsule but continues to be surrounded by an extension of the capsule that forms a tendon sheath.

The biceps tendon and structures of the rotator interval are increasingly recognised as playing an important role in joint stability. In addition to the longhead of biceps tendon, the interval contains the superior glenohumeral ligament (SGHL) and the coracohumeral ligament (CHL) which together form the biceps pulley mechanism. The CHL arises from the base of the coracoid process and forms the roof of the rotator interval. Although it inserts on the greater tuberosity, it also blends with the supraspinatus. A separate component passes more medially inserting onto subscapularis and blending with its fibres. The SGL also forms part of the pulley mechanism passing through the rotator interval, anteromedial to the long head of biceps tendon and inserting onto the humerus in the region of the bicipital groove.

Rotator Cuff Disease

Rotator cuff tendinopathy is defined as collagenous degeneration of the rotator cuff tendons and most commonly involves the supraspinatus tendon. Sporting activity may lead to cuff tendinopathy through overuse or impingement mechanisms. Tendinopathic change may subsequently progress to partial or full thickness tearing of the cuff, although the tendinopathic cuff is painful even in the absence of tearing. There may be associated subacromial or subcoracoid bursitis. Ultrasound and MR imaging are generally the imaging modalities of choice when investigating rotator cuff disease and impingement.

Impingement

Two types of shoulder impingement are recognised and both may be associated with rotator cuff pathology.

1. External impingement refers to impingement of the rotator cuff and overlying bursal structures on the structures of the coracoacromial arch which comprises of the coracoid process, coracoacromial ligament and acromion.
2. Internal impingement refers to the impingement of the undersurface of the rotator cuff on the glenoid labrum and humeral head. Complex mechanisms are involved and the exact pathophysiology remains poorly understood.

Rotator Cuff Tendinopathy and External Impingement

The aetiology of rotator cuff tendinopathy (and subsequent rotator cuff tearing) remains controversial [3, 4]. While it may be that intrinsic factors to the tendon such as over use and reduced vascularity are important, it was Neer who proposed that 95% of all rotator cuff tears are the result of chronic impingement of the cuff between the humeral head and coracoacromial arch [5]. Neer described three clinicopathological stages in the impingement syndrome (Table 5.1). The impingement theory led to the development of subacromial decompression surgery as a successful treatment.

Congenital and acquired morphological abnormalities of the coracoacromial arch can lead to impingement although there is some debate regarding the importance of the morphology of the acromion. Bigliani showed that a hooked shape to the acromion (type III) was more frequently associated with the external impingement process than the curved (type II) or flat (type I) morphologies [6]. This has been contested by others [7] although the confusion may in part be due to the lack of reliability between observers when assessing subacromial morphology [3, 4].

Other coracoacromial arch configurations associated with external impingement include subacromial osteophyte or enthesophyte formation, thickening of the coracoacromial ligament and lateral downsloping of the acromion. However it has been noted that many of the acquired features described may be a consequence of rotator cuff disease rather than a cause [3, 4, 8, 9]. An anterior os acromiale may be unstable and may predispose to impingement [10].

Impingement of the subscapularis tendon between the coracoid process and lesser tuberosity known as subcoracoid impingement has also been described [4]. While this may be due to the congenital configuration of the subcoracoid space it can also be seen after fractures of the coracoid or lesser tuberosity.

Secondary external impingement is due to dynamic narrowing of the subacromial space as a result of micro-subluxation of the humeral head in the glenoid. In contrast to primary external impingement, this form of impingement

Table 5.1 Neer's three stages of external impingement [3–5]

Stage 1
Generally occurring in younger patients. There is bursitis along with oedema and haemorrhage in the subacromial space. Although this stage is reversible reduction in lubrication provided by the bursa may lead to progression to stage 2

Stage 2
Tendinopathy of the rotator cuff (particularly supraspinatus) is seen which may progress to partial thickness tearing

Stage 3
Full thickness tearing of the rotator cuff is seen

occurs in the presence of a normal coracoacromial arch. The pattern of micro-instability seen in secondary external impingement may result from chronic micro-trauma to the static stabilisers such as is seen in overhead throwing athletes [11]. Given that the rotator cuff itself also acts to stabilise the glenohumeral joint, it is easy to see that primary degeneration of the cuff can in itself lead to secondary external impingement [3, 12].

Internal Impingement

The concept of external impingement and its relationship to rotator cuff pathology has already been described. However, a second form of impingement termed internal impingement, generally seen in younger population and amongst athletes, is also recognised. The literature surrounding this form of impingement is confusing and although several internal impingement syndromes have been described the true aetiology of these conditions and their relationship to other biomechanical problems and pathologies in the shoulder is poorly understood [13].

Although precise descriptions of internal impingement vary, two broad types have been described. These are posterosuperior impingement and anterosuperior (anterior) impingement.

Posterior Superior Internal Impingement, Glenohumeral Internal Rotation Deficit and the Peel-Back Lesion

Walch et al. reported internal impingement as occurring in normal shoulders when the posterosuperior rotator cuff (close to the junction of supra and infraspinatus tendons) comes into contact with the posterosuperior glenoid labrum in the Abducted and Externally Rotated (ABER) position (Fig. 5.5). With the arm in this position they noted that the cuff may become entrapped (impinged) between the labrum and greater tuberosity [14]. This is a normal phenomenon and is seen in asymptomatic patients but it was suggested that in throwing athletes injury to the posterosuperior cuff and labrum might occur as a result of the increased frequency and/or force of impingement of the cuff on the posterosuperior glenoid [15, 16]. It has been further hypothesised that overstretching of the anterior capsule during the cocking phase of throwing results in micro-instability further aggravating the impingement. A proposed treatment for the presumed micro-instability leading to this form of impingement is an anterior stabilisation. However, while posterosuperior

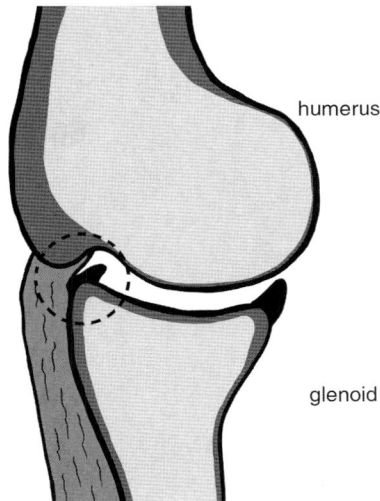

Fig. 5.5 Posterosuperior impingement. In the abducted and externally rotated position the undersurface of the cuff abuts the posterosuperior glenoid. In this position, impingement of cuff tissues and labrum may occur between the greater tuberosity and glenoid (*circle*)

impingement may still be a mechanism of injury to the cuff in the older throwing athlete where hyper-external rotation leads to chronic failure of the anteroinferior capsule, the micro-instability theory of posterosuperior impingement has more recently been questioned. Walch et al. in their original reports found no evidence of instability in the cases they examined under anaesthesia [14]. Their finding was supported in another study that found no correlation between instability and MR imaging evidence of internal impingement leading authors to conclude that anterior stabilisation is inappropriate in these patients [17, 18].

An alternative aetiology to micro-instability for the development of the changes to the cuff and labrum attributed to posterosuperior internal impingement has been put forward. It has been noted that repetitive tensile loading during a thrower's follow-through results in tightening and contracture of the posterior band of the IGHL. This has two key effects:

1. An acquired loss of internal rotation (Glenohumeral Internal Rotation Deficit (GIRD)) observed in throwers.
2. A posterosuperior shift of the contact point of the humerus on the glenoid.

Shift of the contact point of the humerus on the glenoid allows an increase in external rotation at the shoulder joint, but this is at the cost of a loss in internal rotation (GIRD). Furthermore, there is a resulting pseudo-laxity of the anterior IGHL due to the reduced cam effect of the humerus brought about by the posterosuperior shift of the humeral head causing a redundancy of the anteroinferior joint capsule [17, 19] (Fig. 5.6). The pattern of injury seen in patients with glenohumeral internal rotation deficit (GIRD) comprises Superior labral anterior to posterior (SLAP) type II lesions located posteriorly

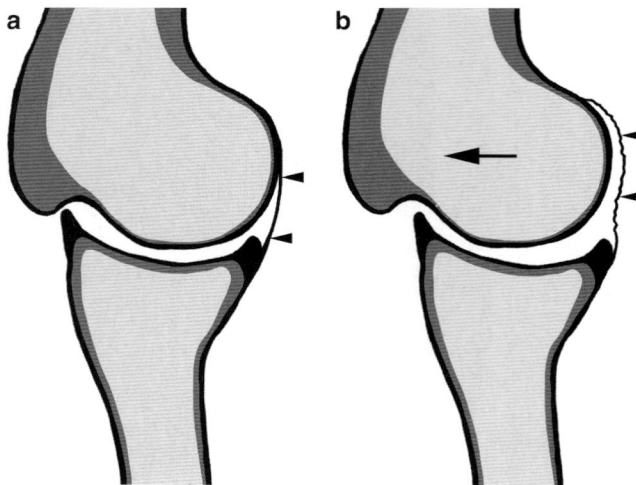

Fig. 5.6 Anterior capsular redundancy. (**a**) Normally in the abducted and externally rotated position the "cam" effect of the humeral head stretches the anterior capsular tissues taut (*arrowheads*). (**b**) If the humeral head is shifted posterosuperiorly relative to the glenoid as occurs with the GIRD phenomenon, and as indicated by the *arrow*, the "cam" effect is lost resulting in anterior capsular redundancy (*arrowheads*)

along with posterior articular surface rotator cuff tears. It is suggested these occur as a result of the hyper-external rotation made possible by the contracted and tightened posterior band of the IGHL through the so-called peel-back mechanism. Hyper-external rotation produces posterosuperior peel-back forces on the biceps–labral complex which can ultimately lead to a type 2 SLAP lesion. The same process brings about an over twisting and eventually tearing of the rotator cuff typically occurring as undersurface partial thickness tearing to the posterior supraspinatus. This combination of findings is known as the peel-back lesion. There may be some aggravation of this process by the abrasive effect of the cuff on the labrum but this is said to be a relatively minor effect and generally occurs in throwing athletes who achieve massive hyper-external rotation typically in excess of 130° [17].

Although the cause of the pathological findings seen in throwers shoulders remains the subject of debate, the combination of imaging findings is well recognised [20, 21]. Ultrasound will demonstrate damage to the rotator cuff in the form of undersurface partial thickness tears but is poorly sensitive to labral injury. MR imaging is able to image both the cuff and labroligamentous structures, including the biceps anchor along with the articular surfaces. The superior labrum should be examined for a posterior (type IIB) SLAP lesion and there may be associated thickening of the posterior capsular structures and posterior band of the IGHL. The cuff may show undersurface tearing as described above while sclerosis and cyst formation of the posterior rim of the glenoid and/or humeral head may also be seen as a result of repetitive contact between the humeral head and glenoid.

The finding of calcification in the region of the posteroinferior labrum is known as the Bennett lesion and is a poorly understood and occasionally symptomatic finding in over arm throwing athletes. It has been associated with the other features of "posterosuperior impingement" but this finding is also seen in asymptomatic athletes, and a cause and effect relationship with internal impingement has not been established. It may alternatively relate to chronic micro-trauma to the posterior labrum and capsule.

Anterosuperior Internal Impingement

Anterosuperior impingement (ASI) has been described as a form of internal impingement occurring in a position of horizontal adduction and internal rotation. In this position, the undersurface of the biceps pulley mechanism and subscapularis tendon may impinge against the anterosuperior glenoid rim [22, 23]. Initial reports suggested that ASI resulted in damage to the subscapularis and pulley mechanism [22], but damage to these structures, and loss of their stabilising function, is now thought to be the cause of ASI rather than the effect [23]. Once impingement occurs there may be progressive damage to these structures and increasing soft tissue injury results in an increasing frequency of ASI [23]. There may also be damage to the anterosuperior labrum as a result of impingement of the anterior cuff on the labrum. From the radiologist's point of view it is important to recognise the association between undersurface tears of subscapularis and supraspinatus, and rotator interval (biceps pulley) tears along with the possibility of labral damage. The combination of rotator cuff tear and labral injury has been termed the SLAC lesion (superior labrum anterior cuff).

Rotator Cuff Tears

Tears of the rotator cuff extending from the bursal surface to articular surface of the tendon are known as full thickness tears and result in an abnormal communication between the glenohumeral joint and the subacromial bursa. Partial thickness tears involve only the bursal or articular surface. Intrasubstance tears may also be seen.

Rotator cuff tears typically start at the anterior edge of supraspinatus, close to its insertion into the humerus, or in the region of the rotator crescent previously described. Having developed the tear may propagate. Initially extension tends to be through the rotator crescent and therefore through the remainder of the supraspinatus and into infraspinatus. The tear may also extend anteriorly through the rotator interval into subscapularis. When the tear only involves part of the supraspinatus tendon retraction of the tendon will be

Table 5.2 Classification of rotator cuff tear size [24]

Small	<1 cm
Medium	1–3 cm
Large	3–5 cm
Massive	>5 cm

Table 5.3 Assessment of partial thickness tears [25]

Grade 1	<3 mm deep
Grade 2	3–6 mm deep (<50% of cuff thickness involved)
Grade 3	>6 mm deep (>50% of cuff thickness involved)

Table 5.4 Classification of biceps pulley lesions [23]

Type 1	Isolated pulley lesion (CHL and/or SGHL) without subscapularis or supraspinatus tear
Type 2	Pulley lesion with partial articular surface supraspinatus tear
Type 3	Pulley lesion with partial articular surface subscapularis tear
Type 4	Pulley lesion with partial articular surface supraspinatus and subscapularis tears

minimal, but once the whole tendon is involved there may be considerable retraction.

The size of rotator cuff tear is normally assessed by measurement of its maximum diameter and classified as small, medium, large or massive (Table 5.2) [24]. Tears may be described as *anterior free edge*, where the tear develops at the anterior edge of supraspinatus; or *mid-substance*, where intact tendon is seen both anterior and posterior to the tear. In the majority of cases, rotator cuff tears develop as a consequence of tendon degeneration and impingement. However, acute trauma can lead to a tendon tear, or not uncommonly to disruption of the kinetic chain as a result of bone avulsion from the greater or lesser tuberosity.

When tears of the infraspinatus or subscapularis are seen there is usually an associated supraspinatus tear. Occasionally isolated tears of the subscapularis or infraspinatus are seen following acute trauma, particularly in athletes where unusual mechanisms of injury may occur.

Partial Thickness Tears

Partial thickness tears of the rotator cuff may be articular surface, bursal surface or interstitial in nature and are said to be more painful than full thickness tears. Articular (undersurface) tears are more common than bursal surface tears. They may arise from acute injury or from chronic microtrauma on a background of tendinopathy resulting from the overuse and impingement mechanisms previously described. Partial thickness tears are more common than full thickness tears and represent a diagnostic challenge to both MR imaging and ultrasound.

The thickness of tendon involvement in partial thickness tears is variable ranging from minimal surface damage through to a near full thickness tear. Partial thickness tears can be graded according to the thickness of tendon involved the tendon (Table 5.3) [25].

A partial thickness tear may extend proximally within the tendon, with a significant intrasubstance component. This is known as *tendon delamination* and presents particular challenges for surgical repair. A delaminating tear extending to the articular surface of supraspinatus has also been termed the *PASTA* lesion (partial articular supraspinatus tendon avulsion).

A *Rim-Rent* tear is described as an articular surface partial thickness tear occurring right at its attachment to the greater tuberosity.

Rotator Interval Tears

The rotator interval, the gap between subscapularis and supraspinatus, contains the long head of biceps tendon. The coracohumeral ligament (CHL) forms the roof of the interval and the superior glenohumeral (SGHL) forms the floor laterally. These structures may be torn as a result of an extension of a rotator cuff tear from the supraspinatus or subscapularis. In addition, tears of the interval may occur as isolated lesions [26–28]. Damage to the rotator interval may be associated with the internal impingement syndromes described earlier.

Tears of the lateral rotator interval will result in disruption of the biceps pulley mechanism leading to biceps instability. Full thickness tears of the rotator cuff extending to the rotator interval are associated with biceps instability. However, it is also important to recognise biceps pulley lesions may occur in isolation or associated with only subtle partial thickness cuff damage. Habermeyer has classified these biceps pulley lesions into four types (Table 5.4) [23]. Occult bicipital instability has been termed the *hidden lesion* by Walch due to the difficulty of detecting this pattern of injury at arthroscopy [29]. Disruption of the biceps pulley mechanism resulting in biceps instability will tend to result in medial subluxation of the biceps out of the bicipital groove. Different patterns of biceps subluxation are seen depending on the structures that have been injured. Four patterns have been described [27, 30]:

1. Intra-articular dislocation with medial displacement of the biceps anterior to the glenohumeral joint space. Here there is disruption of the subscapularis tendon and the SGHL/CHL complex.
2. Disruption of the SGHL/CHL complex but with intact lateral fibres of the CHL resulting in subluxation of the biceps anterior to subscapularis but deep to the lateral components of the CHL.

3. Extra articular subluxation occurring when there is an anterior supraspinatus tendon tear extending into the CHL. Here the long head of biceps will sublux medially to lie superficial to subscapularis.
4. There may be delamination of the deep surface of the subscapularis which is associated with injury to the SGHL/CHL complex and allows subluxation of the biceps tendon into the substance of the subscapularis tear at the site of the delamination.

Calcific Tendinopathy

Intra-tendinous calcium hydroxyapatite deposition can be a feature of tendinopathy, most commonly in the supraspinatus tendon. Deposits may range from small flecks within the tendon through to large foci which may distort the tendon causing impingement or even a block to movement. Calcium deposition can be seen in adjacent soft tissues including the bursa; although this may be the result of a tendinous calcific deposit rupturing into the joint or bursa.

Imaging Findings

Conventional Radiographs

Conventional radiographs do not show the tendons of the rotator cuff themselves but can still prove useful, particularly in the situation of acute trauma. Bone trauma is well demonstrated along with dislocations of the glenohumeral joint. More specifically, in the context of the rotator cuff, avulsion fractures from the greater or lesser tuberosities may be seen. Prior to the widespread availability of cross-sectional imaging techniques conventional arthrography was used for the diagnosis of rotator cuff tears.

Calcium deposition within rotator cuff tendons or the adjacent soft tissues such as the bursa may be shown with conventional radiography.

CT

Although CT itself has little role to play in the investigation of soft tissue rotator cuff pathology, its multi-planar capabilities can be extremely useful when evaluating bone injury to the humeral head. CT arthrography can be used to image the rotator cuff but generally ultrasound and MR imaging are the imaging modalities of choice in this situation.

MR Imaging and MR Arthrography

MR imaging has been extensively used for the assessment of rotator cuff disease and impingement. Bursal fluid is identified using T2w FS or STIR imaging and has been shown to correlate with arthroscopic findings of subacromial bursitis [31]. In clinical practice dynamic assessment of the shoulder with MR imaging is not usually undertaken. However, morphological abnormalities of the coracoacromial arch are readily appreciated on MR imaging such as the configuration of the acromion and coracoacromial ligament. Other features to note include the presence of an os acromiale or undersurface acromial osteophyte/enthesophyte (Fig. 5.7). While these findings are generally best seen on sagittal and coronal oblique imaging, the os acromiale is most easily appreciated on axial imaging and it is important to ensure the acromioclavicular joint has been included on the most superior sections of the axial sequence (Fig. 5.8).

Tendinopathic change in the rotator cuff is seen as thickening of the cuff tendon which takes on an inhomogeneous appearance with increased signal on all sequences (Fig. 5.7). The magic angle effect is a well-recognised MR imaging artefact seen as increased signal on short TE sequences in highly organised linear structures such as tendons when there fibrils are lined close to 55° to B_o of the magnet. The fact that

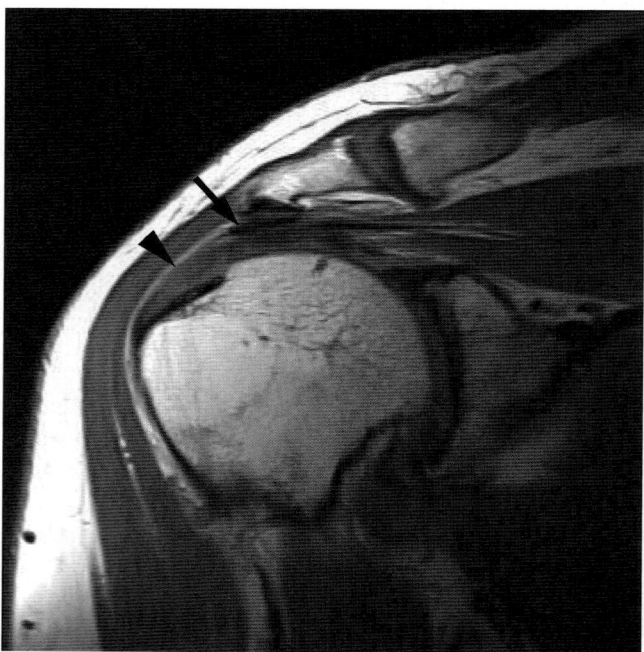

Fig. 5.7 Coronal oblique T1w MR image. Undersurface osteophyte and enthesophyte is seen arising from the acromion and acromioclavicular joint. There is thickening of the coracoacromial ligament (*arrow*). Increased signal is seen in the supraspinatus tendon representing tendinopathic change (*arrowhead*)

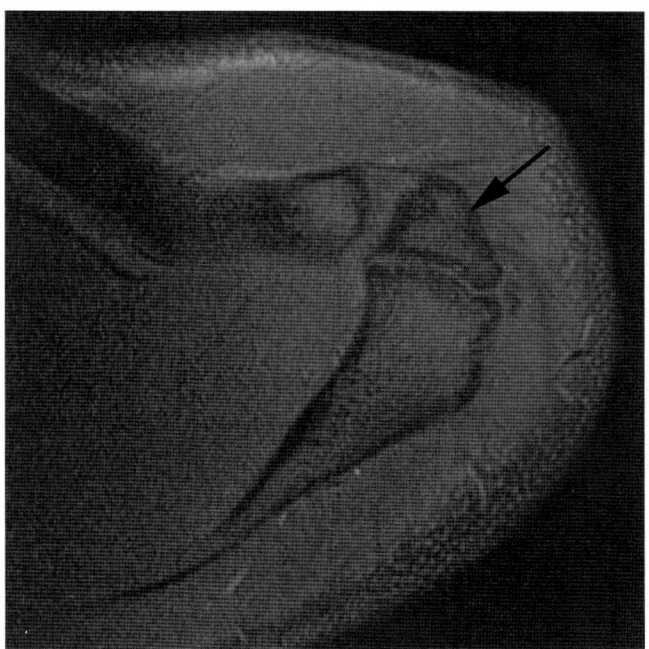

Fig. 5.8 Axial proton density fat-suppressed MR image. This superior axial section is ideal for demonstrating the os acromiale (*arrow*)

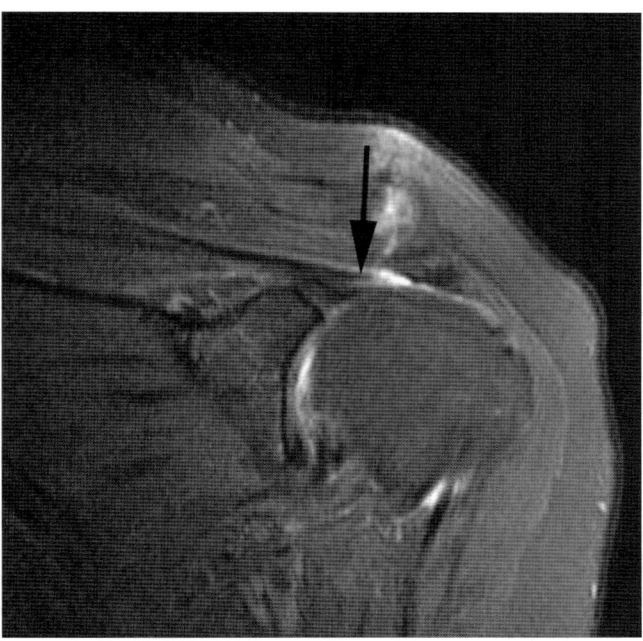

Fig. 5.9 Coronal oblique proton density FS MR image. No supraspinatus tendon is visualised overlying the humeral head due to a full thickness tear. The torn tendon has retracted medially (*arrow*)

the increased signal is seen on all sequences including the long TE sequences implies it is not due to this artefact.

Full thickness tears of the rotator cuff are seen as focal areas of tendon discontinuity (Fig. 5.9). They are easiest to appreciate when the tendon gap is filled with fluid signal intensity but occasionally a gap may be filled with low signal intensity thought to be due to scar tissue [3]. MR arthrography can be considered the gold standard imaging modality for full thickness rotator cuff tears although it is rarely necessary. Contrast will be seen within the subacromial bursa having passed from the glenohumeral joint through the defect in the rotator cuff (Fig. 5.10). For this reason MR arthrography can be helpful in distinguishing a partial thickness tear from a full thickness tear.

Occasionally a rotator cuff tear may communicate with the acromioclavicular joint resulting in cystic expansion of the joint capsule and presenting as a pseudo-tumour on the superior aspect of the ACJ [32]. Here direct communication exists between the glenohumeral joint and ACJ cyst, this has been termed the "geyser" sign.

Articular or bursal partial thickness tears are seen on MR imaging as a focal defect in the tendon filled with joint or bursal fluid (Fig. 5.11a). Granulation tissue may also be present. Fat-suppressed sequences can increase the conspicuity of fluid at the tear site. T2w sequences as opposed to proton density sequences can be particularly helpful in distinguishing increased signal in the tendon due to tendinopathic change from the higher more intense signal seen in a fluid filled tear. If no communication is shown between the intratendinous fluid and either the bursal or articular surface an intrasubstance tear is implied.

MR arthrography offers no advantage over conventional MR imaging for the diagnosis of bursal surface tears. However, contrast extension into articular surface tears may be seen and will improve their conspicuity [33, 34]. MR arthrography can be helpful to distinguish an articular surface partial thickness tear from an intrasubstance tear and a partial thickness tear from a full thickness tear (Fig. 5.12). Visualisation of under surface partial thickness tears may also be improved by scanning the patient with the arm in the ABER position [35]. In this position, the supraspinatus tendon is flaccid and this encourages fluid or contrast from the joint to pass into any undersurface tear (Fig. 5.13). In cases of cuff delamination fluid may be seen tracking proximally along the tendon. In some cases this fluid may extend to the myotendinous junction where a cyst can form within the muscle. This has been termed a "sentinel" cyst and is a secondary sign of the delaminating cuff tear [36] (Fig. 5.11).

MR arthrography is particularly helpful for assessing the structures of the rotator interval and allows demonstration of the components of the biceps pulley mechanism [27, 28, 37]. Bigoni and Chung noted that tears of the rotator interval may not appear as complete disruption of fibres but as thinning, or

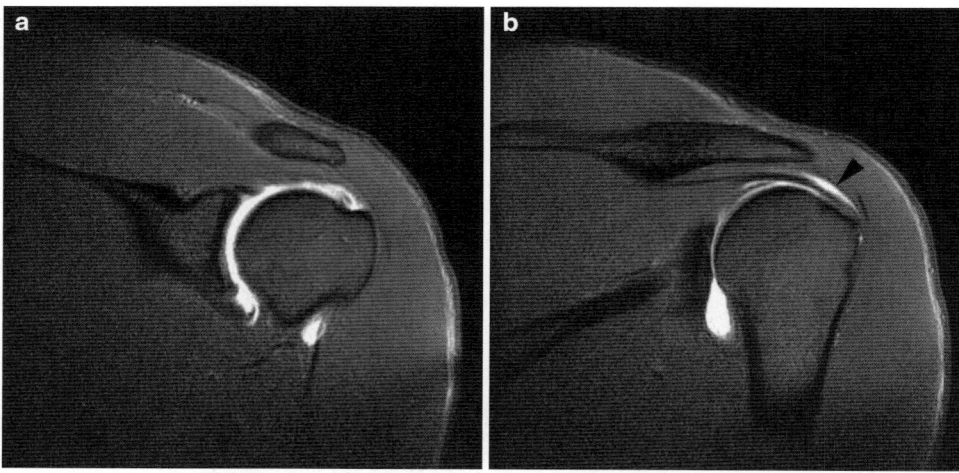

Fig. 5.10 Coronal oblique T1w FS MR arthrogram. (**a**) There is a full thickness tear of supraspinatus. (**b**) A more posterior section shows contrast in the subacromial bursa overlying infraspinatus (*arrowhead*)

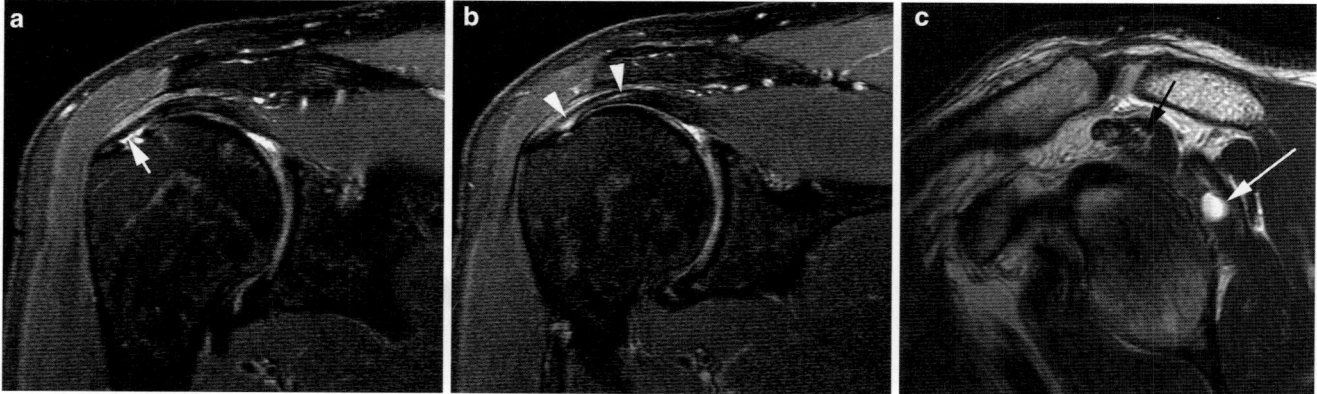

Fig. 5.11 Coronal oblique T2w FS MR images (**a** and **b**) and sagittal T2w MR image (**c**). (**a**) There is an undersurface partial thickness tear of supraspinatus (*arrow*). (**b**) A more posterior image to **a** shows high signal tracking medially along the tendon (*arrowheads*) representing intrasubstance extension of the tear (delamination). (**c**) The sagittal section shows a "sentinel" cyst in the infraspinatus adjacent to the tendon (*white arrow*). Fluid from the tear has tracked along the delaminating tendon to form the intramuscular cyst. Note also the fat atrophy in the supraspinatus muscle (*black arrow*)

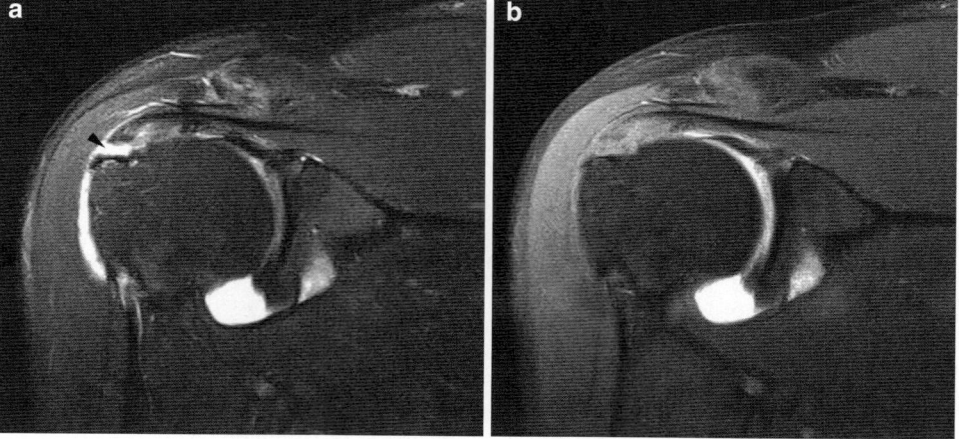

Fig. 5.12 Coronal oblique T2w (**a**) and T1w (**b**) FS MR arthrogram. (**a**) The T2 image shows a tear in the supraspinatus clearly extending to the bursal surface (*arrow*). It is unclear whether the tear is full or partial thickness. (**b**) The T1-weighted image shows there is no passage of contrast from the glenohumeral joint into the subacromial bursa indicating a high grade bursal surface partial thickness tear

Fig. 5.13 Coronal oblique (**a**) and ABER position (**b**) T1w FS MR arthrogram. (**a**) The coronal oblique image shows some minor irregularity to the undersurface of the supraspinatus. (**b**) In the ABER position, the articular surface partial thickness tear with a flap component is better appreciated

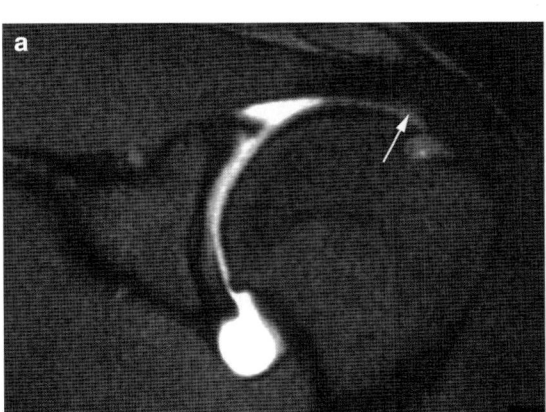
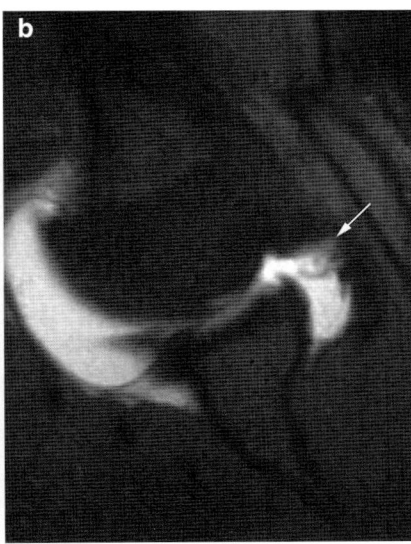

focal discontinuity. They propose that routine MR imaging is unlikely to demonstrate isolated interval tears and optimal imaging requires MR arthrography [37]. Free communication of contrast medium through the interval between the joint and the subacromial bursa, in the absence of a full thickness tear of the cuff tendons, is a useful sign of interval disruption. It is also suggested that subcoracoid bursal collections are a sign of anterior cuff and interval disruption [2].

Calcium deposition within the rotator cuff may be difficult to detect on MR imaging when foci are small. However, larger deposits are seen as decreased signal on all sequences sometimes with surrounding oedema (Fig. 5.14).

In the more chronic stages of rotator cuff tear muscle atrophy may be present. Fat infiltration of the muscles affected can be appreciated on MR imaging along with loss of muscle bulk. Fat atrophy of cuff muscles is an important negative prognostic factor for rotator cuff surgery. Originally the scoring system was developed for assessing fat atrophy on CT by Goutallier et al. (Table 5.5) [38]. However, similar assessments of fat atrophy can be made using MR imaging.

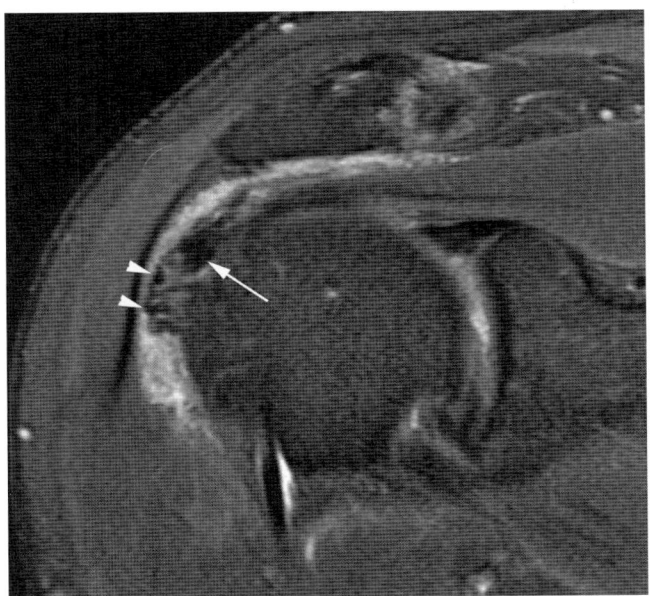

Fig. 5.14 Coronal oblique proton density fat-suppressed MR image. There is extensive calcium deposition in the supraspinatus tendon seen as irregular low reflective material (*arrow*) some of which is extruding into the thickened bursa (*arrowheads*)

Ultrasound

Ultrasound is now widely recognised as a valuable imaging tool for diagnosing rotator cuff pathology. Disadvantages when compared with MR imaging include its operator dependence and inability to assess other important structures of the shoulder including the articular cartilage and the labrum. Nevertheless, it is able to provide high-resolution imaging of the rotator cuff tendons and has the advantage of being able to make a dynamic assessment of the shoulder.

The normal subacromial bursa is identified on ultrasound as a thin low reflective linear structure overlying the rotator cuff tendons. It is separated from the overlying deltoid by a thin hyperechoic line representing the sub-deltoid fat plane (Fig. 5.15). Fluid in the bursa will tend to lie in the more dependent parts of the structure. If excessive probe pressure is used the fluid will be squeezed out of the field of view and not visualised. Bursal inflammation may be seen as more diffuse thickening of the subacromial bursa and both solid and/or fluid elements may be seen with in the bursa (Fig. 5.16a). Dynamic examination is possible and this can help demonstrate fluid in the bursa [39]. A significant disadvantage of ultrasound over MR imaging is its inability to visualise the undersurface of the acromion and ACJ. It is therefore not possible to look for bony structures which may impinge on the bursa and cuff. However, dynamic assessment of the shoulder using ultrasound may help in the demonstration of impingement. A change in the normal convex configuration of the subacromial bursa as it passes under the acromion is said to be a feature of soft tissue impingement and a similar appearance to the bursa may be seen at the coracoacromial ligament, a feature termed the "step sign" by the authors (Fig. 5.17). When the arm is abducted further bunching up of the bursa may be seen as it passes under the coracoacromial ligament or acromion (Fig. 5.16b). As more extreme adduction is achieved the thickened bursa may actually sublux under the coracoacromial arch structures with a palpable clunk. While these signs can be helpful in supporting a diagnosis of impingement they must be correlated with the clinical picture. One small study suggested that while ultrasound was helpful in the diagnosis, 8% of patients showed similar features in the asymptomatic contralateral shoulder [40].

Tendinopathy can also be demonstrated on ultrasound as thickening of the tendon with low reflective change and loss of the normal fibrillar echotexture. It can be helpful to compare the appearances of the tendon with the asymptomatic side [41].

Table 5.5 Goutallier CT scoring of rotator cuff muscle atrophy [38]

Grade 0	No intramuscular fat
Grade 1	Some streaky fat
Grade 2	Fat < muscle
Grade 3	Fat = muscle
Grade 4	Fat > muscle

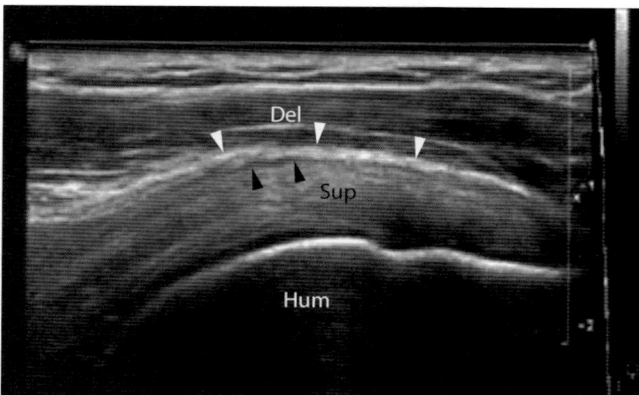

Fig. 5.15 Ultrasound aligned longitudinally along supraspinatus tendon. The normal subacromial bursa is seen as a thin low reflective line (*black arrowheads*) overlying the supraspinatus tendon (Sup). It is separated from the overlying deltoid muscle (Del) by a thin *bright line* representing the subdeltoid fat (*white arrowheads*). *Hum* humerus

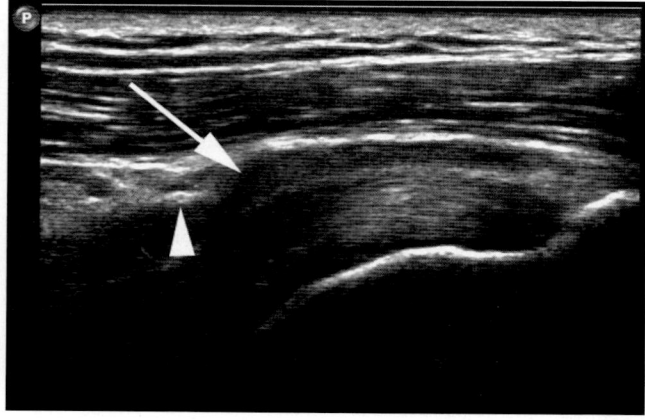

Fig. 5.17 Ultrasound aligned longitudinally along supraspinatus tendon. The thickened subacromial bursa is seen to bulge out (*arrow*) lateral to the coracoacromial ligament (*arrowhead*) forming a step configuration. The step sign

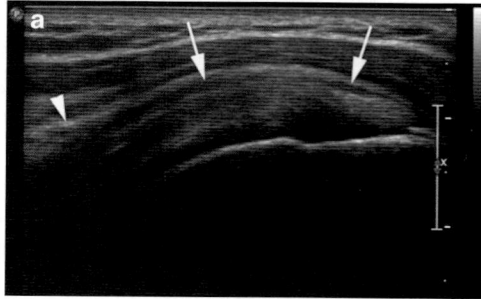 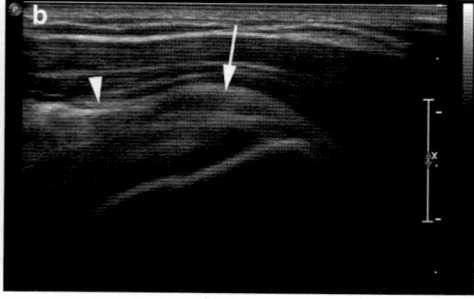

Fig. 5.16 Ultrasound aligned longitudinally along supraspinatus tendon. (**a**) There is a thickened subacromial bursa (*arrows*) indicating bursitis (compare with Fig. 5.15). Note also the heterogeneous appearance to the underlying supraspinatus tendon due to tendinopathic change. The *arrowhead* indicates the coracoacromial ligament. (**b**) When the arm is abducted the bursa bunches up (*arrow*) as it tries to pass under the coracoacromial ligament. A feature of impingement

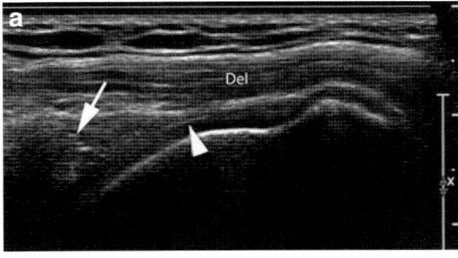
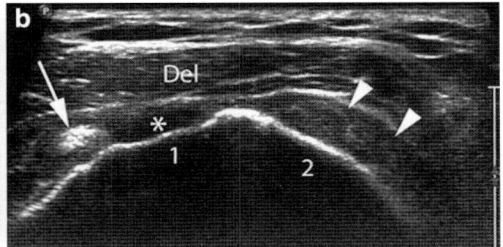

Fig. 5.18 Ultrasound aligned longitudinally (**a**) and transverse (**b**) to the supraspinatus tendon. (**a**) The deltoid muscle (Del) lies directly on the humeral head as it sags through the gap created by the absent supraspinatus. This is a full thickness cuff tear and the retracted tendon is seen on the left of the image (*arrow*). A bright interface from the articular cartilage (*arrowhead*) is seen at one point due to overlying fluid. (**b**) Sectioned transversely across the tear a gap in the rotator cuff is appreciated (*) between the long head of biceps (*arrow*) and the more posterior infraspinatus which is intact (*arrowheads*). The facets on the greater tuberosity for supraspinatus (1) and infraspinatus (2) can be seen

The ultrasound features of rotator cuff tears have been more extensively evaluated. The primary signs of a full thickness cuff tear are:

- Non-visualisation of tendon
- Discontinuity of the tendon filled with fluid, haematoma, prolapsed bursa, peribursal fat or deltoid muscle

Other signs suggestive of a cuff tear include fluid in the subacromial bursa, concavity to the normal convex bursal surface of the cuff and the so-called "cartilage interface sign" where the superficial surface of the articular cartilage on the humeral head is visualised as a brightly echogenic line due to overlying fluid (Fig. 5.18). The conspicuity of a rotator cuff tear can be improved by introducing fluid into the subacromial bursa. However a study by Lee et al. suggests this is generally not necessary [42].

Partial thickness tears of the rotator cuff are more challenging to diagnose. They are seen as abnormal mixed echogenicity or low reflective foci within the tendon substance or as low reflective lesions extending to either the bursal or articular surface (Fig. 5.19). Focal tendon thinning is a further feature [3, 43]. Examination of the myotendinous junction region of infraspinatus and supraspinatus may demonstrate a cyst relating to delamination as can be seen on MR imaging.

Although the structures of the biceps pulley mechanism can be demonstrated on ultrasound the disruption of individual components is difficult to evaluate but biceps subluxation can be detected even when subtle (Fig. 5.20).

Ultrasound is extremely sensitive to the presence of calcification within rotator cuff tendons. The consistency of the calcium can range from a paste like deposition, seen as a mixed echogenicity focus within the tendon with hyperechoic areas, through to more solid calcium flecks seen as brightly echoic foci. Larger deposits of mature calcium hydroxyapatite present a bright surface with posterior acoustic shadowing.

Compared with MR imaging, assessment of fat atrophy using ultrasound is less precise and the subscapularis muscle is not adequately visualised. Nevertheless studies have shown

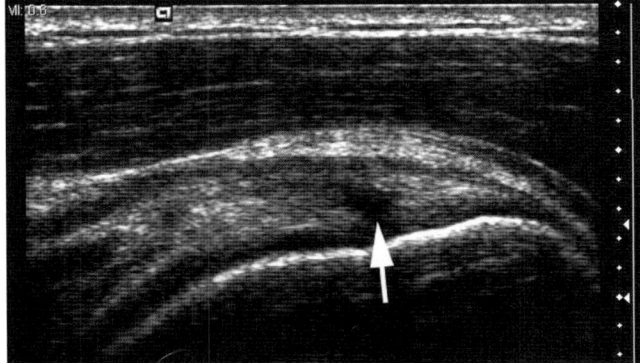

Fig. 5.19 Ultrasound aligned longitudinally along supraspinatus tendon. There is an articular surface partial thickness tear seen as a low reflective area in supraspinatus extending to the articular surface (*arrow*). Note how the normal convex bursal surface is maintained, although some thickening of the subacromial bursa can be appreciated. The location of this tear close to the footprint means it is also known as a "rim-rent" tear

that the grading of fat atrophy in supraspinatus and infraspinatus is feasible and should form part of the routine examination [44, 45].

The Relative Merits of Ultrasound and MR Imaging for Visualising the Rotator Cuff

The choice of modality for imaging of the rotator cuff varies from centre to centre. Both techniques have advantages and disadvantages (Table 5.6). Overall MR imaging is more widely available than ultrasound although this may change in the future as more people become trained to undertake ultrasound. Studies suggest that full thickness tears are reliably shown with both ultrasound and MR imaging and with similar degrees of accuracy [46–48]. Similar accuracy in measuring rotator cuff tears is also found when ultrasound and MR imaging are compared; although both techniques

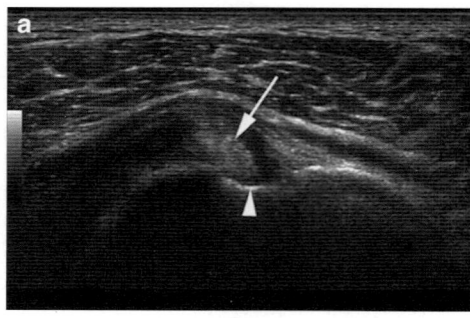 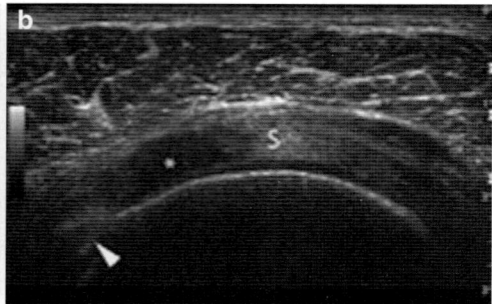

Fig. 5.20 Ultrasound aligned transversely across the bicipital groove (**a**) and more proximally cross the supraspinatus tendon. (**a**) The biceps tendon (*arrow*) is subluxing medially within the bicipital groove (*arrowhead*). (**b**) More proximally a large articular surface (*partial thickness*) tear of supraspinatus is seen (*) as a low reflective area in the tendon between the biceps (*arrowhead*) and remainder of supraspinatus (S)

Table 5.6 Advantages and disadvantages of MR imaging and ultrasound for imaging the rotator cuff and subacromial bursa

	Ultrasound	MR imaging
Advantages	• High resolution demonstrating internal structure of the tendons • Widely available and inexpensive • Easily allows dynamic assessment of the cuff and bursa • Allows assessment of the patient clinically at the time of examination • Portable • Quicker to undertake	• Allows assessment of the entire joint including the articular cartilage labrum • Images more easily understood by referring clinician • Can be done remotely
Disadvantages	• Highly operator dependent • Images can be difficult for referring clinician to understand • Poor visualisation of the undersurface of the coracoacromial arch • Does not visualise other important structures such as the articular cartilage and labrum	• More expensive • Dynamic assessment is more complex • Invasive if combined with arthrography • Maybe contraindicated, e.g. Pacemaker, etc. • Takes longer • Patient may not tolerate so well

tend to underestimate the tear size compared with arthroscopic assessment [48].

Both MR imaging and ultrasound show reduced accuracy in the diagnosis of partial thickness tears but again similar levels of accuracy are seen when the two techniques are compared against each other [49].

Imaging the Postoperative Rotator Cuff (also see Chapter 8)

When imaging the postoperative cuff it is helpful to know what surgical technique has been employed. MR imaging is generally possible with modern suture anchors, but with older metals anchors CT arthrography can be useful. Ultrasound can also useful to demonstrate the integrity of a rotator cuff repair.

Following cuff repair only a minority of cases will demonstrate normal MR imaging [50]; intermediate or low signal in the repaired tendon is a common finding [51]. Susceptibility artefact may be present, and an absence of the normal sub-deltoid fat plane, along with the presence of subdeltoid bursal fluid are normal postoperative findings. MR arthrography is a useful technique for evaluating the rotator cuff but it is important to realise that any repair is not always watertight and leakage of contrast through the cuff is not a sign of repair failure, even for partial thickness tears [50, 51]. Apart from failure of the cuff repair other potential complications include infection, capsulitis and displacement of surgical hardware (Fig. 5.21).

Glenohumeral Instability

Types of Instability and Imaging Modalities

Shoulder instability can be considered in two broad categories.

1. Instability occurring following a traumatic dislocation of the shoulder: This will usually be unidirectional and results from the disruption of the stabilising structures of the glenohumeral joint. This form of instability will generally require surgery.
2. Multidirectional instability occurring without a history of injury: Here there is normally a capsular laxity (which may be congenital) which leads to the instability.

Since the rotator cuff muscles, acting through their tendons, act as a dynamic stabilisers of the joint rotator cuff disruption will lead to shoulder instability. With increasing age the rotator cuff becomes more likely to tear as a result of shoulder dislocation, and in the older athlete with post-traumatic instability the rotator cuff should be the first area of investigation. In this group of patients, ultrasound may be the first line imaging modality following a dislocation if it is available. In the younger patient sustaining a shoulder dislocation it is more likely that there will be a disruption of the static stabilisers. In this situation MR imaging or MR arthrography will be the modality of choice. Because these techniques also allow an assessment of the rotator cuff there is a strong argument that for instability in the athlete they should form the basis of investigation. If for any reason MR imaging is contraindicated, CT arthrography also demonstrates the static stabilisers well and will also identify any full thickness rotator cuff tear [52, 53].

Bone injury to both the humerus and glenoid may be seen following dislocation and conventional radiographs are important. CT allows a multi-planar means of assessing the bone defects, and this may be particularly helpful prior to surgical intervention.

Bankart Lesion and Bankart Variants

Anteroinferior dislocation is the most common pattern of dislocation seen and generally occurs with the arm in the abducted and externally rotated position. The anterior band of the IGHL acts as a check rein to further excursion when the arm is in this position and it is this structure and its attachments that is vulnerable when there is an anteroinferior dislocation.

The IGHL most frequently fails at its attachment to the inferior pole of the glenoid (where it is intimately associated with the labrum). The most common pattern of injury involves detachment of the ligament at glenoid rim along with the labrum and this is referred to as the Bankart lesion (Fig. 5.22a and b). A soft tissue Bankart lesion involves avulsion of the labrum from the glenoid while a bone or osseous Bankart lesion is seen when a fragment of the glenoid rim itself is also avulsed. The presence and size of any bone component to the Bankart is important to record as it will influence the surgical management.

Several variants of the soft tissue Bankart are recognised:

1. The Perthe's lesion

This is a labroligamentous avulsion but the scapular periosteum remains intact and is stripped medially from the anterior

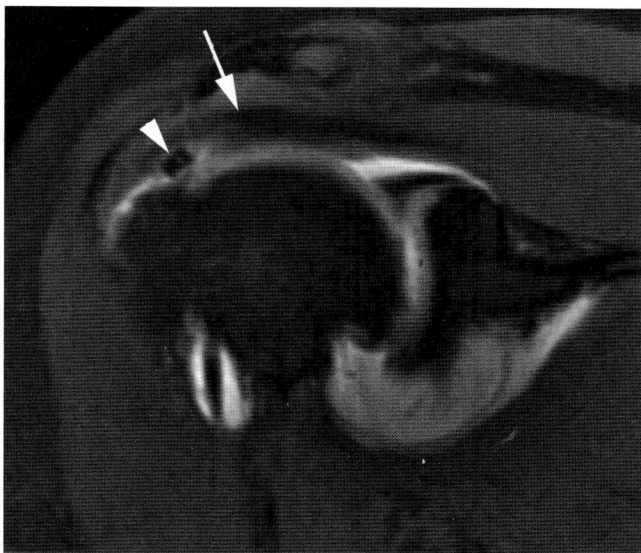

Fig. 5.21 Coronal oblique T1w FS MR arthrogram. The patient has had a rotator cuff repair which has failed with retraction of the cuff (*arrow*). A suture anchor has been displaced into the gap in the cuff (*arrowhead*)

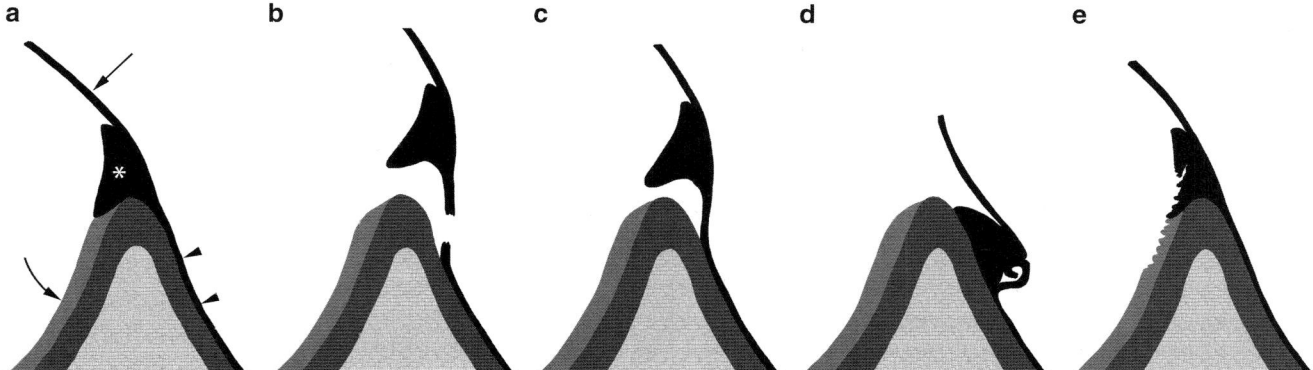

Fig. 5.22 Bankart variants. (**a**) The normal attachment of the labrum (*) and IGHL (*arrow*) to the glenoid is shown diagrammatically (*arrowheads* = periosteum, *curved arrow* = articular cartilage). (**b**) Soft tissue Bankart lesion. Note the tearing of the periosteum. (**c**) Perthe's lesion. The periosteum remains intact. (**d**) ALPSA lesion. (**e**) GLAD lesion

glenoid. The significance of this lesion is that the labrum and ligament may show minimal displacement and the findings on MR imaging can be extremely subtle [54] (Fig. 5.22c).

2. The ALPSA lesion

The ALPSA (anterior labroligamentous periosteal sleeve avulsion) is characterised by the torn labrum being displaced inferomedially by the IGHL and rolling up like a sleeve against the anteroinferior glenoid neck. The labroligamentous complex is displaced medially from the normal position. Healing by fibrosis may occur but the abnormal anatomical location leads to recurrent dislocations (Fig. 5.22d).

3. The GLAD Lesion

The GLAD lesion (glenolabral articular disruption) refers to a partial anteroinferior labral tear associated with a divot in the articular cartilage [55]. This may result from a forced adduction injury and, although it causes pain, it is found in a stable shoulder (Fig. 5.22e).

Less commonly dislocation causes failure of the IGHL at other locations away from the glenoid attachment.

Sites of failure include:

1. The humeral attachment of the ligament. This is known as a HAGL (humeral avulsion of the glenohumeral ligament) lesion. A bone fragment may be avulsed with the ligament and this has been termed a BHAGL (bony humeral avulsion of the glenohumeral ligaments) lesion although this is rare.
2. The mid-substance of the ligament.
3. Very occasionally the glenohumeral ligaments may avulse from the glenoid without associated labral disruption. This has been termed the GAGL (glenoid avulsion the glenohumeral ligament) lesion.

Impaction of the anteroinferior glenoid onto the posterosuperior humerus can cause a compression fracture of the humerus known as a Hill-Sachs fracture. This can increase in size with recurrent dislocations and may cause a dislocated shoulder to lock making relocation extremely difficult. A large Hill-Sachs fracture can also cause locking to occur in extreme abduction and external rotation if the defect engages with the rim of the glenoid.

Posterior Labral Injury

The posterior band of the IGHL will fail in a posterior dislocation and a similar range of injuries to the labrum and glenohumeral ligament is seen.

These include:

1. The reverse Bankart lesion
2. The reverse Hill-Sachs impaction fracture
3. A posterior labrocapsular periosteal sleeve avulsion (POLPSA) lesion, where the posterior capsule and the labrum are stripped away from the glenoid with the periosteum remaining intact
4. The reverse HAGL lesion

Some sporting activities result in chronic damage to the posterior labrum without an acute dislocation. Here recurrent posterior translation of the humeral head on the glenoid, such as occurs in rugby and American football when a tackling opponent is fended off, can lead to chronic posterior labral damage. In this situation posterior subluxation and instability may become a problem [56]. This has also been suggested as the aetiology for the Bennett lesion discussed earlier.

Non-traumatic Multidirectional Instability

Multidirectional instability is usually secondary to capsular laxity. The role of imaging in this situation is limited and its main role is to exclude an acquired cause of the instability. On MR imaging subtle subluxation of the humeral head on the glenoid may be appreciated on the axial views, and occasionally sclerosis at points on the glenoid rim may be detected.

Imaging Findings in Instability

Conventional films are important in the evaluation of any bone injury and remain a key first line investigation. However, appreciation of soft tissue injury requires more sophisticated imaging. While ultrasound is able to visualise the labrum, particularly posteriorly, it struggles to do this consistently. The main role of ultrasound in the investigation of instability is if a rotator cuff tear is the suspected cause. However, in the majority of athletes it is important to look for labroligamentous pathology and MR imaging or MR arthrography are the modalities of choice, particularly given they will also show rotator cuff injury. CT arthrography is useful if MR imaging is contraindicated.

MR Imaging and MR Arthrography

Using fat-suppressed imaging, such as may be used in MR arthrography, can make it difficult to detect small bony components of any Bankart lesion. It is useful to include a non-fat-suppressed axial series as part of the protocol. In the soft tissue Bankart the labrum is completely detached from bony glenoid and fluid or contrast will be seen to separate the labrum from the glenoid (Fig. 5.23). The ALPSA lesion is demonstrated on axial and coronal MR imaging where the displaced anterior labrum will be seen lying medially on the neck of the glenoid (Fig. 5.24). In the chronic situation, variable amounts of fibrosis may be seen. The Perthe's lesion is perhaps the most difficult to identify because in this situation the IGHL and labrum occupy a normal position relative to the underlying glenoid. There may be haemorrhage/oedema at the IGHL attachment site but the most characteristic sign is the presence of subtle linear increased signal intensity at the base of the labrum. This is easier to detect on MR arthrography. MR imaging in the ABER position can be particularly helpful in improving visualisation by applying traction to the labrum through the IGHL opening up the site of detachment (Fig. 5.25). This can also be helpful when looking for the GLAD lesion. When a Bankart lesion is detected it is important to look for associated abnormalities such as a Hill-Sach humeral fracture or articular cartilage damage to be glenoid fossa.

The HAGL lesion can be difficult to detect on conventional MR imaging in the absence of a joint effusion and MR arthrography is particularly useful here. The high false-positive rate has been emphasised [57]. Coronal images normally demonstrate a "U" configuration to the inferior glenohumeral ligaments as they form the axillary pouch. In cases of HAGL lesion, the humeral attachment of the "U" is torn allowing the IGHL to lie more inferiorly giving the ligament a "J"-shaped configuration [58] (Fig. 5.26).

In many cases, conventional MR imaging is able to effectively image shoulder instability, but MR arthrography does increase the conspicuity of the associated lesions and while the literature varies as to whether it is more accurate or not, it can certainly help increase diagnostic confidence. In the context of sports injuries, it is worth noting that Magee et al. showed that in a population of athletes (baseball players) higher diagnostic accuracy was achieved with MR arthrography when compared with conventional MR imaging; the added accuracy of the arthrographic technique was not reproduced to the same extent in a general population [59]. More recently another article has shown that even compared with 3T conventional MR imaging, MR arthrography shows significantly increased sensitivity for the detection of anterior labral tears (along with partial thickness articular surface supraspinatus tears and SLAP tears) [60].

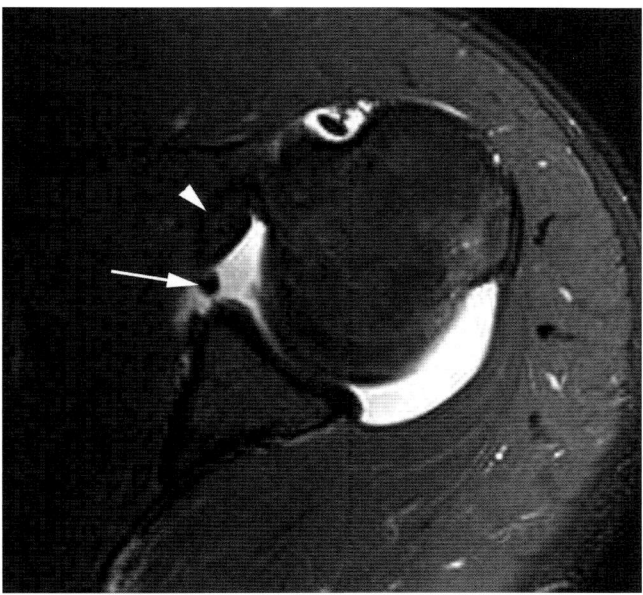

Fig. 5.23 Axial T1w FS MR arthrogram. The labrum is detached from the anterior glenoid (*arrow*) along with the associated anterior band of the IGHL (*arrowhead*). A soft tissue Bankart lesion

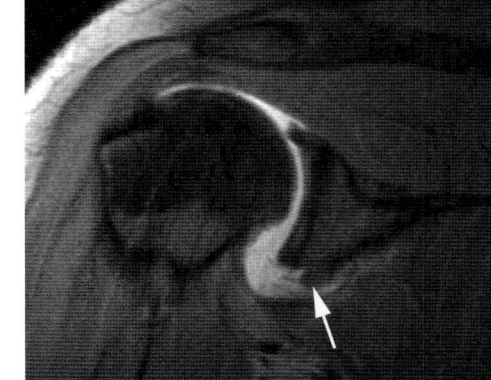
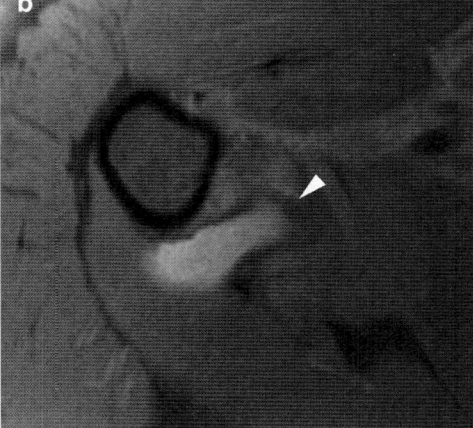

Fig. 5.24 Coronal oblique (**a**) and axial position (**b**) T1w FS MR arthrogram. The abnormally inferior and medially located labrum (*arrow*) and associated IGHL (*arrowhead*) can be appreciated in keeping with an ALPSA lesion

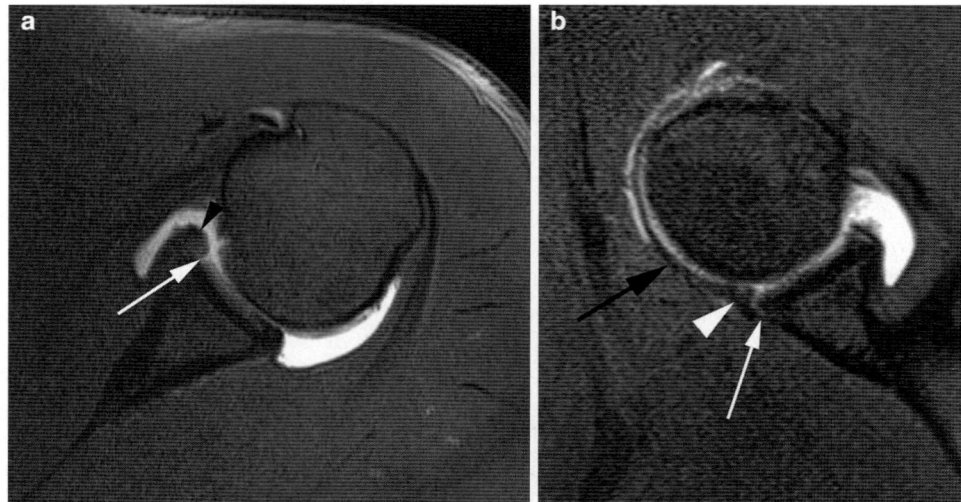

Fig. 5.25 Axial (**a**) and ABER position (**b**) T1w FS MR arthrogram. (**a**) The anterior labrum has an abnormally blunted appearance (*arrowhead*) and there is a fissure between the articular cartilage and the labrum (*arrow*) not normally seen as a normal variant in the anteroinferior labrum. (**b**) The appearances of a Perthe's lesion are much more clearly seen in the ABER position with separation of the labrum (*arrowhead*) from the glenoid due to traction on the anterior IGHL (*black arrow*). Note the intact periosteum (*white arrow*)

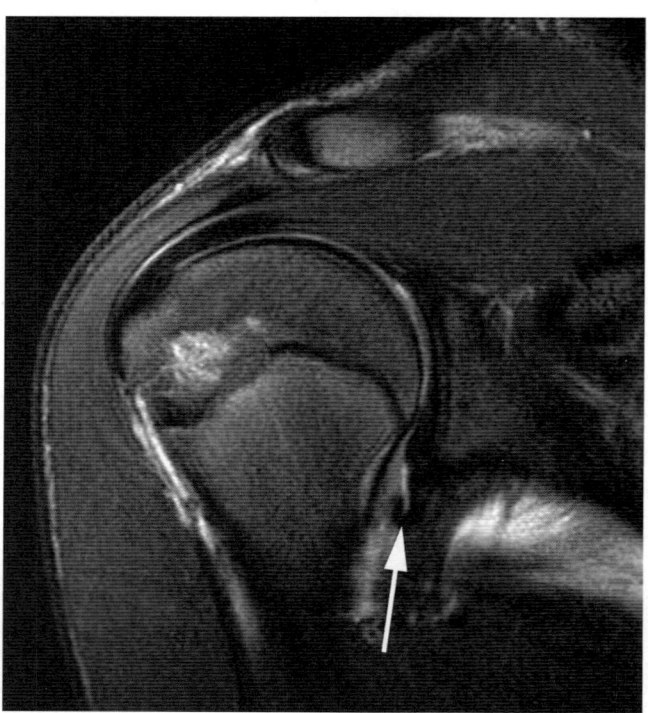

Fig. 5.26 Coronal oblique T2w FS MR image. There is disruption of the anterior band of the IGHL at it humeral origin. The ligament (*arrow*) has displaced inferiorly with a "J" configuration typical for a HAGL lesion

CT and CT Arthrography

CT can be useful for evaluating any bony components to a Bankart lesion and also for accurately assessing the size and location of any Hill-Sach fracture. While in itself it is not helpful for soft tissue Bankart lesions CT arthrography has been extensively used in investigating instability. Although studies tend to suggest that CT arthrography is not as accurate as MR arthrography for diagnosing instability lesions, it does present a viable alternative when MR imaging is contraindicated.

Imaging the Shoulder After Stabilisation Surgery

Following labral repair susceptibility artefact may be seen at the repair site reflecting the presence of suture anchors. There is often capsular thickening present which may be irregular and nodular [51]. Complications include recurrent instability and this may be due either to retearing of the labroligamentous complex or the result of an inadequate repair. The aim of the surgical repair should be to restore the normal anatomical labral alignment. In cases of retearing, the disruption may not occur at the same site as the original surgery. Following the repair, this area may no longer represent a weak point and the point of disruption may move elsewhere, so a HAGL lesion may be seen on re-injury after a successful Bankart repair [61].

SLAP Lesions

The SLAP lesion (Superior Labral Anterior to Posterior) lesion describes a tear of the superior labrum, usually involving the biceps anchor, which may extend into the adjacent labrum anterior and posterior to the biceps tendon, or even into other associated anatomical structures. The young throwing athlete is typically affected presenting with pain, clicking and instability; and the mechanisms of injury include repetitive overhead activity such as is seen in throwing athletes and swimmers. The peel-back mechanism described under the internal impingement section of this chapter is now recognised as important in the aetiology of at least a subset of SLAP lesions, typically giving rise to a posterosuperior labral tear [62]. However, it may well be that different mechanisms of injury result in different types of lesion.

Types of SLAP Lesion

SLAP lesions were first classified into four types based on the work of Snyder et al. [63]. This classification only considered the extent and morphology of the tear as it involved the superior labrum and biceps anchor. It included the type I lesion, seen as fraying of the superior labrum without frank tear or biceps tear. This is a common finding and in many cases is probably age related and seen in asymptomatic subjects. The type II lesion is the most frequent type seen and is associated with tearing of the labrum and biceps anchor from the glenoid. These have been further subdivided into three subgroups according to the location of the labral tear [64]. The type IIA SLAP lesion involves tearing of the anterosuperior labrum while the IIB is a tear of the posterosuperior labrum. The type IIC tear extends both anterior and posterior to the biceps anchor. The location of the subtype of type II tear relates to the mechanism of injury. The posterosuperior (IIB) tear is seen as a result of the peel-back mechanism seen in throwing athletes with GIRD; while the anterosuperior (IIA) tear is commonly associated with articular surface partial thickness tears at the anterior supraspinatus (SLAC lesion). Type III and IV lesions refer to tears with a bucket handle configuration; the type III lesion being a tear of the superior labrum while the type IV extends into the biceps.

Subsequently the classification scheme has been widened to include the so-called extended SLAP tears where the labral tear extends into other structures [65, 66]. A summary of the classification system is given in Table 5.7. Types I to IV remain the same as the original classification system described above. Along with type VI they represent varying degrees of detachment and displacement of the superior labrum, with or without extension into the biceps, and are a cause of shoulder pain that may require surgery. Types III, IV and VI involve displaced labral fragments (bucket handle type configuration).

The remaining types represent tears extending into other structures and can be referred to as extended SLAP tears. Other involved structures may include the anteroinferior labrum (type V), middle glenohumeral ligament (VII) or posteroinferior labrum (VIII). Depending on the nature of the extended tear these may be causes of shoulder instability and will often require surgery.

Table 5.7 Classification of SLAP lesions [63, 64, 67, 75]

Type	Description
I	Fraying of the superior labrum. Seen as part of the normal aging process and may be an incidental finding
II	Tear of the biceps/labral complex. Subdivided into:
	(A) Tear extending into the anterosuperior labrum
	(B) Tear extending into the posterosuperior labrum
	(C) Tear extending into both the anterior and posterior superior labrum
III	Bucket handle tear
IV	Bucket handle tear which extends into biceps tendon
V	SLAP tear extending anteroinferiorly into a Bankart lesion
VI	Flap tear, probably due to a bucket handle tear where the handle has torn
VII	SLAP tear extending into the middle glenohumeral ligament
VIII	SLAP tear extending posteroinferiorly into a reverse Bankart lesion
IX	Tearing of the labrum throughout its circumference
X	SLAP tear associated with a rotator interval tear through SGHL

This extensive classification can seem intimidating and is the source of some confusion, but the key point when reporting is to be sure to describe the extent of the SLAP tear, extension into the biceps and any other structures, and any flipped or free bucket handle component. It is usually easier and more reliable to communicate these observations by describing them rather than worrying about the particular classification.

Imaging Findings

SLAP lesions can be diagnosed with reasonable accuracy using conventional MR imaging but the literature would suggest that MR arthrography is superior, especially in patients with chronic instability [67]. The key feature of a SLAP lesion on MR arthrography is the tracking of contrast into the labral tear (Fig. 5.27). This contrast may extend into the biceps tendon depending on the configuration of the tear. A further feature may be a separated labral fragment as seen in types 3, 4 and 6 (Fig. 5.28). Associated structures should be examined. In particular, extension into the middle glenohumeral ligament, Type VII, may be seen (Fig. 5.27b) or associated inferior labral injury. Associated rotator cuff or interval tears may also be seen.

It is important to recognise the range of normal variants seen in the superior labral region. In particular a sublabral sulcus (discussed earlier) needs to be distinguished from labral tearing. If more than one focus of linear high signal is seen in the labrum it is clearly an indication of the tear rather than a sulcus. It is also important to look at the alignment of any high signal; in the case of a sulcus it should be seen extending medially paralleling the glenoid rim. In the past it has been

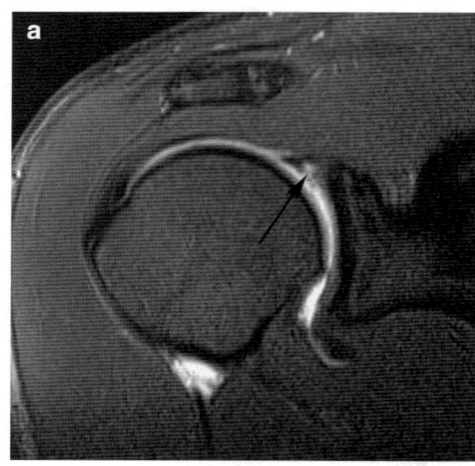 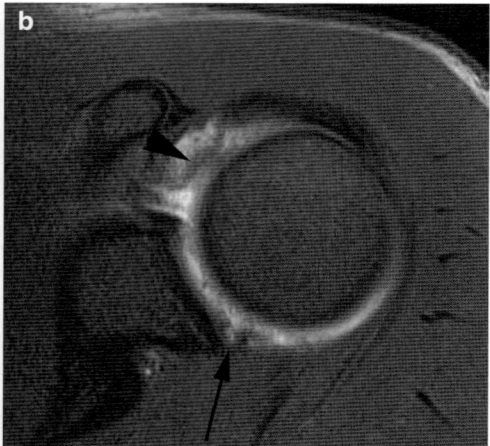

Fig. 5.27 Coronal oblique (**a**) and axial position (**b**) T1w FS MR arthrogram. (**a**) Contrast is seen tracking into the superior labrum (*arrow*) in keeping with a SLAP lesion. Note the irregular margins and wide labral defect in contrast to the appearances of a sublabral sulcus (compare with Fig. 5.1). (**b**) The axial image shows extension of the SLAP tear posteriorly (*arrow*). There is also abnormal increased signal, thickening and irregularity to the middle glenohumeral ligament reflecting extension of the tear into this structure making this a type VII SLAP tear

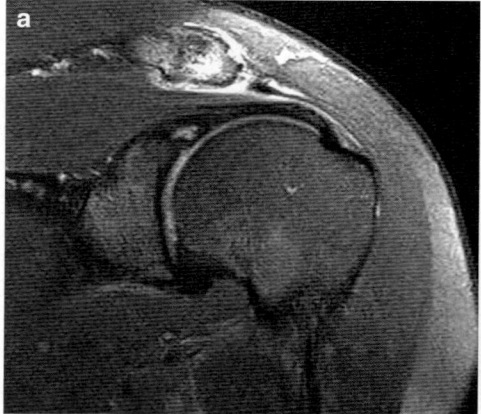 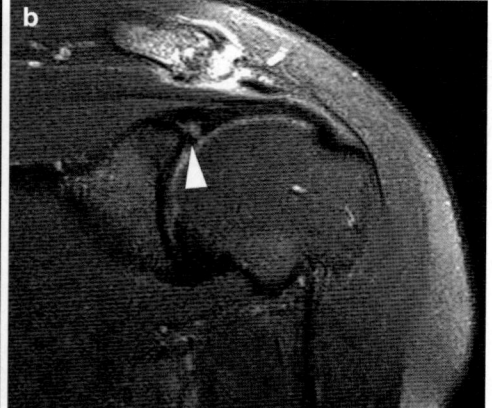

Fig. 5.28 Coronal oblique T1w FS MR arthrogram. (**a**) There is a SLAP lesion with abnormal contrast tracking into the superior labrum. (**b**) A slightly more anterior section shows a separated fragment of labrum (*arrowhead*) which could be followed further on contiguous images before becoming one again with the labrum. Surgically, this was seen to represent the bucket handle flap of a type III SLAP lesion

suggested that linear high signal extending posterior to the biceps anchor is a sign of tear rather than sulcus but a study comparing MR arthrography with arthroscopy found this was unhelpful, as was the shape of any high signal [68]. This study did find that both tearing of the anterosuperior labrum and anteroposterior extension of the high signal on axial images were useful findings seen in SLAP lesions but not sulci.

A second pitfall relates to the oblique anterior course taken by the biceps after it has arisen from the labrum/glenoid. This results in the appearance of a normal cleft which may be seen between the biceps and the labrum and on MR arthrography will contain contrast and should not be mistaken for a tear.

A diagnostic clue to there being a SLAP lesion can be the presence of a paralabral cyst. These may not fill with gadolinium on MR arthrogram but are well shown on T2w imaging and may occasionally be picked up on ultrasound. They usually communicate with the labral tear and often extend into the spinoglenoid notch where they may cause compression of the supraspinatus nerve and associated infraspinatus muscle atrophy. If the cyst extends very anteriorly there may also be atrophy of the supraspinatus.

Miscellaneous Conditions

The Biceps Tendon

The biceps tendon is susceptible to both chronic repetitive injury and to acute disruption. As it passes through the rotator interval the biceps tendon is susceptible to external impingement in the same way as the remainder of the rotator cuff and this may lead to tendinopathy or tearing. There may be associated tenosynovitis. Acute disruption of the biceps tendon most often occurs in association with proximal humeral fractures.

Biceps instability resulting from pulley lesions or rotator interval tears is also associated with biceps tendinopathy. Throwing athletes may also experience biceps tendinopathy resulting from the peel-back mechanism.

MR imaging and ultrasound will readily identify biceps rupture and tendinopathy although ultrasound will not reliably demonstrate the intracapsular portion of the tendon and changes here will be missed. It is important to note that when fluid is seen in the biceps tendon sheath on ultrasound or MR imaging it does not automatically equate to tenosynovitis as the sheath communicates with the joint capsule and any joint effusion will also be seen around the biceps tendon.

Adhesive Capsulitis

Adhesive capsulitis has also been termed frozen shoulder. Contraction of the joint capsule results in severely limited movement of the glenohumeral joint. The condition may arise spontaneously and is often preceded by trauma or surgery. The condition is easily identified at arthrography where the low capacity of the joint will be appreciated as contrast is introduced. Indeed, one treatment for adhesive capsulitis is a distension arthrogram where the capsule is distended with fluid to the point of rupture. It is currently thought that the condition has an autoimmune aetiology.

Ultrasound may show no anatomical abnormality although during the dynamic stages of the examination the condition can often be diagnosed due to the severe limitation to movement at the glenohumeral joint and absence of other causes. Synovitis and a joint effusion may be seen. One study has suggested echogenic material can be seen in the rotator interval and this may be hypervascular, although in the authors' experience this is not a reliable sign [69]. Findings on MR imaging include thickening of the IGHL and capsular structures along with synovial hypertrophy in the axillary pouch (Fig. 5.29). Jung et al. suggest a thickening of the axillary pouch capsule and synovium in excess of 3 mm as helpful in the diagnosis on MR arthrography, although on conventional MR imaging 4 mm may be a better cut off [70, 71]. Soft tissue thickening in the rotator interval may also be seen and obliteration of the fat triangle behind the coracoid process on sagittal oblique imaging is reported as a helpful sign [72].

The Acromioclavicular Joint

The ACJ is vulnerable to acute injury in contact sports and injury ranges from sprains of the acromioclavicular ligament to complete disruption of the joint resulting in separation.

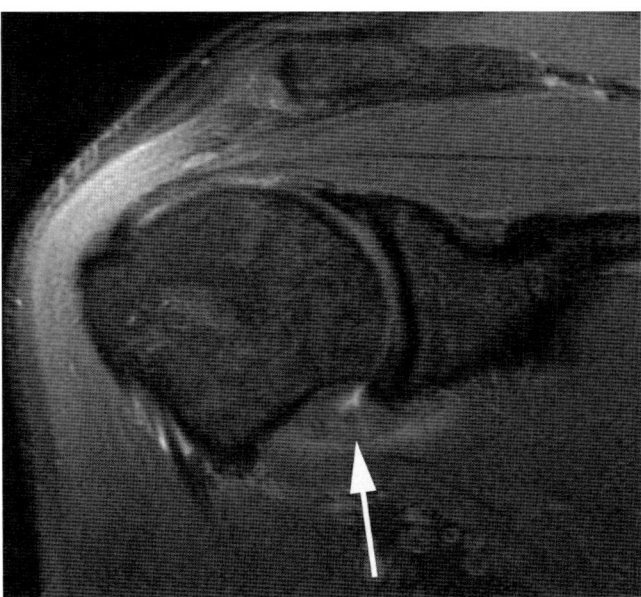

Fig. 5.29 Coronal oblique T2w FS MR image. There is gross thickening of the synovium and capsule of the axillary recess with loss of capsular volume. The findings are typical for adhesive capsulitis

Integrity of the joint is maintained by acromioclavicular ligaments along with ligaments running from the coracoid process to the acromion and clavicle. Progressive disruption of these ligaments results in varying degrees of acromioclavicular separation:

Stage 1: A sprain of the acromioclavicular ligaments without tear. Radiographs will be unremarkable but the ligaments will show abnormal oedematous change on MR imaging along with a joint effusion. A joint effusion and capsular thickening may be noted on ultrasound.

Stage 2: Disruption of the acromioclavicular ligaments with intact coracoclavicular ligaments. Radiographs will show some separation of the ACJ without widening of the gap between the coracoid and clavicle. Ligament disruption will be demonstrated on ultrasound and MR imaging.

Stage 3: Disruption of both the acromioclavicular and coracoclavicular ligaments. Widening of the ACJ is more marked and there will be inferior subluxation of the acromion with widening of the coracoclavicular space seen on both plain film and MR imaging.

Conventional radiographs of the contralateral shoulder can be helpful for comparison and weight-bearing films can be particularly useful to distinguish between the different stages of ligament disruption on plain film.

Osteolysis of the lateral clavicle may be seen following trauma such as described above. It may also occur as a consequence of repetitive low-grade injury and is classically described in weightlifters. The osteolysis will be demonstrated on plain films (Fig. 5.30), but changes are also described on

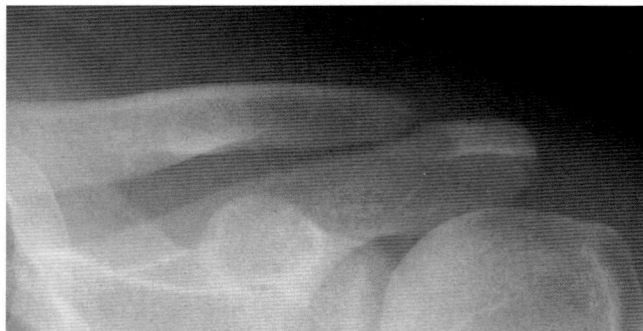

Fig. 5.30 AP radiograph of the ACJ. There is resorption of the lateral end of the clavicle in this boxer with clavicular osteolysis

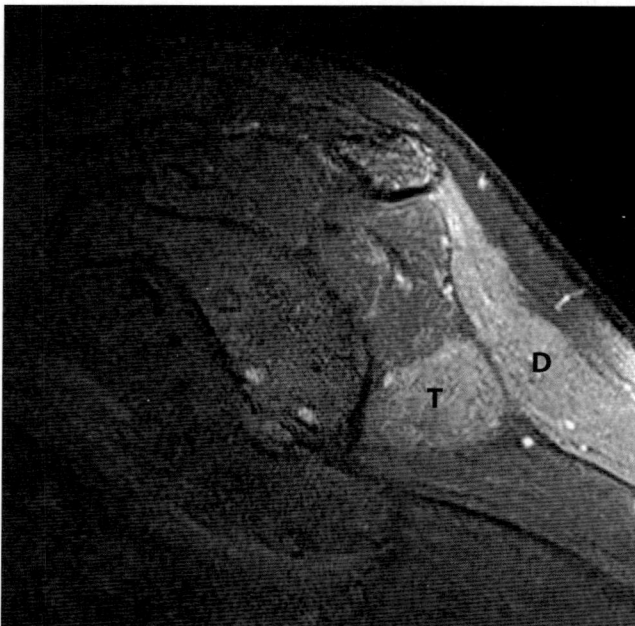

Fig. 5.31 Sagittal oblique T2w FS MR image. There is abnormal increased signal seen in the deltoid (D) and teres minor (T) muscle bellies when compared with the adjacent musculature. This developed in a throwing athlete as a result of repetitive stretching leading to the build up of scar tissue in the quadrilateral space compromising the axillary nerve

MR imaging where findings include soft tissue swelling, bone marrow oedema in the distal clavicle and cortical irregularity [73].

Nerve Entrapments

Entrapment of the suprascapular nerve by a paralabral cyst in the spinoglenoid notch has already been mentioned as an occasional feature of SLAP lesions. There will be denervation change in infraspinatus and, with more proximal entrapment, supraspinatus. This is seen as fat atrophy or in the more acute stages as oedematous change, within the muscles (Fig. 5.31). Occasionally a similar syndrome can arise in athletes as a result of repetitive stretching. Entrapment of the axillary nerve (supplying the deltoid and teres minor) can occur in the quadrilateral space. This space is bounded superiorly by the teres minor, inferiorly by the teres major, laterally by the humerus and medially by the long head of triceps. The axillary nerve passes through the space along with the posterior circumflex humeral vessels. The most common cause of entrapment here is trauma, particularly following humeral fracture. However, hypertrophy of the teres minor muscle can also produce axillary nerve entrapment. Inferior glenoid labral cysts associated with labral tearing have also been described in the quadrilateral space [74].

References

1. Burkhart SS, Esch JC, Jolson RS (1993) The rotator crescent and rotator cable: an anatomic description of the shoulder's "suspension bridge". Arthroscopy 9(6):611–616
2. Grainger AJ, Tirman PF, Elliott JM, Kingzett-Taylor A, Steinbach LS, Genant HK (2000) MR anatomy of the subcoracoid bursa and the association of subcoracoid effusion with tears of the anterior rotator cuff and the rotator interval. AJR Am J Roentgenol 174(5):1377–1380
3. Campbell RS, Dunn A (2008) External impingement of the shoulder. Semin Musculoskelet Radiol 12(2):107–126
4. Fritz RC (2002) Magnetic resonance imaging of sports-related injuries to the shoulder: impingement and rotator cuff. Radiol Clin North Am 40(2):217–234, vi
5. Neer CS 2nd (1983) Impingement lesions. Clin Orthop Relat Res (173):70–77
6. Bigliani LU, Levine WN (1997) Subacromial impingement syndrome. J Bone Joint Surg 79(12):1854–1868
7. Morrison DS, Frogameni AD, Woodworth P (1997) Non-operative treatment of subacromial impingement syndrome. J Bone Joint Surg 79(5):732–737
8. Uhthoff HK, Hammond DI, Sarkar K, Hooper GJ, Papoff WJ (1988) The role of the coracoacromial ligament in the impingement syndrome. A clinical, radiological and histological study. Int Orthop 12(2):97–104
9. Ozaki J, Fujimoto S, Nakagawa Y, Masuhara K, Tamai S (1988) Tears of the rotator cuff of the shoulder associated with pathological changes in the acromion. A study in cadavera. J Bone Joint Surg 70(8):1224–1230
10. Neer CS 2nd (1984) Rotator cuff tears associated with os acromiale. J Bone Joint Surg 66(8):1320–1321
11. Jobe FW, Kvitne RS, Giangarra CE (1989) Shoulder pain in the overhand or throwing athlete. The relationship of anterior instability and rotator cuff impingement. Orthop Rev 18(9):963–975
12. Mehta S, Gimbel JA, Soslowsky LJ (2003) Etiologic and pathogenetic factors for rotator cuff tendinopathy. Clin Sports Med 22(4):791–812
13. Grainger AJ (2008) Internal impingement syndromes of the shoulder. Semin Musculoskelet Radiol 12(2):127–135
14. Walch G, Boileau P, Noel E, Donnell S (1992) Impingement of the deep surface of the supraspinatus tendon on the posterosuperior glenoid rim: an arthroscopic study. J Shoulder Elbow Surg 1:238–245
15. Jobe CM (1995) Posterior superior glenoid impingement: expanded spectrum. Arthroscopy 11(5):530–536

16. Jobe CM (1996) Superior glenoid impingement. Current concepts. Clin Orthop Relat Res (330):98–107
17. Burkhart SS, Morgan CD, Kibler WB (2003) The disabled throwing shoulder: spectrum of pathology Part I: pathoanatomy and biomechanics. Arthroscopy 19(4):404–420
18. Halbrecht JL, Tirman P, Atkin D (1999) Internal impingement of the shoulder: comparison of findings between the throwing and nonthrowing shoulders of college baseball players. Arthroscopy 15(3):253–258
19. Burkhart SS, Lo IK (2007) The cam effect of the proximal humerus: its role in the production of relative capsular redundancy of the shoulder. Arthroscopy 23(3):241–246
20. Kaplan LD, McMahon PJ, Towers J, Irrgang JJ, Rodosky MW (2004) Internal impingement: findings on magnetic resonance imaging and arthroscopic evaluation. Arthroscopy 20(7):701–704
21. Giaroli EL, Major NM, Higgins LD (2005) MRI of internal impingement of the shoulder. AJR Am J Roentgenol 185(4):925–929
22. Gerber C, Sebesta A (2000) Impingement of the deep surface of the subscapularis tendon and the reflection pulley on the anterosuperior glenoid rim: a preliminary report. J Shoulder Elbow Surg 9(6):483–490
23. Habermeyer P, Magosch P, Pritsch M, Scheibel MT, Lichtenberg S (2004) Anterosuperior impingement of the shoulder as a result of pulley lesions: a prospective arthroscopic study. J Shoulder Elbow Surg 13(1):5–12
24. Post M, Silver R, Singh M (1983) Rotator cuff tear. Diagnosis and treatment. Clin Orthop Relat Res (173):78–91
25. Ellman H (1990) Diagnosis and treatment of incomplete rotator cuff tears. Clin Orthop Relat Res (254):64–74
26. Le Huec JC, Schaeverbeke T, Moinard M, Kind M, Diard F, Dehais J et al (1996) Traumatic tear of the rotator interval. J Shoulder Elbow Surg 5(1):41–46
27. Morag Y, Jacobson JA, Shields G, Rajani R, Jamadar DA, Miller B et al (2005) MR arthrography of rotator interval, long head of the biceps brachii, and biceps pulley of the shoulder. Radiology 235(1):21–30
28. Weishaupt D, Zanetti M, Tanner A, Gerber C, Hodler J (1999) Lesions of the reflection pulley of the long biceps tendon. MR arthrographic findings. Invest Radiol 34(7):463–469
29. Walch G, Nove-Josserand L, Levigne C, Renaud E (1994) Tears of the supraspinatus tendon associated with "hidden" lesions of the rotator interval. J Shoulder Elbow Surg 3(6):353–360
30. Bennett WF (2001) Subscapularis, medial, and lateral head coracohumeral ligament insertion anatomy. Arthroscopic appearance and incidence of "hidden" rotator interval lesions. Arthroscopy 17(2):173–180
31. Morag Y, Jacobson JA, Miller B, De Maeseneer M, Girish G, Jamadar D (2006) MR imaging of rotator cuff injury: what the clinician needs to know. Radiographics 26(4):1045–1065
32. Tshering Vogel DW, Steinbach LS, Hertel R, Bernhard J, Stauffer E, Anderson SE (2005) Acromioclavicular joint cyst: nine cases of a pseudotumor of the shoulder. Skeletal Radiol 34(5):260–265
33. Palmer WE, Brown JH, Rosenthal DI (1993) Rotator cuff: evaluation with fat-suppressed MR arthrography. Radiology 188(3):683–687
34. Flannigan B, Kursunoglu-Brahme S, Snyder S, Karzel R, Del Pizzo W, Resnick D (1990) MR arthrography of the shoulder: comparison with conventional MR imaging. AJR Am J Roentgenol 155(4):829–832
35. Tirman PF, Bost FW, Steinbach LS, Mall JC, Peterfy CG, Sampson TG et al (1994) MR arthrographic depiction of tears of the rotator cuff: benefit of abduction and external rotation of the arm. Radiology 192(3):851–856
36. Kassarjian A, Torriani M, Ouellette H, Palmer WE (2005) Intramuscular rotator cuff cysts: association with tendon tears on MRI and arthroscopy. AJR Am J Roentgenol 185(1):160–165
37. Bigoni BJ, Chung CB. MR imaging of the rotator cuff interval. Magn Reson Imaging Clin North Am 12(1):61–73, vi
38. Goutallier D, Postel JM, Lavau L, Bernageau J (1999) Impact of fatty degeneration of the supraspinatus and infraspinatus muscles on the prognosis of surgical repair of the rotator cuff. Rev Chir Orthop Reparatrice Appar Mot 85(7):668–676
39. Farin PU, Jaroma H, Harju A, Soimakallio S (1990) Shoulder impingement syndrome: sonographic evaluation. Radiology 176(3):845–849
40. Bureau NJ, Beauchamp M, Cardinal E, Brassard P (2006) Dynamic sonography evaluation of shoulder impingement syndrome. AJR Am J Roentgenol 187(1):216–220
41. Beggs I (2004) Alternative imaging techniques. Magn Reson Imaging Clin N Am 12(1):75–96, vi
42. Lee HS, Joo KB, Park CK, Kim YS, Jeong WK, Park DW et al (2002) Sonography of the shoulder after arthrography (arthrosonography): preliminary results. J Clin Ultrasound 30(1):23–32
43. van Holsbeeck MT, Kolowich PA, Eyler WR, Craig JG, Shirazi KK, Habra GK et al (1995) US depiction of partial-thickness tear of the rotator cuff. Radiology 197(2):443–446
44. Khoury V, Cardinal E, Brassard P (2008) Atrophy and fatty infiltration of the supraspinatus muscle: sonography versus MRI. AJR Am J Roentgenol 190(4):1105–1111
45. Strobel K, Hodler J, Meyer DC, Pfirrmann CW, Pirkl C, Zanetti M (2005) Fatty atrophy of supraspinatus and infraspinatus muscles: accuracy of US. Radiology 237(2):584–589
46. Hodler J, Terrier B, von Schulthess GK, Fuchs WA (1991) MRI and sonography of the shoulder. Clin Radiol 43(5):323–327
47. Swen WA, Jacobs JW, Algra PR, Manoliu RA, Rijkmans J, Willems WJ et al (1999) Sonography and magnetic resonance imaging equivalent for the assessment of full-thickness rotator cuff tears. Arthritis Rheum 42(10):2231–2238
48. Bryant L, Shnier R, Bryant C, Murrell GA (2002) A comparison of clinical estimation, ultrasonography, magnetic resonance imaging, and arthroscopy in determining the size of rotator cuff tears. J Shoulder Elbow Surg 11(3):219–224
49. Kenn W, Hufnagel P, Muller T, Gohlke F, Bohm D, Kellner M et al (2000) Arthrography, ultrasound and MRI in rotator cuff lesions: a comparison of methods in partial lesions and small complete ruptures. Rofo 172(3):260–266
50. Spielmann AL, Forster BB, Kokan P, Hawkins RH, Janzen DL (1999) Shoulder after rotator cuff repair: MR imaging findings in asymptomatic individuals – initial experience. Radiology 213(3):705–708
51. Ruzek KA, Bancroft LW, Peterson JJ (2006) Postoperative imaging of the shoulder. Radiol Clin North Am 44(3):331–341
52. Rafii M, Minkoff J (1998) Advanced arthrography of the shoulder with CT and MR imaging. Radiol Clin North Am 36(4):609–633
53. Rafii M, Minkoff J, Bonamo J, Firooznia H, Jaffe L, Golimbu C et al (1988) Computed tomography (CT) arthrography of shoulder instabilities in athletes. Am J Sports Med 16(4):352–361
54. Wischer TK, Bredella MA, Genant HK, Stoller DW, Bost FW, Tirman PF (2002) Perthes lesion (a variant of the Bankart lesion): MR imaging and MR arthrographic findings with surgical correlation. AJR Am J Roentgenol 178(1):233–237
55. Neviaser TJ (1993) The GLAD lesion: another cause of anterior shoulder pain. Arthroscopy 9(1):22–23
56. Mair SD, Zarzour RH, Speer KP (1998) Posterior labral injury in contact athletes. Am J Sports Med 26(6):753–758
57. Melvin JS, Mackenzie JD, Nacke E, Sennett BJ, Wells L (2008) MRI of HAGL lesions: four arthroscopically confirmed cases of false-positive diagnosis. AJR Am J Roentgenol 191(3):730–734
58. Bui-Mansfield LT, Taylor DC, Uhorchak JM, Tenuta JJ (2002) Humeral avulsions of the glenohumeral ligament: imaging features and a review of the literature. AJR Am J Roentgenol 179(3):649–655
59. Magee T, Williams D, Mani N (2004) Shoulder MR arthrography: which patient group benefits most? AJR Am J Roentgenol 183(4):969–974

60. Magee T (2009) 3-T MRI of the shoulder: is MR arthrography necessary? AJR Am J Roentgenol 192(1):86–92
61. Schippinger G, Vasiu PS, Fankhauser F, Clement HG (2001) HAGL lesion occurring after successful arthroscopic Bankart repair. Arthroscopy 17(2):206–208
62. Grossman MG, Tibone JE, McGarry MH, Schneider DJ, Veneziani S, Lee TQ (2005) A cadaveric model of the throwing shoulder: a possible etiology of superior labrum anterior-to-posterior lesions. J Bone Joint Surg 87(4):824–831
63. Snyder SJ, Karzel RP, Del Pizzo W, Ferkel RD, Friedman MJ (1990) SLAP lesions of the shoulder. Arthroscopy 6(4):274–279
64. Morgan CD, Burkhart SS, Palmeri M, Gillespie M (1998) Type II SLAP lesions: three subtypes and their relationships to superior instability and rotator cuff tears. Arthroscopy 14(6):553–565
65. Beltran J, Jbara M, Maimon R (2003) Shoulder: labrum and bicipital tendon. Top Magn Reson Imaging 14(1):35–49
66. Mohana-Borges AV, Chung CB, Resnick D (2003) Superior labral anteroposterior tear: classification and diagnosis on MRI and MR arthrography. AJR Am J Roentgenol 181(6):1449–1462
67. Chang D, Mohana-Borges A, Borso M, Chung CB (2008) SLAP lesions: anatomy, clinical presentation, MR imaging diagnosis and characterization. Eur J Radiol 68(1):72–87
68. Jin W, Ryu KN, Kwon SH, Rhee YG, Yang DM (2006) MR arthrography in the differential diagnosis of type II superior labral anteroposterior lesion and sublabral recess. AJR Am J Roentgenol 187(4):887–893
69. Lee JC, Sykes C, Saifuddin A, Connell D (2005) Adhesive capsulitis: sonographic changes in the rotator cuff interval with arthroscopic correlation. Skeletal Radiol 34(9):522–527
70. Emig EW, Schweitzer ME, Karasick D, Lubowitz J (1995) Adhesive capsulitis of the shoulder: MR diagnosis. AJR Am J Roentgenol 164(6):1457–1459
71. Jung JY, Jee WH, Chun HJ, Kim YS, Chung YG, Kim JM (2006) Adhesive capsulitis of the shoulder: evaluation with MR arthrography. Eur Radiol 16(4):791–796
72. Mengiardi B, Pfirrmann CW, Gerber C, Hodler J, Zanetti M (2004) Frozen shoulder: MR arthrographic findings. Radiology 233(2):486–492
73. Yu YS, Dardani M, Fischer RA (2000) MR observations of posttraumatic osteolysis of the distal clavicle after traumatic separation of the acromioclavicular joint. J Comput Assist Tomogr 24(1):159–164
74. Robinson P, White LM, Lax M, Salonen D, Bell RS (2000) Quadrilateral space syndrome caused by glenoid labral cyst. AJR Am J Roentgenol 175(4):1103–1105
75. Maffet MW, Gartsman GM, Moseley B (1995) Superior labrum-biceps tendon complex lesions of the shoulder. Am J Sports Med 23(1):93–98

Chapter 6
Elbow Injuries

Kenneth S. Lee, Michael J. Tuite, and Humberto G. Rosas

Introduction

Elbow injuries in sports are growing as the number of athletes of all ages and skill levels participating in overhead throwing activities continue to rise. Twenty-five percent of all sports injuries include the elbow, wrist, or forearm [1]. Over 14 million people play tennis, 3 million play racquetball [2], and 2 million children play little league baseball in the United States [3] every year. Overhead throwing motion seen in baseball pitching, serving in tennis, throwing in American football, or overhead spiking in volleyball cause elbow injuries from repetitive valgus stress producing lateral elbow compression, medial soft tissue stretching, and posterior impingement [1]. Bone and soft tissue injuries of the elbow are mainly from overuse (Table 6.1), the most common injury seen in 50% of athletes being lateral epicondylosis (tennis backhand) [4]. Overuse injuries are related to suboptimal mechanics, improper equipment, and deconditioned state [4], which is especially seen in the "weekend warrior." Other causes of elbow pain include medial epicondylosis, collateral ligament damage, triceps or biceps injury, nerve entrapment, or degenerative change.

As athletes vary in skill level and age, from children to the elderly, different injury patterns can be seen. Injury patterns in children can be complex due to the ordered appearance of secondary ossification centers and fusion with the epiphysis. In children, the epiphyseal plate is weaker than its surrounding tendon and ligament structures predisposing to epiphyseal plate injuries. This is distinct from adults, or the skeletally mature, where the tendon and ligament structures are more likely to be injured. Acute osseous or chondral injuries can also occur. It is important for coaches, parents, and physicians to understand the biomechanics of elbow injuries for accurate diagnosis and proper prevention or rehabilitation. Treatment is usually conservative with surgery reserved for recalcitrant cases. Magnetic resonance (MR) imaging, computed tomography (CT), and ultrasound (US) play vital roles in helping to diagnose the various elbow injuries.

Epidemiology

Over the last three decades, child participation in sports has been on the rise. In the UK, 75% of children between ages 5 and 15 participate in an organized sport [1, 5]. Many children undergo year round training and are encouraged to start at an early age, probably due to the "get them while they are young" philosophy. By the time some children reach their teens, training per week can reach up to 20 h or more [1].

Unlike children, adults present with tendinous and ligamentous injury related to sporting activity. About 30–50% of recreational tennis players will get "tennis elbow." [6] About one-third of these players will present with severe symptoms that can interfere with their activities of daily living. Interestingly, novice players are more likely to develop lateral epicondylosis than expert tennis players [6]. This may be related to equipment, technique, and physical conditioning.

Anatomy and Biomechanics

Knowledge of elbow anatomy and its complex biomechanical properties is important for proper diagnosis and treatment. It is also important to realize that stress distribution occurs across the radiohumeral and ulnohumeral joints. Flexion–extension occurs at the ulnohumeral joint and supination–pronation movements at the proximal radio-ulnar joint. The normal range of motion of the elbow joint is −15° to 0° in full extension to 150° in full flexion [1] and 75° of pronation to 85° of supination [7]. The functional range of motion in daily living is about 30–130° of flexion [7]. The bony anatomy is the primary stabilizer of the joint (Fig. 6.1) at ranges less than 20° of flexion and greater than 120° of flexion. The primary stabilizers of the joint between 20 and

Kenneth S. Lee (✉)
Department of Radiology, University of Wisconsin School of Medicine & Public Health, University of Wisconsin Hospital & Clinics, Madison, WI, USA
e-mail: klee2@uwhealth.org

120° are its soft tissue structures, such as the anterior joint capsule, the ulnar collateral ligament (UCL) complex, and the lateral collateral ligament complex. Dynamic stabilization is achieved by different structures at different positions of the elbow joint.

The ulnar collateral ligament complex is made of three bundles: the anterior, posterior, and transverse bundles.

Table 6.1 Common overuse injuries of the elbow

Overuse injury	Sport activity	Mechanism of injury
Lateral epicondylosis (tennis elbow)	Racquet sports	Backhand with extension
Medial epicondylosis (golfer's elbow), ulnar collateral ligament sprain, ulnar nerve entrapment, pronator syndrome, radiocapitellar DJD, triceps injuries	Baseball, American football, golf, volleyball, javelin	Valgus stress with throwing
Distal biceps tendinopathy	Bowling, weight lifting, rock climbing, canoeing	Forced extension with flexed elbow
Ulnar nerve entrapment	Skiing, weight lifting	Traction injury
Triceps tendinopathy	Gymnastics, boxing	Forceful repetitive extension
Radial tunnel syndrome	Swimming, golf, bowling, rowing, weight lifting	Repetitive supination–pronation with injury to the posterior interosseous nerve

The anterior bundle is the most important stabilizer against valgus stress and is made of two bands: anterior and posterior bands. The anterior band plays a role in stabilization at lesser degrees of flexion, while the posterior band acts at higher degrees of elbow flexion. The anterior band is more likely to be injured while the elbow is in the extended position. The adjacent muscles help to provide dynamic stability to valgus stress: pronator teres, flexor digitorum superficialis, and flexor carpi ulnaris. When the medial UCL is compromised, the radial head provides secondary stability to valgus stress [7].

The lateral collateral ligament complex provides stability of the lateral elbow and is made of three structures: the radial collateral ligament, lateral ulnar collateral ligament, and the accessory lateral collateral ligament. The lateral UCL is the primary stabilizer against rotatory subluxation of the ulnohumeral joint. Injury to the lateral UCL causes posterolateral rotatory instability. The radial collateral ligament provides secondary stability.

In children and adolescents, it is important to understand the ordered progression of the secondary ossification centers around the elbow. Different injury patterns are seen in children and adolescents than in skeletally mature adults because the physeal plate is the structure of least resistance to injury. Essentially, there are six secondary ossification centers that demonstrate a chronological sequence of ossification. Many radiologists and clinicians rely on the mnemonic C-R-I-T-O-E to help remember this sequence: capitellum, radial head, internal (medial epicondyle), trochlea, olecranon, and external (lateral epicondyle). In general, the first ossification center appears around 1–2 years of age with each of

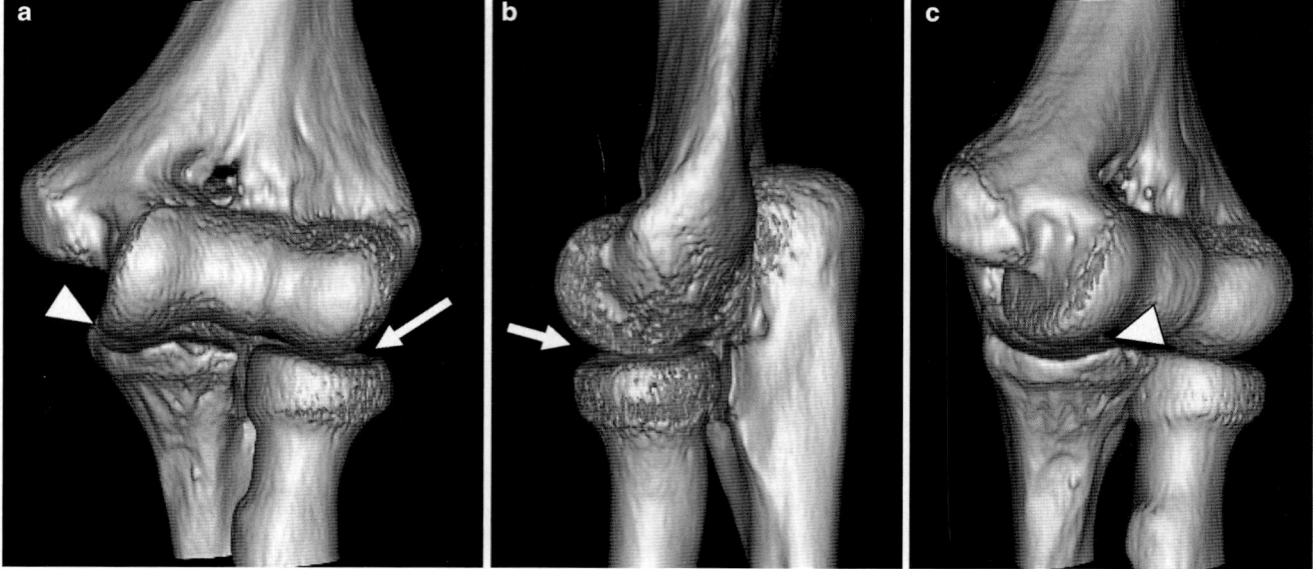

Fig. 6.1 Normal bony anatomy of the elbow joint. Three-dimensional CT rendering (Vitrea) of the anterior elbow (**a**), lateral view of the lateral elbow (**b**), and oblique view of the medial elbow (**c**) show the normal relationship of the radiocapitellar (*arrow*) and ulnotrochlear (*arrowhead*) joints

the remaining five appearing about every 2 years. Ossification is usually complete with fusion of the apophyses by the mid-teen years [1].

The biomechanics involved in the overhead throwing motion is also important in understanding the various causes of elbow injuries. Baseball or football overhead throwing generates a great amount of valgus stress and extension forces. Its complex movement has been extensively studied and can be divided into six phases: wind up, stride, cocking, arm acceleration, arm deceleration, and follow through. The windup phase starts as the pitcher shifts their weight to their back foot and ends as the front knee reaches maximal elevation. The stride phase then starts as the pitcher moves their front foot forward toward the catcher as the two arms move apart and downward. The cocking phase starts when the front foot hits the ground and the arm then reaches maximum external rotation. The acceleration phase occurs between maximum external rotation until ball release. The arm deceleration phase is defined as the moment of ball release until the arm reaches maximal internal rotation. Lastly, the follow through phase is when the shoulder reaches maximal internal rotation and ends when the pitcher regains a balanced position. The greatest torque occurs during the arm cocking, acceleration, and deceleration phases.

Diagnostic Imaging

Diagnostic imaging can help clinicians diagnose sports-related injuries of the elbow. Most injuries are from chronic overuse rather than acute injuries. Standard radiography should be the initial imaging modality used and should never be substituted for the more costly advanced imaging modalities. In general, MR imaging is very useful in the setting of the injured athlete, with appropriate adjunctive studies using ultrasound or CT in select cases.

Magnetic Resonance Imaging

MR imaging is a valuable tool for diagnosing sports-related injuries of the elbow. Its advantages include bone marrow edema sensitivity as well as soft tissue and cartilaginous structure evaluation. The large field of view makes MR imaging particularly useful in diagnosing vague or diffuse elbow pain. MR imaging also provides exquisite anatomic detail and pathology, enabling clinicians and surgeons to quickly diagnose injuries, plan for rehabilitation or preoperative assessment.

Sports-related injuries of the elbow are well imaged with noncontrast MR imaging; the goal is to establish MR imaging sequences that allow for fast image acquisition to optimize patient comfort and relevant diagnostic information. Specific elbow MR imaging protocols used by the authors include:

1. Axial T2w FS images
2. Sagittal T2w FS images
3. Coronal proton-density-weighted FS images

Additional sequences for epicondylitis/MCL/RCL tears also include:

1. Axial proton-density-weighted FS images
2. Coronal T1w images
3. Coronal inversion recovery (STIR) images

Additional sequences for osteochondritis dissecans (OCD), loose body, biceps/triceps tears, or nerve impingement include:

1. Axial T1w images
2. Sagittal T1w images

MR arthrography has shown to be useful for loose body evaluation and partial tears of the medial ulnar collateral ligament. The authors' standard MR arthrography protocol includes:

1. Axial T1w images
2. Sagittal T1w FS images
3. Coronal T1w FS images
4. Sagittal T2w FS images
5. Coronal T2w FS images

Computed Tomography

Computed tomography (CT) is a useful tool in evaluating for loose bodies, soft tissue calcifications, or fractures. The advantages of CT include quick scan time, little motion artifact, and accessibility. A clear disadvantage is the use of ionizing radiation.

The CT protocol used by the authors includes:

1. Place marker on pain site
2. Obtain scout image
3. 0.6 mm thin section axial images
4. Reformat in sagittal and coronal planes

Musculoskeletal Ultrasound

Musculoskeletal ultrasound is well-suited for the evaluation of sports-related elbow injuries. It offers focused, high resolution imaging of tendon, ligaments, and nerve structures. Its advantages include safe nonionizing radiation, accessibility, and cost effectiveness. Another unique advantage is its ability for dynamic assessment of tendon and ligament structures such as in cases of partial tears of the medial UCL. It is also easy to assess the contralateral side as a control. Ultrasound can also be useful in therapeutic guided injections.

Common Sports Injuries

Sports-related injuries of the elbow can be divided into two broad categories: acute and the far more common chronic overuse injuries. Both will be discussed here, along with the biomechanics of the injury and typical imaging findings. However, general terminology related to elbow injuries can be confusing and often used interchangeably in the literature. Kraushaar and Nirschl [6, 8] have suggested four stages of injury. Stage I is described as an acute injury, termed *epicondylitis* that causes inflammation. Stage II is related to a chronic overuse pattern of repetitive microtrauma that causes structural changes, referred to as *epicondylosis*. This stage affects many athletes and can lead to prolonged symptoms and decreased athletic performance [6]. Stage III is a partial tear with an ineffective healing response (i.e., scarring and calcification), and is termed *epicondylalgia*. Stage IV is a complete tear.

Chronic Overuse Injuries

The most common mechanism by which we see chronic overuse injuries of the elbow involves the overhead throwing motion. Presentation to the orthopedic clinic is on the rise because of the growing popularity of sports that require this repetitive motion, such as in tennis, racquetball, American football, volleyball, handball, or javelin throwing [6]. The overhead throwing motion involves a constellation of movements at the elbow joint, which include valgus stress (velocity: 900°/s) [1, 9], medial stretching, lateral compression, and posterior impingement [1]. Different injuries occur with differences in sporting activity, biomechanics, and age.

Lateral Epicondylosis

Lateral epicondylosis is commonly referred to as "tennis elbow." It is the most common cause of elbow pain in skeletally mature athletes occurring in over 50% of tennis players [4], mainly from the backhand motion. It is characterized as repetitive microtrauma with mucoid degeneration of the common extensor tendon where it attaches to the lateral epicondyle of the humerus. The mechanism of injury is a forceful torquing of the extensor muscles of the wrist affecting the tendinous insertion onto the lateral epicondyle, usually involving the lateral aspect of the tendon formed by the extensor carpi radialis brevis. There is also variable involvement of the extensor digitorum communis, extensor carpi radialis longus, and extensor carpi ulnaris tendons [6, 10–12].

Lateral epicondylosis will result in weakness and suboptimal athletic performance. The differential diagnosis includes lateral ulnar collateral ligament (UCL) tear, intraarticular loose bodies, degenerative change, and nerve entrapment. Diagnosis is often made clinically. However, ultrasound or MR imaging may be useful in evaluating nonspecific lateral elbow pain, or in those athletes recalcitrant to conservative management in helping to evaluate extent of tissue damage. [13] The normal common extensor tendon demonstrates a tight fibrillar pattern on high resolution ultrasound [14]. A pathologic tendon may demonstrate hypoechogenicity, increase in caliber, fiber disruption, or hyperemia upon Doppler interrogation [15, 16]. MR imaging shows the normal common extensor tendon as a homogeneous low signal T1 and T2w structure. In epicondylosis, the extensor tendon may increase in caliber and demonstrate increased signal intensity on both T1 and T2w images (Fig. 6.2), which correlates histopathologically as mucoid degeneration and neovascularization. Many athletes with lateral epicondylosis may present with a thinned common extensor tendon with fluid-like signal intensity on T2w imaging [13] (Fig. 6.3). Concomitant injury to the lateral UCL should also be considered.

Medial Epicondylosis

Medial epicondylosis is commonly referred to as "golfer's elbow." It is characterized by pain from the common flexor tendon origin at the medial epicondyle of the humerus. The mechanism of injury is from repetitive pronation and wrist flexion with eventual pathologic changes occurring between the pronator teres and flexor carpi radialis origin. Field and Savoie [4] found this to be especially seen in tennis players that rely heavily on top spin forehand strokes which involves forced pronation. Less common sites of involvement include the flexor carpi ulnaris, palmaris longus, and flexor sublimis origins [17]. The differential diagnosis of medial epicondylosis also includes medial ulnar collateral ligament injury, ulnar nerve injury or entrapment, and medial elbow joint pathology. [4] However, medial-sided elbow pain may be confounded by two or more causes. For example, Nirschl [17] found that 60% of patients that had surgery for medial epicondylosis also had a positive Tinel sign of ulnar neuropathy [17].

Once clinically suspected, ultrasound is a well-suited modality for a quick and focused exam of the common flexor tendon origin. In medial epicondylosis, the common flexor tendon may exhibit hypoechogenicity, loss of the normal

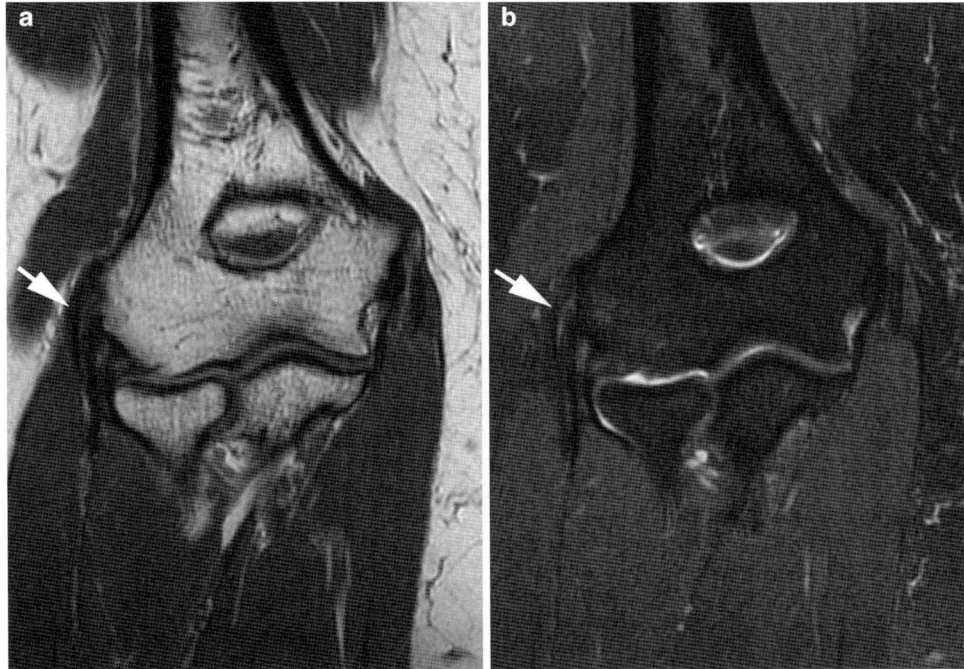

Fig. 6.2 Lateral epicondylosis in a 55-year-old male recreational tennis player with chronic lateral elbow pain. Coronal T1w FSE image (**a**) and coronal T2w FS FSE image (**b**) images show thickening and increased signal of the common extensor tendon origin (*arrow*) (courtesy of Dr. Jean-Pierre Phancao of National Orthopedic Imaging Associates, San Francisco, California)

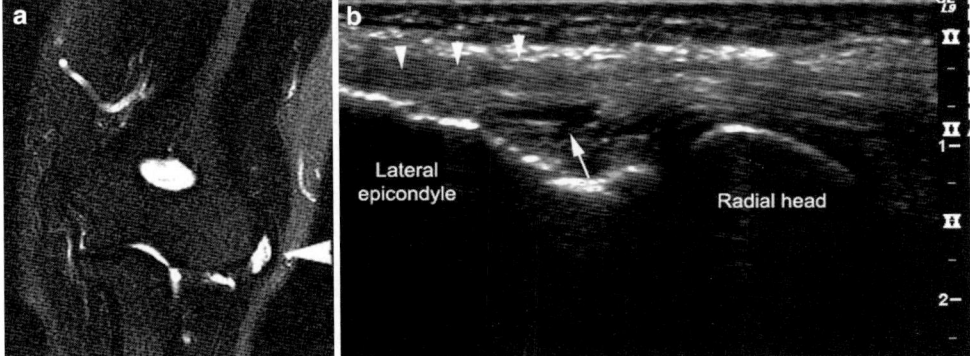

Fig. 6.3 Lateral epicondylosis in a 45-year-old female with chronic lateral elbow pain. Coronal T2w FS FSE image (**a**) shows fluid-intense signal (*arrowhead*) and thinning of the common extensor tendon origin representing an area of collagen disruption. Ultrasound long-axis view of the lateral elbow (**b**) nicely correlates with MR image findings of collagen disruption of the deep surface (*arrow*) of the common extensor tendon origin (*arrowheads*)

fibrillar pattern, increased caliber, and hyperemia from neovascularization on Doppler interrogation [15]. MR imaging may be helpful in those that pose a clinical diagnostic dilemma of medial elbow pain, which require a larger field of view, soft tissue, bone marrow, or joint evaluation. The normal MR imaging appearance of the common flexor tendon is a homogeneous low signal T1 and T2w structure (Fig. 6.4). Similar to the pathologic mucoid degenerative changes seen for lateral epicondylosis, the common flexor tendon in medial epicondylosis may demonstrate thickening with increased signal intensity on both the T1 and T2w images (Fig. 6.5).

Medial Ulnar Collateral Ligament Injury

Medial ulnar collateral ligament (UCL) injury is a less common disorder from repetitive forced valgus stress on the medial ligaments that results in pain and can lead to a significant decrease in athletic performance. First described by Timmerman and Andrews [18], it is most commonly associated with the overhead motion of baseball pitching, resulting in injury of the anterior bundle, which is the primary stabilizer to valgus stress. The mechanism of injury involves forceful valgus stress during overhead throwing, medial

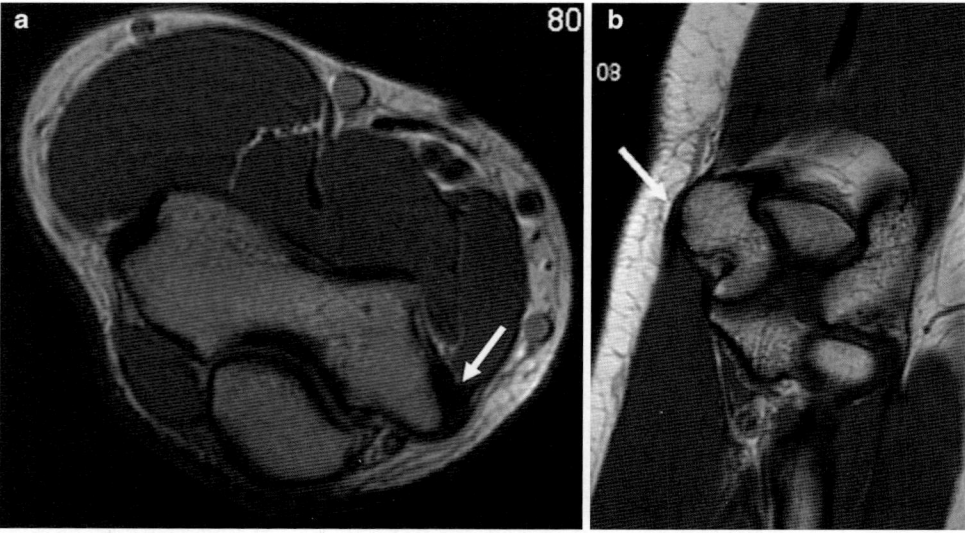

Fig. 6.4 Normal MR imaging appearance of the common flexor tendon origin. Axial T1w FSE image (**a**) and coronal T1w FSE image (**b**) show homogeneously low signal of the normal common flexor tendon origin (*arrow*)

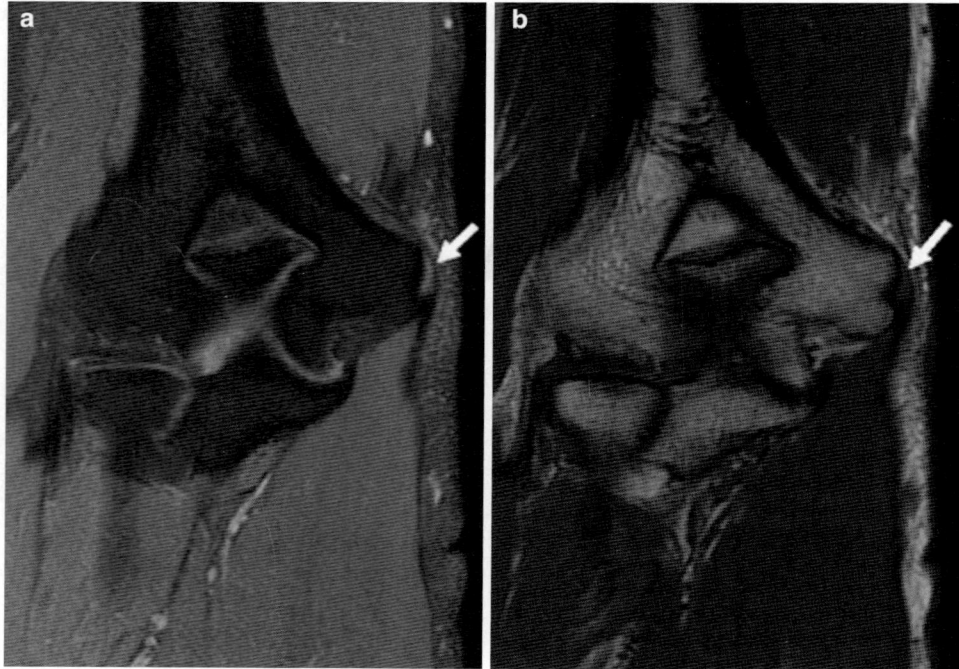

Fig. 6.5 Medial epicondylosis in a 39-year-old male golfer with aggravating medial elbow pain. Coronal fat-suppressed, PD-weighted, (**a**) and coronal T1w FSE (**b**) images show increased signal intensity involving the common flexor tendon origin (*arrow*)

stretching of the soft tissue, and posterior impingement [11, 19]. Once the anterior bundle is compromised, the radial head becomes the secondary restraint to valgus stress. However, with repetitive abnormal stress, valgus instability will result in intraarticular damage to the joint and degenerative osteophyte formation. It is important to note that 40% of patients with medial UCL instability will also develop ulnar nerve traction injury [4, 20].

Full thickness tears of the medial UCL are uncommon; rather injury to the medial UCL usually involves the deep capsular layer of the anterior bundle. Ultrasound and MR arthrogram may help in the diagnostic workup. High resolution ultrasound can offer a quick assessment to medial UCL damage [15] (Fig. 6.6). The anterior bundle will appear heterogenous to hypoechoic with loss of the normal fibrillar pattern. One of the advantages of ultrasound is its dynamic capability.

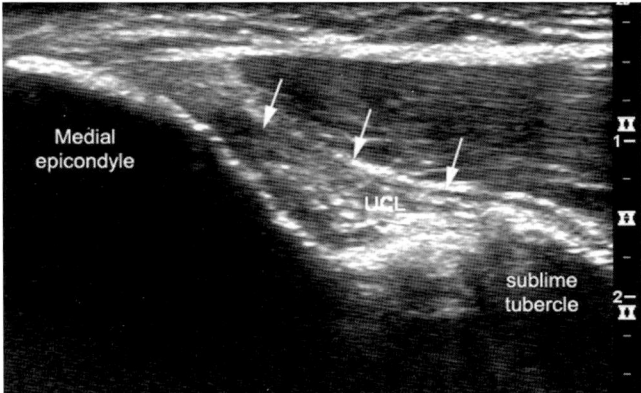

Fig. 6.6 Normal longitudinal ultrasound of the medial ulnar collateral ligament. Long-axis ultrasound of the medial elbow shows a normal tight fibrillar pattern to the anterior bundle of the ulnar collateral ligament (*arrows*)

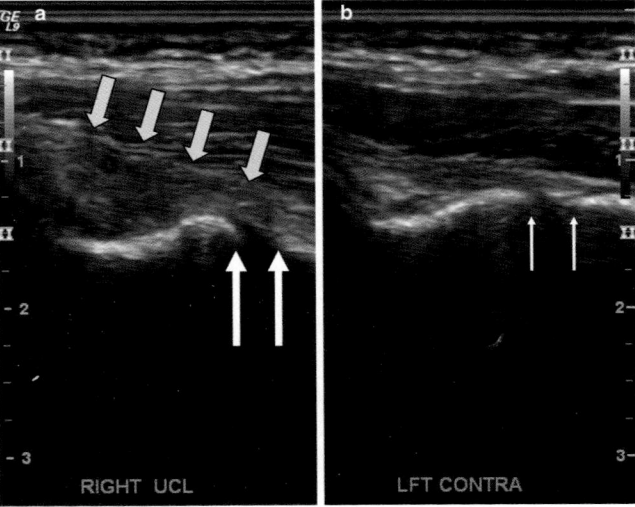

Fig. 6.7 Ultrasound assessment of the medial UCL. Long-axis ultrasound of the medial elbow shows loss of the normal fibrillar structure of the injured UCL (*arrows*) of the right elbow (**a**) compared to the normal left (**b**). In addition, dynamic assessment can show asymmetric widening (>1.0 mm) [21] between the abnormal (**a**) (*large double arrow*) and contralateral (**b**) (*small double arrow*) ulnotrochlear joint

De Smet and Winters [21] showed that dynamic ultrasound evaluation during valgus stress placed on the flexed elbow can demonstrate asymmetric widening of the ulnohumeral joint compared to the normal contralateral side (Fig. 6.7). This correlates with Timmerman and Andrews' findings [18, 22] during arthroscopic evaluation of widening of the ulnohumeral joint from a tear of the deep layer of the UCL while it remained intact externally.

MR imaging evaluation is also well-suited for UCL assessment. The best sequence to evaluate the medial UCL is the coronal T1w and proton-density-weighted images [13]. The anterior bundle is a thin low signal intensity structure extending

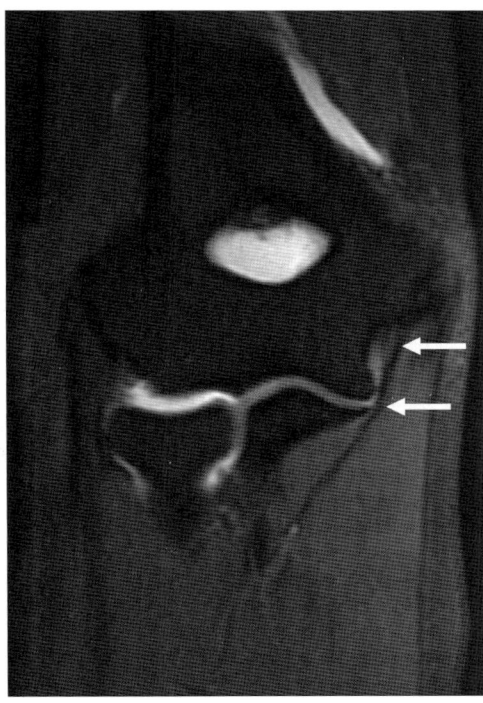

Fig. 6.8 Normal MR arthrogram appearance of the medial ulnar collateral ligament. Coronal T1w FS MR arthrogram image of the elbow shows an intact medial ulnar collateral ligament (*arrow*). No extravasation of intraarticular contrast

from the medial humerus, just anterior to the common flexor tendon origin, and inserts on a tubercle of the medial margin of the coronoid process called the sublime tubercle (Fig. 6.8). A full thickness tear will demonstrate a high intensity signal surrounding a disrupted and wavy ligament (Fig. 6.9). MR imaging is 100% sensitive and specific for detecting full thickness tears. However, partial tears of the UCL may be best evaluated with MR arthrography. Intraarticular gadolinium seen interposed between the distal UCL detachment and the adjacent sublime tubercle in partial tears is diagnostic and referred to as the "T-sign" [22] (Fig. 6.10).

Medial Epicondyle Apophysitis (Little Leaguer's Elbow)

Sports-related elbow injuries in the pediatric population has grown in prevalence, particularly in throwing sports such as in little league baseball where an estimated 2 million children participate in every year. "little leaguer's elbow" was first described by Brogden and Crow in 1960 [3] as a medial epicondyle fracture in an adolescent baseball pitcher. However, little league elbow has now been used to refer to a constellation of sports-related elbow injuries in the growing child athlete aged 8–16 years [23, 24]. It is important to understand that specific types of elbow injuries in a growing

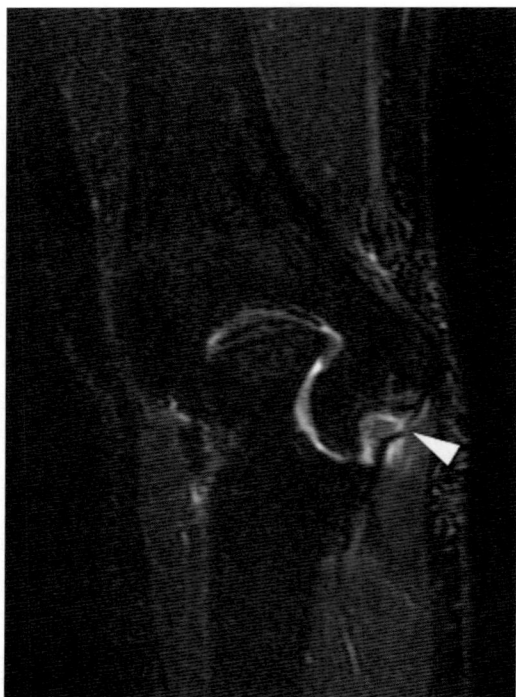

Fig. 6.9 Full thickness tear of the medial ulnar collateral ligament (UCL) in a 23-year-old baseball pitcher. Coronal fat-suppressed T2w FSE image demonstrates a full thickness defect of the UCL (*arrowhead*), wavy appearance of the distal portion, and surrounding edema

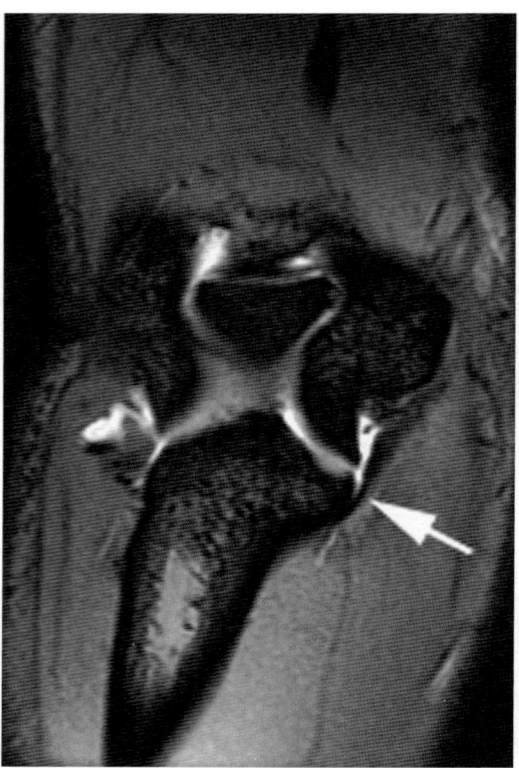

Fig. 6.10 Partial thickness tear of the anterior bundle of the ulnar collateral ligament. Coronal gradient echo image shows intraarticular gadolinium interposed between the distal portion of the anterior bundle of the UCL and sublime tubercle. No extravasation of contrast indicating integrity of the superficial layer

athlete occur at different stages of maturation of the well known and predictable sequence of the six secondary ossification centers [3, 24, 25]. The most common injury pattern seen in children is medial epicondyle apophysitis. The mechanism of injury is from repetitive forced valgus stress derived from the early and late cocking phases of overhead throwing [3]. In children, the point of least resistance to valgus stress overload is the medial epiphyseal growth plate, thus causing apophysitis in this age group. As the child matures to adolescence, the apophysis no longer remains the weakest link and instead avulsion fractures, partial or complete, become more prevalent. Radiographs are invaluable in detecting asymmetric apophyseal widening or fragmentation of the secondary ossification center [25]. MR imaging may also be helpful in detecting physeal injury in little leaguer's elbow (Fig. 6.11) as well as avulsion fractures.

Osteochondritis Dissecans

With chronic repetitive valgus overload, lateral-sided elbow injuries become more prevalent such as osteochondritis dissecans (OCD) of the capitellum. The mechanism of injury relates to the compressive forces derived from the late cocking and early acceleration phases of throwing [3] seen in baseball pitchers and water polo [26] players. This injury can also be seen in gymnasts [27] during handstands which generate radiocapitellar overload with weight-bearing on the extended elbow. It is the leading cause of permanent elbow disability in adolescent athletes [3]. OCD of the capitellum is characterized as a focal subchondral bone lesion which may demarcate to become fragmented and unstable. Unrecognized lesions may progress to severe symptoms of decreased range of motion, locking, instability of the radial head, and flexion contracture of greater than 15° [3, 13].

In contrast, osteochondrosis of the capitellum, called Panner's disease, is the most common cause of chronic lateral-sided elbow pain in athletes under the age of 10 [3]. It is characterized by minimal flattening of the subchondral bone plate of the capitellum. Unlike OCD of the capitellum, Panner's disease is considered a self-limiting condition that does not lead to long-term sequelae of joint deformity. Radiographic evaluation may show diffuse fragmentation of the capitellar epiphysis. Although some controversy exists, most authors believe that the two conditions share the same cause [13].

MR imaging is well-suited for evaluating OCD of the capitellum. OCD of the capitellum has a spectrum of findings from early subchondral marrow changes not seen radiographically to unstable lesions [28, 29]. Typical findings include a crescentic area of high T2 and low-to-intermediate

Fig. 6.11 Medial epicondyle apophysitis (little leaguer's elbow). Coronal (**a**) and axial (**b**) T2w FS FSE image shows diffuse edema involving both the medial epicondyle apophysis (*arrow*) and the physis (*arrowhead*)

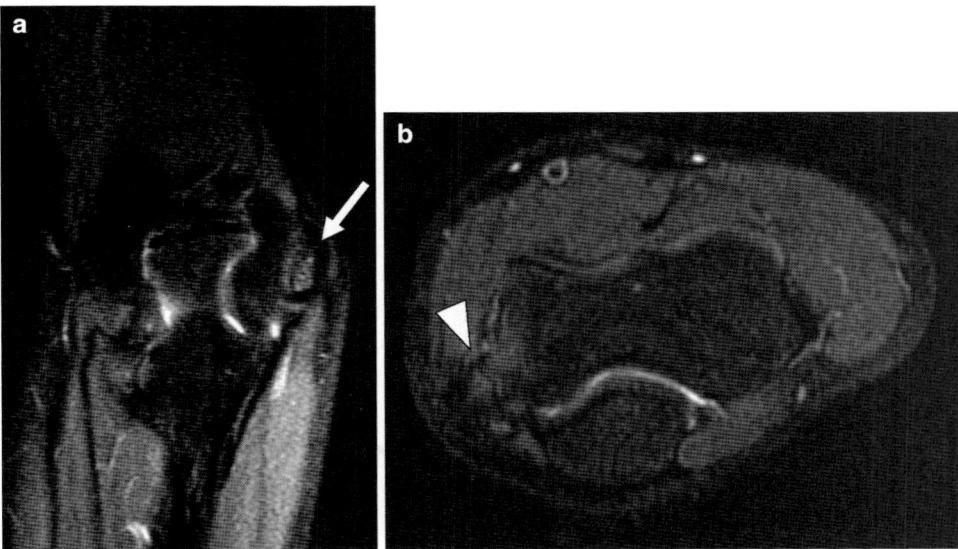

Fig. 6.12 Osteochondritis dissecans in a 14-year-old male baseball player with lateral elbow pain. Sagittal T1w FSE image (**a**) shows low signal defect in the capitellum (*arrow*). Sagittal T2w FS FSE image (**b**) of the same slice shows a focal area of high signal in the capitellum (*arrow*)

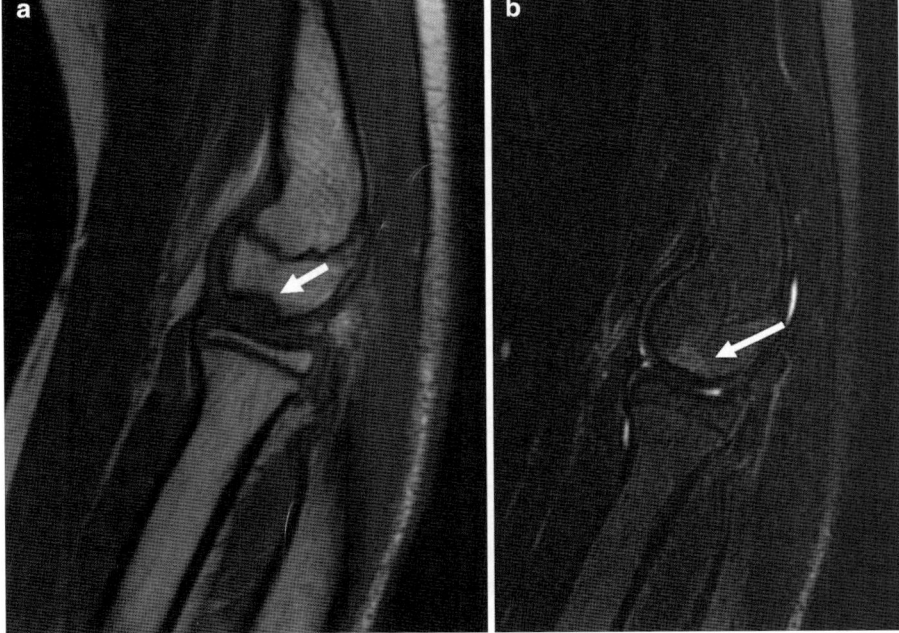

T1 signal abnormality of the subchondral bone of the anterolateral capitellum [28] (Fig. 6.12). Unstable lesions can demonstrate findings of linear high T2 signal intensity cleft between the fragment and bone (Fig. 6.13), full thickness irregularity of cleft in the adjacent cartilage, and/or intraarticular loose bodies [28]. MR imaging is excellent for early detection in radiographically occult lesions and for characterization of stable or unstable OCD to help guide management.

Degenerative Joint Disease/Intraarticular Loose Bodies

Repetitive overhead movements can result in intraarticular injuries. Once the primary stabilizers of the elbow joint such as ligamentous and capsular restraints break down, the bony articulations bear more stress. For example, with compromise of the medial UCL, more stress is transferred to the radiocapitellar bony articulation resulting in abnormal compression

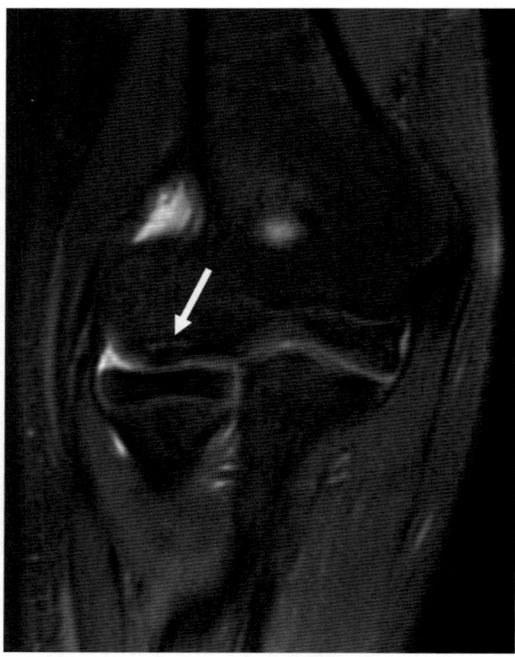

Fig. 6.13 Unstable OCD in a 13-year-old male baseball pitcher. Coronal T1w FS MR arthrogram image shows gadolinium-intense crescentic signal (*arrow*) undercutting the OCD fragment

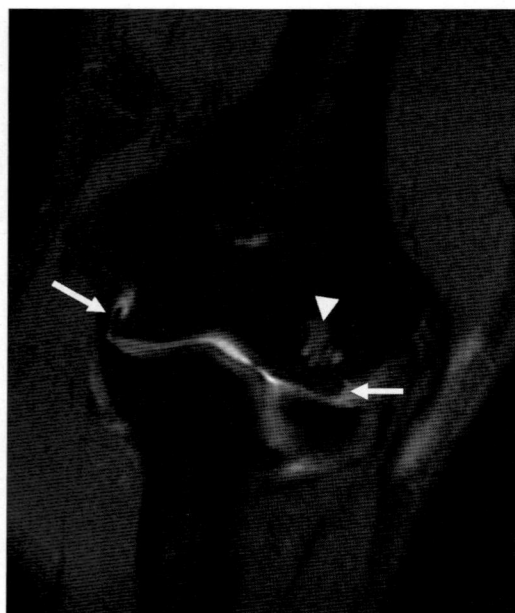

Fig. 6.14 Degenerative joint disease in 56-year-old male. Coronal T2 FS MR arthrogram image shows ulnotrochlear and radiocapitellar joint osteophytes (*arrows*). There is also degenerative subchondral edema of the capitellum (*arrowhead*)

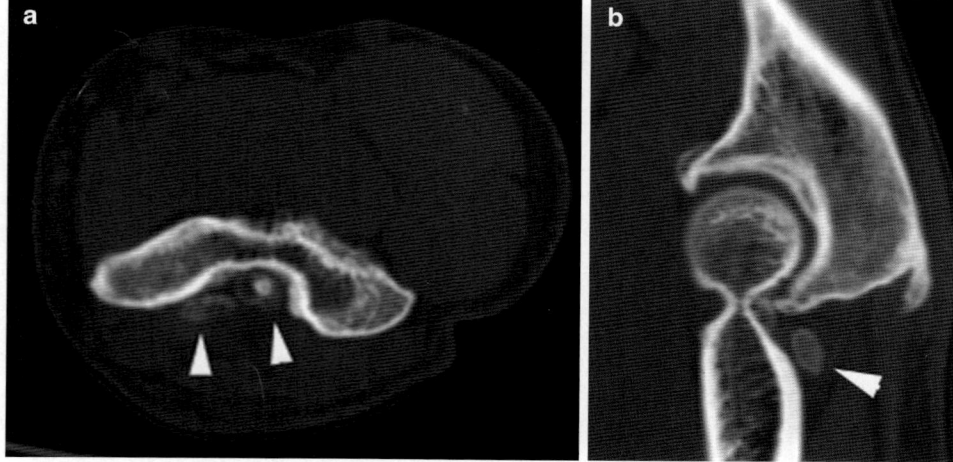

Fig. 6.15 Intraarticular loose bodies of the elbow in a 50-year-old male with locking symptoms. Axial (**a**) and sagittal (**b**) computed tomography images show multiple ossified loose bodies in the olecranon fossa

of the articular surface and eventual development of posteromedial gutter osteophytosis and loose body formation [11]. Older athletes participating in overhead motion seen in tennis serves also develop degenerative change, which causes pain posteriorly, stiffness, and locking from loose body formation (Fig. 6.14). Intraarticular loose bodies may be cartilaginous, ossified bodies, or bony fragments [13]. Loose bodies may also be located in either the coronoid or olecranon fossa, which often makes detection difficult. CT is well-suited to demonstrate intraarticular loose bodies, but may be difficult to detect chondral bodies (Fig. 6.15). However, MR imaging is superior for soft tissue and bone marrow assessment and can be a useful tool in detecting chondral or ossified loose bodies, especially with the addition of intraarticular contrast (Fig. 6.16). MR imaging can also be useful for diagnosing early degenerative change of articular cartilage loss, subchondral edema, and osteophyte formation.

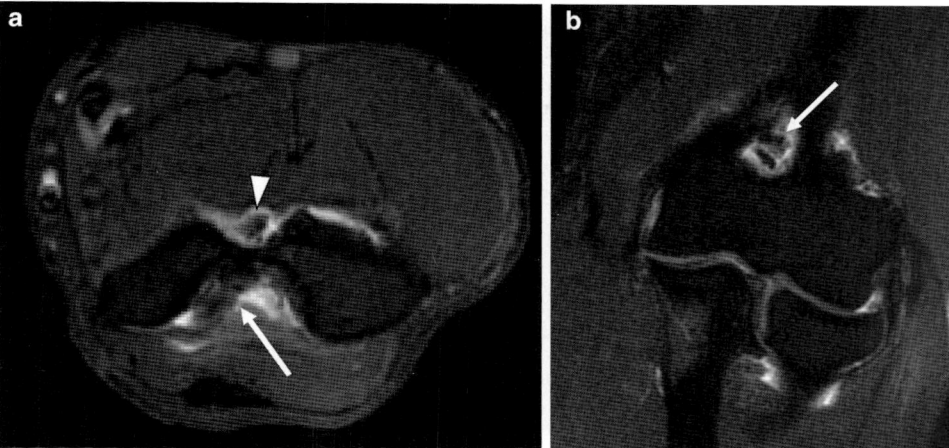

Fig. 6.16 Intraarticular loose bodies in 56-year-old male. Axial (**a**) and coronal (**b**) T1w FS MR arthrogram images show intraarticular loose bodies in the olecranon fossa (*arrow*) and coronoid fossa (*arrowhead*)

Nerve Entrapments

Upper extremity weakness, hand pain, and numbness are common presenting symptoms to the clinician. Onset is usually insidious and not associated with a traumatic event [4, 20, 30]. Often confused with musculoskeletal injuries, entrapment neuropathies of the ulnar, radial, or median nerves or their branches are an important cause to consider in the athlete. One study showed that 23–64% of hand pain and numbness was attributable to entrapment neuropathies in wheelchair athletes [6].

As previously mentioned, Nirschl et al. found that 60% of patients who had surgery for medial epicondylosis also had a positive Tinel sign of ulnar neuropathy [17]. Ulnar nerve entrapment can be an isolated or concominant cause of medial-sided elbow pain. MR imaging and US are useful in evaluating for ulnar neuritis. The normal MR imaging appearance of nerves demonstrates a low-to-intermediate signal intensity on all pulse sequences [13]. With inflammation from impingement, the nerve can become hyperintense on T2-weighted (Fig. 6.17) or short tau inversion recovery (STIR) images. The inflamed nerve can also be increased in caliber with surrounding soft tissue edema or adjacent bone marrow edema. High resolution ultrasound is a useful focused exam for ulnar neuritis [31]. The normal sonographic appearance of a nerve is an echogenic, fasciculated structure, seen both in the transverse and coronal planes. In cases of entrapment, the nerve may become enlarged, edematous and hypoechoic [31]. The length of the nerve can be evaluated using an extended field of view image capture. This capability is also useful in discerning caliber change in entrapment neuropathies; the nerve is thicker and hypoechoic proximal to the site of entrapment [31]. Another useful application of ultrasound is its dynamic evaluation for ulnar nerve subluxation. The transducer is placed in the transverse plane over

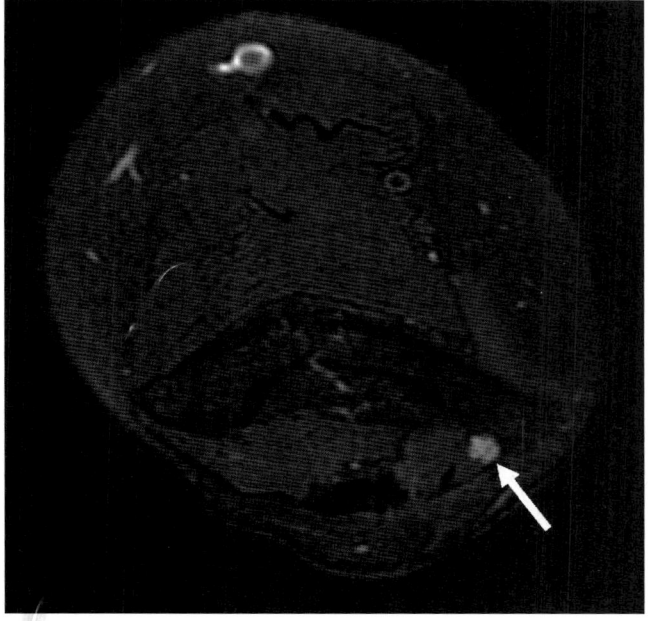

Fig. 6.17 Ulnar neuropathy in a 27-year-old female with medial elbow pain and forearm weakness. Axial T2w FS FSE image shows high signal intensity of the ulnar nerve (*arrow*) just proximal to the cubital tunnel

the cubital tunnel and with elbow motion from neutral to flexed position, ulnar nerve subluxation out of the cubital tunnel can be observed [32].

Less common entrapment neuropathies include "resistant tennis elbow," which may be due to entrapment of the posterior interosseous nerve, a branch of the radial nerve [6]. This entity causes lateral-sided elbow pain and weakness and is often confused with lateral epicondylosis. Radial tunnel syndrome is characterized as entrapment of the deep branch of the radial nerve, most commonly at the Arcade of Frohse just proximal to the supinator [33, 34]. It can be seen in athletes

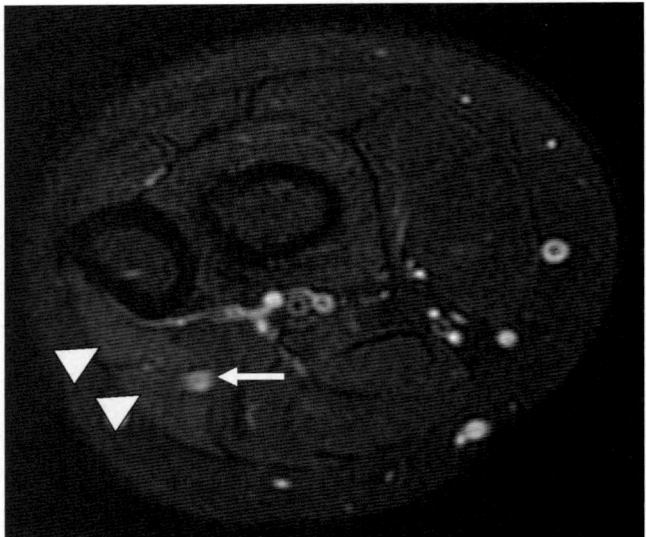

Fig. 6.18 Early denervation edema. Axial T2w FS FSE image of the forearm shows high signal denervation edema of the flexor carpi ulnaris and flexor digitorum profundus muscles (*arrowhead*). Ulnar nerve remains high in signal intensity (*arrow*)

involved in racquet or overhead throwing sports. It is often confused with "tennis elbow," but differs by symptoms lasting greater than 6 months despite conservative treatment [6]. Pronator syndrome is caused by median nerve entrapment distal to the elbow between the two pronator heads. It can be seen in athletes involved in tennis or overhead motion sports, and manifests as anterior pain and distal paresthesia worsened with resisted pronation.

Although MR imaging is less useful in evaluating radial or median neuropathies than the more superficially located ulnar nerve, MR imaging may be useful in detecting the sequela of chronic nerve entrapment [13]. The superior soft tissue characterization of MR imaging enables one to evaluate muscle signal changes of denervation of the forearm, especially the late stages of fatty infiltration and atrophy but also early denervation muscle edema (Fig. 6.18). These are best seen on STIR or T2w images with fat saturation for denervation changes and T1w images for fatty infiltration and atrophy. MR imaging is also useful in evaluating for possible space-occupying lesions that may be the cause of entrapment. High resolution ultrasound can also be used to evaluate the radial and median nerves, but is operator-dependent [31].

Acute Injuries

Fractures

Sports-related fractures about the elbow are not uncommon. In children, acute fractures comprise a significant portion of all sports-related injuries. Houshian et al. [5]

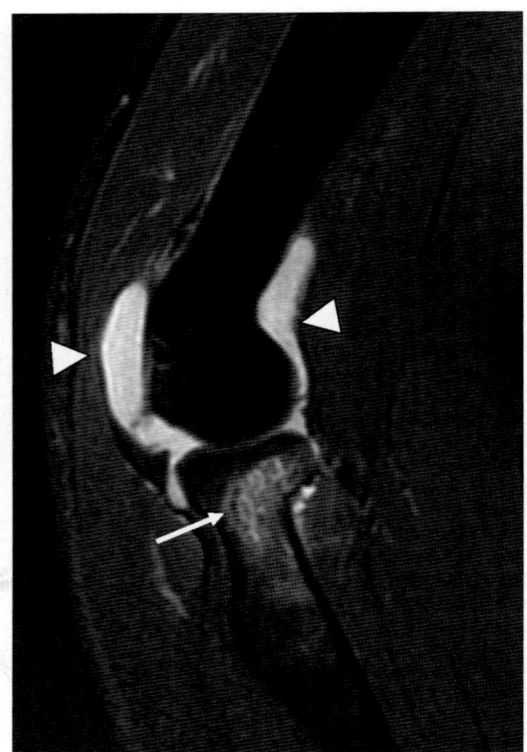

Fig. 6.19 Nondisplaced radial head fracture in 25-year-old male after fall; radiographs were negative (not shown). Sagittal T2w FS FSE image shows low signal linear fracture involving the radial head (*arrow*) that extended to the articular surface (not shown) with surrounding marrow edema. Joint effusion is also seen (*arrowheads*)

found that close to 50% of all elbow fractures in children were a result of sports or equipment-related activities. These include stress injury to the physis of the medial epicondylar apophysis in little leaguer's elbow, avulsion fracture of the medial epicondyle in adolescent pitchers, and olecranon growth plate fractures in gymnasts [27] and wrestlers [1]. Olecranon tip fractures can be seen in baseball pitchers, likely from repetitive impingement of the posteromedial olecranon process [10]. MR imaging is especially useful in radiographically occult fractures, such as a nondisplaced radial head (Fig. 6.19) or olecranon fractures (Fig. 6.20). MR imaging may also be useful in detecting stress injuries about the elbow in the "weekend warrior," such as olecranon stress fractures in tennis players [35, 36]. It is also helpful for clinicians in planning management based on staging criteria.

Distal Biceps Injury

Distal biceps tendon injuries consist of either partial or complete tears at or near its insertion onto the radial tuberosity. It is most often associated with a single acute traumatic event with an audible popping sound and intense pain [6]. The mechanism of injury is usually forced extension

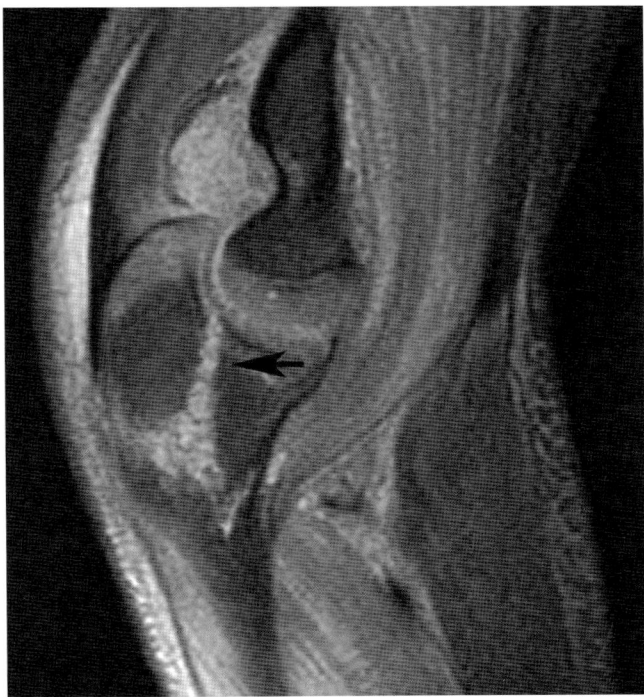

Fig. 6.20 Intraarticular fracture of the olecranon in 18-year-old female after fall. Sagittal fat-suppressed short tau inversion recovery image shows a T-shaped high signal intensity fracture of the olecranon (*arrows*). There is also a joint effusion (*arrowhead*)

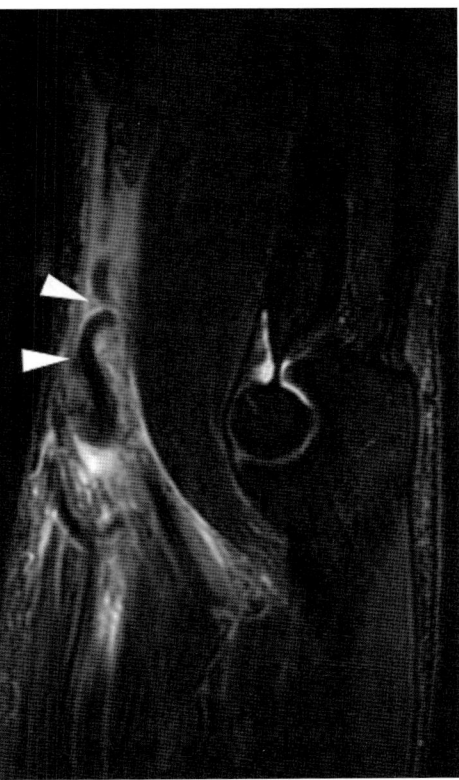

Fig. 6.21 Acute full thickness tear of the distal biceps tendon in 23-year-old weightlifter. Sagittal T2w FS MR image shows the retracted and wavy distal end of the torn biceps tendon (*arrowheads*). There is also surrounding soft tissue edema and hemorrhage

with the elbow flexed at 90° [7]. It commonly involves the dominant side, mostly in males, and between the ages of 40–60 years [13]. Distal biceps tendon ruptures are often clinically apparent with an associated tear of the bicipital aponeurosis (lacertus fibrosus), resulting in proximal retraction into the arm, swelling, and ecchymosis. However, without disruption of the bicipital aponeurosis, biceps tendon tears may be difficult to assess clinically. For this reason, MR imaging is used to evaluate for distal biceps tendon tears. Partial or complete tears will demonstrate high T2 signal intensity in the region of the tear, as well as surrounding soft tissue edema and associated bone marrow edema of the radial tuberosity [37]. Axial and sagittal MR images are the best views to evaluate for tendon tears and retraction in full thickness ruptures [13] (Fig. 6.21). Partial tears may be associated with radiobicipital bursitis [38] (Fig. 6.22). Ultrasound is also useful in evaluating for radiobicipital bursitis [39].

Triceps Injury

Partial tears or complete ruptures of the triceps tendon are rare [6]. It usually occurs as a result of a fall on an outstretched hand, less commonly from a direct blow or from a forced flexion [34]. The location of triceps tendon tears is usually at or near its olecranon process attachment. MR imaging is useful in detecting triceps tendon tears and degree of retraction in cases of complete rupture [13, 40] (Fig. 6.23). Partial tears will manifest as high T2 signal abnormality involving the triceps tendon, usually best seen in the sagittal plane. MR imaging may also help to evaluate for bone marrow edema or associated injuries to the elbow joint. Ultrasound may also help to provide a quick assessment of the triceps tendon. Its normal fibrillar pattern would be discontinuous.

Conclusion

Sports-related elbow injuries are growing in prevalence across all age groups, from children in little league to the "weekend warrior" adult athlete. This demands both clinician and radiologist to recognize the importance of efficient and accurate diagnosis for proper management to prevent long-term disability and to decrease time away from the sport. Accurate diagnosis requires a proper knowledge of the complex anatomy of the elbow and a thorough understanding of the underlying biomechanics of sports-related injuries. In addition, understanding the capabilities and limitations of the various imaging modalities will facilitate a quick, accurate, and cost-effective diagnosis.

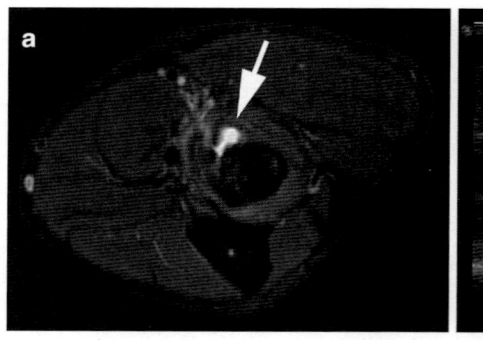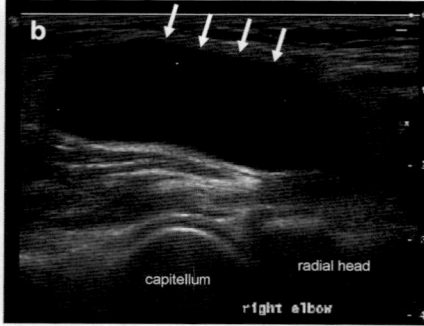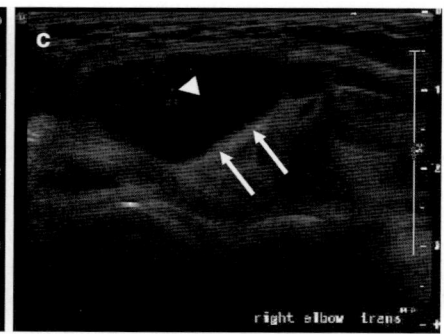

Fig. 6.22 Radiobicipital bursitis in 27-year-old male with high-grade partial tear of the distal biceps tendon. Axial T2w FS FSE image (**a**) shows fluid-signal bursal fluid adjacent to the radial tuberosity (*arrowhead*). There is marked attenuation of the distal biceps tendon at the radial tuberosity (*arrow*) with adjacent high signal intensity in the soft tissue (*double arrowhead*) consistent with high-grade tear (courtesy of Dr. Jean-Pierre Phancao of National Orthopedic Imaging Associates, San Francisco, California). Longitudinal (**b**) and transverse (**c**) ultrasound images in a different patient show a large amount of fluid in the radiobicipital bursa (*arrows*) surrounding an intact distal biceps tendon (*arrowhead*)

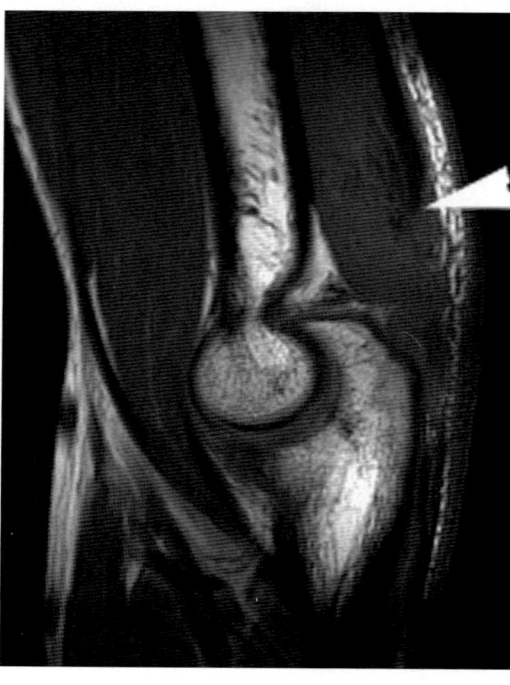

Fig. 6.23 Acute rupture of the triceps tendon in a 16-year-old male after skateboarding accident. Sagittal T1w FSE image shows the retracted end of the triceps tendon (*arrowhead*) from the distal attachment of the olecranon

References

1. Magra M, Caine D, Maffulli N (2007) A review of epidemiology of paediatric elbow injuries in sports. Sports Med 37(8):717–735
2. Koplan JP, Siscovick DS, Goldbaum GM (1985) The risks of exercise: a public health view of injuries and hazards. Public Health Rep 100(2):189–195
3. Klingele KE, Kocher MS (2002) Little league elbow: valgus overload injury in the paediatric athlete. Sports Med 32(15):1005–1015
4. Field LD, Savoie FH (1998) Common elbow injuries in sport. Sports Med 26(3):193–205
5. Houshian S, Mehdi B, Larsen MS (2001) The epidemiology of elbow fracture in children: analysis of 355 fractures, with special reference to supracondylar humerus fractures. J Orthop Sci 6(4): 312–315
6. Hume PA, Reid D, Edwards T (2006) Epicondylar injury in sport: epidemiology, type, mechanisms, assessment, management and prevention. Sports Med 36(2):151–170
7. Frostick SP, Mohammad M, Ritchie DA (1999) Sport injuries of the elbow. Br J Sports Med 33(5):301–311
8. Kraushaar BS, Nirschl RP (1999) Tendinosis of the elbow (tennis elbow). Clinical features and findings of histological, immunohistochemical, and electron microscopy studies. J Bone Joint Surg Am 81(2):259–278
9. Bylak J, Hutchinson MR (1998) Common sports injuries in young tennis players. Sports Med 26(2):119–132
10. Albright JA, Jokl P, Shaw R, Albright JP (1978) Clinical study of baseball pitchers: correlation of injury to the throwing arm with method of delivery. Am J Sports Med 6(1):15–21
11. Fleisig GS, Barrentine SW, Escamilla RF, Andrews JR (1996) Biomechanics of overhand throwing with implications for injuries. Sports Med 21(6):421–437
12. Kijowski R, Tuite M, Sanford M (2004) Magnetic resonance imaging of the elbow. Part I: normal anatomy, imaging technique, and osseous abnormalities. Skeletal Radiol 33(12):685–697
13. Tuite MJ, Kijowski R (2006) Sports-related injuries of the elbow: an approach to MRI interpretation. Clin Sports Med 25(3): 387–408, v
14. Connell D, Burke F, Coombes P et al (2001) Sonographic examination of lateral epicondylitis. AJR Am J Roentgenol 176(3):777–782
15. Kijowski R, De Smet AA (2006) The role of ultrasound in the evaluation of sports medicine injuries of the upper extremity. Clin Sports Med 25(3):569–590, viii
16. Levin D, Nazarian LN, Miller TT et al (2005) Lateral epicondylitis of the elbow: US findings. Radiology 237(1):230–234
17. Nirschl RP (1988) Prevention and treatment of elbow and shoulder injuries in the tennis player. Clin Sports Med 7(2):289–308
18. Timmerman LA, Andrews JR (1994) Undersurface tear of the ulnar collateral ligament in baseball players. A newly recognized lesion. Am J Sports Med 22(1):33–36
19. Kooima CL, Anderson K, Craig JV, Teeter DM, van Holsbeeck M (2004) Evidence of subclinical medial collateral ligament injury and posteromedial impingement in professional baseball players. Am J Sports Med 32(7):1602–1606
20. Glousman RE (1990) Ulnar nerve problems in the athlete's elbow. Clin Sports Med 9(2):365–377

21. De Smet AA, Winter TC, Best TM, Bernhardt DT (2002) Dynamic sonography with valgus stress to assess elbow ulnar collateral ligament injury in baseball pitchers. Skeletal Radiol 31(11):671–676
22. Timmerman LA, Schwartz ML, Andrews JR (1994) Preoperative evaluation of the ulnar collateral ligament by magnetic resonance imaging and computed tomography arthrography. Evaluation in 25 baseball players with surgical confirmation. Am J Sports Med 22(1):26–31, discussion 2
23. Kocher MS, Waters PM, Micheli LJ (2000) Upper extremity injuries in the paediatric athlete. Sports Med 30(2):117–135
24. Benjamin HJ, Briner WW Jr (2005) Little league elbow. Clin J Sport Med 15(1):37–40
25. Hang DW, Chao CM, Hang YS (2004) A clinical and roentgenographic study of Little League elbow. Am J Sports Med 32(1):79–84
26. Krijnen MR, Lim L, Willems WJ (2003) Arthroscopic treatment of osteochondritis dissecans of the capitellum: report of 5 female athletes. Arthroscopy 19(2):210–214
27. Maffulli N, Chan D, Aldridge MJ (1992) Overuse injuries of the olecranon in young gymnasts. J Bone Joint Surg Br 74(2):305–308
28. Kijowski R, De Smet AA (2005) MRI findings of osteochondritis dissecans of the capitellum with surgical correlation. AJR Am J Roentgenol 185(6):1453–1459
29. Kijowski R, De Smet AA (2005) Radiography of the elbow for evaluation of patients with osteochondritis dissecans of the capitellum. Skeletal Radiol 34(5):266–271
30. Cain EL Jr, Dugas JR, Wolf RS, Andrews JR (2003) Elbow injuries in throwing athletes: a current concepts review. Am J Sports Med 31(4):621–635
31. Bianchi S (2008) Ultrasound of the peripheral nerves. Joint Bone Spine 75(6):643–649
32. Jacobson JA, Jebson PJ, Jeffers AW, Fessell DP, Hayes CW (2001) Ulnar nerve dislocation and snapping triceps syndrome: diagnosis with dynamic sonography – report of three cases. Radiology 220(3):601–605
33. Ferdinand BD, Rosenberg ZS, Schweitzer ME et al (2006) MR imaging features of radial tunnel syndrome: initial experience. Radiology 240(1):161–168
34. Rettig AC (1998) Elbow, forearm and wrist injuries in the athlete. Sports Med 25(2):115–130
35. Coel M, Yamada CY, Ko J (1993) MR imaging of patients with lateral epicondylitis of the elbow (tennis elbow): importance of increased signal of the anconeus muscle. AJR Am J Roentgenol 161(5):1019–1021
36. Patten RM (1995) Overuse syndromes and injuries involving the elbow: MR imaging findings. AJR Am J Roentgenol 164(5):1205–1211
37. Ho CP (1995) Sports and occupational injuries of the elbow: MR imaging findings. AJR Am J Roentgenol 164(6):1465–1471
38. Williams BD, Schweitzer ME, Weishaupt D et al (2001) Partial tears of the distal biceps tendon: MR appearance and associated clinical findings. Skeletal Radiol 30(10):560–564
39. Sofka CM, Adler RS (2004) Sonography of cubital bursitis. AJR Am J Roentgenol 183(1):51–53
40. Kijowski R, Tuite M, Sanford M (2005) Magnetic resonance imaging of the elbow. Part II: abnormalities of the ligaments, tendons, and nerves. Skeletal Radiol 34(1):1–18

Chapter 7
Hand and Wrist Injuries

Philip J. O'Connor

Introduction

In comparison to lower limb injury, wrist and hand injury in sport is relatively uncommon accounting for only 3–9% of all sports injury [1].

It however has much greater relevance in some sports particularly where the incidence of injury is increased (golf, tennis, snowboarding and contact sports) or the impact of wrist and hand dysfunction on performance is high. Preservation of hand and wrist function is also vital to activities of daily life and early accurate diagnosis and treatment of sports-related wrist and hand injury will have clear patient benefits beyond sport.

History and physical examination remain the mainstay of diagnosis. There is however a broad spectrum of sports injury of the wrist and hand from acute high impact to overuse injury of the bones and soft tissues that can occur in a wide variety of sporting activities [2–8]. The clinical presentation and clinical findings in these conditions often substantially overlap and as in all areas of modern medicine imaging is becoming an increasingly important part of the clinical assessment. To understand wrist and hand injury a clear understanding of some complex anatomy, biomechanics and injury mechanisms is required. This chapter will deal with the wrist and hand detailing the anatomy, biomechanics, injury patterns and imaging approaches and findings in sports injury of the hand and wrist.

Wrist Anatomy

Osseous Anatomy

The distal radius and ulna articulate with the proximal row of the carpi (Fig. 7.1). The radial styloid lies on the lateral side of the distal radius and represents the most distal point of the radius and the origin of the radial collateral ligament of the wrist. The distal articular surface of the radius is divided into two portions by a central ridge, often this is only faintly visible but can be more prominent creating radial and ulnar facets to the distal radial articulation. The ulnar facet should articulate with the lunate and the radial portion articulates with the scaphoid. The distal radius has a prominent dorsal tubercle called Lister's tubercle. This is an important landmark when defining the tendon anatomy of the extensor tendon compartments of the wrist with extensor compartment 3 lies on the ulnar aspect of this tubercle. The distal ulna lies in a notch on the medial border of the distal radius, the ulnar notch. The distal ulnar is normally within 2-mm length difference from the distal articular surface of the radius. Differences in the length of the ulna is termed ulnar variance and can be either positive (ulna longer than the radius) or negative (ulna shorter than the radius). Alteration in ulnar variance is important to wrist function and has clear association with carpal injury. Positive ulnar variance is associated with impaction injury between the distal ulna and the carpi and injury to the triangular fibrocartilagenous complex. Negative ulna variance is associated with Keinbock's disease (avascular necrosis of the lunate) which is thought to have an increased incidence in some sports. Negative ulna variance is thought to be a factor in developing Keinbock's because of increased osseous loading of the radial portion of the wrist resulting from ulna shortening (Fig. 7.2) [9]. The distal ulna also has a boney prominence on its medial side, the ulna styloid process, this is the peripheral attachment of the triangular fibrocartilage. The medial aspect of the distal ulna also contains a groove for the sixth extensor tendon compartment, the extensor carpi ulnaris (ECU) tendon.

The proximal and distal rows of the carpi are shown in figure and consist of eight separate bones acting as two separate functional biomechanical units (Fig. 7.1). They are firmly bound together by intrinsic check reign ligaments and guided by complex extrinsic ligaments. The proximal row consists of the scaphoid, lunate, triquetral and pisiform (this is a sesamoid bone lying within the flexor carpi ulnaris tendon). The scaphoid, lunate and triquetral are the main functional unit of the proximal carpal row and are unusual in that they have no tendon attachments. As such they have no capacity for

Philip J. O'Connor (✉)
Department of Musculoskeletal Radiology, Leeds Teaching Hospitals, Chapeltown Road, Leeds, LS7 4SA, UK
e-mail: philip.o'connor@leedsth.nhs.uk

independent movement and act entirely as what is in effectively a functional buffer or spacer between the distal carpal row and distal radius and ulna. The scaphoid acts as a key link between the distal and proximal row rotating during ulna and radial deviation of the wrist and bearing substantial load when the wrist is stressed. As a result, it is a common site of bony injury in the proximal row. The distal row articulates with the base of the metacarpals. The trapezium has a saddle-shaped articulation with the base of the first metacarpal; as a result, even minor subluxation can result in substantial articular incongruence and dysfunction. The trapezoid lies on the medial aspect of the trapezium and fits into a deep notch in the second metacarpal base. The capitates articulates predominantly with the third metacarpal base but also has articular relations with the second and fourth metacarpals. On the dorsal aspect of the third metacarpal base there is a common accessory ossicle termed the os styloideum. This is susceptible to both traction or impaction injury and can be a symptomatic normal variant of the wrist [10, 11].

Anatomy of the Wrist Joint Compartments

The wrist joint is divided into a series of compartments which normally do not communicate:

1. The radiocarpal compartment
2. The distal radioulnar compartment
3. The midcarpal compartment
4. The pisotriquetral compartment
5. The common carpometacarpal compartment
6. The first carpometacarpal compartment
7. The intermetacarpal compartment

The Radiocarpal Compartment

The proximal surface of the radiocarpal compartment is formed by the distal radial articular cartilage and the triangular fibrocartilage complex (TFCC) which overlies the distal ulna. The distal margins are formed by the scaphoid, lunate and the triquetral bones. These bones form a smooth C-shaped articular surface, the so-called greater arc of the wrist (Fig. 7.3). These bones are closely bound by the intrinsic ligaments of the wrist, tears of these ligaments cause malalignment and disruption of the greater arc of the wrist. The triangular fibrocartilage complex separates this compartment from the distal radioulnar joint. The wrist joint is capable of a wide range of movements, to allow

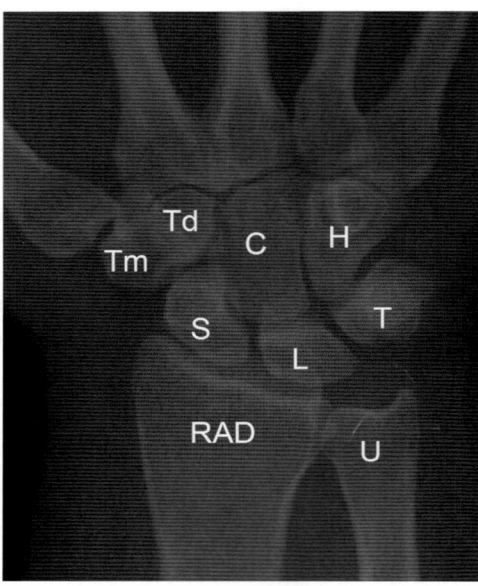

Fig. 7.1 DP radiograph of the wrist showing the relations of the carpal bone. *RAD* radius, *U* ulna, *S* scaphoid, *L* lunate, *T* triquetral, *Tm* trapezium, *Td* trapezoid, *C* capitate, *H* hamate

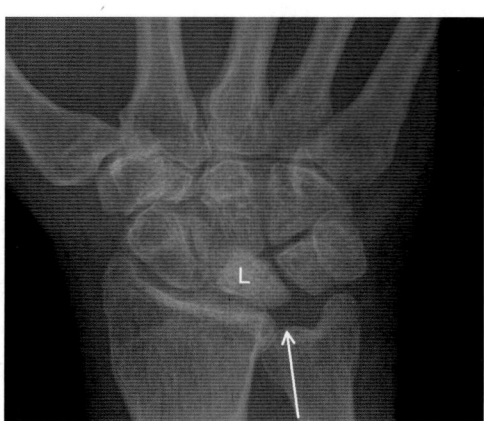

Fig. 7.2 DP radiograph of wrist showing a patient with negative ulna variance (*arrow*) and avascular necrosis of the lunate (L)

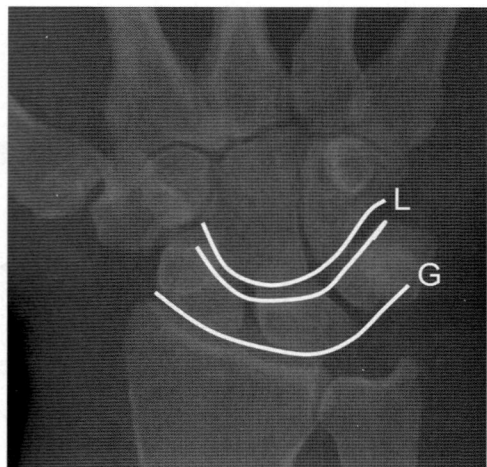

Fig. 7.3 DP radiograph showing greater (G) and lesser (L) arcs of the wrist

for this there are substantial capsular recesses most marked over the dorsal aspect of this compartment, at ultrasound these can be clearly visualized and can mimic pathology.

The Distal Radioulnar Compartment

This compartment is L shaped, proximally it is bounded by the articular cartilage surface of the dials ulnar and the ulnar notch of the radius. Distally lies the triangular fibrocartilage complex which extends from the base of the ulnar styloid to the ulnar notch of the distal radius. The principle movement occurring at this joint is pronation and supination where rotation of the radius occurs around the ulnar which should remain centred in the ulnar notch of the distal radius.

The Midcarpal Compartment

This compartment lies between the proximal and distal carpal rows, the articular surfaces of the proximal row in this compartment form a smooth arc called the lesser arc of the wrist (Fig. 7.3). Any disruption of this line indicates incongruence of the proximal row intercarpal relations, ligament derangement and possible instability. The joint space of the midcarpal compartment is widest over its ulnar aspect at the articulation of the triquetral and hamate. The radial aspect of this compartment is where the scaphoid articulates with the trapezium and trapezoid, this is a common site for developing osteoarthritis and this area is often referred to as the STT joint or complex.

The Pisotriquetral Compartment

The pisiform is a sesamoid bone lying within the flexor carpi ulnaris tendon sheath. It articulates with the triquetrum, there is considerable potential for movement in the pisotriquetral joint and to allow for this there is a sizeable synovial recess present over the proximal aspect of this articulation. This compartment can communicate with the wrist joint.

The Common Carpometacarpal Compartment

This compartment lies between the second to fifth metacarpal bases and the distal carpal row. The joint line of this compartment is somewhat convoluted but should remain the same width throughout (Fig. 7.4). Any variation in joint space could indicate dislocation or fracture dislocation. The synovial cavity of this compartment extends between the metacarpal bases and between the carpal bones of the distal row. There are three main articulations with this compartment; the trapezoid – second metacarpal, the capitates – third metacarpal and the hamate – fourth and fifth metacarpal.

The First Carpometacarpal Compartment

This is a saddle-shaped articulation between the trapezium and the first carpometacarpal. Its saddle-shaped articular surfaces mean that even minor degrees of malalignment following trauma produce considerable articular incongruence. It also makes radiographic imaging and injection of this joint more difficult even with imaging guidance.

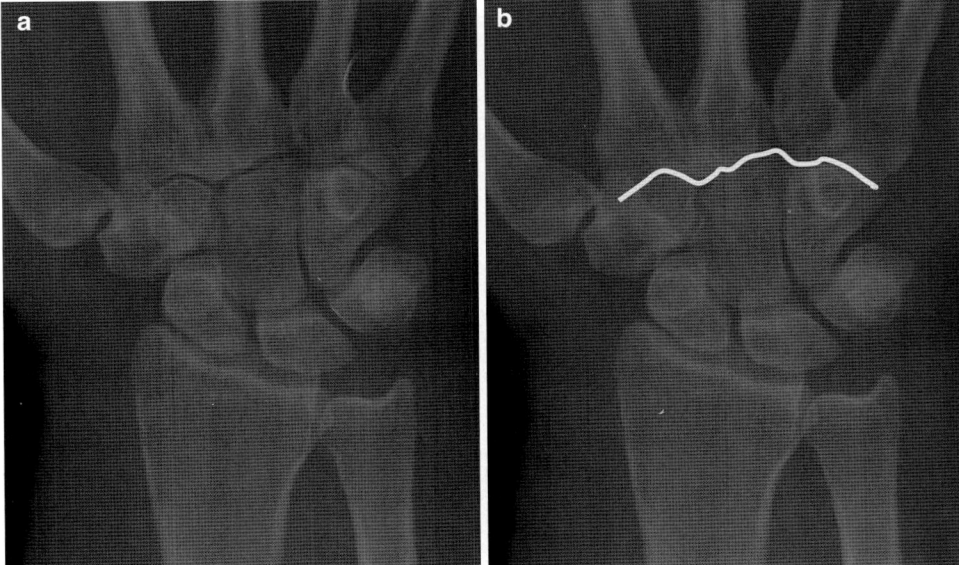

Fig. 7.4 (a and b) DP radiograph of the wrist. The second to fifth carpometacarpal joint should be uniformly congruent with the same width of joint space throughout. The joint line is marked with the *white line* in **b**

The Intermetacarpal Compartments

These are three synovial compartments that lie between the metacarpal bases, they frequently communicate with the common carpometacarpal compartment and are common sites of involvement in early inflammatory arthritides.

Soft Tissue Anatomy

Ligaments

Intrinsic or Interosseous ligaments

The bones of the proximal carpal row are joined by two interosseous ligaments.

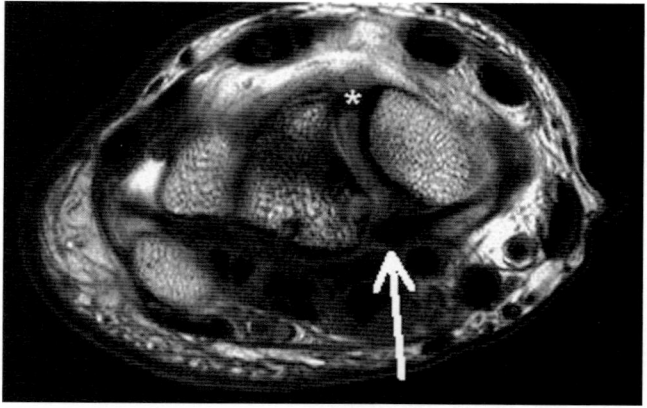

Fig. 7.5 Axial T2w MR scan of the wrist showing the dorsal (*asterisk*) and volar (*arrow*) of the interosseous scapholunate ligament

The scapholunate and triquetrolunate ligaments tightly bind the scaphoid, lunate and triquetrum over the proximal aspect of their articulations. The ligaments are C-shaped when imaged in the sagittal plane and extend from the palmar to dorsal aspects of these articulations. They have a central membranous portion with dorsal and volar thickenings of the ligament (Fig. 7.5). The dorsal component is the strongest portion of these ligaments with the central membranous portion relatively weak [12]. The lunate insertion of these ligaments is strong and in young individuals where avulsion fractures are more common avulsion of the lunate insertion of the scapholunate ligament is seen. The imaging appearances of these ligaments are best appreciated on MR arthrography and can vary from linear to a somewhat triangular appearance (Fig. 7.6). Development of multichannel dedicated wrist coils and the move to higher field strengths has greatly improved the MR visualization of the wrist and there is debate as to whether MR arthrography is necessary to accurately visualize derangement of these ligaments. The scapholunate ligament is weaker than then the lunatotriquetral ligament and as a result is injured more frequently. Both ligaments are flexible and can up to double in length prior to failure. When these ligaments are torn there is communication between the radiocarpal and midcarpal joint spaces allowing contrast or fluid within these compartments to flow freely. Disruption of the scapholunate ligament allows widening of the scapholunate space, in normality this space should measure proximally less than 2 mm on a dorsopalmar radiograph. If the space measures over 4 mm there is definite scapholunate dissociation, if it measures between 2 and 4 mm there is potential scapholunate dissociation and correlation with clinical signs and symptoms and other imaging is advised.

The distal carpal row contains three interosseous ligaments between the hamate, capitates and the trapezoid–trapezium complex. The ligaments do not fully extend from the dorsal

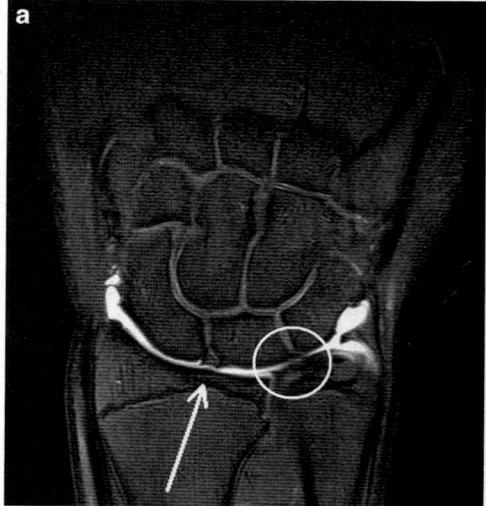
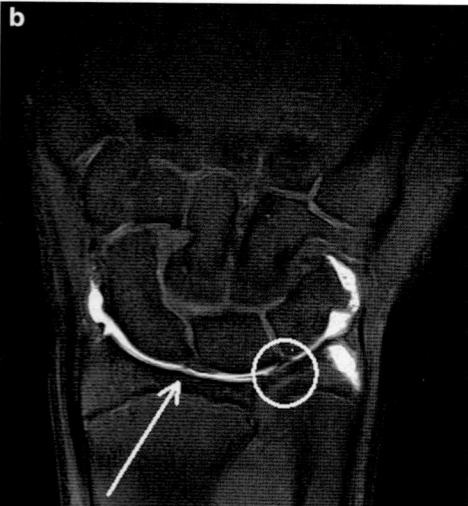

Fig. 7.6 Coronal T1 fat-saturated MR arthrogram of the wrist. (**a**) This shows normal appearances with a triangular configuration of the scapholunate (*arrow*) and linear configuration to the triquetrolunate ligament (*circled*). (**b**) This shows the opposite of **a** with normal variation. The scapholunate (*arrow*) has a linear configuration with a triangular configuration of the triquetrolunate ligament (*circled*)

to palmar aspects of these joints explaining the frequent communication between midcarpal and common metacarpal compartments in normality. These ligaments are strong and are rarely injured.

Extrinsic Ligaments

These ligaments are mainly divided into dorsal and volar ligament groups. The volar ligaments are stronger and are more significant stabilizers of wrist motion. Their relative strength however means they are less commonly injured. These ligaments are focal thickenings of the joint capsule and as such are difficult to visualize consistently with ultrasound, MR and even MR arthrography.

Volar

There are three volar ligaments on the radial aspect of the wrist joint; the radioscaphocapitate, the radiolunatotriquetral and the radioscapholunate ligaments.

- The strong radioscaphocapitate ligament arises from the volar aspect of the radial styloid, courses distal over a groove on the volar aspect of the scaphoid waist to it attachment on the centre of the volar surface of the capitates (Fig. 7.7). This ligament acts a fulcrum about which the scaphoid rotates during wrist motion, disruption of this ligament will result in abnormal scaphoid movement. This ligament is a primary stabilizer of the midcarpal compartment.
- The radiolunatotriquetral ligament is a large ligament arising from the volar lip of the radial styloid next to the origin of the radioscaphocapitate ligament. This broad ligament passes over the volar aspect of the lunate to its insertion on the triquetrum and acts as a support or sling to the lunate.
- The radioscapholunate ligament arises from the midportion of the distal radius over its volar aspect and inserts on the base of the scaphoid and lunate (Fig. 7.7). Its fibres reinforce the volar aspect of the interosseous scapholunate ligament and carry the neurovascular supply to scapholunate interosseous membrane. Disruption of this ligament in combination with the interosseous scapholunate ligament will result in scapholunate dissociation.

There are two main volar extrinsic ligaments over the ulnar aspect of the wrist.

These arise from the volar aspect of the triangular fibrocartilage complex and the base of the ulnar styloid. These course distally to insert on the lunate and triquetrum and are termed the Ulnolunate and ulnotriquetral ligaments, respectively. They form part of the triangular fibrocartilage complex and will be discussed further later.

Dorsal

The Dorsal extrinsic carpal ligaments are focal thickening of the joint capsule mainly on the radial aspect of the wrist joint. They form a V-configuration with the base of the V centred on the dorsal aspect of the triquetrum (Fig. 7.8). The radiolunatotriquetral ligament arises from the dorsal aspect of the distal radius close to Lister's tubercle adjacent to the extensor retinaculum, the dorsal carpal ligament extends from the triquetrum distally where it blends with the capsule of the wrist joint. Traction injury to these ligaments is the cause of the classic triquetral avulsion fracture seen dorsally on lateral radiographs of the wrist (Fig. 7.9). Occasionally proximal damage can occur at the origin of the radiolunatotriquetral ligament which can be associated with extensor retinacular disruption.

The Triangular Fibrocartilage Complex

The TFCC overlies the distal ulnar and is a key stabiliser of the distal radioulnar joint. In addition, the TFCC acts as a buffer between the distal ulnar and the carpi and has complex anatomy. The components of the TFCC are the fibrocartilagenous articular disc, the meniscus homologue,

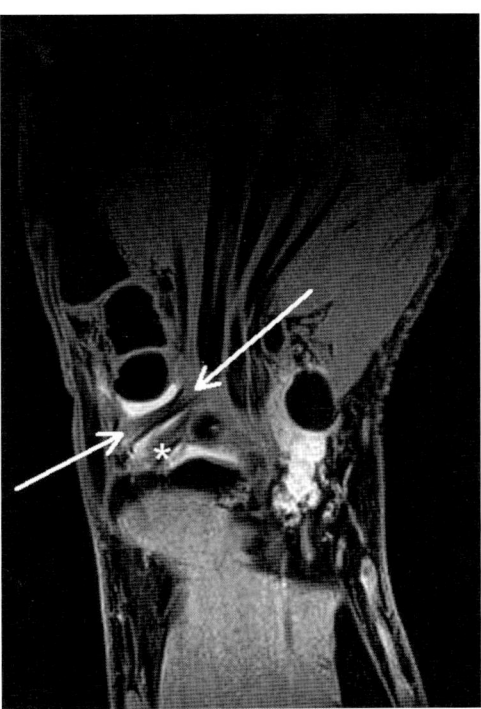

Fig. 7.7 Coronal T1 gradient echo sequence of wrist showing the volar radioscaphocapitate (*arrows*) and the radioscapholunate (*asterisk*) ligaments

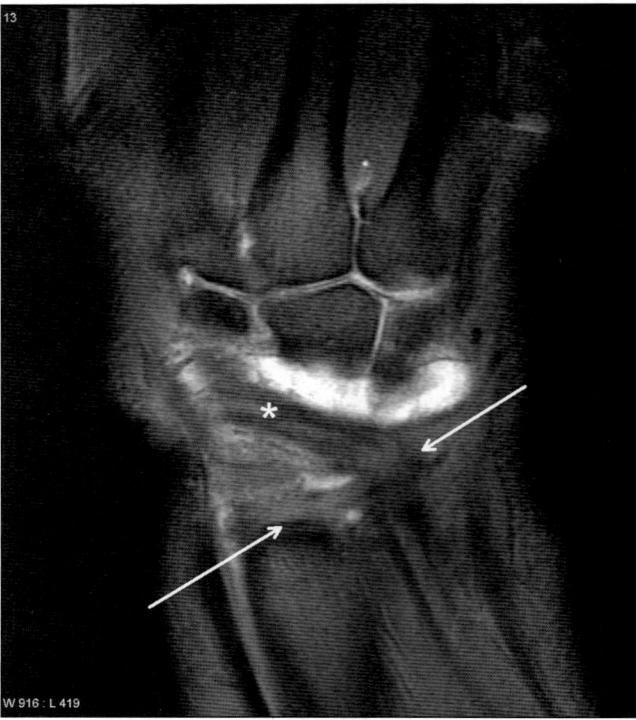

Fig. 7.8 Coronal T1 FSE MR arthrogram of wrist showing the dorsal extrinsic ligaments. The radiolunatotriquetral (*arrows*) and the dorsal carpal ligament (*asterisk*) are normally well seen on MR

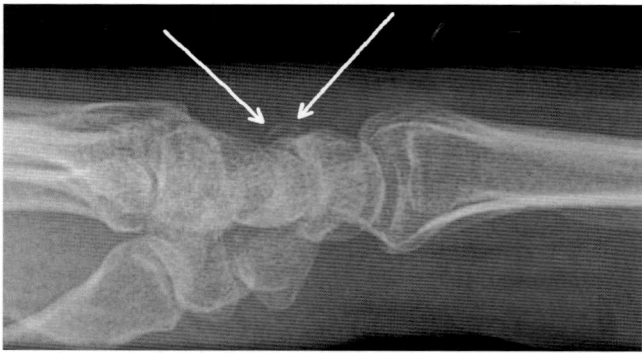

Fig. 7.9 Lateral radiograph of wrist showing the classic dorsal avulsion fracture of the triquetral (*arrows*)

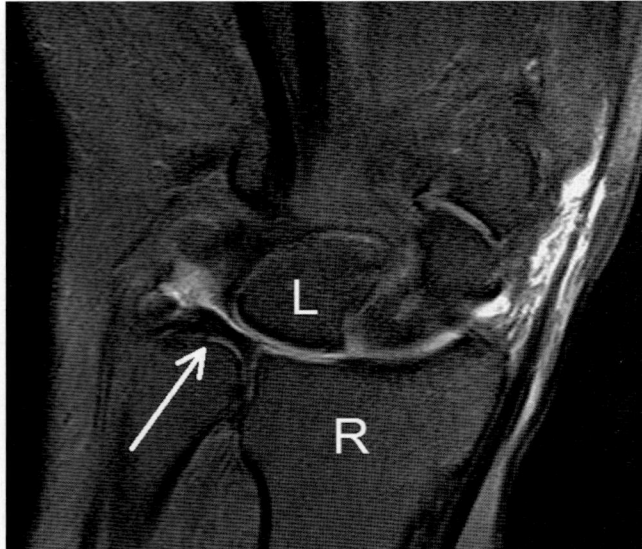

Fig. 7.10 Coronal PD fat-saturated MR scan of wrist showing the normal appearances of the TFCC (*arrows*)

the ulnocarpal ligaments, dorsal and volar radioulnar ligaments and ECU sheath.

Its main component is a fibrocartilagenous disc, this disc is thicker over its ulnar portion with a thinner membranous portion close to it radial insertion on the ulnar notch of the distal radius (Fig. 7.10). The disc varies in thickness from 5 to 2 mm with its blood supply arising from its periphery fed by the ulna artery via its radiocarpal branches and the dorsal and palmar branches of the anterior interosseous artery. As a result of this peripheral supply the membranous portion is less well vascularized, this limits the healing potential of membranous portion damage. Asymptomatic fenestration of perforation of the membranous portion is common past middle age. The disc inserts medially at the base of the ulnar styloid at the fovea and is attached. The ligaments of the TFCC act to stabilize and reinforce the margins of the fibrocartilagenous disc. On the volar aspect lie the strong ulnotriquetral and the weaker ulnolunate ligaments with an attachment of the TFCC also to the triquetrolunate interosseous ligament present on its volar aspect. Damage to the TFCC is as a result linked to triquetrolunate ligament injury. There are also transversely orientated volar and dorsal radioulnar ligaments which with the ECU tendon sheath help stabilize the disc relative to the distal ulnar and DRUJ. In addition to these ligaments is the meniscus homologue which is a combination of loose areolar tissue and the ulnar collateral ligament which form a peripheral soft tissue attachment of the disc. This is frequently associated with a large pre-styloid synovial recess arising from the radiocarpal compartment which can give confusing appearances when fluid filled or distended at arthrography.

Tendon and Soft Tissue Anatomy

The muscles of the forearm that move the hand and wrist all pass through fibro-osseous tunnels around the wrist joint. As such they have associated tenosynovial sheaths and are grouped by the differing tenosynovial sheaths they share/occupy.

The Extensor Compartment

The extensor tendons share six separate tenosynovial sheaths number 1–6 from radial to ulna. Lister's tubercle is a key landmark for identifying the extensor compartments. When viewed in the axial plane, the third extensor compartment containing extensor pollicis longus lies just on the ulna or medial aspect of Lister's tubercle (Fig. 7.11). Compartment 2 is the next radial compartment containing the tendons of extensor carpi radialis longus and brevis with compartment 1 containing Abductor pollicis longus and extensor pollicis brevis. This is the compartment involved in DeQuervain's tenosynovitis and frequently contains internal septae and accessory tendons. This normal variation becomes more apparent when there is tenosynovitis and the fluid and inflammation increase conspicuity of the structures. The superficial sensory branch of the radial nerve passes over extensor compartment 1 at the level of the radial styloid, this can be clearly visualized at ultrasound and should be identified and avoided when performing imaging-guided injections for De Quervain's tenosynovitis. The nomenclature and order of these radial extensor tendons can be remembered easily as from extensor pollicis Longus in compartment 3 they are alternately named brevis, longus, brevis and longus. So the order of tendons from extensor compartment 3–1 is extensor pollicis longus, extensor carpi radialis brevis, extensor carpi radialis longus, extensor pollicis brevis, abductor pollicis longus.

Extensor compartment 4 is large containing the extensor digitorum and extensor indicis tendons. This compartment has a thick fibrocartilagenous retinaculum that is hoop shaped and inserts onto the distal radius adjacent to Lister's tubercle with the radiolunatotriquetral ligament. This retinaculum can mimic tenosynovitis on ultrasound as it appears as a hypoechoic rim surrounding the tendons. Its tapered morphology on longitudinal scans distinguishes it from true tenosynovitis. The retinaculum itself constrains the tendons preventing bowstringing of the extensor tendons, this also gives an unusual appearance to extensor digitorum tenosynovitis as the fluid and inflamed tenosynovium is compressed by the retinaculum giving a characteristic dumbbell appearance on longitudinal scans. This can be confusing when first visualized, especially as ultrasound. Extensor compartment 5 is a small compartment containing extensor digitorum minimis with extensor compartment 6 containing extensor carpi ulnaris. This is a large tendon that lies within a notch on the medial aspect of the distal ulna. The structural integrity of the tendon and its tunnel is essential for normal mechanics and function without pain. This tendon sheath is approximately 5 cm in length with the fibro-osseous tunnel measuring 1.5 cm in length, it is anchored to the distal ulna by a subsheath on its deep portion. It is the complex interactions between the overlying extensor retinaculum, the ECU tendon sheath, its subsheath and the underlying TFCC which combine to allow normal forearm and wrist function.

The Flexor Compartment

On the volar aspect of the wrist lies the flexor compartment flexor, this is divided into two main fibro-osseous tunnels the carpal tunnel and Guyon's canal by the flexor retinaculum.

The flexor retinaculum or transverse carpal ligament is a broad sheet of fibrous tissue that forms the roof of the carpal tunnel (Fig. 7.12). Proximally it connects the scaphoid tubercle and pisiform and distally the trapezium and hook of the hamate. The retinaculum varies in configuration, proximally the retinaculum is more bowed and is convex on its volar aspect, distally it becomes more flattened.

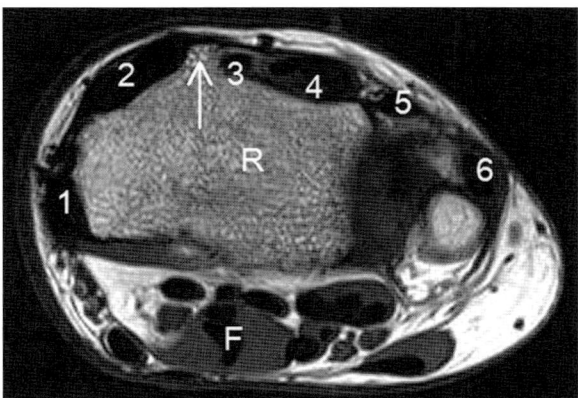

Fig. 7.11 Axial T1w MR scan of the wrist showing the anatomy of the six extensor compartments (numbered). Lister's tubercle (*arrow*) serves as a useful landmark for identifying the position of compartments 2 and 3 when assessing either MR or ultrasound scans. *R* radius, *F* flexor digitorum superficialis

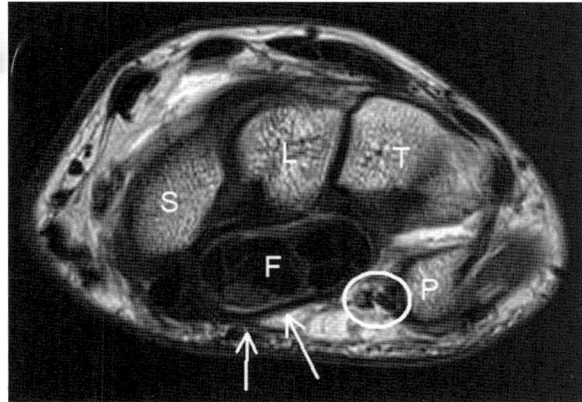

Fig. 7.12 Axial T1w MR scan through the proximal carpal row showing the ulna neurovascular bundle in Guyon's canal (*circled*) and the carpal tunnel containing the finger flexors (F). The roof of the carpal tunnel, the flexor retinaculum (*arrows*), is clearly visualized. *S* scaphoid, *L* lunate, *T* triquetral, *P* pisiform

Within the carpal tunnel lie the long flexor tendons of the fingers and the median nerve. The relative positions of these structures vary as they move from proximal to distal in the carpal tunnel. Proximally the carpal tunnel is bounded by the scaphoid, capitates, lunate and trapezium. The median nerve at this level lies just deep to the flexor retinaculum anterior to the deep and superficial flexors of the fingers. The flexor pollicis longus tendon lies lateral to the flexor digitorum tendons. More distally the carpal tunnel is bounded by the hamate, capitates, trapezoid and trapezium with the retinaculum having a more flattened configuration. The median nerve has a more flattened configuration in the distal carpal tunnel, the median nerve is mobile within the carpal tunnel, proximally it lies anterior to the flexor indicis tendon and distally it lies on the ulnar aspect of flexor indicis. Contraction of the flexors or wrist flexion produces ulna shift of the median nerve with the nerve lying between the second and fifth superficial flexor tendons.

Guyon's canal is a fibro-osseous tunnel approximately 4 cm in length extending from the pisiform to the hypothenar eminence (Fig. 7.12). Its ulna border is formed by the pisiform and hook of hamate, its floor by the flexor retinaculum and its roof by the superficial flexor retinaculum and pisohamate interosseous ligament. The tunnel contains the ulna nerve, ulna artery and their two accompanying veins.

Nerve Anatomy

Ulnar Nerve

The ulna nerve passes down the ulna aspect of the elbow between the two heads of flexor carpi ulnaris and just below elbow, it sends branches to flexor carpi ulnaris and ulnar half of flexor digitorum profundus. It passes down forearm deep to FCU, and then enters Guyon's canal. It gives off its dorsal sensory branch about 5 cm proximal to the pisiform with a deep motor branch passing through Guyon's canal adjacent to the hook of the hamate. The deep branch innervates the hypothenar muscles and third and fourth lumbricals, adductor pollicis, all interossei, and deep head of flexor pollicis brevis. The arrangement of these branches help the clinician define the level of entrapment deepening on whether FDP is involved (elbow) there is dissociated sensory and motor dysfunction (Guyon's canal).

Median Nerve

The median nerve passes down the forearm positioned between the deep and superficial flexor compartment. As the nerve approaches the carpal tunnel it becomes more superficial lying on the volar aspect of the flexor tendons. Once it emerges from the carpal tunnel into the palm the median nerve divides into its digital branches. A high division of the median nerve is a relatively common finding and is associated with a persistent median artery.

Radial Nerve

At the level of the elbow the radial nerve divides into the posterior interosseous and superficial radial nerve. The superficial radial nerve passes down the forearm deep to brachioradialis, 8 cm from the wrist the nerve emerges from underneath brachioradialis to pass over the superficial aspect of extensor compartment 1 at the level of the radial styloid. This nerve is to be avoided when performing DeQuervain's tenosynovitis therapeutic injections. The nerve provides sensory innervation to the dorsum of thumb, first web space and hand as far as the middle of ring finger. This excludes the subungual region of the thumb which is supplied by the median nerve.

Hand Anatomy

Tendon Anatomy

There are two main muscles responsible for finger flexion, flexor digitorum profundus (FDP) and superficialis. They form relatively thick tendons in the distal forearm with FDP as one would expect lying deep to the flexor digitorum superficialis (FDS). FDP passes through the carpal tunnel into the palm and extends to insert into the base of the distal phalanx. The superficialis tendon follows the same course into the finger but divides into two at the level of the proximal interphalangeal joint with each slip passing around FDP to insert onto the middle phalanx. This results in unusual appearances as the two slips of FDS pass around FDP especially at ultrasound where anisotropy from tendon passing in differing directions can give the artefactual appearance of tendon damage. The differing insertion of FDP and FDS give very differing function with FDP solely responsible for flexion of the distal interphalangeal joint and both tendons contributing to flexion and the PIPJ and MCPJ.

The flexor tendons are guided by a series of fibrocartilagenous retinaculae or pulleys reinforcing their palmar aspect that prevent bowstringing of these tendons. These structures are small but easily visualized with modern ultrasound equipment, they are difficult to demonstrate in normals with MR.

The pulleys are divided into annular and cruciform pulleys and are numbered accordingly. The cruciform pulleys are weaker and functionally less important than the annular pulleys. There are five annular pulleys that are numbered A1–A5 [13]. These pulleys have a characteristic hypoechoic appearance at ultrasound and should be of uniform thickness holding the tendons closely apposed to the adjacent bone. Two of these pulleys warrant particular discussion [14, 15]. The A1 pulley lies over the palmar aspect of the flexor tendon at the level of the metacarpal head. Abnormal thickening of this pulley or the adjacent tendon sheath is responsible for triggering of fingers. The A2 pulley lies on the palmar aspect of the flexor tendons at the level of the midproximal phalanx. This pulley is the most frequently disrupted pulley and when torn allows separation of the tendon away from the underlying proximal phalanx. Demonstration of this required both static and dynamic scanning with ultrasound, the modality of choice.

The extensor tendons of the fingers occupy extensor compartment 4 at the level of the wrist. There are four tendons at this level, distal to the wrist the extensor tendons merge with the deep fascia at the level of the metacarpal head to form the extensor expansion. The extensor tendon divides into three components at the level of the PIPJ. The central component inserts at the base of the middle phalanx with the two lateral components passing distally to insert onto the dorsal aspect of the base of the distal phalanx. The little finger has its own extensor tendon (extensor compartment 5) and also receives a slip tendon from extensor digitorum. Short tendons from the interossei and lumbricals also insert onto the extensor expansion.

The osseous anatomy of the hand is relatively straight forward with each finger having metacarpal, proximal, middle and distal phalanges. The thumb differs slightly having only a proximal and distal phalanx. These are connected by a series of synovial joints. The metacarpophalangeal joint synovial joints have a thin dorsal capsule separated from the overlying extensor tendon by a thin bursa. This is not fluid filled in normal patients. Each metacarpophalangeal joint has a palmar and two collateral ligaments. The palmar ligament has a strong insertion on the phalangeal base with a relatively weak proximal insertion on the metacarpal neck. This ligament blends with the collateral and the transverse palmar ligaments and lies deep to the flexor tendons. Movements at the finger metacarpophalangeal joints are relatively complex with flexion–extension, abduction–adduction and limited rotation all possible. The range and degree of movement requires complex ligamentous constraints and the lack of intrinsic osseous stability renders these joint liable to dislocation and subluxation. The thumb has less range of movement than the fingers with only flexion–extension movements that occurs at 90° to the plane of flexion–extension in the fingers.

The interphalangeal joints are also synovial and also have a palmar and two collateral ligaments reinforcing the fibrous capsule. The volar plate is a fibrocartilagenous disc reinforcing the volar aspects of capsular insertions of the interphalangeal joints of the hand and foot. They lie deep to the flexor tendons and can be both disrupted themselves or involved in avulsion fractures of the phalanges during dislocation or subluxation.

The ulna collateral ligament of the thumb metacarpophalangeal joint lies deep to the adductor aponeurosis of the thumb. The thumb adductor inserts at the base of the proximal phalanx with fibres extending dorsally to form this aponeurosis. This is an important relationship when considering injury of the ulna collateral ligament.

The Biomechanics of the Wrist

Approximately half of flexion–extension movement occurs at the radiocarpal joint and half at the midcarpal joint. Movements between radial and ulna deviation involve flexion of the scaphoid during radial deviation with the scaphoid engaging the scaphoid fossa of the distal radial articular surface. In ulna deviation, there is extension of the scaphoid with the lunate engaging the lunate fossa of the distal radial articular surface. This extension of the scaphoid helps visualize the scaphoid waist on PA radiograph; hence, the inclusion of an ulnar deviation angled view of the wrist in scaphoid series radiographs. The triquetrum has similar movements to those of the scaphoid during radial and ulna deviation although the degree of movement is much less. The lunate controls these movements and a degree of elasticity in the interosseous ligament connecting the lunate to the scaphoid and triquetrum is required to allow this degree of movement.

The biomechanics of the wrist ligaments during movement are complex. Both ligament groups are important contributors to wrist stability, the extrinsic ligaments are relatively stiff compared to the intrinsic ligaments with intrinsics having more elastic potential under load capable of stretching to greater length before disruption or permanent deformity occurs. The volar radiocarpal and the interosseous ligaments are the most important contributors to carpal stability. Derangement of either the intrinsic or extrinsic ligaments can result in instability and disruption of normal carpal relations. This is described in detail in the carpal instability and in the interosseous ligament sections but briefly involves the wrist assuming an instability pattern characterized by either dorsal or volar tilt of the lunate and derangement of the greater and or lesser arcs of the wrist where there is disruption of the interosseous ligaments.

Wrist Pathology

Scaphoid Fractures

Fracture of the scaphoid is the commonest wrist fracture most frequently resulting from a fall onto an outstretched hand. Scaphoid fractures are of concern because the unusual blood supply arrangements of the scaphoid. The scaphoid vascular supply runs principally from distal to proximal within the bone thus fracture of the scaphoid waist has a significant incidence of avascularity of the proximal fragment. This can result in an increased incidence of non-union and avascular collapse of the proximal fragment. Collapse is associated with an increased incidence of radioscaphoid arthritis and non-union is linked with ongoing wrist dysfunction and potential instability. Early diagnosis and effective immobilization helps reduce these complications. Contact sports such as rugby, American football or martial arts are most common linked with scaphoid injury though catching sports like cricket or baseball also have a higher incidence of scaphoid fracture [1, 16–18].

Fracture of the scaphoid waist is the commonest site account for 60% of fracture with 20% occurring in the distal and proximal poles, respectively. Distal fractures have the lowest incidence of avascular necrosis with the incidence rising for more proximal fractures. The overall incidence of AVN is 10–15%.

Radiographs are the initial modality of choice with a scaphoid series including DP, lateral and ulna deviation and angled views to view the scaphoid at as near to 90° from its long access as possible. No visible fracture on the initial radiographs, does not exclude significant scaphoid injury and in the presence of clinical suspicion follow-up radiographs at 10–14 days or alternative imaging such as MR are indicated. Limited protocol MR will demonstrate scaphoid fracture to good effect (Fig. 7.13). Scintigraphy can also be used but is generally reserved for patients with negative serial radiographs and persisting symptoms at 6 weeks. CT is of value in assessing fracture healing and developing non-union. Post-intravenous gadolinium scanning can be of value in demonstrating viability in the proximal pole in fractures (Fig. 7.14). Avascularity of the proximal pole is a key factor in developing non-union. The key indicator of developing non-union is sclerosis developing around the fracture site without bridging bone. Interosseous ligament injury can also occur in association with scaphoid fracture, this can be demonstrated at MR but may also require MR arthrography for assessment/diagnosis.

Stress fractures of the scaphoid related to sports have been described, these involve relative high force repetitive activity such as gymnastics or shot-putt [16].

Hamate Fracture

Hamate fractures are seen quite frequently in sports [1, 2, 19–22]. It is important to differentiate between body of hamate and hook of hamate fractures as they have quite different aetiologies. Body of hamate fractures occur in association with fracture dislocations of the fourth and fifth metacarpal bases. A direct blow to the metacarpals is the commonest mechanism of injury seen in punching and contact sports. In assessing these fractures it is important to ensure congruence of the joint space of the entire carpometacarpal joint space (Fig. 7.15). Fractures of the body of the hamate are difficult to diagnose with radiography and cross-sectional imaging with

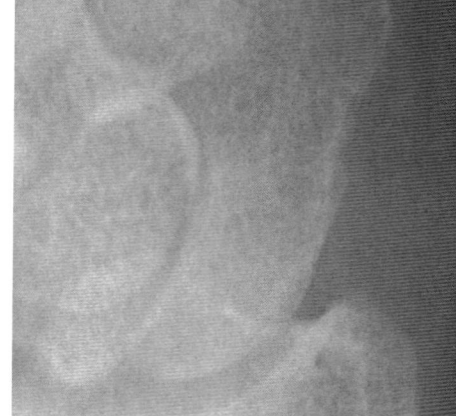
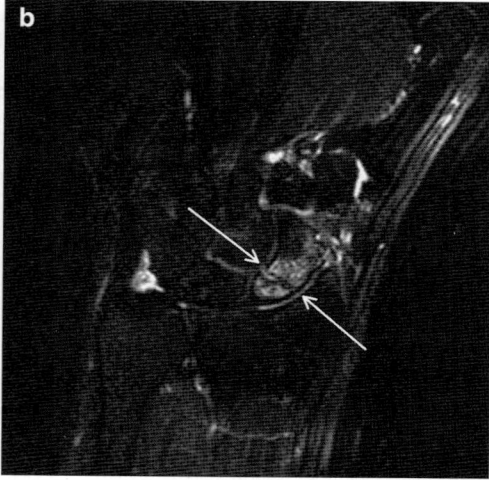

Fig. 7.13 (a) Radiograph of scaphoid in trauma patient showing no visible fracture. (b) T2 fat-suppressed MR of the same patient where a complete fracture of the proximal scaphoid waist (*arrows*) is seen surrounded by marked bone and soft tissue oedema

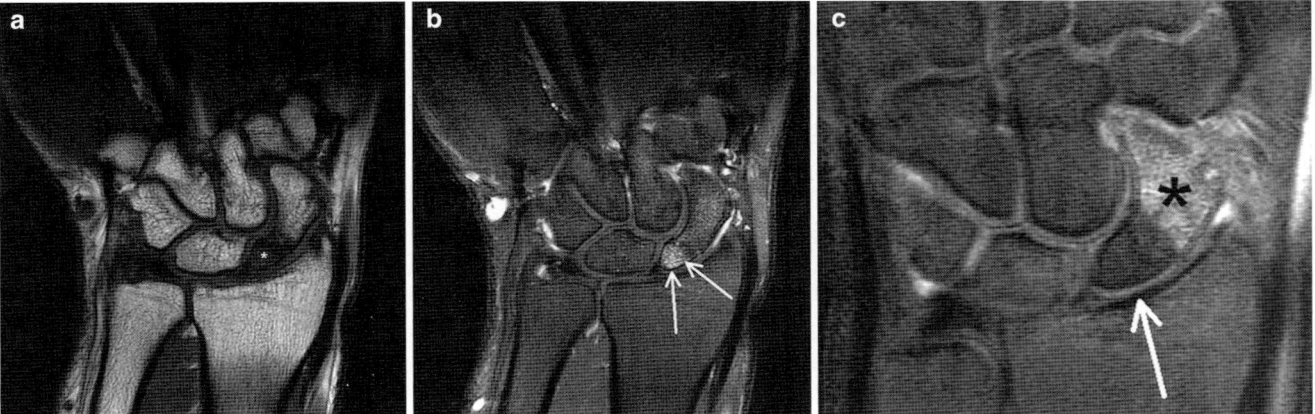

Fig. 7.14 MR scans assessing proximal pole vascularity. (**a**) T1-weighted MR scans show uniformly decreased signal in the proximal fracture fragments (*asterisk*). (**b**) Viable proximal pole showing enhancement in the proximal pole fragment on the post-gadolinium scans (*arrows*). (**c**) Non-viable proximal pole with no enhancement proximally on the post-gadolinium scans (*arrows*) and clear enhancement distal to the fracture site (*asterisk*)

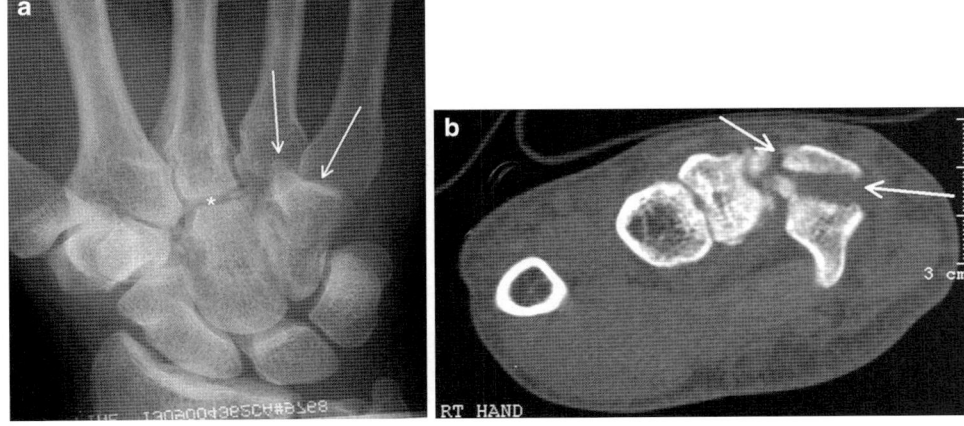

Fig. 7.15 (**a**) DP radiograph of the wrist showing normal congruence of the radial aspect of the carpometacarpal joints (*asterisk*) with loss of joint space in the forth and fifth carpometacarpal joints. (**b**) Axial CT of same patient showing fracture dislocation of the forth and fifth carpometacarpal joints with fracture of the Hamate body (*arrows*)

CT or MR is frequently required. Assessments of the degree of angulation, comminution and articular incongruence or subluxation are the important imaging findings.

Hook of hamate fractures are different, they can occur as a result of direct injury following a fall onto the outstretch hand or fall on the hand while holding an object but is also seen in particular sporting activities. Racquet, club or bat sports are the most common associations with impaction of the grip of the racquet or club on the hamate resulting in osseous injury. This can be either acute following a single traumatic event or chronic resulting stress fracture. These fractures are difficult to diagnose clinically and are important as they have a high incidence of complication. There is a substantial risk of osteonecrosis and non-union in these fractures, this combined with the close relations of the hook of hamate with the ulna neurovascular structure can result in ulna nerve dysfunction of damage to the ulna artery (Fig. 7.16). Racquet sports differ from other sports in their side distribution. Racquet sports cause impact of the grip against the hook of hamate of the *dominant* hand where as in golf, baseball and hockey the club will impact against the hamate in the *non-dominant* hand [1, 2, 20, 23, 24].

Fracture Dislocation of the Wrist

Fracture dislocations of the wrist are high-energy injuries involving complex fracture patterns and malalignment of the carpi. Cycling, motorsport and contact sports are

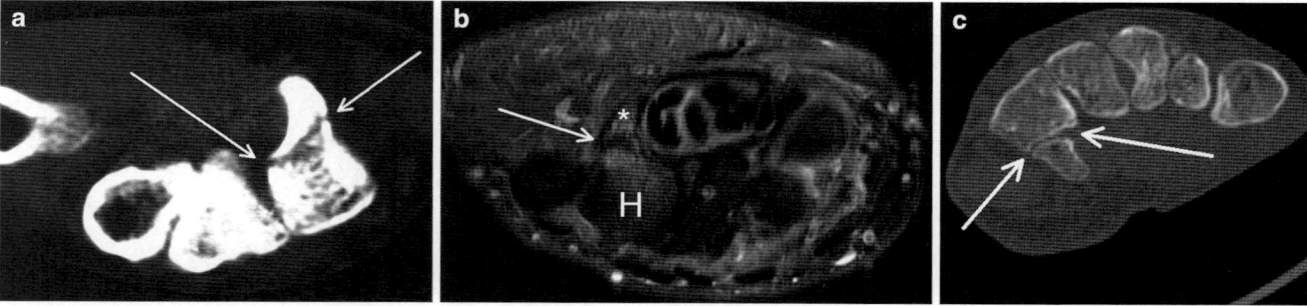

Fig. 7.16 (a) Axial CT showing fracture through the base of the hook of hamate (*arrows*). (b) T2 fat-saturated axial MR showing acute fracture (*arrow*) at the base of the hook of hamate (*asterisk*) surrounded by bone marrow and soft tissue oedema. *H* hamate. (c) Axial CT scan showing established non-union in a hook of hamate fracture with clearly defined sclerotic margins (*arrows*)

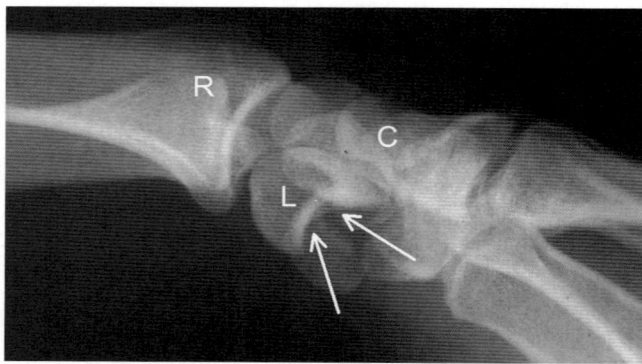

Fig. 7.17 Lateral view of the wrist showing the empty distal articular surface of the lunate (*arrows*) with dorsal displacement of the capitates (C) in perilunate dislocation. *R* radius

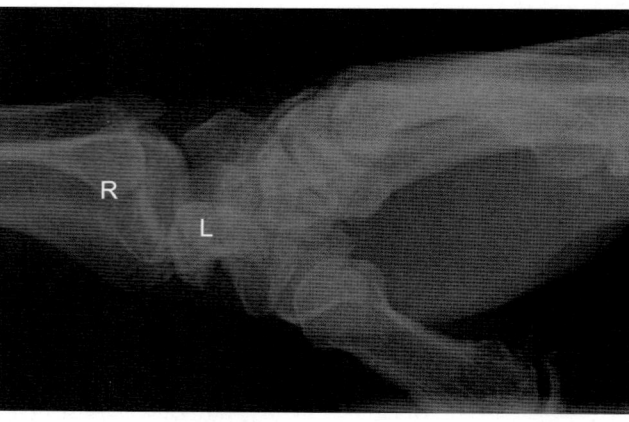

Fig. 7.18 Lateral radiograph of wrist showing lunate dislocation. In comparison to Fig. 7.21 the lunate (L) has turned through nearly 90° typical of lunate dislocation. *R* radius

the most frequent associated sports. The nomenclature of fracture dislocation follows midcarpal relations and specifically the alignment of the lunate and capitate. Perilunate dislocation represents dislocation occurring at the midcarpal joint level with the lunate remaining normally aligned with the distal radius. The capitate and distal row are normally displaced dorsally with volar angulation of the lunate present, the degree of lunate angulation is usually mild compared to lunate dislocation and the capitates shifts dorsally relative to the distal radius on the lateral projection (Fig. 7.17). In lunate dislocation the lunate is dislocated in a volar direction and is normally angulated to 90° with relatively normal alignment of the capitate and distal radius on the lateral view (Fig. 7.18). Lunate dislocation normally results from an axial loading injury with failure of the dorsal radiocarpal ligaments allowing volar displacement of the lunate. Perilunate and lunate dislocations are associated with fractures; perilunate dislocation is normally accompanied by complex fractures of the carpi forming arcs of derangement across the proximal and distal carpal row and the distal radius and ulna. The nomenclature is descriptive

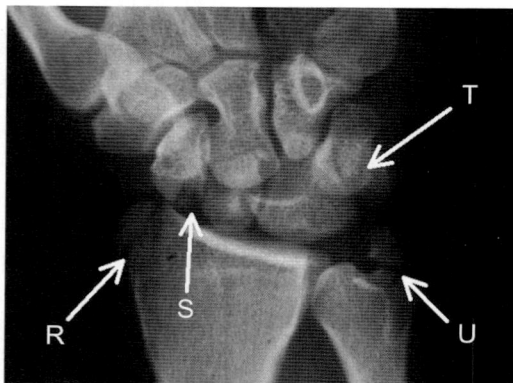

Fig. 7.19 Trans-radial (R) trans-scaphoid (S) trans-triquetral (T) trans-ulna (U) perilunate dislocation

and involves the names of all the fractured bones preceded by "trans" followed by perilunate fracture dislocation. Thus the fracture in Fig. 7.19 would be termed a "trans-radial trans-scaphoid trans-triquetral trans-ulna perilunate fracture dislocation," simple!

Other Wrist fractures

The most common fractures around the wrist affect the distal radius and ulna occurring approximately ten times more frequently than carpal bone fractures. These classically result from axial compression during a fall onto the outstretched hand with the pattern of fracture varying with the exact position of the wrist at impact. Clearly, these can occur in any sport but contact and high-speed sports on hard surfaces will result in a higher incidence of these injuries. There are various eponyms for different types of fractures with distal radial fractures most commonly result from falling onto a pronated dorsiflexed hand. When assessing wrist fractures it is vital to appreciate the degree of articular surface involvement and malalignment present and to look for any associated interosseous ligament damage. Ligamentous and TFCC injuries can accompany distal radial fractures in up to 50% of cases.

The Colles' fracture is a transverse fracture of the distal radius extending from the volar aspect to the dorsal distal radius associated with an ulna styloid fracture in about 50% of cases. The fracture is associated with dorsal angulation of the distal radial articular surface and a degree of radial shortening producing a classic "dinner fork" deformity of the wrist. The fracture is associated with complication most frequently resulting from malunion with persisting deformity limiting function in the wrist, carpal tunnel syndrome, reflex sympathetic dystrophy, flexor tendon entrapment and secondary ulna impaction syndrome are all recognized complications.

The Smith's fracture is very similar to a Colles' fracture but with volar rather than dorsal angulation. The appearance on the PA radiograph is remarkably similar and assessment of the lateral view is important in differentiating these fractures. The smith's fracture has similar complication to a Colles' fracture and carries a higher incidence of extensor tendon injury.

A Barton's fracture is actually a form of fracture dislocation involving the dorsal rim of the distal radius. This classically occurs with axial compression of the wrist in pronation and dorsiflexion as would occur in a deceleration injury when holding a steering wheel or handle bars. The larger the fracture fragment the greater the degree of instability present and the higher the likelihood of internal fixation being required. The reverse Barton's fracture is actually more common than the dorsal fracture, which can be considered a variant of the Smith's fracture.

True dislocation of the radiocarpal joint is relatively rare and although it can be an isolated finding it is usually associated with either a Barton's or reverse Barton's fracture.

Fracture of the distal radial styloid can occur as either an avulsion injury or be related to direct impaction. This fracture is also known as the Chauffeur's fracture and resulted from the kick back of the starting handle of old cars. The fracture tends to be somewhat oblique and as such can be difficult to demonstrate on a PA and lateral view of the wrist alone. Fortunately, these patients normally have tenderness in the anatomical snuffbox and scaphoid series films are normally obtained allowing fracture diagnosis. This is however still one of the review areas within the wrist for fractures along with the scaphoid, capitates and hamate. This fracture is associated with scapholunate ligament injury particularly when the fracture line runs close to the scapholunate interspace (Fig. 7.20) [25].

The Galeazzi fracture is the combination of a distal radial fracture and dislocation of the distal radioulnar joint. This occurs because the radius and ulna form an osseous ring. The analogy often used is that of a polo mint that has similar mechanical properties to a ring of bone in terms of rigidity. It is very difficult to break this ring in only one place thus when there is one break there should usually be a second disruption present within this ring. In the Galeazzi fracture the fracture is accompanied not by a second fracture but by dislocation of the distal ulna. Radiographs are usually taken of the forearm rather than the wrist itself and the patient has most pain related to the radial fracture site. Particular attention needs to be paid to the wrist appearances and formal views of the wrist are advised with early recourse to cross-sectional imaging when required.

Other isolated fractures of the capitate, lunate, pisiform, trapezium and trapezoid are rare and are more frequently

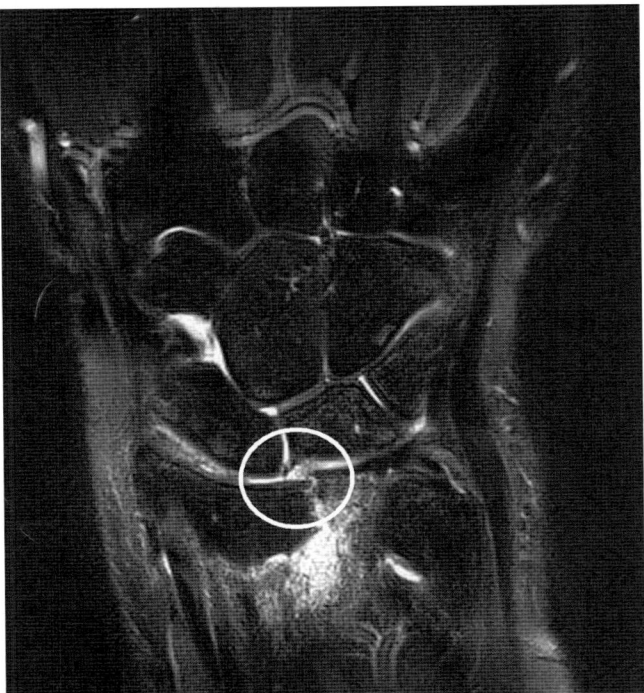

Fig. 7.20 MR scan showing distal radial styloid fracture associated with scapholunate ligament tear (*circled*)

seen in high-energy injury with complex greater arc fracture dislocations. The increasing use of MR in patients with suspected bone or ligament injury fractures has lead to increased awareness of these injuries. Capitate fracture, in particular, can occur as an isolated injury. They are particularly difficult to demonstrate radiographically, require careful assessment of the radiographs and cross-sectional imaging is frequently required where there is borderline radiographic abnormality.

Ligament Injury

Scapholunate Ligament Injury

The scapholunate ligament has surprisingly complex functionality for such a small ligament. It has a short strong dorsal, weaker volar and a weakest central thin membranous component controlling movement between the scaphoid and lunate. The dorsal component is the key link between the scaphoid and lunate during flexion and extension movement with the volar portion controlling more rotation of the scaphoid relative to the lunate. There is a disparity between the degrees of movement between the scaphoid and lunate in flexion; from neutral the lunate flexes by 30° compared to 60° of scaphoid flexion. Extension on both bones is similar at about 30°. The scaphoid flexes during flexion and radial deviation of the wrist. Imagine the trapezium moving proximally towards the radius in radial deviation, the scaphoid has to flex its distal pole out of the way to allow this movement to occur. Both the volar and dorsal portion of the ligament is required to maintain normal biomechanics of the scapholunate unit [26].

Disruption normally relates to a single traumatic event which most frequently occurs following a fall onto the outstretch hand in hyperextension and pronation. An ulna-deviated position also places the ligament at greater risk of damage, patients with negative ulna variance and lunatotriquetral coalition are also at greater risk of scapholunate ligament injury.

In the acute phase patients present with an acutely painful swollen wrist, chronic cases present more with signs and symptoms of secondary carpal instability.

The radiographic features are widening of the scapholunate interspace measured over its proximal aspect. Less than 2 mm is normal. Greater than 4 mm indicates ligament disruption. Two to four millimetre widening indicate borderline widening warranting further investigation especially when there is evidence of a Dorsal intercalated segment instability pattern (see carpal instability below). This used to be known as the "Terry Thomas" sign but this name has now been sadly superseded by the names "Madonna" or "Letterman" sign (Fig. 7.21).

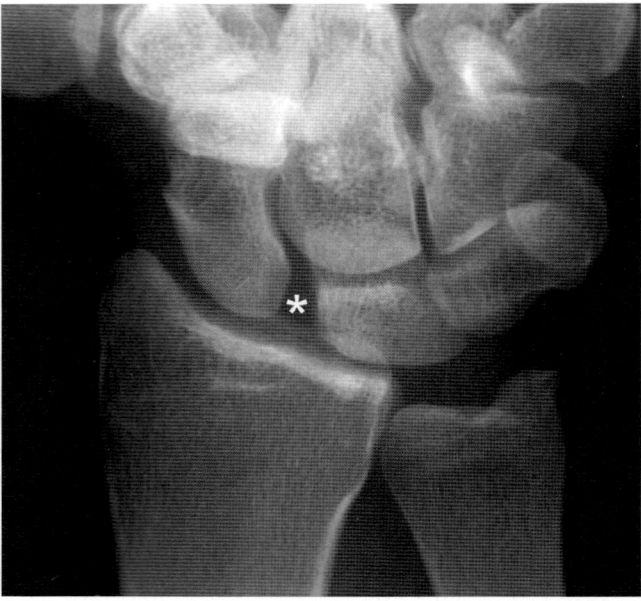

Fig. 7.21 DP radiograph of the wrist demonstrating widening of the scapholunate interspace (*asterisk*), the "Terry Thomas" sign

Further investigation can be with stress radiographs, fluoroscopy, conventional arthrography, MR or MR arthrography. Radiographs or fluoroscopic images taken in differing positions and under stress either from clenched fist or distraction fluoroscopy should demonstrate the same scapholunate distance throughout movement, variation in the width of the scapholunate interval is a strong indicator of ligament derangement. Arthrography can be performed via a variety of approaches, the commonest injection site are the dorsal aspect of the scaphoid avoiding the dorsal trim of the radius and the dorsal aspect of the lunate. Injection are usually performed with a 23-gauge needle and a mix of iodinated contrast and long-acting local anaesthetic, the local anaesthetic is to help determine whether the abnormality seen is symptomatic or not. Asymptomatic abnormalities are seen in the interosseous ligaments and TFCC, failure of the patients symptoms to improve for 5–6 h post-injection when there is long-acting local anaesthetic around the abnormality suggests it may not be responsible for the patient's pain. The author would not advise injecting more than 3 ml of this contrast mix as overfilling of the joint synovial recesses can limit visualization of the interosseous ligament areas (Fig. 7.22). When MR or CT arthrography is being performed more injectate can be injected as the cross-sectional nature of the MR and CT gives good visualization regardless of the amount of contrast in the recesses (Fig. 7.23). If the recesses are over filled at arthrography a distraction view is useful to pull contrast back into the main joint space. Arthrography is considered the technique of choice for demonstrating ligament tears and should include pre- and post-contrast views which

7 Hand and Wrist Injuries

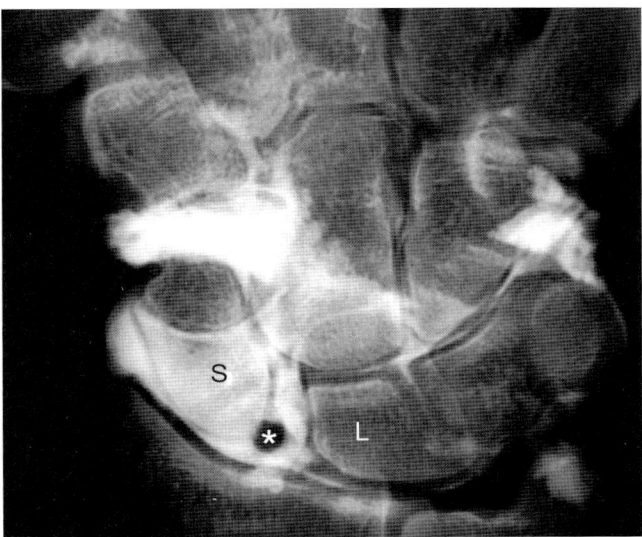

Fig. 7.22 Conventional arthrography showing increased separation of the scaphoid (S) and lunate (L). Contrast has flowed freely into the midcarpal compartment with the torn end of the scapholunate ligament clearly visible (*asterisk*)

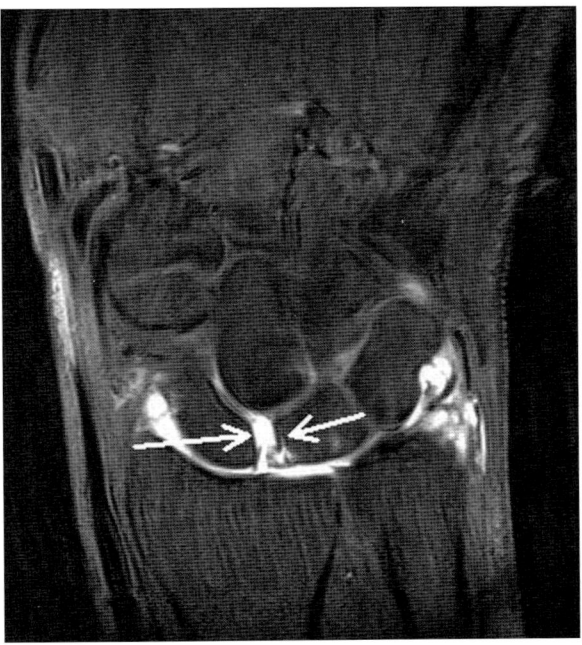

Fig. 7.23 Coronal T1 fat-saturated MR arthrography image showing contrast flowing between the radiocarpal and midcarpal compartments through a widened scapholunate interspace (*arrows*). The redundant torn scapholunate ligament is visible in this interspace proximally

include PA, lateral, ulna deviation, radial deviation and distraction views. MR arthrography is currently considered the gold standard though developments in coil technology with the introduction of high-quality eight-channel wrist coils and increasing availability of 3T scanners conventional MR is showing increasing promise in the detection of significant scapholunate injury [27].

The normal dorsal component of the scapholunate ligament can be visualized with ultrasound in 78% of normal patients where it appears as a bright linear structure over the dorsal aspect of the scapholunate [28, 29]. There is little data available to assess how well ultrasound would perform in detecting abnormalities of the scapholunate ligament though given its limited access it is unlikely to be of significant value.

Although MR will not help determine the clinical relevance of a ligament deficiency the developments in coil technology and a move to 3T imaging allow improved resolution of the interosseous images in non-arthrographic studies. The coronal plane is the most useful with the normal scapholunate ligament visualized connecting the proximal aspects of the lunate and scaphoid. Sagittal sequences are also useful in demonstrating the thickened dorsal and volar components and any associated instability pattern. At MR the scapholunate ligament is seen as a triangular or linear structure, it is generally of low signal though can show increased signal on gradient echo images. There is normal variation to the scapholunate with both linear and even somewhat circular appearances described. T1 and STIR or T2 fat-suppressed sequences are advised, PD fat-suppressed sequences and T1 gradient echo sequences can be of value though undercutting of the scapholunate insertions by articular cartilage can give rise to diagnostic confusion. Abnormality of the ligament is best demonstrated in the presence of effusion where an arthrographic effect helps diagnosis. This is most likely to be present in the acute phase of injury. Fluid outlining a defect within the ligament or diffuse high signal and or enhancement within or around the ligament are signs of derangement. Avulsion of the ligament can also be seen, the fracture fragments are small and exceptionally difficult to appreciate on radiographs and cross-sectional imaging with either CT or MR is usually required (Fig. 7.24). Scapholunate dissociation is not entirely the result of scapholunate ligament derangement, it is possible to tear all or a portion of the scapholunate without having the wrist to assume an instability pattern. Disruption of the extrinsic ligaments is also important in the development of widening of the scapholunate interval and the development of an associated DISI deformity.

Triquetrolunate Ligament Tears

The triquetrolunate ligament is divided in to three parts – anterior intermediate and posterior – has the opposite relative strengths of its component when compared to the scapholunate ligament. The volar portion is the strongest with a weaker dorsal component. The intermediate membranous portion has

Fig. 7.24 (a) T2-weighted fat-saturated coronal MR showing radiocarpal and midcarpal effusion with marked oedema in the lunate and distal ulna (*arrows*). (b) T1w scan showing the avulsion fractures of the lunate at the scapholunate insertion (*arrow*). There is also a fracture visible at the base of the ulna styloid

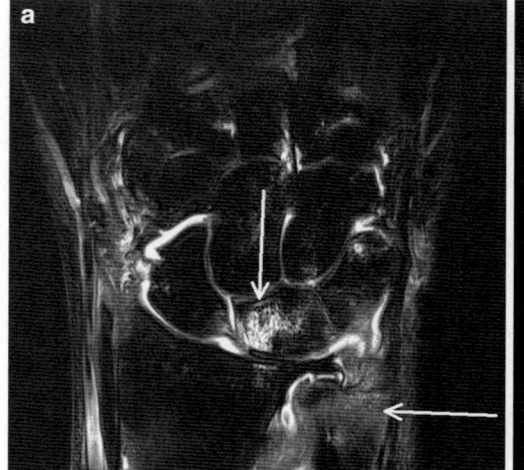
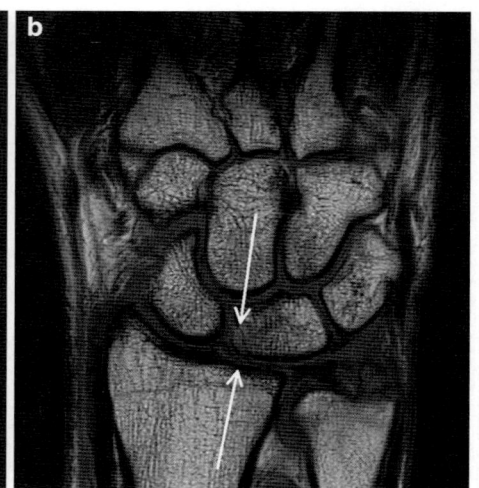

Fig. 7.25 (a) Radial deviation DP radiograph showing a step in the lesser arc at the triquetrolunate interspace. *L* lunate, *T* triquetral. (b) Conventional arthrogram showing contrast flowing from the ulnocarpal space into the midcarpal compartment (*arrows*) in keeping with disruption if the triquetrolunate ligament

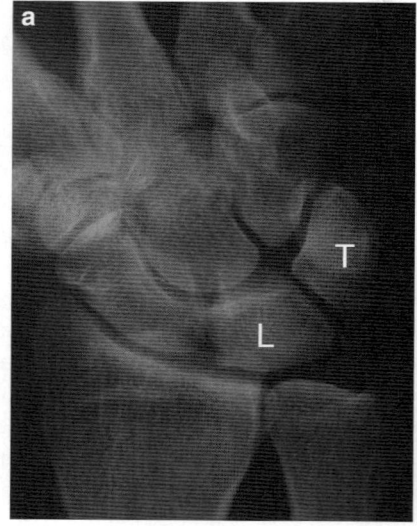
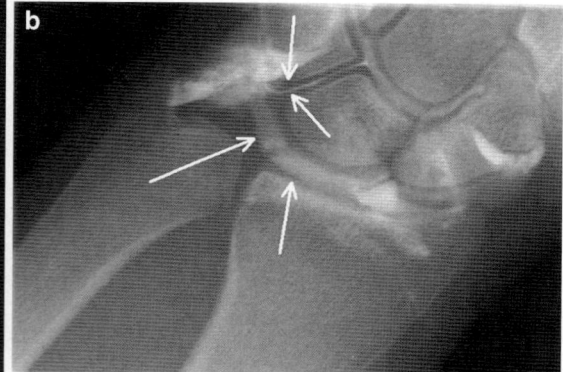

virtually exactly the same strength as those of the scapholunate ligament.

The triquetrolunate ligament can be disrupted in isolation or can be injured in association with other injuries such as fracture dislocation, TFCC tears and ulna abutment syndromes. As with the scapholunate the normal triquetrolunate ligament can be seen at MR imaging. It has a somewhat variable appearance with low signal intensity on T1 and T2 and PD fat-suppressed sequences and intermediate signal on gradient echo. Imaging of ligament tears can be inferred by demonstrating abnormal widening of the triquetrolunate interspace on static plain films of dynamic fluoroscopy (Fig. 7.25a). Arthrography of the radiocarpal compartment should not communicate with the midcarpal space in normality. Contrast extending through the triquetrolunate interspace into the midcarpal space occurs with triquetrolunate tears (Fig. 7.25b). Occasionally, overfilling of the recesses can make assessment of the route taken by the contrast to reach the midcarpal compartment difficult. In these cases, distraction views can be of value in pulling contrast back into the radiocarpal and midcarpal compartments from the recesses can show whether there is any intact ligament in

7 Hand and Wrist Injuries

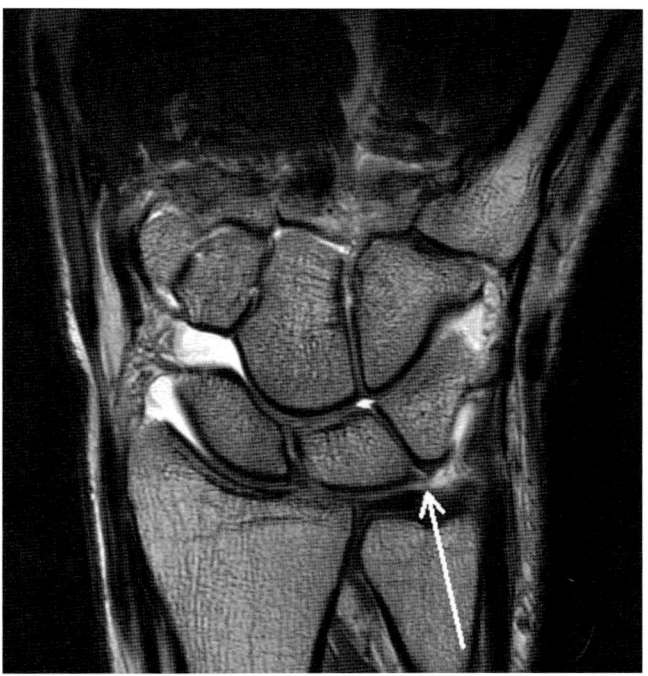

Fig. 7.26 Coronal T2w scan showing a tear of the triquetrolunate ligament (*arrow*)

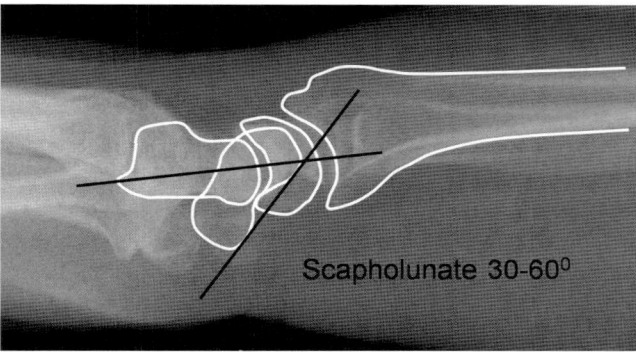

Fig. 7.27 Lateral radiograph of wrist with superimposed line drawing to show the normal scapholunate angle

the proximal triquetrolunate interspace. Alternatively, cross-sectional imaging with CT or MR if dilute gadolinium has been mixed with the iodinated contrast will be of value in demonstrating ligamentous disruption. Non-arthrographic MR can demonstrate triquetrolunate tears though not as well as it does scapholunate damage. As with the scapholunate ligament non-arthrographic MR is most effective in the acute phase utilizing the arthrographic effect of joint effusion (Fig. 7.26).

Wrist Instability

Carpal instability can be classified into dissociated and non-dissociated types and can be either static or dynamic [30]. In static instability there is permanent malalignment of the Carpi which will be demonstrated on non-dynamic imaging modalities such as radiography, CT or MR. Dynamic instability occurs when the carpi adopt an instability pattern only during specific movement, usually ulna to radial deviation, which will only be detecting all cases by dynamic screening of the wrist or kinematic MR.

In wrist instability there is derangement of the normal ligamentous supports of the wrist allowing malalignment of the carpi to develop. There are several distinct patterns of instability that can develop; these include dorsal and volar intercalated segment instability, ulna translocation and midcarpal instability.

Dorsal and volar intercalated segment instability occurs as a result of ligamentous injury to the scapholunate or triquetrolunate ligament combined with extrinsic ligamentous damage. The intercalated segment is the proximal row and is unusual as it has no tendon insertion making it entirely dependent of its articulations for movement; it acts as a spacer between the distal carpal row and the radius and ulna guiding the complex movement achievable by the wrist. Ligamentous failure around this intercalated segment allows dorsal or volar angulation of this segment associated with proximal migration of the capitates towards the forearm. Assessment of the presence or absence of an intercalated segment instability pattern requires and understanding of the normal carpal angles. A well-positioned lateral view is required to assess carpal angles, well-positioned means the radial styloid should lie at the midpoint of the distal radial articular surface, the wrist should be held in neutral with particularly no radial deviation or extension of the wrist. Radial deviation is particularly important as in this position there is scaphoid flexion mimicking dorsal intercalated segment instability. They can be distinguished by the fact that with radial deviation artefact there is no dorsal shift of the capitate relative to the distal radius.

The normal scapholunate angle in neutral position measures between 30 and 60° [31]. This is measured between a line drawn perpendicular to a line paralleling the distal lunate articular surface and a tangential line connecting the convexities of the proximal and distal scaphoid (Fig. 7.27). With Dorsal intercalated segment instability (DISI) there is dorsal tilt of the lunate relative to the scaphoid with the angle measuring greater than 80°. In volar intercalated segment instability (VISI) the converse occurs, there is volar tilt of the lunate relative to the scaphoid resulting in a scapholunate angle of less than 20°. DISI deformity in trauma most commonly results from scapholunate ligament derangement and VISI deformity from triquetrolunate ligament disruption. The commonest cause in the general population, however, is arthropathy with both deformities particularly common in inflammatory wrist arthropathy. Rheumatoid, gout and pyrophosphate arthropathy are the most common inflammatory aetiologies. These instability patterns can be either static or dynamic in nature. Static deformity is present at all time and will be detectable on well-positioned radiographs. Dynamic instability occurs only during loading or particular movements and can be more difficult to diagnose. The wrist often assumes a momentary instability pattern during wrist movement with pain and an audible/palpable clunk. This clunk can occur when the wrist moves into an unstable configuration or during relocation when normal alignment is achieved. These dynamic instabilities are more difficult to diagnose and are best demonstrated with fluoroscopic imaging during movement. Radial-ulna deviation movement of the wrist is the best positioning for assessment with PA and lateral-screening fluoroscopy. This can be performed as a preliminary screening prior to performing arthroscopy. The abnormal configuration can be recorded as can variation in the scapholunate and the triquetrolunate articular interspaces, assessment of abnormality in these interspaces and the greater or lesser arcs help distinguish dissociated from non-dissociated instability. Non-dissociative instability results from extrinsic ligamentous injury with intact intrinsic ligaments and is sometimes termed midcarpal instability. It is much less common than dissociative instability and is generally treated conservatively with rest and support.

Extrinsic ligament assessment is possible with MR though its accuracy and clinical role are not firmly established. Demonstration of major disruption of the extrinsic ligaments is possible and these are relatively frequently associated with other capsule of soft tissue injuries. Extensor retinacular injury in particular is seen to be associated with forced hyperextension injury of the wrist with retinacular avulsion and avulsion of the radial origin of the radiolunatotriquetral extrinsic ligament.

Other instability patterns have been described in the wrist and the nomenclature is somewhat confusing and variable. Ulna translocation is an instability pattern where there is ulna shift of the carpi on the distal radius with more than 50% of the lunate overhanging the ulna margin of the radius. This instability pattern is unusual following trauma and is not usually seen as a result of sporting injury, arthropathy especially inflammatory arthropathies such as rheumatoid are the most common aetiologies.

Triangular Fibrocartilage Complex Injury

Dysfunction and disruption of the TFCC is a common cause of ulna-sided wrist pain. It commonly occurs following a fall onto the outstretched pronated hand. In sport, it occurs in contact sports associated with frequent hand offs (rugby, American football) or axial loading of the pronated wrist (martial arts, gymnastics)

The TFCC represents a functional buffer between the distal ulnar and the carpi and is an important stabilizer of the ulna aspect of the wrist. Abnormalities are classified according to the Palmer classification [32] which splits them into two broad groups, acute or type 1 and chronic or type 2 injuries. The chronic type 2 injuries are those seen in association with ulna abutment syndromes. Patients can present with either pain and swelling alone (this tends to be the case with lesions of the fibrocartilagenous disc alone) or with instability symptoms related to abnormal movement of the ulnocarpal compartment or DRUJ. Pain and tenderness is usually located immediately distal to the ulna articular surface, pain is exacerbated by ulnar deviation especially in pronation where there is relative elongation of the ulna relative to the radius. An inflammatory element to the patient's pain may well also be present with a secondary local synovitis giving night pain and morning exacerbation. There can also be symptoms related to associated injuries such as triquetrolunate ligament disruption and extensor carpi ulnaris injury. Tears of the TFCC are seen more in advancing age [33] and in asymptomatic volunteers [34–37], close correlation of any imaging abnormality in the TFCC with the clinical setting and the use of local anaesthetic with arthrographic contrast with a symptom log is vital. Assessment of the integrity of the TFCC with non-arthrographic MR is possible and large tears and their associated ligamentous derangements, ulna variance bone changes and synovitis can be demonstrated [38]. The reading radiologist most watch for undercutting of the radial insertion of the TFCC with articular cartilage, this is a normal variant and does not represent avulsion or injury of the radial attachment. Altered signal can also be seen within the TFCC as a result of degeneration and altered signal within the TFCC does not necessarily mean there is a physical defect or biomechanical dysfunction present. These changes are seen more commonly with increasing age [39, 40]. In pre-operative assessment cases, MR arthrography remains the imaging technique of choice.

The Palmer classification separates tear by site as well as chronicity with type 1 tears acute and all type 2 tears chronic. The Palmer classification can be assessed effectively with MR [38].

Type 1A tears occur within the membranous portion of the TFCC and are the most frequent asymptomatic abnormalities seen. These tears are rarely functionally important and symptomatic treatment of any associated synovitis can be of value. Oblique and more complex tears can be associated with displaced flaps of articular disc and secondary mechanical symptoms and tend to be of more significance than perforations (Fig. 7.28).

Type 1B tears are an avulsion injury of the periphery of the TFCC at its insertion on the ulna styloid and are associated

Fig. 7.28 (a) Coronal T1 fat-saturated MR arthrography showing type 1A pin point perforation of the membranous portion of the TFCC (*arrows*). (b) Coronal T1 fat-saturated MR arthrography showing type 1A tear. This tear is complex with a sizeable tear of the membranous TFCC with flap extension extending medially (*arrows*)

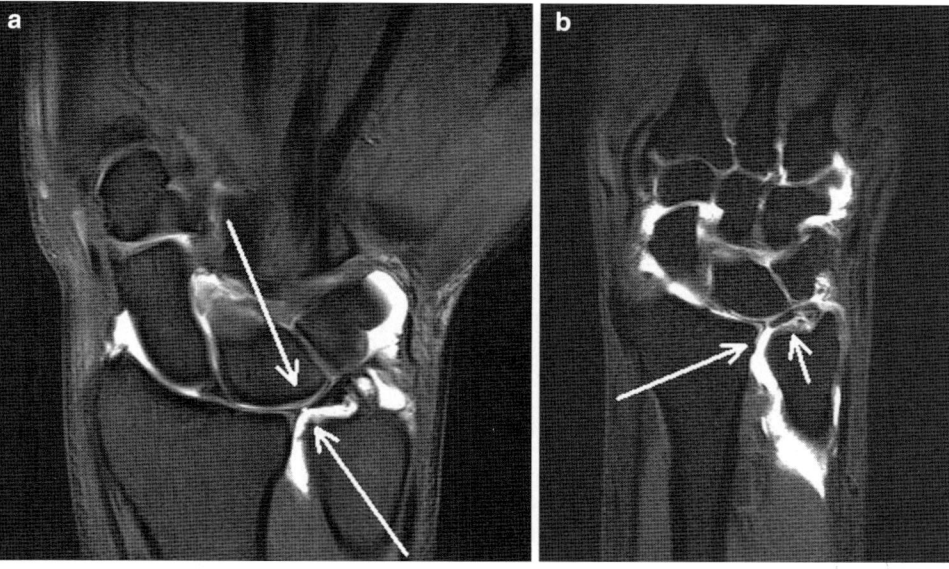

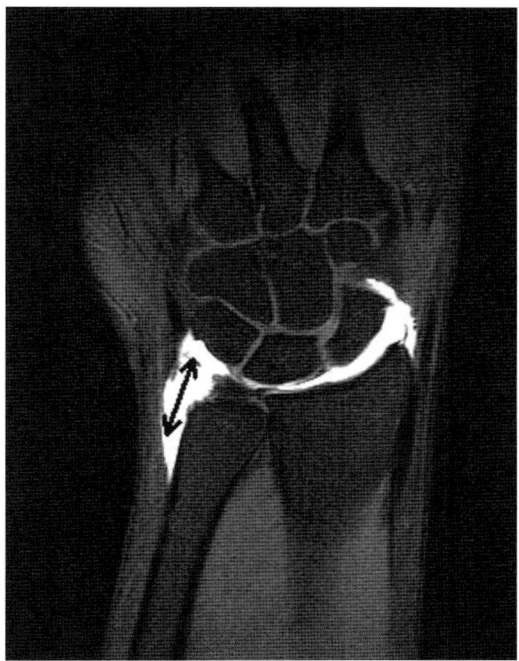

Fig. 7.29 Peripheral injury of the TFCC with contrast flowing freely over the medial border of the ulna (*double-headed arrow*)

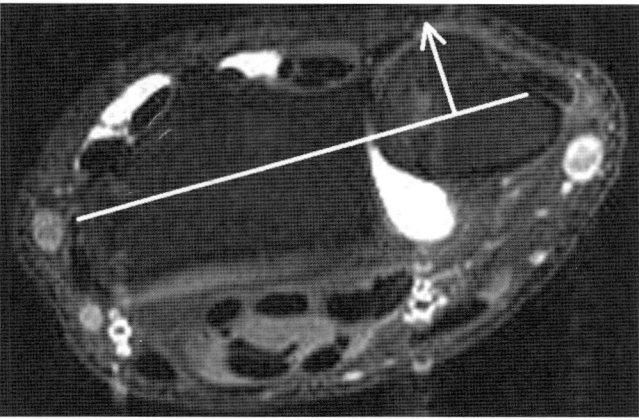

Fig. 7.30 Axial MR arthrography T1 fat-saturated image in a patient with TFCC disruption. There is dorsal subluxation of the distal ulna relative to the radius (*arrow*)

with fracture of the ulna styloid base (Fig. 7.29). These have an association with instability of the distal radioulnar joint.

Type 1C tears involve disruption of the distal insertion of the ulnolunate and ulnotriquetral ligaments and are again associated with distal radioulnar instability (Fig. 7.30).

Type 1D tears are the rarest acute injury and are avulsion of the radial insertion of the TFCC.

The types of degenerative or type 2 tears described by the Palmar classification is slightly different. These tears are seen in association with ulna abutment syndromes and are classified with developing progressive damage and arthropathy change.

Type 2A injury is an evidence of ulna abutment with thinning and irregularity of the central portion of the TFCC without perforation (Fig. 7.31).

Type 2B change is the combination of 2A change with chondromalacia of the lunate or distal ulna articular cartilage.

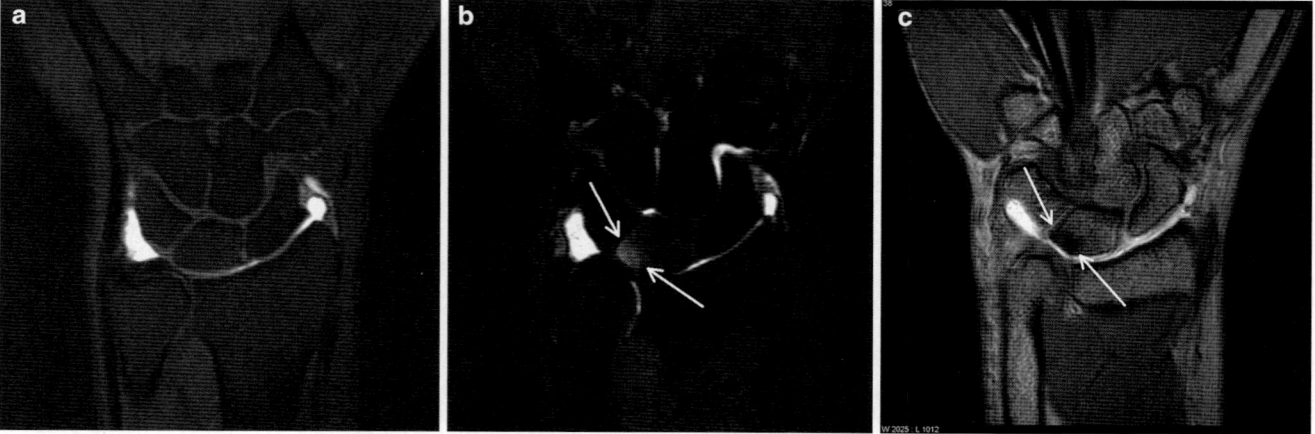

Fig. 7.31 (a) T1 fat-saturated MR arthrogram image showing thinning of the TFCC with no velar evidence of abutment. (b) The T2 fat-saturated image in the same position shows oedema in the ulna portion of the proximal lunate (*arrows*) typical for ulna abutment. (c) Gradient echo sequence susceptibility clearly demonstrates the subchondral abutment change in the lunate (*arrows*)

In type 2C there is perforation of the TFCC with the defects tending to be larger than those seen in acute injury.

In 2D lesions there is the presence of 2C lesion combined with triquetrolunate ligament tear and in type 2E there is osteoarthosis of the DRUJ and ulnocarpal compartment.

Degenerative type 2 lesions of the TFCC are more common than acute injuries with degenerative tears tending to be more rounded with smoother margins than acute tears. Differentiating degenerative change in the fibrocartilagenous disc from tears on conventional MR is difficult, increased signal on T2 fat-saturated sequences or fluid signal extending from DRUJ to ulnocarpal compartment when effusion is present gives most diagnostic confidence. The sensitivity of conventional MR is relatively low with high specificity [41] though sensitivity and specificity has been reported as high as 84 and 100% for 3T scanning [27]. It should be borne in mind that this latter study is an early report with a small highly selected patient group, selection included knowledge of the MR findings in the decision to operate which was one of the inclusion criteria and as such there will be an artificially high incidence of MR lesions and disease in the study population increasing diagnostic confidence, further work is required. MR arthrography in comparison has been thoroughly evaluated with sensitivity and specificity of 75–94% and 80–89% [42, 43]. With sensitivities and specificities of this order it is clear that MR and MR arthrography cannot replace arthroscopy, they do however contribute to patient care and alter management in the majority of cases [44].

It is recommended that arthrography be performed with radio/ulnocarpal injection initially, distal radioulnar joint injection should only be performed after this when there is a specific clinical question about the integrity of the TFCC [45].

Ulna Abutment Syndrome

Ulna abutment is a degenerative condition resulting from boney impaction of the ulna aspect of the wrist with soft tissue and articular surface damage centred around the TFCC, distal ulna articular surface, triquetrum and the lunate. Plain radiographs may demonstrate positive ulnar variance though this is not a pre-requisite, ulna abutment can occur in patients with normal ulna variance though is exceptionally rare where there is negative ulna variance [32]. The ulna lengthens relative to radius in pronation, as a result ulna abutment typically produces recurrent symptoms most marked in the pronated ulna-deviated position. Advanced cases can be demonstrated on plain radiography with subchondral degenerative changes including sclerosis and cyst formation. For early diagnosis MR is required and will demonstrate bone marrow oedema and sclerosis with lunate cartilage damage and soft tissue inflammatory changes centred around any TFCC damage (Fig. 7.31). Inflammatory change in the bone marrow with overlying cartilage damage on the ulna aspect of the lunate is the commonest MR finding [46]. Treatment is usually conservative through steroid injection which can be of value in managing an acute flare up. In resistant cases arthroscopic debridement of the TFCC or even ulna osteotomy can be required.

This condition should be differentiated from ulna impingement syndrome, this is a condition associated with negative ulna variance to the point where the distal ulna does not articulate with the glenoid notch associated with formation of a scalloped concavity on the ulna border of the distal radius. It is associated with a similar clinical presentation to ulna impaction syndrome though movement are particularly aggravated by pronation–supination movements [47, 48].

Distal Radioulnar Joint

Given its bony anatomy this joint has very little inherent stability relying heavily on its adjacent soft tissues. Key soft tissue stabilizers are the joint capsule, the interosseous membrane and TFCC, the forearm muscles especially pronator quadratus provide dynamic stability. The ulna is relatively fixed with the radius rotating around the ulna during pronation–supination movements. When the radius dislocates relative to the ulna but the injury is described in relation to the ulna's position.

Dorsal dislocation of the DRU joint is common and results from fall on pronated hand. It involves disruption of the dorsal radioulnar ligament of the TFCC and dorsal capsule of DRU joint.

Volar dislocation of the joint usually results from a forced supination injury or direct blow to the dorsum of the forearm.

Radiography may suggest features of instability with widening of radioulnar joint and dislocation though positioning is difficult with artefactual malalignment relatively easy to reproduce. A well-positioned lateral view should project the radial styloid at the midpoint of the distal radial articular surface, if this is the case dorsal or volar displacement of the ulna can be assessed, without good positioning radiography must be interpreted only with caution. Cross-sectional imaging with CT or MR will often be required. Axial scans should demonstrate the ulna lying centrally within the sigmoid notch of the distal radius, subluxation and subtle malalignment can be seen. These latter changes can be seen as a normal variant and comparison with the asymptomatic side, if there is one, is advised [49].

An ulna styloid fracture with detachment of the ulna styloid process from the shaft may result in destabilization of the DRUJ.

Sports Injuries and Imaging in Children

Hand and wrist injuries are common in patients with immature skeleton [50–54]. The weak link in the kinetic chain in young patients is the growth plate with ligament and tendon injury which is rare. The growth plate can be damaged by either chronic repetitive trauma or high-energy single injury. The distal radius and ulna growth plate is the most frequent site of injury. Acute trauma results in typical Salter Harris type injuries with chronic repetitive damage producing an unusual chronic Salter Harris type 1 fracture. This is characterised by sclerosis around a widened irregular growth plate associated with some minor periosteal new bone formation (Fig. 7.32). This latter injury occurs as a result of either contact from inadvertent sports injury mainly resulting from falls or from the particular sports themselves such as gymnastics

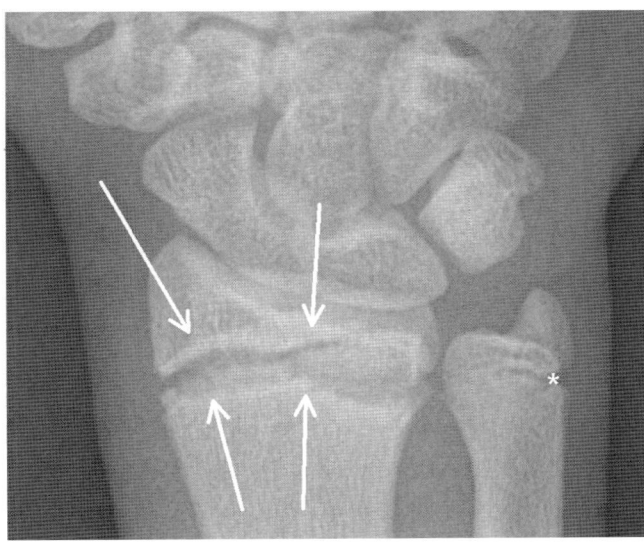

Fig. 7.32 DP radiograph of wrist showing typical appearances of gymnasts' wrist. There is widening, irregularity and sclerosis of the distal radial growth plate (*arrows*) in keeping with chronic Salter Harris one injury. There is also minor involvement of the distal ulna growth plate (*asterisk*)

where athletes spend much of their time weight bearing on their hands [55–58]. Falling onto the outstretched hand tends to occur more commonly in certain sports and is more significant on hard surfaces; basketball, rugby and soccer are all common sports for wrist injuries. Some sports having a high incidence of falls such as skating, snowboarding and skateboarding. In snowboarding and skateboarding there is a tendency to fall on one's wrist more than the other, often resulting in asymmetrical of unilateral change. This chronic injury is usually treated conservatively and settles well with rest and training regime modification.

One other use for MR imaging of the hand and wrist mainly adolescents is MR bone age assessment. This is particularly important in soccer where children are grouped and compete by age and in large events in countries where age documentation is less strict and forged documents common. There is an incentive for older children to play in younger age groups to attract the attention of club scouts and potential contracts. Using ionizing radiation to age these children is clearly unethical as there is no medical indication for the exposure. MR bone ageing looking at hand and wrist growth plates is one potential solution to this difficult problem.

Tenosynovitis of the Wrist

The anatomy of the extensor and flexor compartments ate the level of the wrist is complex. As the tendon groups are relatively constrained by retinaculae and undertake complex movements they are prone to developing overuse and sports-related injury. Tendinopathy of these tendon groups is unusual as is tendon disruption. These are normally only seen in patients with systemic diseases such as inflammatory arthropathy or in cases where there is an external influence on tendon integrity such as a screw head or lacerating injury. The predominant finding is that of tenosynovitis which presents as focal pain and swelling associated with crepitus. Crepitus relates to abnormal movement of the tendon through it tendon sheath and can be a symptom experienced by the patient, palpable or audible during movement depending on severity. The long extensor tendons of the fingers are particularly prone to developing tenosynovitis at the level of the wrist and occurs with repetitive or unusual activity involving the wrist. Wrist-intensive sports including racquet and bat, golf and gymnastic are more likely to develop tenosynovial disease [2, 59–64]. The imaging features are those of inflammatory change in the tenosynovial sheath adjacent to soft tissues. This is demonstrated as high signal encircling the tendon on T2-weighted fat-saturated MR and hypoechogenicity surrounding the tendons on ultrasound (Fig. 7.33). Differentiating effusion from tenosynovitis is important as tendon sheaths often contain small amount of effusion in normality. Demonstrating power Doppler signal within a tendon sheath or gadolinium enhancement at MR helps differentiate. The distribution of inflammatory change in the tendon sheath can be confusing as a result of the retinaculae, synovitis and effusion tends to accumulate either side of the retinaculum giving a dumbbell appearance to the tendon sheath that when seen for the first time is confusing.

Several of the tendon groups that develop tenosynovitis around the wrist warrant discussion as separate entities.

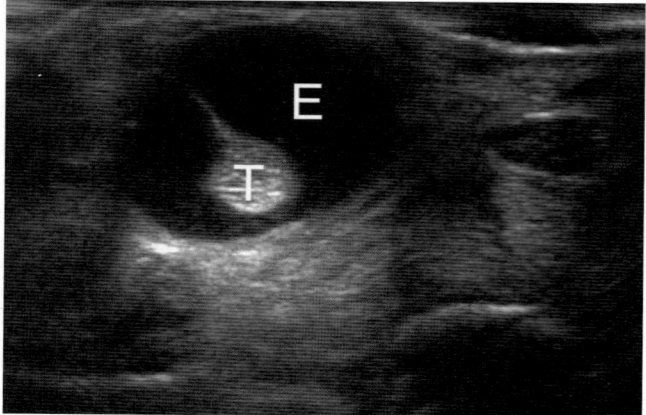

Fig. 7.33 Transverse sonogram showing tenosynovitis with a large amount of effusion (E) present around the tendon (T) but within the tendon sheath. Fluid is differentiated from synovitis by its compressibility and lack of vascularity on power Doppler examination

De Quervain's Tenosynovitis

De Quervain's stenosing tenosynovitis is a stenosing tenosynovitis of extensor compartment 1 of the wrist. It affects the tendons of the abductor pollicis longus (APL) and extensor pollicis brevis (EPB) muscles though there are frequently accessory tendons and fibrous septae present in this compartment [62, 64]. These accessory tendons and septae are not well visualized normally but become visible in the presence of tenosynovitis. The classical presentation is pain over the radial aspect of the wrist, aggravated by thumb movements during pinching, grasping, or lifting. It can occur in a number of different sports as a result of overuse such as rowing, golf or in the dominant hand in racquet sports. It is also more prevalent in office and manual workers and during pregnancy. There is swelling and tenderness over the radial aspect of the wrist with crepitus sometimes palpable adjacent to the radial styloid. Other clinical sign's include reproduction of the patient's pain during ulna deviation with the finger gripping the thumb against the palm. This is known as Finklestein's test and passively loads the tendons of extensor compartment 1. The imaging findings are a combination of retinacular abnormality, tendinopathy and tenosynovitis. Tenosynovitis is characterized by hypoechoic, hypervascular tissue with the tendon sheath at ultrasound or increased signal around the tendons on T2 fat sat or STIR MR scans. The retinaculum can be thickened and there can be enlargement and neovascularity of the tendons [65, 66]. The tendon and retinacular enlargement can be difficult to appreciate without comparison with the contra lateral side and is one of the key advantages of ultrasound imaging. The condition is a stenosing tenosynovitis and thickening and narrowing of the compartment and tendon enlargement can both be contributory factors. Tenosynovial sheath effusion is not a major feature of DeQuervain's. Injection treatment is common [67] though siting the needle effectively can be difficult. Ultrasound guidance is advised for injection with the deep aspect of the Tendon sheath, the target of choice. This has two main advantages. Deep injection is the easiest approach for achieving intrasheath injection and also reduces the risk of any subcutaneous fat atrophy and depigmentation that can occur with more superficial injections.

Extensor Carpi Ulnaris Tenosynovitis

This tendon occupies extensor compartment 6 and is a tendon that becomes a disease in several sporting activities. It is well described in tennis, golf and rugby league [2, 59, 61, 63, 68, 69] and is slightly different to other tendon problems around the wrist as it is prone to both instability and tenosynovitis. The mechanisms for developing sports injury of ECU are normally overuse for tenosynovitis with instability the result of either overuse or single traumatic injury. ECU injury in rugby results from ball carrying in ulnar deviation, supination and flexion, the position in which the ECU is most unstable and vulnerable to sheath injury. Sheath injury is seen more commonly in rugby league than rugby union as the ball must be retained in the tackle as opposed to union where the ball is released.

Tenosynovitis images in a similar way to the other tendons around the wrist (see above). Sheath abnormalities are more difficult to diagnose and vary in severity from complete disruption and dislocation of the tendon from the ECU groove to subtle subluxation during pronation–supination movements. Complete disruption is relatively easy to demonstrate with MR and shows malalignment of the tendon within its groove associated with surrounding high signal on T2-weighted sequences. Subtle changes are more difficult to demonstrate and require scanning of the ECU in neutral, prone and supine positioning. This is best performed at ultrasound and comparison with the contra lateral side is advised as a degree of subluxation out of the groove in supination is seen as a normal variant [70].

Intersection Syndrome

Intersection syndrome of the wrist occurs commonly in sports that require frequent wrist movements such as rowers (where it is referred to as "teno"), canoeists and weight lifters and can be confused with tenosynovitis [59]. It presents with swelling and post-exertional pain on the radial aspect of the wrist approximately 5 cm proximal to the radial styloid associated with crepitus. The diagnosis is normally clinical with imaging rarely required for diagnosis. The pathology is a friction syndrome occurring between the extensor compartments 1 and 2 and presents radiologically as tenosynovitis of both sheaths with an adventitial bursa present between the two compartments at the level of intersection. Treatment is usually conservative with modification of training or activity, ice and strapping. Occasionally guided steroid injection can be used for specific training or competition needs.

Other common sites of tenosynovitis of the wrist include the extensor pollicis longus as it passes around Lister's tubercle and extensor carpi ulnaris. These usually follow repetitive wrist motion and are readily confirmed on US.

Dorsal Impingement of the Distal Radius

Also known as gymnast's wrist this is an overuse syndrome resulting from repetitive hyperextension and loading of the wrist [8]. It results in soft tissue and bone change as is so often the case with impingement syndromes. The soft tissue changes result from entrapment of the dorsal capsule between the distal radius and the extensor carpi radialis brevis tendon sheath causing focal synovitis and inflammatory change over the dorsal aspect of the distal radius which can become chronically thickened and scarred similar to the meniscoid lesion seen in ankle impingement syndromes. Secondary reactive bone oedema is also seen over the dorsal aspect of the distal radius. Treatment is usually conservative with rest and sometimes steroid injections, arthroscopic debridement is reserved for resistant cases [8, 71]. Dorsal impingement of the extensor digitorum group and the extensor retinaculum has been described as a cause for similar soft tissue changes to those described above, they again result from repetitive wrist extension with an axial loading and should be included in the differential diagnosis of dorsal wrist pain in athletes [72].

Hammer Hand Syndrome

Also known as hypothenar hammer syndrome this condition is commonly seen in manual workers and result from repetitive trauma to the ulna border of the wrist. The butt of a hammer or the use of high-force vibration hand tools (such as a jack hammer) are common causes and it also seen in a sporting setting. Similar to hook of hamate injury (with which it is associated) it is seen in the dominant hand for racquet and bat sports and in the non-dominant hand in golf. Cyclists also have a propensity to developing this condition as a result of pressure from the handle bars of the bike. Soft tissue damage occurs at the level of the hamate centred on the Guyon's canal affecting the ulna neurovascular bundle [73]. Damage is usually the result of repetitive force though has been described following single traumatic events. The clinical presentation is of pain, sensory loss, weakness and local tenderness over the hypothenar eminence. The imaging findings depend on the degree of soft tissue damage present. The commonest imaging findings are in the ulna artery, damage to the media of the ulna artery result in thrombosis of this vessel best demonstrated with Doppler ultrasound, MR or MR arthrography [19, 74]. More severe damage results in intimal damage and is associated with aneurismal dilatation of the ulna artery (Fig. 7.34).

Ulna nerve dysfunction can also be seen in this condition [75]. Ulna nerve impairment occurring at this level is far less common than ulnar nerve neuropathy resulting from elbow disease. Pure motor neuropathies are the most common (>50%), followed by mixed sensory and motor ($\approx$33%), and most rarely, pure sensory lesions with imaging showing oedema and inflammation of the tissues within the Guyon's canal and compression of or increased signal within the deep terminal branch of the ulna nerve.

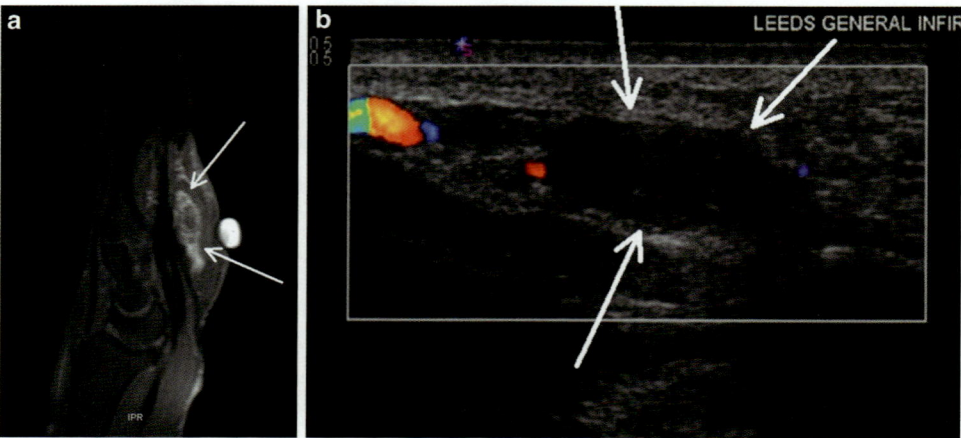

Fig. 7.34 (a) Sagittal T1 fat-saturated post-iv gadolinium scan of the wrist. This demonstrates dilatation of the ulna artery with central non-enhancement in a patient with a thrombosed aneurismal ulna artery (*arrows*) as part of Hammer hand syndrome. (**b**) Longitudinal ultrasound showing the thrombosis of the dilated ulna artery depicted in **a** containing thrombus and no flow on colour Doppler (*arrows*)

Carpal Tunnel Syndrome

Carpal Tunnel Syndrome is an entrapment neuropathy of the median nerve in the carpal tunnel. There are a large variety of causes with progressive disease potentially resulting in substantial impairment of the thumb and hand function. The usual presentation is that of insidious onset pain and variable neurological symptoms, worse at overnight or first thing in the morning. Many cases are idiopathic though conditions such as diabetes, hypothyroidism, flexor tenosynovitis, previous wrist trauma, pregnancy or carpal tunnel mass lesion are recognized causes. Sensory symptoms typically precede the development of motor impairment. Carpal tunnel syndrome is seen in a number of sports [3, 59, 75, 76].

The role of imaging can be in confirming the presence of carpal tunnel syndrome by demonstrating, wasting of the nerve in the carpal tunnel or proximal swelling of the nerve. At MR imaging inflammatory change and focal swelling of the median nerve itself can also be seen. The main role of imaging, however, is to demonstrate distinct abnormalities within the carpal tunnel itself that are potentially treatable without carpal tunnel release such as a lipoma or tenosynovitis of the flexor tendons. Tenosynovitis is the most frequent underlying abnormality seen in CTS; rheumatoid, gout, pyrophosphate are the commonest aetiologies. Imaging can also be of value in identifying patients with anatomical variants such as a high division of the median nerve which can be associated with a persistent median artery.

Wrist Ganglia

Ganglia are the most frequent mass lesion seen around the hand and wrist. They are synovial-lined cystic swellings present slightly more frequently in middle-aged women. They contain jelly-like fluid under tension and with wrist ganglia having a variety of aetiologies. They usually communicate with an adjacent joint, tendon sheath or ligament [77–79]. Neural ganglia are seen elsewhere in the body and result from decompression of fluid down articular branch of a peripheral nerve, they have been reported in the ulna nerve in and around Guyon's canal. There is a unifying theory of neural ganglia that they all arise from decompression of joint fluid down small articular branches of peripheral nerves [80].

Tendon sheath ganglia are most common in the fingers associated with the flexor tendons and are termed "seed ganglia." These are small lesions that are typically asymptomatic and only infrequently require treatment. They can occur close to the pulleys especially the A2 pulley but rarely effect tendon movement. The lesions are well defined and have characteristic hypoechogenicity at ultrasound and arise from the tendon sheath itself. They do not move with either passive or active tendon movements. The differential diagnosis for these seed ganglia is focal pigmented villonodular synovitis or giant cell tumour of the tendon sheath. These are solid hypervascular lesions arising from the tendon sheath that can be confused clinically with ganglia. Ganglia normally fluctuate in size somewhat and have no vascularity on Doppler examination [81, 82]. Giant cell tumours are markedly hypervascular solid lesions on with a history of continuous progressive enlargement.

The dorsal occult ganglion is an important cause of dorsal wrist pain. It has a different aetiology to the other ganglia around the wrist resulting from myxoid degeneration of either the scapholunate ligament or triquetrolunate ligaments [78, 83]. They occur at the fibrocartilagenous insertion of these ligaments dorsally and as such these ganglia often have both intraosseous and extra osseous components. The ganglions arise close to the extensor compartment 4 (extensor digitorum) and can present either as a palpable abnormality or focal pain. Ultrasound imaging can demonstrate a fluid filled hypoechoic lesion and correlate the abnormality with symptoms. It can also show erosion of the adjacent bone indicative of intraosseous extension. The lesions can vary in appearance from completely hypoechoic fluid to septated lesion containing echogenic material, ganglia should not demonstrate vascularity on power Doppler examination. The contents of ganglia are usually jelly-like fluid and contain calcification no calcification, a minimum of a 19G needle is required for aspiration. MR can also show these lesions effectively and has the advantage of demonstrating any synchronous intra-articular or intraosseous pathology or extension. The ganglion usually demonstrates uniformly high signal on T2-weighted or STIR sequences with intermediate signal on T1 imaging. Post-gadolinium scanning is rarely required though can help distinguish focal synovitis or mass lesion from a ganglion, ganglia should show little or no enhancement [83].

Ganglia are a common asymptomatic finding and close correlation between the abnormality and the patient's symptoms is required, this is one area where ultrasound is particularly effective and carries an advantage over MR. Most lesions will settle spontaneously but occasionally intervention is required. This can be undertaken in a variety of ways with guided injection of steroids (be careful to avoid depo products that carry a higher incidence of lipoatrophy and depigmentation), fenestration of the lesion and surgical removal. All are associated with a substantial recurrence rate with surgery having the lowest rate of 15%. Imaging is of value in demonstrating the relationship of the ganglion to any nearby neurovascular structures and in identifying the neck and tissue of origin of the ganglion to allow effective tying off of the neck during excision of the lesion.

Finger Pathology

Finger Tenosynovitis

Tenosynovitis is a common inflammatory process of the hand and is usually as a result of repetitive activities and sport. However, this can also occur in systemic inflammatory joint disease such as rheumatoid arthritis.

During the acute stage, there is an accumulation of peritendinous fluid and thickening of the tendon. In the chronic stage, there is thickening of the tendon and synovial sheaths with formation of cysts and nodules.

Clinically, flexor tenosynovitis is present if passive flexion of a finger exceeds active flexion. Crepitus may be palpated over the palm as the fingers are extended and flexed.

US may demonstrate the synovial thickening and fluid as hypoechoic regions surrounding the echogenic tendon.

Power Doppler can distinguish thickened synovium from fluid by depicting flow in the vascularised synovium. Aspiration of fluid and steroid injection may be performed if required.

Pulley Disruption

Disruption of the cruciate and annular pulleys of the fingers are common in sport. The injuries tend to acute or acute on chronic injury and are seen in high-energy-resisted finger extension injury. The most frequent mechanism seen in sport are climbers and in rugby where the tackler is holding the opponents shirt.

As you will remember there are five annular (A1–A5) pulleys and three cruciform (C1–C3) ligaments in each finger from neck of metacarpal and ends at distal phalanx. These lie on the palmar aspect of the flexor tendons and are key stabilizers of the flexor tendons preventing them from bow stringing away from the underlying bone during active flexion [13].

Injuries usually affect the A2–A4 pulleys in the middle and ring fingers with the A2 pulley most commonly affected [84, 85].

Onset is usually acute and is associated with a sensation of something tearing and sometimes a popping sensation of noise. Swelling and focal pain and tenderness on the palmar aspect of the injured pulley ensues and persists. As expected, radiography is negative though is often required to exclude any underlying bony injury.

Direct imaging of the pulleys themselves is now possible using high resolution ultrasound and modern MR coil technology. Disruption of the pulley itself is seen as thickening and inflammatory changed centred on the pulley itself. Secondary signs of pulley injury ore anterior displacement of the flexor tendon away from the underlying phalanx with fluid signal on T2-weighted sequences interposed between the tendon and bone [86–88]. Ultrasound is also good at visualizing the secondary features of pulley injury and has the added advantage of being dynamic [14, 89]. Scanning with the hand flat, the potentially damaged pulley should be visualized as the patient flexes the finger against resistance. During this the tendon will be seen to pull away from the underlying bone and fluid will pool between the tendon and bone confirming pulley disruption (Fig. 7.35).

Trigger Finger

This condition is also known as stenosing tenosynovitis of the finger and is characterized by a specific abnormal movement of the flexor tendon of the finger called triggering.

Triggering is where the tendon becomes stuck when moving from the fully flexed to the extended position. The tendon can only be released by short flexion extension movement of wiggling the finger. The condition can be progressive and on occasions can lead to fixed flexion deformity.

It is most common in the ring finger and thumb of middle-aged patients and is associated with diabetes, rheumatoid and deposition diseases that affect tendons such as gout and amyloid.

The abnormality is normally located close to the A1 pulley. Thickening of the pulley itself to the adjacent tendon sheath can be seen with focal peritendinous inflammatory change described.

Catching of the flexor tendon as it moves passed the A1 pulley can be demonstrated at ultrasound as can thickening of the pulley or adjacent sheath and tendon [90, 91].

Treatment is usually conservative with rest, ice and splinting. In resistant cases imaging-guided treatment with either dry needling of the peritendinous thickening or nodule [92] with or without local steroid injection is commonly undertaken, occasionally operative release is required.

Boxer's Knuckle

Boxer's knuckle occurs as a result of repetitive or isolated injury to the sagittal bands of the extensor retinaculum. These occur most commonly in punching sports such as boxing, martial arts and other contact sports but can also occur with prolonged gripping (such as golf or tennis). The extensor hood is made up of two transverse ligaments which serve to stabilize the extensor tendon during flexion at the knuckle.

The ligaments are most susceptible to injury during full flexion with the radial band of the second and third finger most commonly disrupted. This allows ulna shift of the extensor tendon during flexion. The patient presents with pain and soft tissue swelling over the dorsal aspect of the knuckle which can be chronic or related to acute injury. The abnormal movement of the tendon can be difficult to detect clinically especially in the acute phase, imaging can be of value in such cases. MR demonstrates ulna shift of the extensor tendon and soft tissue inflammation centred on the extensor hood. Ultrasound has the added advantage of being able to scan the tendon dynamically throughout flexion extension movement [93]. Severe derangement of the extensor hood can extend right through the dorsal capsule into the metacarpophalangeal joint (Fig. 7.36).

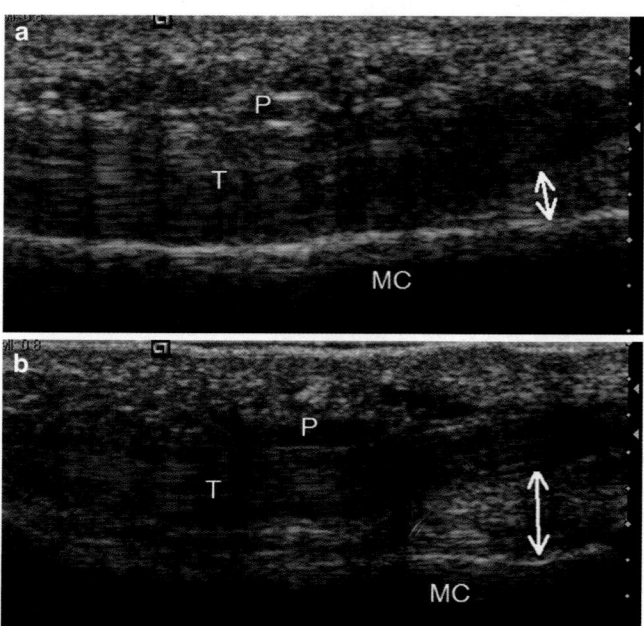

Fig. 7.35 Longitudinal ultrasound scans at the level of the A2 pulley. (**a**) Shows normal appearances of the A2 pulley (P) with normal distance (*double-headed arrow*) between the flexor tendon (T) and the underlying phalanx (MC). (**b**) There is disruption of the pulley with thickening of the pulley (P) and increased separation of the tendon away from the underlying bone (*double-headed arrow*).

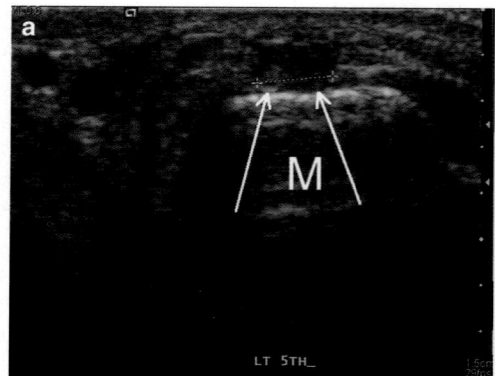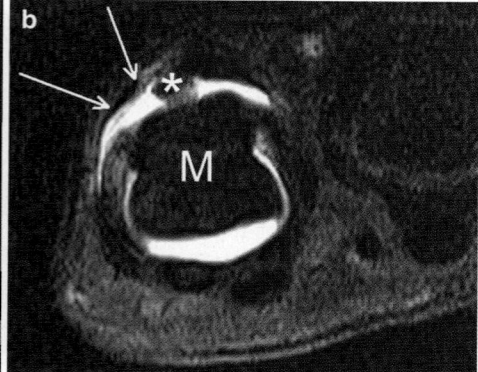

Fig. 7.36 (**a**) Transverse ultrasound of the dorsal fifth metacarpal head in a boxer. There is a defect present in the dorsal hood (*arrows* and measured) allowing radial subluxation of the extensor tendon off the metacarpal head (M). (**b**) MR arthrogram of the same case showing the dorsal hood and capsular defect (*arrows*) with slight radial shift of the extensor tendon (*asterisk*)

Mallet Finger

Mallet finger describes injury to the extensor tendon insertion on the distal phalanx. This can either be an avulsion fracture of the lateral slip insertions or disruption of the tendons themselves. This injury results in inability to extend the distal interphalangeal joint (DIPJ) and produces a characteristic deformity with flexion of the DIPJ without flexion at the proximal interphalangeal joint (PIPJ). The aetiology is a direct blow to the finger tips and is commonly seen in most catching sports. Those sports using hard balls such as baseball or cricket have a higher incidence of extensor tendon injury.

The diagnosis is clinical with imaging required to identify the presence or absence of a fracture, the severity of fracture and in the absence of fracture the site of extensor tendon disruption. The deformity is virtually impossible to reproduce in normality thus when demonstrated radiographically is related to extensor tendon injury rather than the result of radiographic positioning. The radiographs are the mainstay of fracture imaging with the degree of articular involvement bets assessed on the lateral view. Greater than 30% involvement of the articular surface warrants consideration for open reduction and fixation (Fig. 7.37). The extensor tendons are extremely thin and difficult to demonstrate at both ultrasound and MR. In the presence of disruption ultrasound is the modality of choice for demonstrating the site of tear and the position of the tendon ends Dynamic scanning is vital both with passive (moves the distal tendon) and active movement of the extensor tendon (moves the proximal tendon) required for diagnosis.

Bennett's Fracture

The Bennett's fracture is a common fracture dislocation of the first carpometacarpal bone. It results from axial loading of a partially flexed thumb. The base of the metacarpal is displaced in a dorsal and radial direction. This associated with an avulsion fracture of the volar and ulna border of the metacarpal base. The fracture fragment varies in size, when interpreting the imaging one must remember this is a fracture dislocation. The avulsion fragment is normally aligned and the usually larger portion of the metacarpal is subluxed/dislocated. Given that the first carpometacarpal joint is a saddle-shaped bone any minor malalignment results in substantial articular incongruity, as a result open reduction and fixation is frequently required.

Volar Plate Injury

Volar plate injury in the hand normally results from forced hyperextension of the fingers. In sport this occurs as a result of contact or catching injury. The volar aspects of the metacarpophalangeal joint and interphalangeal joints are reinforced by a fibrocartilagenous plate that has a strong distal osseous insertion. Trauma can result in either disruption or avulsion of this plate and is usually seen in the setting of severe dorsal subluxation or dislocation of these joints (Fig. 7.38). The patients present with persisting pain post-injury and sometimes symptoms suggestive of instability. At imaging, the volar plate has typical appearances of fibrocartilage being low signal on T2-weighted MR scanning difficult to discriminate the plate from the adjacent tendon. With injury the plate demonstrates increased signal either within the plate itself or at the site of bone avulsion, if present [86, 94]. Treatment is usually conservative though operative repair may be required when larger avulsion fragments are present.

Ulna Collateral Ligament Injury of the Thumb

Injury of the ulnar collateral ligament of the thumb can be seen as a result of both chronic and acute injury. Acute injuries are most common in sport associated with forced flexion of the thumb seen most commonly in skiers and cyclists.

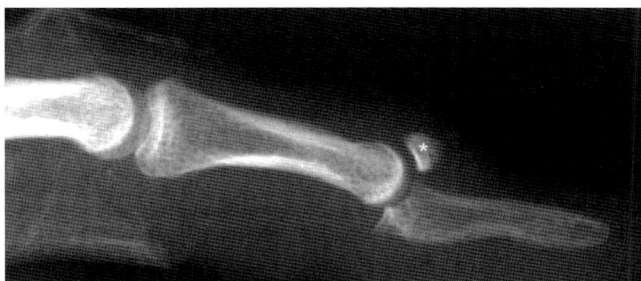

Fig. 7.37 Mallet finger with a large avulsion fracture (*asterisk*) associated with subluxation to the extent that the middle phalanx articulates with the donor site rather than the articular surface

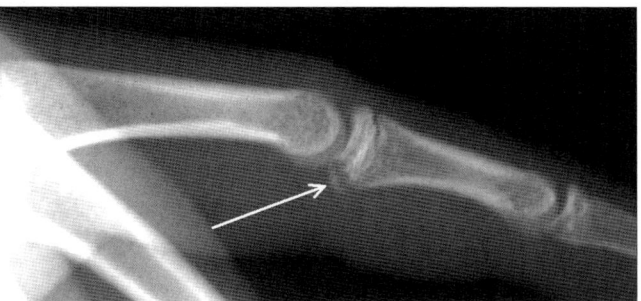

Fig. 7.38 Volar plate avulsion fracture (*arrow*)

Chronic injury was first described as a repetitive strain injury to the UCL from repeated twisting movement of the hand while wringing the necks of small animals, the so-called gamekeeper's thumb.

The ulna collateral ligament lies on the ulna aspect of the first metacarpophalangeal joint just deep to the insertion of the adductor aponeurosis of the thumb. An appreciation of this close relationship and the ability to visualize the adductor aponeurosis is key to effective imaging of ulna collateral ligament injury. The adductor aponeurosis images as a thin low signal band approximately 1.5 cm wide over the ulna aspect of the ulna collateral ligament at the level of the MCPJ. Avulsion injuries are usually seen at the distal insertion of the UCL and are well visualized with radiography. Disruption of the ulna collateral ligament itself causes fibres derangement and thickening of the tendon. This can be visualized indirectly with stress radiography though direct imaging of the ligament with either MR or ultrasound is required. With full thickness disruption of the UCL the proximal portion of the ligament can become displaced proximal to the adductor aponeurosis which then becomes a barrier to effective healing of the UCL, this is called a "Stener" lesion and is an indication for operative repair [95]. Imaging with ultrasound allows appreciation of the thickened proximal portion of the UCL trapped proximal to the thin adductor aponeurosis (Fig. 7.39). MR has been shown to be more reliable in the identification of this bunched up thickened proximal fragment though recently dynamic scanning during small thumb flexion extension movements has improved visualization of the adductor aponeurosis which moves separate to UCL during this movement. This should improve diagnostic accuracy of ultrasound.

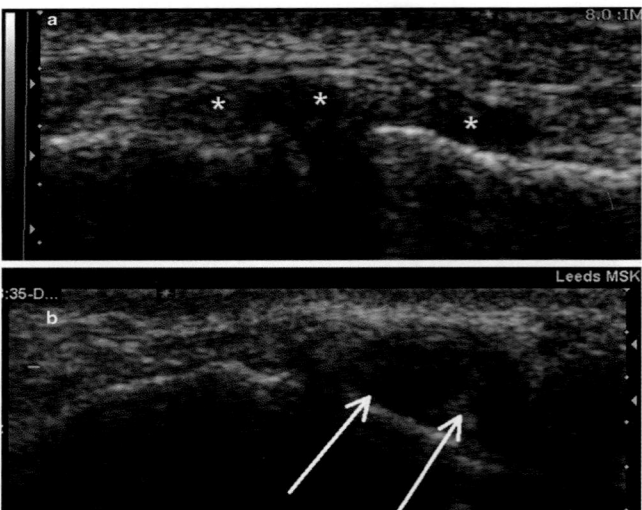

Fig. 7.39 Longitudinal ultrasounds of the ulna collateral ligament of the thumb. (**a**) Normal ulna collateral ligament of the thumb (*asterisks*). The ligament should be of uniform thickness throughout. (**b**) Stener lesion of the the UCL with marked bunching up of the proximal fibres (*arrows*) trapped by the overlying adductor aponeurosis

Boxer's Fracture

The boxer's fracture is an impaction injury of the fifth metacarpal neck as a result of punching injury. Bone breaks in different ways dependant on the forces applied, compression and twisting of bone produce spiral fractures that can be the hardest fractures to visualize radiographically. Their oblique path can be virtually invisible on two views and routinely when this injury is suspected we perform DP, lateral and oblique view of the hand. The aim of imaging is to diagnose the presence or absence of a fracture and to document the degree of shortening, angulation and intra-articular extension present.

Interestingly, professional boxers are taught to punch with maximal force passing through the third metacarpal so a true boxer should really fracture this bone first. The fifth metacarpal fracture could be termed the amateur boxer's fracture. Boxing has also been associated with high-force avulsion injury to the extensor carpi radialis brevis tendon insertion [96].

Fracture Dislocations of the Carpometacarpal Joints

Fracture dislocation of the carpometacarpal joints are generally the result of a high-energy injury. Punching injury is the most common mechanism and there is a strong association between CMC fracture dislocation and metacarpal shaft and neck fractures. Fracture of the adjacent wrist bones is also common. The lesion should be suspected when there is incongruity of the CMC joint space on the DP view of the wrist or fracture of an isolated third or fourth metacarpal without evidence of damage to the other metacarpal. Cross-sectional imaging is required when these fractures are demonstrated radiographically and frequently demonstrates more extensive damage than was suspected radiographically. As such, it is advised that the radiologist has a relatively low threshold for recourse to cross-sectional imaging as these injuries are associated with substantial morbidity and frequently require operative intervention.

References

1. Geissler WB (2001) Carpal fractures in athletes. Clin Sports Med 20:167–188
2. Jacobson JA, Miller BS, Morag Y (2005) Golf and racquet sports injuries. Semin Musculoskelet Radiol 9:346–359
3. Masmejean EH, Chavane H, Chantegret A, Issermann JJ, Alnot JY (1999) The wrist of the formula 1 driver. Br J Sports Med 33:270–273
4. McCarroll JR (2001) Overuse injuries of the upper extremity in golf. Clin Sports Med 20:469–479

5. Rettig AC (2004) Athletic injuries of the wrist and hand: part II: overuse injuries of the wrist and traumatic injuries to the hand. Am J Sports Med 32:262–273
6. Rooks MD (1997) Rock climbing injuries. Sports Med 23:261–270
7. Theriault G, Lachance P (1998) Golf injuries. An overview. Sports Med 26:43–57
8. Webb BG, Rettig LA (2008) Gymnastic wrist injuries. Curr Sports Med Rep 7:289–295
9. Kristensen SS, Thomassen E, Christensen F (1986) Ulnar variance in Kienbock's disease. J Hand Surg Br 11:258–260
10. Conway WF, Destouet JM, Gilula LA, Bellinghausen HW, Weeks PM (1985) The carpal boss: an overview of radiographic evaluation. Radiology 156:29–31
11. Maquirriain J, Ghisi JP (2006) Acute os styloideum injury in an elite athlete. Skeletal Radiol 35:394–396
12. Sokolow C, Saffar P (2001) Anatomy and histology of the scapholunate ligament. Hand Clin 17:77–81
13. Doyle JR (1988) Anatomy of the finger flexor tendon sheath and pulley system. J Hand Surg Am 13:473–484
14. Hauger O, Chung CB, Lektrakul N et al (2000) Pulley system in the fingers: normal anatomy and simulated lesions in cadavers at MR imaging, CT, and US with and without contrast material distention of the tendon sheath. Radiology 217:201–212
15. Lee JC, Healy JC (2005) Normal sonographic anatomy of the wrist and hand. Radiographics 25:1577–1590
16. Hanks GA, Kalenak A, Bowman LS, Sebastianelli WJ (1989) Stress fractures of the carpal scaphoid. A report of four cases. J Bone Joint Surg Am 71:938–941
17. Heckmann A, Lahoda LU, Alkandari Q, Vogt PM, Knobloch K (2008) C-type scaphoid fracture in a elite power lifting. Sportverletz Sportschaden 22:106–108
18. Hosey RG, Hauk JM, Boland MR (2006) Scaphoid stress fracture: an unusual cause of wrist pain in a competitive diver. Orthopedics 29:503–505
19. Blum AG, Zabel JP, Kohlmann R et al (2006) Pathologic conditions of the hypothenar eminence: evaluation with multidetector CT and MR imaging. Radiographics 26:1021–1044
20. David TS, Zemel NP, Mathews PV (2003) Symptomatic, partial union of the hook of the hamate fracture in athletes. Am J Sports Med 31:106–111
21. Evans MW Jr (2004) Hamate hook fracture in a 17-year-old golfer: importance of matching symptoms to clinical evidence. J Manipulative Physiol Ther 27:516–518
22. Evans MW Jr, Gilbert ML, Norton S (2006) Case report of right hamate hook fracture in a patient with previous fracture history of left hamate hook: is it hamate bipartite? Chiropr Osteopat 14:22
23. Batt ME (1993) Golfing injuries. An overview. Sports Med 16:64–71
24. Murray PM, Cooney WP (1996) Golf-induced injuries of the wrist. Clin Sports Med 15:85–109
25. Mann FA, Wilson AJ, Gilula LA (1992) Radiographic evaluation of the wrist: what does the hand surgeon want to know? Radiology 184:15–24
26. Short WH, Werner FW, Green JK, Masaoka S (2002) Biomechanical evaluation of ligamentous stabilizers of the scaphoid and lunate. J Hand Surg Am 27:991–1002
27. Magee T (2009) Comparison of 3-T MRI and arthroscopy of intrinsic wrist ligament and TFCC tears. AJR Am J Roentgenol 192:80–85
28. Griffith JF, Chan DP, Ho PC, Zhao L, Hung LK, Metreweli C (2001) Sonography of the normal scapholunate ligament and scapholunate joint space. J Clin Ultrasound 29:223–229
29. Jacobson JA, Oh E, Propeck T, Jebson PJ, Jamadar DA, Hayes CW (2002) Sonography of the scapholunate ligament in four cadaveric wrists: correlation with MR arthrography and anatomy. AJR Am J Roentgenol 179:523–527
30. Cassidy C, Ruby LK (2003) Carpal instability. Instr Course Lect 52:209–220
31. Larsen CF, Mathiesen FK, Lindequist S (1991) Measurements of carpal bone angles on lateral wrist radiographs. J Hand Surg Am 16:888–893
32. Friedman SL, Palmer AK (1991) The ulnar impaction syndrome. Hand Clin 7:295–310
33. Fortems Y, De Smet L, Dauwe D, Stoffelen D, Deneffe G, Fabry G (1994) Incidence of cartilaginous and ligamentous lesions of the radio-carpal and distal radio-ulnar joint in an elderly population. J Hand Surg Br 19:572–575
34. Kirschenbaum D, Sieler S, Solonick D, Loeb DM, Cody RP (1995) Arthrography of the wrist. Assessment of the integrity of the ligaments in young asymptomatic adults. J Bone Joint Surg Am 77:1207–1209
35. Romaniuk CS, Butt WP, Coral A (1995) Bilateral three-compartment wrist arthrography in patients with unilateral wrist pain: findings and implications for management. Skeletal Radiol 24:95–99
36. Brown JA, Janzen DL, Adler BD et al (1994) Arthrography of the contralateral, asymptomatic wrist in patients with unilateral wrist pain. Can Assoc Radiol J 45:292–296
37. Cantor RM, Stern PJ, Wyrick JD, Michaels SE (1994) The relevance of ligament tears or perforations in the diagnosis of wrist pain: an arthrographic study. J Hand Surg Am 19:945–953
38. Oneson SR, Scales LM, Timins ME, Erickson SJ, Chamoy L (1996) MR imaging interpretation of the Palmer classification of triangular fibrocartilage complex lesions. Radiographics 16:97–106
39. Mikic Z, Somer L, Somer T (1992) Histologic structure of the articular disk of the human distal radioulnar joint. Clin Orthop Relat Res 29–36
40. Mikic ZD (1978) Age changes in the triangular fibrocartilage of the wrist joint. J Anat 126:367–384
41. Hobby JL, Tom BD, Bearcroft PW, Dixon AK (2001) Magnetic resonance imaging of the wrist: diagnostic performance statistics. Clin Radiol 56:50–57
42. Meier R, Schmitt R, Christopoulos G, Krimmer H (2003) [TFCC-lesion. MR arthrography vs. arthroscopy of the wrist]. Unfallchirurg 106:190–194
43. Joshy S, Ghosh S, Lee K, Deshmukh SC (2008) Accuracy of direct magnetic resonance arthrography in the diagnosis of triangular fibrocartilage complex tears of the wrist. Int Orthop 32:251–253
44. Hobby JL, Dixon AK, Bearcroft PW et al (2001) MR imaging of the wrist: effect on clinical diagnosis and patient care. Radiology 220:589–593
45. Maizlin ZV, Brown JA, Clement JJ et al (2009) MR arthrography of the wrist: controversies and concepts. Hand (N Y) 4:66–73
46. Imaeda T, Nakamura R, Shionoya K, Makino N (1996) Ulnar impaction syndrome: MR imaging findings. Radiology 201:495–500
47. Cerezal L, del Pinal F, Abascal F, Garcia-Valtuille R, Pereda T, Canga A (2002) Imaging findings in ulnar-sided wrist impaction syndromes. Radiographics 22:105–121
48. Bell MJ, Hill RJ, McMurtry RY (1985) Ulnar impingement syndrome. J Bone Joint Surg Br 67:126–129
49. Staron RB, Feldman F, Haramati N, Singson RD, Rosenwasser M, Esser PD (1994) Abnormal geometry of the distal radioulnar joint: MR findings. Skeletal Radiol 23:369–372
50. Emery KH (2006) Imaging of sports injuries of the upper extremity in children. Clin Sports Med 25:543–568, viii
51. Hagel B (2005) Skiing and snowboarding injuries. Med Sport Sci 48:74–119
52. Kraus R, Szalay G, Meyer C, Kilian O, Schnettler R (2007) Distal radius fracture – a goalkeepers' injury in children and adolescents. Sportverletz Sportschaden 21:177–179
53. Macgregor DM (2003) Don't save the ball! Br J Sports Med 37:351–353

54. Zimmermann R, Rudisch A, Fritz D, Gschwentner M, Arora R (2007) MR imaging for the evaluation of accompanying injuries in cases of distal forearm fractures in children and adolescents. Handchir Mikrochir Plast Chir 39:60–67
55. Caine DJ, Nassar L (2005) Gymnastics injuries. Med Sport Sci 48:18–58
56. DiFiori JP (2006) Overuse injury and the young athlete: the case of chronic wrist pain in gymnasts. Curr Sports Med Rep 5:165–167
57. DiFiori JP, Mandelbaum BR (1996) Wrist pain in a young gymnast: unusual radiographic findings and MRI evidence of growth plate injury. Med Sci Sports Exerc 28:1453–1458
58. Dobyns JH, Gabel GT (1990) Gymnast's wrist. Hand Clin 6:493–505
59. Bilic R, Kolundzic R, Jelic M (2001) Overuse injury syndromes of the hand, forearm and elbow. Arh Hig Rada Toksikol 52:403–414
60. du Toit P, Sole G, Bowerbank P, Noakes TD (1999) Incidence and causes of tenosynovitis of the wrist extensors in long distance paddle canoeists. Br J Sports Med 33:105–109
61. Guerini H, Drape JL, Le Viet D et al (2007) Imaging of wrist injuries in athletes. J Radiol 88:111–128
62. Ilyas AM, Ast M, Schaffer AA, Thoder J (2007) De quervain tenosynovitis of the wrist. J Am Acad Orthop Surg 15:757–764
63. Rettig AC (1994) Wrist problems in the tennis player. Med Sci Sports Exerc 26:1207–1212
64. Rossi C, Cellocco P, Margaritondo E, Bizzarri F, Costanzo G (2005) De Quervain disease in volleyball players. Am J Sports Med 33:424–427
65. Glajchen N, Schweitzer M (1996) MRI features in de Quervain's tenosynovitis of the wrist. Skeletal Radiol 25:63–65
66. Klug JD (1995) MR diagnosis of tenosynovitis about the wrist. Magn Reson Imaging Clin N Am 3:305–312
67. Richie CA 3rd, Briner WW Jr (2003) Corticosteroid injection for treatment of de Quervain's tenosynovitis: a pooled quantitative literature evaluation. J Am Board Fam Pract 16:102–106
68. Montalvan B, Parier J, Brasseur JL, Le Viet D, Drape JL (2006) Extensor carpi ulnaris injuries in tennis players: a study of 28 cases. Br J Sports Med 40:424–429, discussion 429
69. Wiesler ER, Lumsden B (2005) Golf injuries of the upper extremity. J Surg Orthop Adv 14:1–7
70. Pfirrmann CW, Theumann NH, Chung CB, Botte MJ, Trudell DJ, Resnick D (2001) What happens to the triangular fibrocartilage complex during pronation and supination of the forearm? Analysis of its morphology and diagnostic assessment with MR arthrography. Skeletal Radiol 30:677–685
71. Henry M (2008) Arthroscopic management of dorsal wrist impingement. J Hand Surg Am 33:1201–1204
72. VanHeest AE, Luger NM, House JH, Vener M (2007) Extensor retinaculum impingement in the athlete: a new diagnosis. Am J Sports Med 35:2126–2130
73. Jagenburg A, Goyen M, Hirschelmann R, Carstens IM, Kroger K (2000) Hypothenar hammer syndrome: causes, sequelae and diagnostic aspects. Rofo 172:295–300
74. Winterer JT, Ghanem N, Roth M et al (2002) Diagnosis of the hypothenar hammer syndrome by high-resolution contrast-enhanced MR angiography. Eur Radiol 12:2457–2462
75. Akuthota V, Plastaras C, Lindberg K, Tobey J, Press J, Garvan C (2005) The effect of long-distance bicycling on ulnar and median nerves: an electrophysiologic evaluation of cyclist palsy. Am J Sports Med 33:1224–1230
76. Hsu WC, Chen WH, Oware A, Chiu HC (2002) Unusual entrapment neuropathy in a golf player. Neurology 59:646–647
77. Dias JJ, Dhukaram V, Kumar P (2007) The natural history of untreated dorsal wrist ganglia and patient reported outcome 6 years after intervention. J Hand Surg Eur Vol 32:502–508
78. Magee TH, Rowedder AM, Degnan GG (1995) Intraosseus ganglia of the wrist. Radiology 195:517–520
79. Wright WC, Griffiths HJ (2002) Radiologic case study. Wrist instability, volar intercalary segmental instability, and ganglion cysts. Orthopedics 25(906):995–996
80. Wang H, Terrill RQ, Tanaka S, Amrami KK, Spinner RJ (2009) Adherence of intraneural ganglia of the upper extremity to the principles of the unifying articular (synovial) theory. Neurosurg Focus 26:E10
81. Teefey SA, Dahiya N, Middleton WD, Gelberman RH, Boyer MI (2008) Ganglia of the hand and wrist: a sonographic analysis. AJR Am J Roentgenol 191:716–720
82. Wang G, Jacobson JA, Feng FY, Girish G, Caoili EM, Brandon C (2007) Sonography of wrist ganglion cysts: variable and noncystic appearances. J Ultrasound Med 26:1323–1328, quiz 1330–1321
83. Goldsmith S, Yang SS (2008) Magnetic resonance imaging in the diagnosis of occult dorsal wrist ganglions. J Hand Surg Eur Vol 33:595–599
84. Bollen SR (1990) Injury to the A2 pulley in rock climbers. J Hand Surg Br 15:268–270
85. Rooks MD, Johnston RB 3rd, Ensor CD, McIntosh B, James S (1995) Injury patterns in recreational rock climbers. Am J Sports Med 23:683–685
86. Clavero JA, Alomar X, Monill JM et al (2002) MR imaging of ligament and tendon injuries of the fingers. Radiographics 22:237–256
87. Gabl M, Lener M, Pechlaner S, Lutz M, Rudisch A (1996) Rupture or stress injury of the flexor tendon pulleys? Early diagnosis with MRI. Handchir Mikrochir Plast Chir 28:317–321
88. Parellada JA, Balkissoon AR, Hayes CW, Conway WF (1996) Bowstring injury of the flexor tendon pulley system: MR imaging. AJR Am J Roentgenol 167:347–349
89. Cresswell TR, Allott C, Auchincloss JM (1998) Colour Doppler ultrasound in the diagnosis, management and follow-up of a digital flexor pulley injury. J Hand Surg Br 23:655–657
90. Smith RD, O'Leary ST, McCullough CJ (1998) Trigger wrist and flexor tenosynovitis. J Hand Surg Br 23:813–814
91. Guerini H, Pessis E, Theumann N et al (2008) Sonographic appearance of trigger fingers. J Ultrasound Med 27:1407–1413
92. Paulius KL, Maguina P (2009) Ultrasound-assisted percutaneous trigger finger release: is it safe? Hand (N Y) 4:35–37
93. Lopez-Ben R, Lee DH, Nicolodi DJ (2003) Boxer knuckle (injury of the extensor hood with extensor tendon subluxation): diagnosis with dynamic US – report of three cases. Radiology 228:642–646
94. Masson JA, Golimbu CN, Grossman JA (1995) MR imaging of the metacarpophalangeal joints. Magn Reson Imaging Clin N Am 3:313–325
95. Stener B (1963) Skeletal injuries associated with rupture of the ulnar collateral ligament of the metacarpophalangeal joint of the thumb. A clinical and anatomical study. Acta Chir Scand 125:583–586
96. Breeze SW, Ouellette T, Mays MM (2009) Isolated avulsion fracture of the extensor carpi radialis brevis insertion due to a boxer's injury. Orthopedics 32:210

Chapter 8
Postoperative Imaging in Sports Medicine

Ali Naraghi and Lawrence M. White

Introduction

With advances in surgical and arthroscopic techniques, an increasing number of patients are undergoing operative treatment of sports injuries. Following such procedures a proportion of patients may present with residual or recurrent symptoms. These symptoms may be related to failed surgery, a new injury or a complication of prior surgery. Imaging is being increasingly used in this patient group to elucidate the cause of potential symptoms and for documentation of surgical success or failure.

Postoperative imaging poses unique challenges in sports medicine imaging. The interpreting radiologist must first be cognizant that the patient has had previous surgery, as this may not be in the provided history. Interpretation also requires knowledge of the commonly used surgical techniques and their potential complications. Surgery also results in morphological changes to normal structures, which may simulate pathological processes and may be misinterpreted as a recurrent lesion if conventional diagnostic criteria are employed. Bulk orthopaedic hardware can also result in substantial imaging-related artefacts obscuring and distorting the area of interest. Even in the absence of bulk orthopaedic hardware, microscopic metallic debris shed from surgical instruments may result in extensive MR imaging artefact. This may necessitate modification of imaging protocols in the postoperative setting.

Surgical intervention is most commonly performed in the knee and shoulder and these will form the basis of this chapter. Depending on the procedure performed and the nature of the postoperative symptoms, the full range of imaging studies including conventional radiography (CR), ultrasound (US), computer tomography (CT) and magnetic resonance (MR) imaging may be utilized and provide complimentary information. In our experience, MR imaging with its excellent soft tissue evaluation and multiplanar capability forms the cornerstone for advanced imaging evaluation of the postoperative patient by allowing global assessment of soft tissue and osseous structures.

Optimisation of Imaging Techniques in the Postoperative Patient

Presence of postoperative metal hardware results in imaging-related artefact, which may obscure adjacent anatomy or mimic pathological changes. This is particularly the case with CT and MR imaging. Modification of imaging parameters and appropriate positioning of the extremity can reduce the degree of artefact around metal hardware.

With CT the degree of metal artefact is related to the hardware thickness and density composition through which the X-ray beam must cross. Therefore, positioning the patient within the CT gantry such that the X-ray beam is perpendicular to the smallest diameter of the hardware will help reduce the degree of artefact [1]. Increasing the peak tube voltage and tube current also helps to reduce artefact. With modern multislice scanners, reducing the pitch to less than 1 results in overlapping slices which increases the effective milliampere-seconds (mAs) [2]. Soft tissue algorithms and multiplanar reformations may also further allow better visualization of bony and soft tissue structures around metal implants. With smaller hardware, however, the use of bony algorithm may still be advantageous [1].

The degree of metal related artefact on MR imaging is related to the composition of the hardware, its orientation relative to the main magnetic field and the pulse sequence parameters utilized for image acquisition. Titanium implants cause less distortion and artefact than steel or cobalt implants due to their reduced ferromagnetic characteristics. The hardware geometry also has important implications with regards to the degree of artefact. Linear implants produce fewer

Lawrence M. White (✉)
Division of Musculoskeletal Radiology, Department of Medical Imaging, Mount Sinai Hospital, University of Toronto, 600 University Avenue, Toronto, ON M5G 1X5, Canada
e-mail: lwhite@mtsinai.on.ca

artefacts than those with complex or spherical geometry. Aligning the hardware with the main magnetic field similarly helps to reduce the degree of artefacts on MR imaging.

The choice of pulse sequences and imaging parameters is crucial to minimizing image distortion and artefact on MR imaging. Even in the absence of bulk metal hardware there can be extensive artefact on postoperative MR images (Fig. 8.1). Gradient-echo images which lack a 180° refocusing pulse are inherently prone to intravoxel dephasing and loss of signal, and in general should be avoided in postoperative imaging. Gradient-echo images may be useful, however, to identify microscopic metallic debris if there is doubt as to whether the patient has had surgery. Fast-spin echo sequences, using multiple 180° refocusing pulses, minimize the signal loss caused by inhomogeneities in the local magnetic field induced by metal hardware. The reduction in artefact is further maximized by increasing the echo train length and reducing the interecho spacing. Fast-spin echo images suffer from misregistration artefact which is inversely proportional to the frequency-encoding gradient strength and is manifested in the frequency-encoding direction. Using a higher frequency-encoding gradient strength (corresponding to use of a widened/higher imaging receiver bandwidth), and orienting the frequency-encoding direction along the length of the hardware help to reduce metal related artefacts [3]. Reducing slice thickness and increasing matrix size also helps to reduce the degree of image distortion [3]. Spectral fat saturation techniques are dependent on a homogenous local magnetic field and in the presence of metal inhomogeneous fat-suppression results [4]. Short-tau inversion recovery sequences are less susceptible to field inhomogeneities and are better suited to imaging around bulk metal hardware, as are water-fat separation strategies (e.g. Dixon imaging techniques).

Postoperative Imaging of the Knee

Postoperative Imaging in Meniscal Surgery

As the natural history of total meniscectomy has been towards premature chondral loss and degenerative change, the fundamental principle in modern meniscal surgery is to preserve as much meniscal tissue as possible whilst addressing the tear and restoring meniscal morphology. This may be achieved by partial meniscectomy or when possible by meniscal repair. The tear pattern and presence of vascularity are critical for determining the optimal treatment. Tears amenable to repair include linear oblique or vertical tears through the peripheral vascular or "red zone" of the meniscus, typically within 3 mm of the meniscocapsular junction. Tears through the "red-white zone," typically between 3 and 5 mm from the meniscocapsular junction have variable vascularity, whereas those through the "white zone" demonstrate poor healing unless vascularity is demonstrated at surgery [5]. Partial meniscectomy is used for treatment of complex, degenerative tears or avascular tears. The aim at partial meniscectomy is to resect the unstable tear component without sacrificing stable meniscal tissue.

Symptoms following partial meniscectomy or repair may be due to residual or recurrent tear at the site of prior surgery, a meniscal tear at a new location or other chondral or ligamentous injury.

MR Imaging

If the relevant history has not been provided there may be clues on MR imaging, which may help in establishing whether there has been previous surgery. Arthroscopy leaves

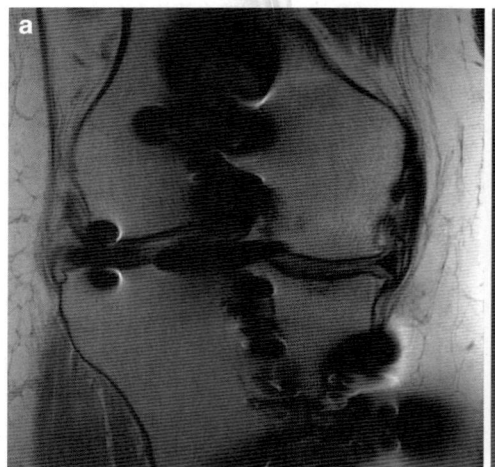
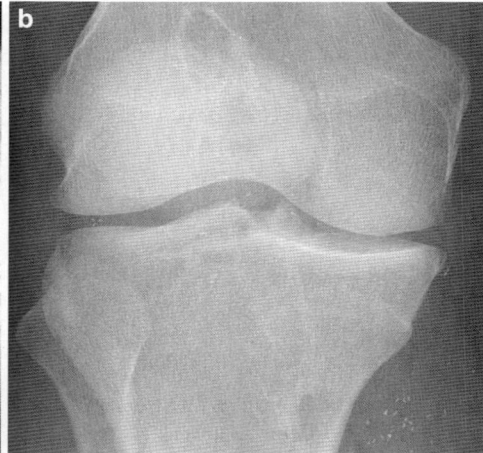

Fig. 8.1 Coronal intermediate-weighted FSE MR image (**a**) following ACL reconstruction shows extensive susceptibility artefact. Corresponding conventional radiograph (**b**) shows numerous tiny metallic fragments as source of artefact

a variable thickness linear low signal intensity scar may be seen within Hoffa's fat pad. A further clue that may focal thickening of the edge of the patellar tendon (Fig. 8.2). Typically, there is little or no artefact in the region of the meniscus to alert the reader, unless meniscal repair has been attempted with a fixation device.

The utility and diagnostic criteria of MR imaging for meniscal tears in virgin menisci are well established with an accuracy of over 90% [6]. Diagnostic criteria include intrameniscal signal extending to an articular surface (grade III signal) seen on at least two slices on a short TE sequence, alteration of meniscal morphology, loss of meniscal volume or demonstration of a displaced fragment. Applying these criteria after meniscal surgery yields modest results for detection of residual or recurrent tears [5, 7–9]. There are several reasons to account for this. First, a healing tear, either following conservative treatment or repair, will show increased signal intensity on short TE sequences corresponding to fibrovascular tissue during the healing phase [5, 7, 10]. These tears may be stable at arthroscopy but signal changes may be evident even at 1 year postsurgery [5, 7]. Second, following partial meniscectomy areas of intrasubstance signal change, classified as grade I or grade II on preoperative MR imaging, may extend to the neo-articular surface and simulate grade III signal following resection of subjacent unstable meniscal tissue. This phenomenon of "signal conversion" may result in a false-positive diagnosis of a meniscal tear using preoperative criteria of meniscal pathology. Finally, the anatomic appearances of menisci may be highly variable following surgery. Morphology is dependent on the location and type of previous tears and the technique used to treat them. Surgery may result in meniscal distortion or blunting as a normal postoperative finding and therefore diagnosis of a residual or recurrent tear cannot be based on alteration of normal virgin meniscal morphology.

Accuracy of MR imaging in diagnosing meniscal tears following surgery appears to be related to the amount of meniscal tissue that has been resected [11]. Where there has been resection of <25% of the meniscus, MR imaging demonstrates accuracy rates of 89–100% utilizing the traditional criteria of grade III signal on short TE sequences [9]. Where >25% has been resected the presence of grade III signal on short TE sequences is of limited diagnostic utility. Accuracy rates of 50–65% have been recorded for conventional MR imaging depending on the degree of resection, the lower figure representing the accuracy in those with >75% of the meniscus resected [9]. Similarly, contour abnormality is of limited accuracy in the diagnosis of a tear in patients with more significant partial meniscectomy with an accuracy rate of only 67–68% [11] (Fig. 8.3). Traditional diagnostic criteria of a meniscal tear can still be applied for diagnosis of tears in part of the meniscus where surgery has not been performed but this is dependent on access to prior surgical reports and preoperative imaging.

Suggested modified criteria for diagnosis for postoperative meniscal tear include an area of fluid signal intensity extending onto the articular surface on T2w images (Figs. 8.4 and 8.5), identification of a displaced meniscal fragment (Fig. 8.6) or meniscal fragmentation [7]. As identification of fluid signal

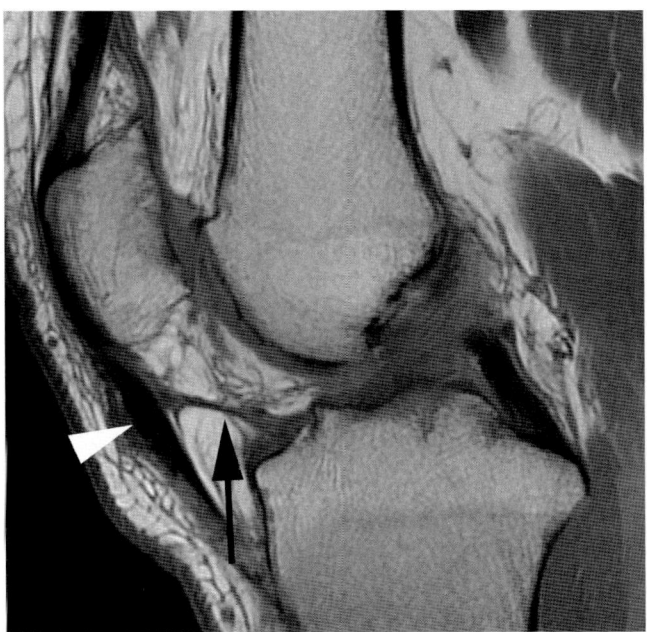

Fig. 8.2 Sagittal proton-density knee MR image following arthroscopy shows linear low signal intensity scar through Hoffa's fat (*arrow*) with adjacent thickening of patellar tendon (*arrowhead*)

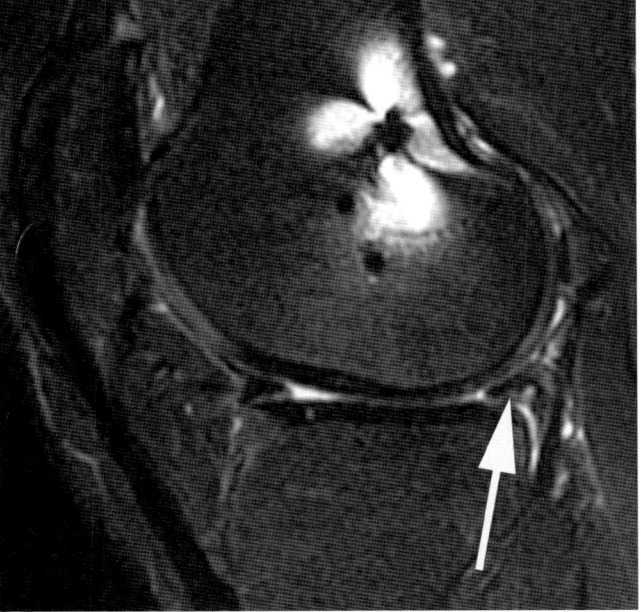

Fig. 8.3 Sagittal T2 FS MR image following partial meniscectomy shows a diminutive and irregular posterior horn (*arrow*). Repeat arthroscopy did not show evidence of a meniscal tear

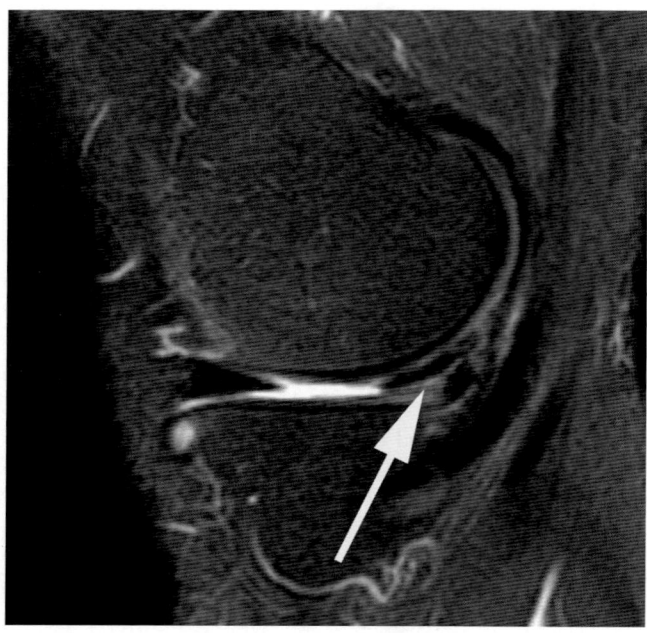

Fig. 8.4 Sagittal T2 FS MR image of the medial compartment after prior partial meniscectomy shows oblique posterior horn undersurface high T2 signal cleft (*arrow*) consistent with a residual or recurrent tear cleft

intensity is critical to diagnosing a recurrent tear, it is worthwhile obtaining T2w images in both the sagittal and coronal planes. The addition of fat saturation increases the conspicuity of the fluid signal and may be helpful. Another potentially useful sign following meniscal repair is widening of the cleft on serial examinations [12]. The identification of fluid within a tear cleft has a high specificity (88–92%) but a low sensitivity (41–69%) [7–9]. However, in applying these diagnostic criteria it must be remembered that fluid signal may be seen within a healing cleft without signifying a residual tear within the first 12 weeks flowing meniscal repair [7].

Identification of fluid signal within a tear is likely related to imbibition of joint fluid into a tear gap. In an attempt to utilize this mechanism, MR arthrography has been used for evaluation of recurrent tears. The benefits of direct MR arthrography are likely related to joint distension, increased intra-articular pressure and bathing the meniscus completely in a diluted gadolinium mixture. In addition, T1w imaging has a higher signal-to-noise ratio and may be advantageous for detection of tear clefts.

Meniscal tears at MR arthrography are diagnosed on the basis of a cleft of similar signal intensity as intra-articular

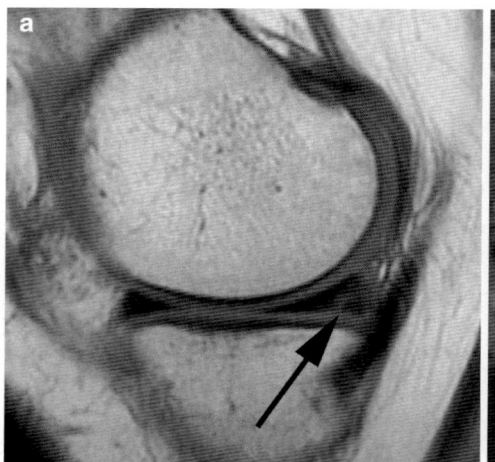
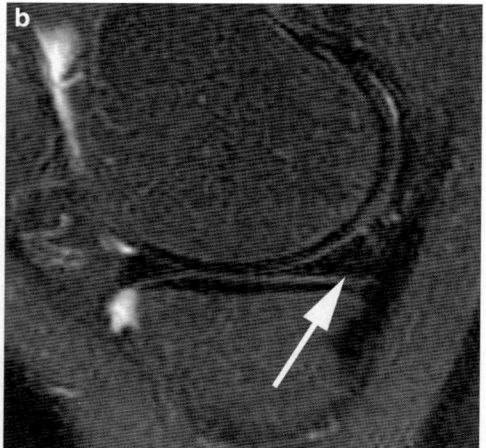

Fig. 8.5 Sagittal proton-density (**a**) and T2 FS (**b**) MR images in a patient with prior meniscal repair shows persistent undersurfacing cleft on the short TE sequence (*black arrow*) with a normal appearance on the T2w image (*white arrow*). Arthroscopy demonstrated a healed tear

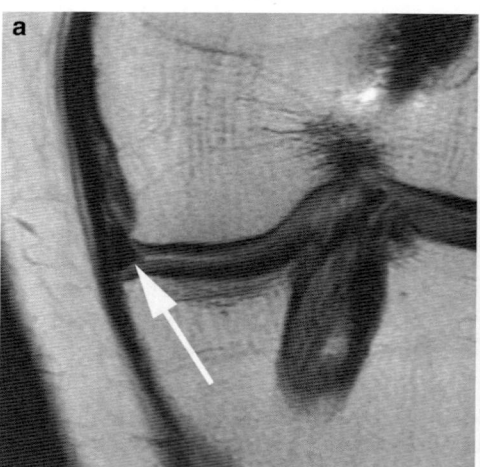
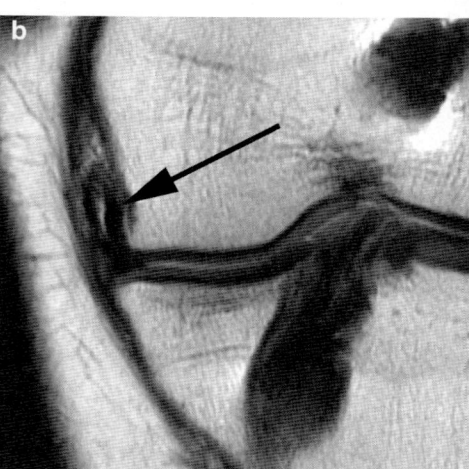

Fig. 8.6 Coronal intermediate-weighted knee MR image (**a**) in a patient with previous ACL reconstruction and partial medial meniscectomy resulting in a diminutive body of the medial meniscus (*white arrow*). Follow-up MR image (**b**) following a repeat injury shows flipped meniscal fragment into the medial gutter (*black arrow*) consistent with recurrent tear

racy of 85–94%, a sensitivity of 90–91% and a specificity of 78–100% [16]. Healing fibrovascular tissue within a tear cleft may show enhancement but this gradually diminishes with progressive healing on successive examinations, both in terms of signal change and size [17].

Computer Tomography

CT arthrography has been utilized for detection of tears in virgin menisci with a sensitivity and specificity over 90%. CT arthrography has a sensitivity of 100% but a specificity of 78% in detection of recurrent or residual meniscal tears. The lower specificity is likely related to the high spatial resolution of CT arthrography identifying small foci of intrameniscal contrast that may represent stable partial thickness tears. Using the criteria of contrast extending throughout the height or depth of the meniscus for a full thickness tear or at least a third of the height or depth of the meniscus for an unstable partial thickness tear, the specificity of CT arthrography improves to 89% but with a lower sensitivity of 93% [18].

Postoperative Imaging of the Knee Ligaments

The Postoperative ACL

Of all the knee ligaments, the ACL is the one most commonly ruptured. Up to 25% of patients may present postoperatively with symptoms of knee pain, persistent instability or loss of terminal extension and may be referred for further imaging assessment following ACL reconstructive surgery.

ACL reconstructive techniques can be broadly categorized into extra-articular and intra-articular techniques. The former are largely historical involving the iliotibial tract or the pes anserinus tendon being rerouted to prevent anterior tibial subluxation due to limited success and development of newer arthroscopically assisted intra-articular techniques. The intra-articular techniques most commonly utilize autograft but other potential graft choices include allograft and synthetic grafts. Bone-patellar tendon-bone (BPTB) and hamstring autografts are now the most commonly used ACL reconstruction constructs. Achilles tendon and fascia lata grafts are less commonly used. The use of synthetic grafts such as knitted Dacron and expanded polytetrafluoroethylene (Gore-Tex) has been limited due to problems related to high rates of graft rupture, graft stretching and foreign body reaction [19] (Fig. 8.8).

With the BPTB ACL reconstruction, the central third of the patellar tendon is harvested with bone plugs from the tibial tuberosity and the patella. Stabilization within the femoral and

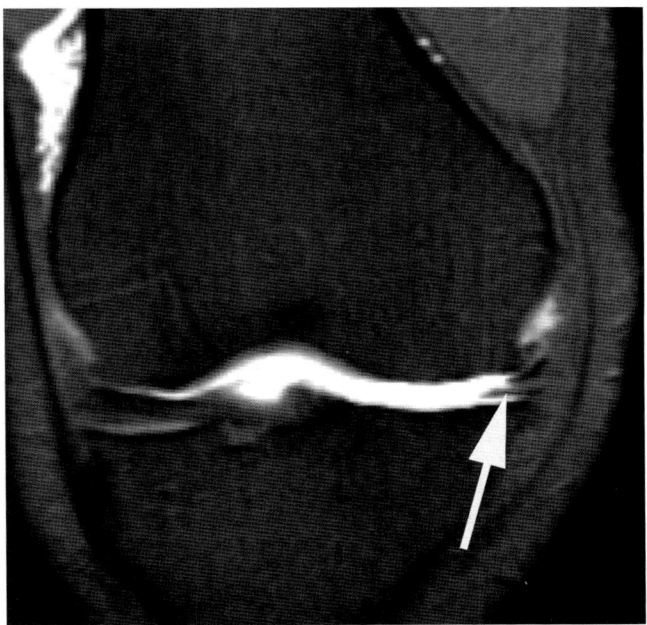

Fig. 8.7 Coronal T1 FS MR arthrographic image following partial meniscectomy in a patient with recurrent symptoms shows imbibition of gadolinium into a recurrent tear cleft in the medial meniscus body (*arrow*)

gadolinium (Fig. 8.7). Several studies directly comparing conventional MR imaging and MR arthrography in each patient have demonstrated higher accuracy rates with MR arthrography in patients with previous meniscal surgery [9, 13, 14]. Studies by Applegate et al. and Sciulli et al. demonstrated overall accuracy of 66–77% for conventional MR imaging and 88–93% for MR arthrography. MR arthrography does not appear to have an advantage over conventional MR imaging for detection of recurrent tears in the subset of patients where <25% of the meniscus has been resected with an accuracy of 89% for both techniques [9, 14]. In another study, whereby patients were randomised to either conventional MR imaging or MR arthrography, there were no statistically significant differences between the two techniques [15].

The drawbacks of direct MR arthrography include its invasive and time-consuming nature. To avoid its drawbacks, indirect MR arthrography has been recommended by some investigators for evaluation of the postoperative meniscus. The technique consists of intravenous injection of 0.1 mmol/kg of gadolinium followed by 20–30 min of gentle exercise before T1w imaging. The potential drawback of indirect MR arthrography in comparison with direct MR arthrography is the lack of joint distension [15] and potential enhancement of vascular and fibrovascular postoperative changes. Diagnosis of a meniscal tear is based on demonstration of areas of signal intensity similar to gadolinium. Indirect MR arthrography shows similar accuracy rates to direct MR arthrography and superior results to conventional MR imaging with an accu-

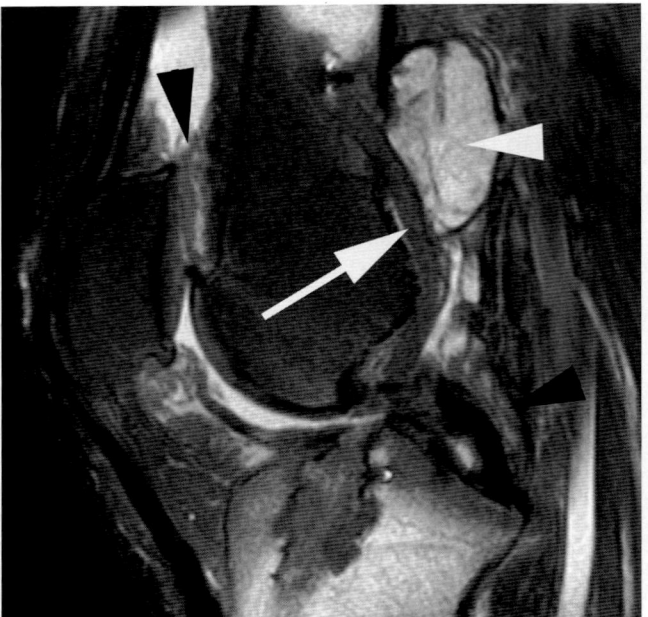 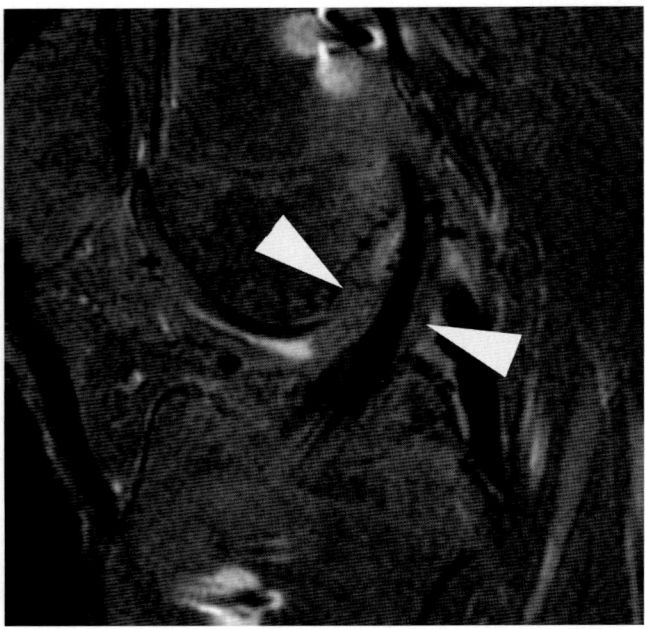

Fig. 8.8 Sagittal T2 FS knee MR image in a patient with prior ACL reconstruction utilizing Gore-Tex graft (*arrow*) shows foreign body reaction. There is a large complex fluid collection posterior to the graft (*white arrowhead*) and synovitis anteriorly and adjacent to the PCL (*black arrowheads*)

Fig. 8.9 Sagittal proton-density knee MR image in a patient with a hamstring ACL graft 3 months postsurgery. The graft is intact but there is periligamentous synovial proliferation (*arrowheads*) which resolved on a subsequent MRI

tibial tunnels is accomplished with interference screws until stable osseous engagement of the bone plugs is achieved. The osseous fixation of the reconstruction graft allows for early return to physical activity, a potential advantage of the BPTB graft. The major disadvantages of this approach are potential complications related to the harvest site including anterior knee pain, patellar tendon rupture and patellar fracture.

Hamstring tendon grafts consist of the resected distal tendons of semitendinosus and gracilis. The tendons are sutured together, doubled up and sutured again to increase the graft strength as a result of its four-bundle configuration. Some surgeons favour hamstring grafts because of a lack of anterior knee symptoms following surgery, faster harvesting and preparation, and the need for a smaller harvest site incision.

Normal postoperative ACL graft appearance is dependent on the graft type used and the interval between surgery and imaging. During the immediate postoperative period the graft should exhibit uniform low signal intensity on all pulse sequences similar to the native PCL [20]. With time the graft undergoes a process of necrosis, revascularization, cellular proliferation and remodelling, collectively termed "ligamentization" of the graft [21]. During this period, the strength of the graft is diminished and the graft demonstrates alteration in signal intensity. These changes are typically seen between 3 and 12 months result in a somewhat inhomogeneous appearance to the graft with increased signal intensity particularly on T1 and T2w acquisitions [22]. This may make assessment of graft integrity difficult [22]. The signal changes, which should never be as bright as fluid on T2w sequences, are thought to be related to the adjacent synovial proliferation [23] (Fig. 8.9) although there is some debate as to whether these changes may partially reflect subclinical impingement of the graft [24, 25]. Typically by 12–18 months the graft assumes its normal signal intensity similar to the native ACL [19]. Recent studies have shown that persistent variable degrees of intrinsic T2-weighted signal intensity change may be visualized in asymptomatic patients with stable ACL grafts at long-term follow-up [26]. In contrast, fluid signal intensity T2 signal traversing the cross-sectional area of the graft and discontinuity of graft fibres are reliable features of graft tearing.

Graft harvest sites may also show morphological changes in asymptomatic individuals. With BPTB grafts, osseous defects are visible in the anterior aspect of the lower patella and the tibial tuberosity. These changes are best visualized on sagittal and axial images (Fig. 8.10). The patellar tendon initially demonstrates a longitudinal defect of its central third spanning the entire length of the tendon (Fig. 8.11). The defect is typically evident even 1 year postsurgery although by 18–24 months the central defect within the patellar tendon may fill with scar tissue and may be indistinguishable on imaging from the normal tendon. The tendon may also appear thickened and of increased signal intensity particularly on short TE sequences [27].

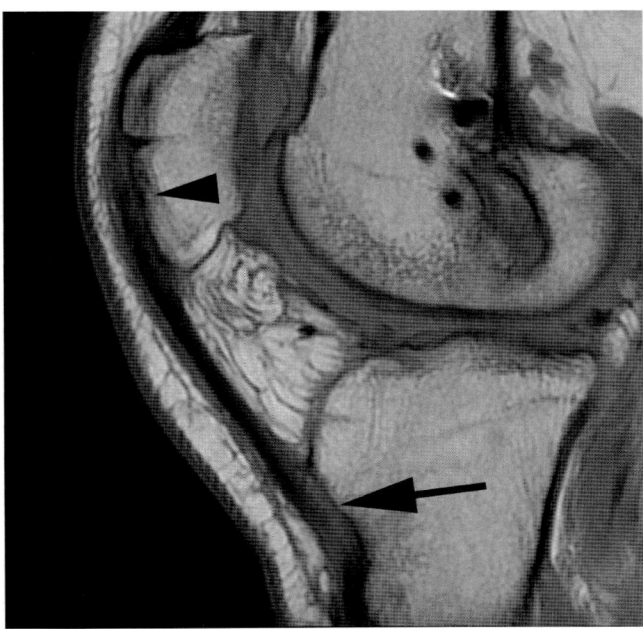

Fig. 8.10 Sagittal proton-density MR image following BPTB ACL reconstruction. Osseous defects are seen anteriorly in relation to the patella (*arrowhead*) and the tibial tuberosity (*arrow*) at the sites of bone plug harvest

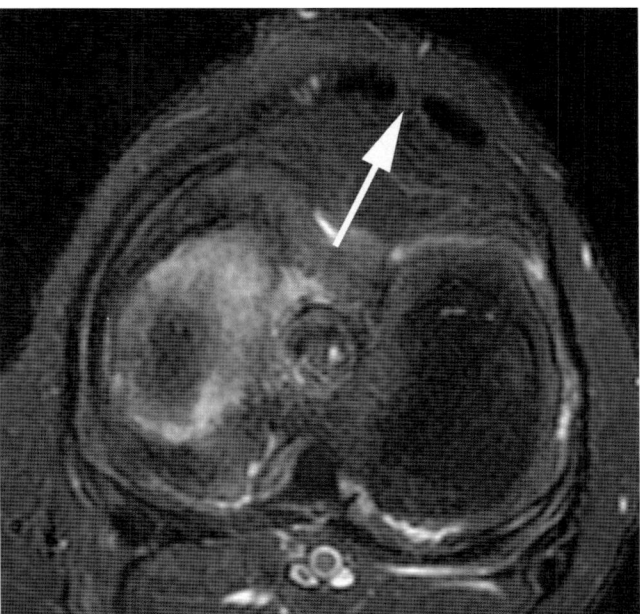

Fig. 8.11 Axial T2 FS MR image following of the patellar tendon shows normal postoperative appearances with a central defect at the harvest site (*arrow*)

The tendons at the site of harvest of the hamstring graft have been shown to regenerate and regain much of their original strength [28]. In the first postoperative month the harvest tracks exhibit tubular fluid signal intensity. With time and progressive regeneration of the tendon low signal intensity tendinous structures are seen in the expected location of the semitendinosus and gracilis tendons although they may be left without their distal attachment (Fig. 8.12).

Technical factors critical to achieving a successful surgical outcome following ACL reconstruction include isometric graft placement, avoiding graft impingement and providing adequate fixation of the graft. These factors as well as graft integrity and potential complications must be assessed on postoperative imaging.

Isometric graft positioning is principally dependent on the location of the femoral tunnel which should simulate the origin of the native ACL as closely as possible. The optimum femoral tunnel opening corresponds closely to the intersection of the roof of the intercondylar notch and the posterior femoral cortex (Fig. 8.13). This allows the graft to maintain constant length and tension during knee motion. A tunnel opening more anteriorly onto the intercondylar roof may potentially predispose to instability. A more posteriorly placed tunnel may result in a posterior femoral cortex fracture. On coronal images or anteroposterior knee radiographs the femoral tunnel should open above the lateral femoral condyle, at 1 o'clock (left knee) and 11 o'clock (right knee). In an attempt to better simulate native ACL biomechanics, control pivot shift and transverse plane rotary movements, a variety of double bundle ACL techniques, reconstructing the anteromedial and posterolateral bundles have been described. These can result in a variable number of femoral and tibial tunnels.

Avoidance of graft impingement is thought to be a more important factor in the outcome of ACL reconstruction than maintaining isometry and is primarily related to correct positioning of the tibial tunnel. Graft impingement initially presents with limitation of knee extension, which may be followed by subsequent graft failure. The tibial tunnel opening is assessed on lateral knee radiographs or sagittal MR images and should be completely located posterior to a line tangential to the intercondylar notch roof (Blummensaat's line) (Fig. 8.14). This relationship is reliant on the knee being extended at the time of imaging as the orientation of Blummensaat's line will be altered with knee flexion [19]. Tibial tunnel position can also be assessed relative to the anteroposterior diameter of the proximal tibia. The ideal position of the centre of the tibial tunnel has been described as 42% of the sagittal distance from the anterior tibial plateau. A tibial tunnel that lies partially or completely anterior to Blummensaat's line or lies 30% of less of the sagittal distance from the anterior tibial plateau is prone to roof impingement during knee extension [29] (Fig. 8.15). In contrast, posterior positioning of the tibial tunnel may predispose to ACL instability. On coronal images or anteroposterior radiographs the tibial tunnel should open onto the intercondylar eminences

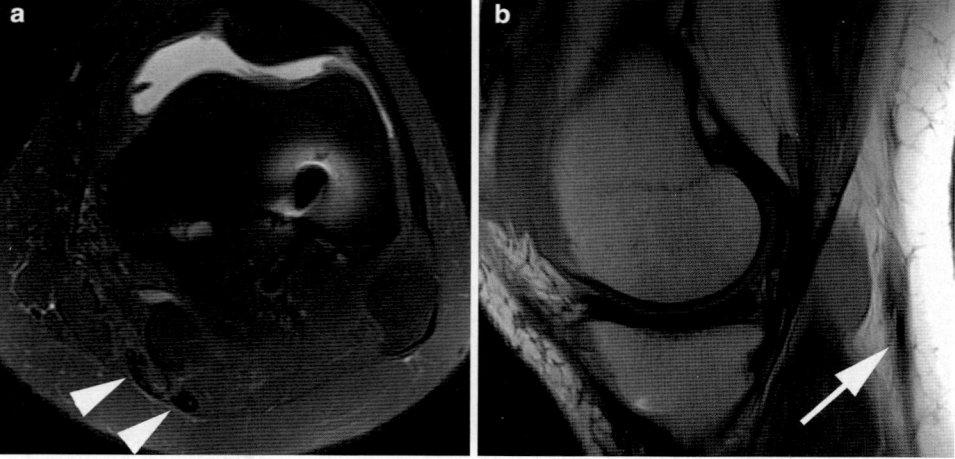

Fig. 8.12 Axial T2 FS MR image (**a**) in a patient with a hamstring ACL graft shows regeneration of the distal gracilis and semitendinosus tendons (*arrowheads*). Sagittal proton-density image (**b**) shows the tendons to be located more posteriorly than normal in the popliteal fossa (*arrow*)

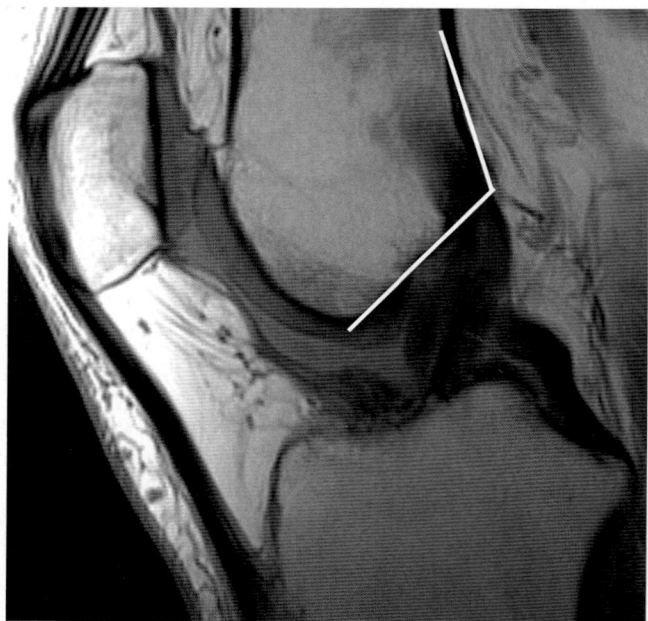

Fig. 8.13 Sagittal proton-density MR image demonstrates the optimal positioning of the femoral tunnel at the junction of the roof of the intercondylar notch and the posterior femoral cortex (*white lines*)

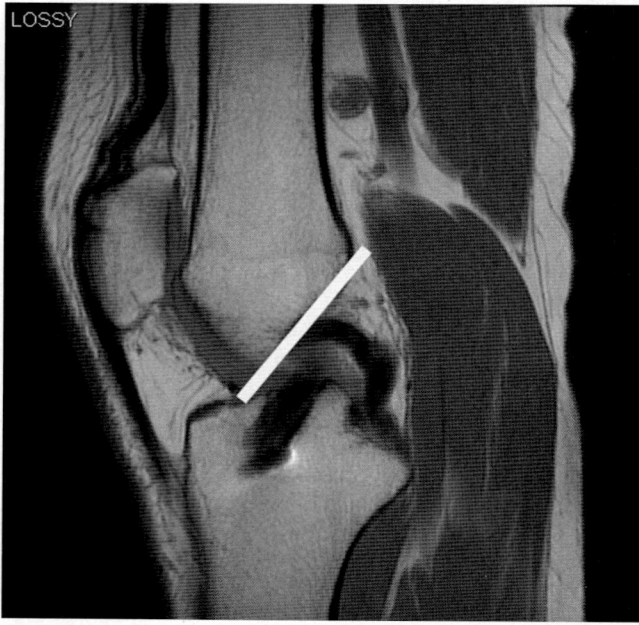

Fig. 8.14 Sagittal proton-density MR image shows the optimal position of the tibial tunnel, lying posterior to a line tangentional to the roof of the intercondylar notch (*white line*)

at 60° to the articular surface. A more vertical graft, exceeding 75°, may result in impingement of the graft onto the PCL during knee flexion, limiting flexion and resulting in high tension and stretching of the graft [30].

In addition to direct visualization of the graft reconstruction tunnels, MRI allows for visualization of the course of an ACL graft, notch osteophytes (Fig. 8.16) and the direct relationship of the ACL graft to the roof and lateral wall of the intercondylar notch. Intra-articular osseous excrescences at the femoral and tibial tunnel openings may also impinge on the graft particularly during knee flexion [19]. In impingement, the graft may be seen to have an angulated course in the region of the distal intercondylar roof resulting in a posterior convexity to the distal graft in contrast to the normal grafts that appear straight with the knee extended. An impinged graft may also exhibit focally increased signal intensity on short TE and T2w images [20, 29] (Fig. 8.17). The graft signal changes with roof impingement may resemble changes seen in the first postoperative year during the "ligamentization" process and therefore additional features such as tunnel

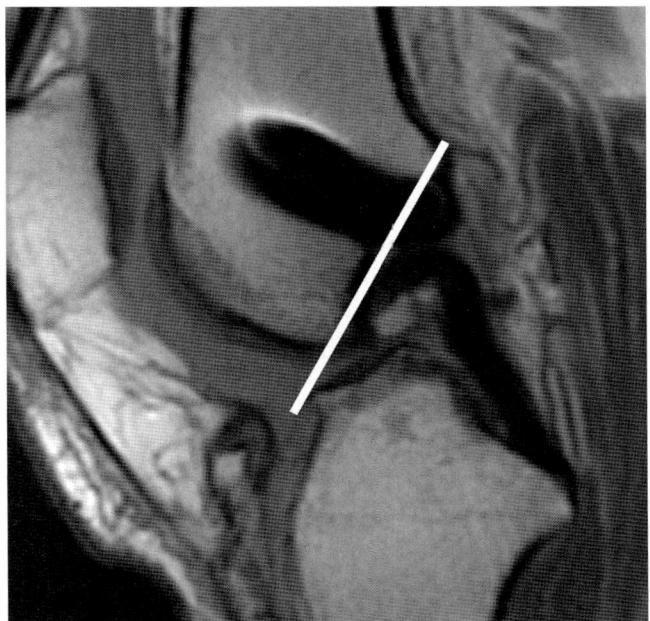

Fig. 8.15 Sagittal proton-density MR image in a patient with a ruptured ACL graft shows the tibial tunnel to lie completely anterior to Blumensaat's line (*white line*)

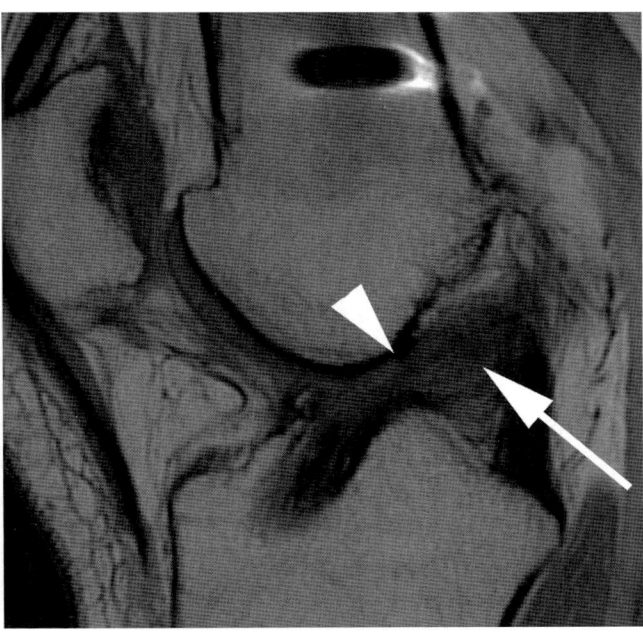

Fig. 8.17 Sagittal proton-density MR image showing ACL graft impingement. The tibial tunnel lies anterior to Blumensaat's line. The graft shows heterogeneous increased signal (*arrow*) and is kinked distally, abutting the roof of the intercondylar notch (*arrowhead*)

In an attempt to prevent impingement some surgeons routinely perform a notchplasty whereby a thin rim of the distal roof and lateral wall of the intercondylar notch are resected. This is manifested on MR imaging as a lateral wall that demonstrates a concave or scalloped contour towards the intercondylar notch (Fig. 8.18). Initially the resected margin may show an indistinct appearance but invariably by 6 months following surgery the margins show linear low signal intensity with recortication and fibrosis [31]. In some instances, however, the fibrotic tissue may hypertrophy and result in mass effect and late impingement on the graft [32].

Loss of knee extension clinically resembling graft impingement may also be seen with localized arthrofibrosis or cyclops lesions [33]. Cyclops lesions may occur in 10% of patients with ACL reconstruction [33] with symptomatic lesions being present in up to 3% of ACL reconstruction patients [34]. Histologically, these nodules are a combination of fibrotic, synovial and osseous tissues [34]. Foci of arthrofibrosis may be entrapped between the distal femur and the proximal tibia, resulting in an inability to gain full extension. MRI has a sensitivity and specificity of 85% for detection of arthrofibrosis [33] demonstrating a soft tissue nodule of low T1 and predominantly low T2 signal intensity typically located within the intercondylar notch anterior to the distal ACL (Fig. 8.19). In a normal postoperative knee joint fluid within the intercondylar notch should extend onto the anterior surface of the graft. In a knee with arthrofibrosis extra tissue is seen between the graft and the joint fluid.

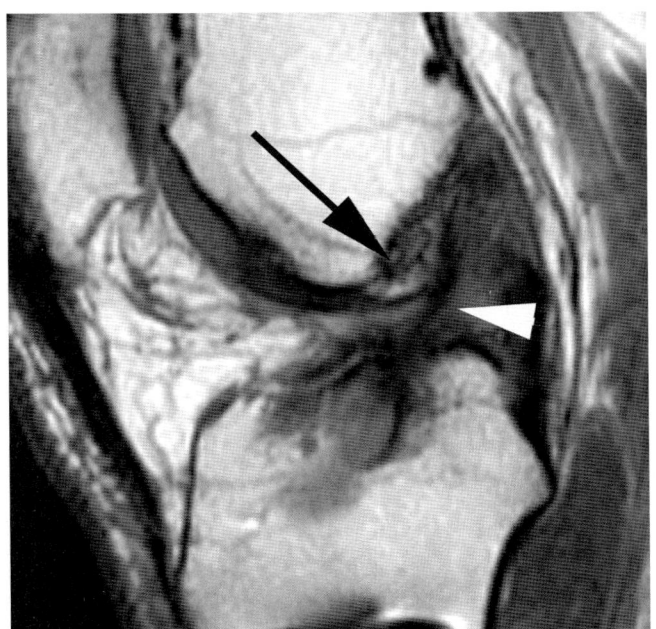

Fig. 8.16 Sagittal proton-density MR image of a patient with clinical graft impingement shows a large notch osteophyte (*arrow*) abutting an attenuated ACL graft (*arrowhead*)

position, graft morphology and swelling, notch morphology as well as the time interval from surgery should be taken into account before attributing signal changes to impingement.

Recurrent instability following ACL graft reconstruction may be related to suboptimal tunnel positioning as discussed above, improper tensioning of the graft, graft failure or stretching. Graft failure may be of insidious onset secondary to graft impingement or of acute onset following recurrent injury. ACL grafts are most prone to recurrent injury during the first few months following surgery when the "ligamentization" process results in structural weakening of the graft. By 12 months after surgery the graft has been shown to have similar biomechanical strength to the native ACL. Complete graft tearing is diagnosed based on demonstration of discontinuity of graft fibres (Fig. 8.20) and extension of fluid into the tear gap on T2w images. The coronal plane is particularly useful for demonstrating graft discontinuity [35]. One study has shown an accuracy of 100% for detection of graft tears with conventional MR imaging [36] whilst another showed a sensitivity of 50% and specificity of 100% for full thickness tears and a sensitivity of 36% and specificity of 80% for all tears [35]. Demonstration of partial thickness tears is particularly problematic on conventional MR imaging with a limited accuracy. Identification of continuous fibres on coronal images has a 100% negative predictive value for discriminating between an intact graft and graft tears (partial and full thickness) [35]. Signs such as extension of fluid into a tear gap and alteration of the thickness of the graft may be seen in cases of complete as well as partial thickness tears whilst altered signal intensity and posterior bowing of the graft may also be seen in asymptomatic cases as well as in those with mechanical impingement. Ancillary signs of ACL insufficiency such as anterior translation of the tibia in relation to the femur greater than 7 mm, buckling of the PCL and uncovering of the posterior horn of the lateral meniscus may also be positive in such cases but are of limited sensitivity although relatively high specificity [35]. Studies using MR arthrography have cited a sensitivity of 100% and specificity of 89–100% for detection of ACL graft tears [37]. Some patients may present with signs and symptoms of ACL instability but with an apparent morphologically intact graft. Instability in such cases may be related to improper tensioning of the graft, progressive graft stretching, or insufficient graft fixation.

A variety of fixation devices have been utilized in ACL reconstruction. These can be divided into direct fixation devices such as interference screws, staples and crosspins or indirect fixation devices, most commonly used with

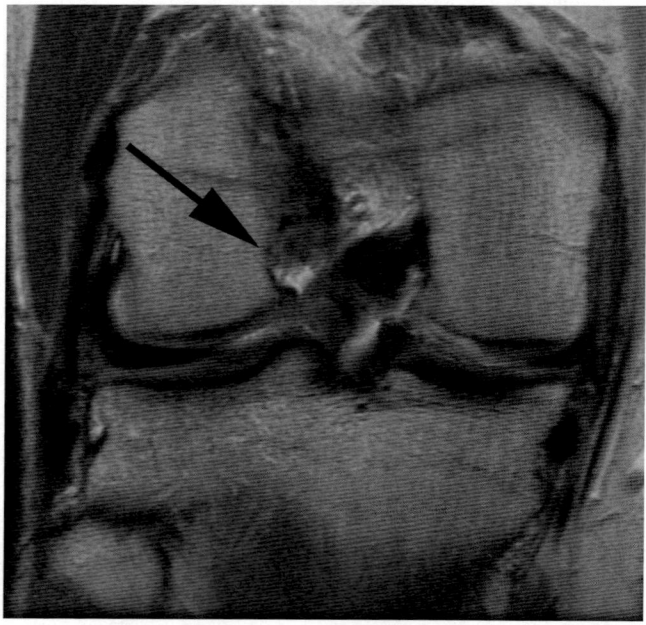

Fig. 8.18 Coronal intermediate-weighted MR image in a patient with previous notchplasty shows characteristic scalloped appearances of the intercondylar notch lateral wall

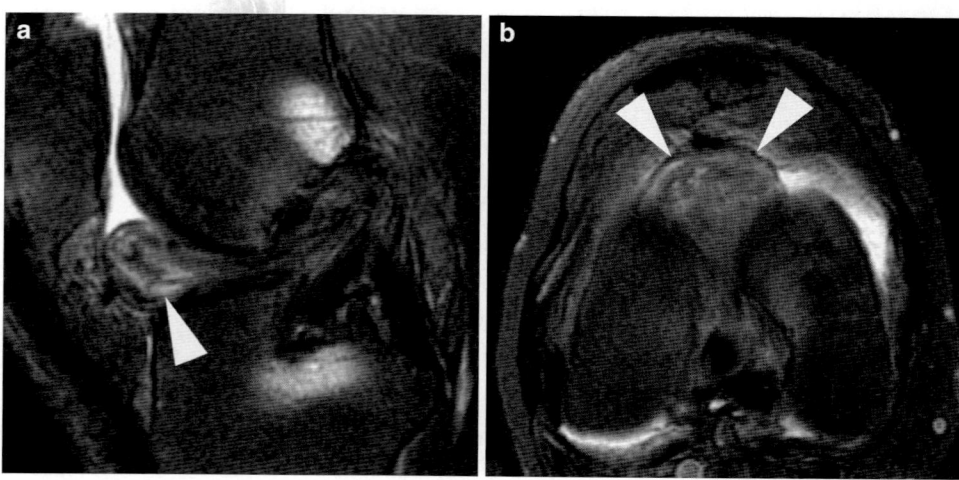

Fig. 8.19 Sagittal (**a**) and axial (**b**) T2 FS MR images in a patient with arthrofibrosis shows heterogeneous, but predominantly low signal cyclops lesion (*arrowheads*)

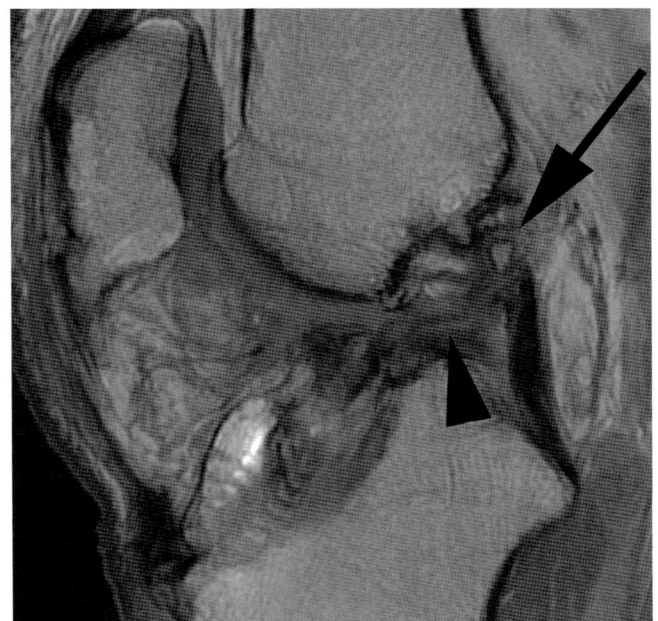

Fig. 8.20 Sagittal proton-density MR image in a patient with ACL graft rupture shows non-visualization of the graft proximally (*arrow*) with an abnormal horizontal course to the distal graft (*arrowhead*)

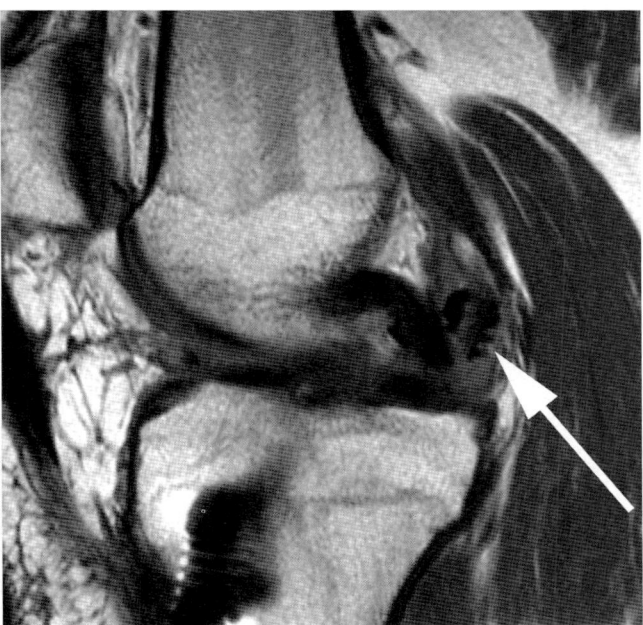

Fig. 8.21 Sagittal proton-density MR image following BPTB ACL reconstruction shows a fractured bioabsorbable interference screw (*arrow*) dislodged from the femoral tunnel

hamstring grafts, such as endobuttons and endopearls. Fixation devices such as interference screws may be metallic or bioabsorbable in nature with the latter having the advantage of limited MR imaging-related artefacts. Potential complications related to fixation hardware include malpositioning of screws or pins causing impingement or fracture, or displacement of screws or crosspins which may result in loss of adequate fixation or mechanical symptoms related to a loose fragment (Fig. 8.21).

A further late complication of ACL grafts, on average occurring 3.5 years after reconstruction, includes development of tunnel or graft ganglion cysts [38]. Ganglion cysts are more commonly encountered with hamstring grafts and endobuttons and may be seen in the setting of cystic degeneration or partial tears of the graft. The tibial tunnel is the most commonly affected site of ganglion cystic change (Fig. 8.22). The ganglion cyst may extend through the intra-articular opening of the tunnel or may extend distally into the subcutaneous tissues, where it may present clinically as a palpable mass. Tunnel ganglion cysts may cause tunnel widening which may lead to graft instability and/or failure. However, the presence of a small amount of fluid within the hamstring graft or the tunnel is normal particularly during the first year postoperatively and of no consequence, typically resolving over time.

Postoperative imaging may also exhibit complications related to the graft donor site, especially with BPTB grafts. Conventional radiography is typically sufficient for the

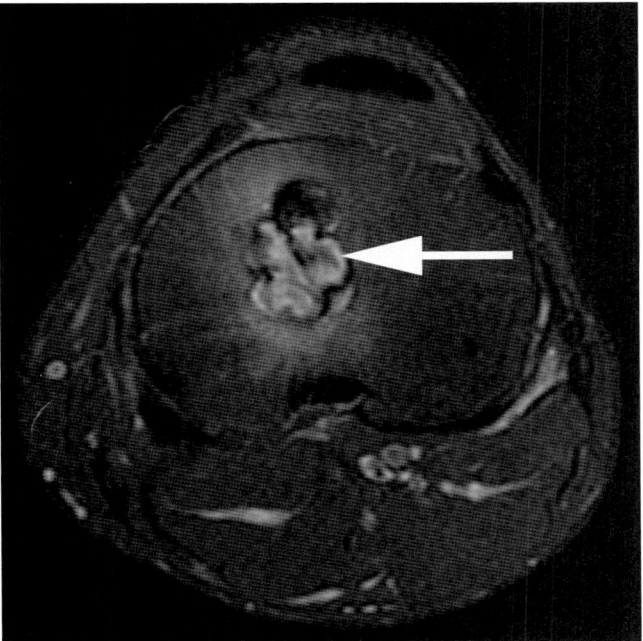

Fig. 8.22 Axial T2 FS MR image through the proximal tibia following ACL reconstruction shows a tibial tunnel with a lobulated contour and fluid signal consistent with a tunnel ganglion cyst (*arrow*)

diagnosis of patellar fractures (Fig. 8.23). Thickening of the patellar tendon beyond 18 months may reflect an inflammatory response [39]. Similarly, patellar tendon ruptures

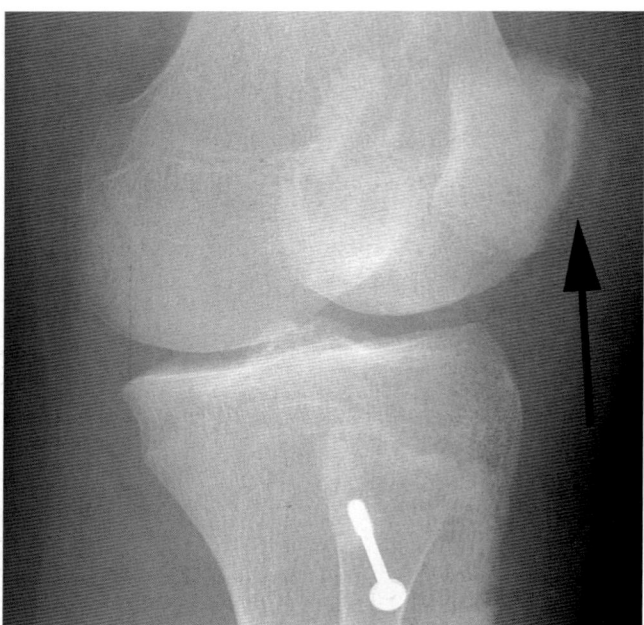

Fig. 8.23 External oblique knee radiograph obtained following BPTB ACL reconstruction demonstrates a patellar fracture (*arrow*)

in comparison with ACL reconstructions. Double bundle techniques have been developed whereby a further femoral tunnel is also placed [41]. Tibial fixation may be achieved either through tibial tunnels or through a tibial inlay technique. The long intraosseous tunnels result in a "killer turn" for the graft to negotiate at the opening onto the posterior tibia, which may cause problems with graft tensioning and ligament failure. With the tibial inlay technique, which is a combined arthroscopic and open procedure, a unicortical window is created in the posterior tibia and a bone plug is placed within the trough and secured with a screw and washer. Choice of graft material for PCL reconstruction includes autograft tissue including BPTB, quadriceps or hamstrings and allograft tissue including tibialis anterior and posterior tendons as well as the Achilles tendon.

Radiological assessment of PCL reconstructions has not been as widely studied as ACL reconstructions. The optimal femoral tunnel position is along the anterior 25% of the roof of the intercondylar notch. More posterior positioning of the femoral tunnel may result in residual instability. The tibial tunnel opening should be situated posteriorly in the midline adjacent to the posterior root of the medial meniscus. With the tunnel technique there is therefore the potential for anterior placement of the tibial tunnel which may result in poor graft function (Fig. 8.24). This problem is eliminated with the tibial inlay technique which are typically

secondary to biomechanical weakening postharvest are equally well demonstrated on ultrasound and MR imaging.

PCL Reconstruction

Athletic injuries account for 40% of PCL injuries, the majority occurring in contact sports [39, 40]. The majority of isolated PCL injuries are low-grade partial tears which may be treated conservatively. However, conservative treatment of high-grade injuries may lead to early degenerative change. Surgery may be considered in individuals with insertional avulsive injury, acute or chronic multiligamentous injuries and in those with isolated PCL injury who have failed rehabilitation and present with pain and instability limiting activity and lifestyle.

As the isometric point of the native PCL footprint is small and the majority of the femoral attachment is non-isometric, the aim of the femoral tunnel placement is to replicate the position of the native PCL attachment rather than replicating the isometric point. The femoral tunnel is typically placed at the 1 o'clock position (right knee) and 11 o'clock (left knee) using interference screw fixation [41]. The PCL consists of two bundles, the stronger anterolateral bundle and smaller posteromedial bundle. Single bundle techniques, which reconstruct the anterolateral bundle, fail to replicate normal PCL biomechanics and have poor results

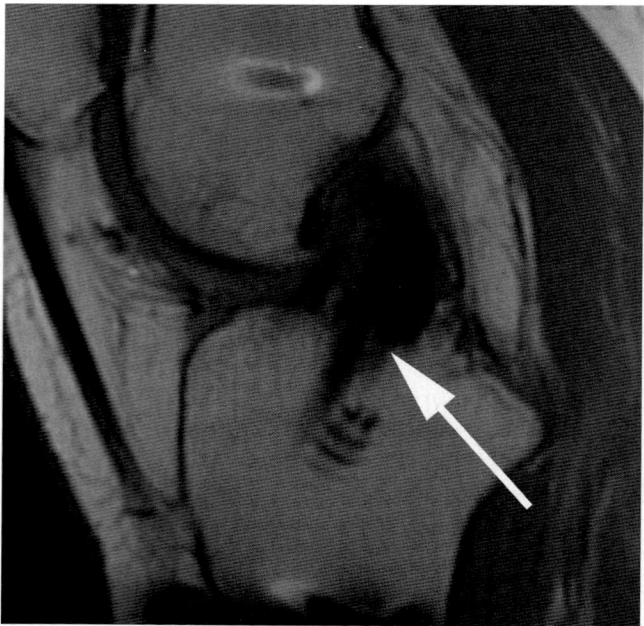

Fig. 8.24 Sagittal proton-density MR image in a patient with residual instability following PCL reconstruction. The tibial tunnel is located too anteriorly (*arrow*)

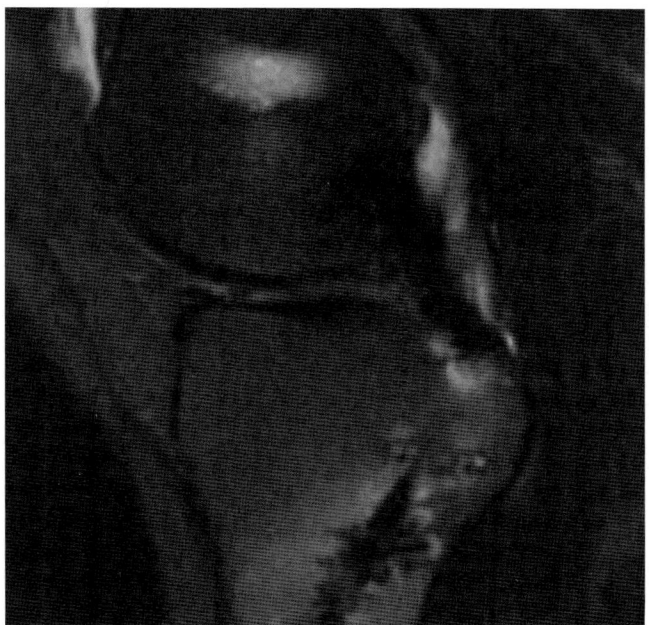 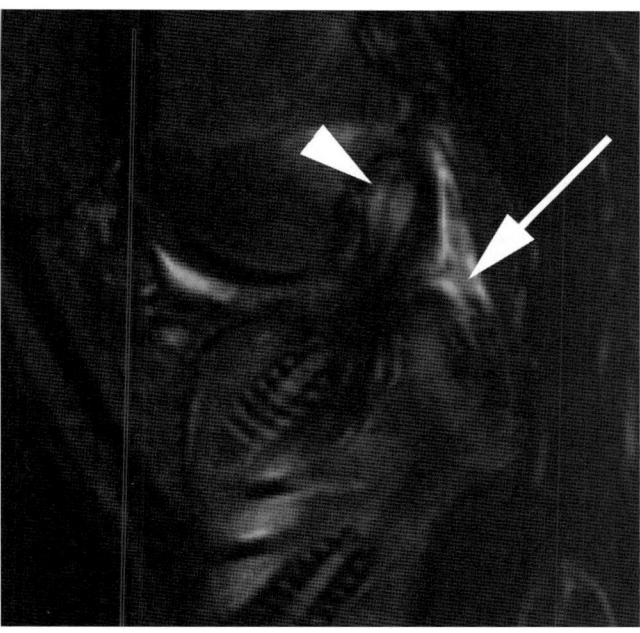

Fig. 8.25 Sagittal T2 FS MR image of a patient with prior PCL reconstruction shows normal PCL graft with diffuse low signal intensity. The tibial tunnel is well located

Fig. 8.26 Sagittal T2 FS MR image of the knee in a patient with multiligamentous reconstruction shows ruptured PCL graft with non-visualization of the graft (*arrow*). The ACL graft shows some expansion and fluid signal proximally (*arrowhead*)

associated with greater MR imaging artefact from fixation screws and staples which may impair visualization of the distal PCL graft.

The normal PCL graft should have uniform low signal on all MRI pulse sequences although it appears to undergo a similar synovialization process to the ACL illustrating inhomogeneity and mild signal change during the first year [42]. On long-term follow-up the graft demonstrates low signal intensity on all pulse sequences (Fig. 8.25). The contour of the normal PCL graft may range from mildly curved to straight. As with ACL reconstruction, graft rupture is manifested by fibre discontinuity and extension of fluid into the gap (Fig. 8.26). Small amounts of fluid signal intensity may be seen extending longitudinally in between the bundles of a hamstring graft without signifying pathology. PCL graft reconstruction may also lead to arthrofibrosis anterior to the graft construct which may be visualized on postoperative MR imaging studies.

Collateral Ligament Repairs

As with PCL injuries, collateral ligament injuries are rarely surgically treated as they are often partial injuries that respond well to non-operative treatment. Even grade III injuries may be treated conservatively. With medial collateral ligament injuries, surgical treatment is reserved for athletes, patients with complete tears causing instability or chronic tears which have failed to respond to conservative treatment. In such instances where surgery is required, the ligament is typically repaired with sutures and staples rather than reconstructed.

With posterolateral corner injuries, early treatment of complete tears is recommended. Within the first 2–3 weeks primary repair may be undertaken but thereafter reconstructive techniques are typically required in those with grade III injuries. Treatment of posterolateral corner injury is especially important in ACL or PCL reconstructions as failure to address posterolateral instability has been recognized as an important cause of reconstruction failure. Primary repair techniques address avulsions with transossoeus tunnels or screw fixation. Repairs may need to be augmented using the iliotibial band or the biceps femoris. Reconstructive techniques in delayed cases may be anatomic or non-anatomic with the former being preferred. Anatomic techniques use semitendinosus autograft or allograft or an Achilles allograft combined with capsular repair or posterolateral capsular shift to reconstruct the popliteus, the fibular collateral and popliteofibular ligaments [43].

MR imaging evaluation of posterolateral corner and medial collateral ligament repairs and reconstructions have not been extensively studied. Screws and staples may result in artefact obscuring the reconstructed ligaments. With ligamentous repairs, the ligaments may initially demonstrate abnormal signal intensity and diffuse thickening. Such thickening invariably persists although the signal intensity diminishes with time.

Imaging Following Cartilage Repair Procedures

As articular hyaline cartilage has a limited healing capacity, a variety of procedures have been developed to treat focal full thickness cartilage injuries. These techniques include simple debridement, marrow stimulation techniques, osteochondral autologous transplantation (OAT), autologous chondrocyte implantation (ACI) and osteochondral allograft fixation. There is no agreement regarding the optimum technique and the choice of technique largely depends on the size and location of the lesion, patient age, whether a prior repair procedure has been attempted and surgeon experience. Any predisposing factors such as instability, presence of meniscal tears and alignment abnormalities also need to be identified preoperatively and addressed either prior to, or concomitant with an attempted cartilage repair procedure.

In our clinical practise, the most commonly implemented sequences for evaluation of articular cartilage pre and postoperatively include fast-spin echo (FSE) intermediate-weighted sequence without fat-suppression, T2w FS images and T1w FS three-dimensional spoiled gradient-echo (SPGR) images. The FSE sequences are advantageous for showing signal abnormalities within articular cartilage and also allow assessment of menisci and ligaments. The three-dimensional SPGR images are typically acquired in the sagittal plane but can be reconstructed in other planes. The technique has the advantage of thinner slices but as gradient-echo acquisition is prone to susceptibility artefact from metal hardware or microscopic metallic debris and is of limited accuracy for assessment of other structures.

Marrow Stimulation

Marrow stimulation techniques refer to a range of procedures including abrasion arthroplasty, subchondral drilling and microfracture. Although the details and technical aspects of these procedures differ, the basic premise is similar with debriding the area of cartilage defect and penetrating the subchondral bone using burrs, drills or picks to cause bleeding and release of pleuripotential stem cells. The ensuing clot differentiates and forms fibrocartilage repair tissue [44]. These techniques are often viewed as a reasonable initial step in treatment of smaller chondral injuries [45]. The main disadvantage of marrow stimulation techniques is that the resultant repair tissue is composed of fibrocartilage, which does not have the same mechanical properties as the native hyaline cartilage.

MR imaging following marrow stimulation techniques typically shows subchondral oedema changes. These diminish over several months, although in symptomatic patients the subchondral changes may progress. The chondral defect fills with an intermediate signal intensity tissue [45] (Fig. 8.27). In the early postoperative period, a 100% fill may not be achieved but by 12 months following surgery the aim is for 100% fill with a smooth articular surface without evidence of flaps or fissures. Imaging correlates of a poor outcome include poor defect fill with cartilage flap tears and fissuring.

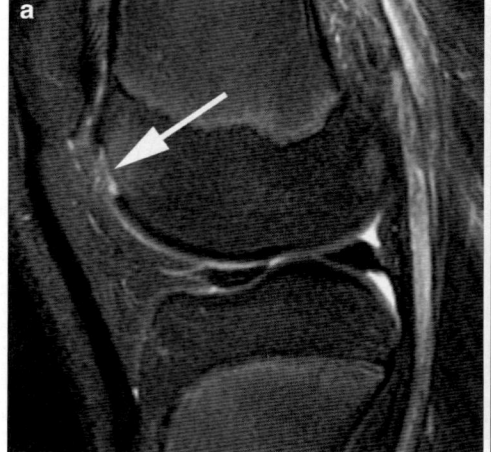
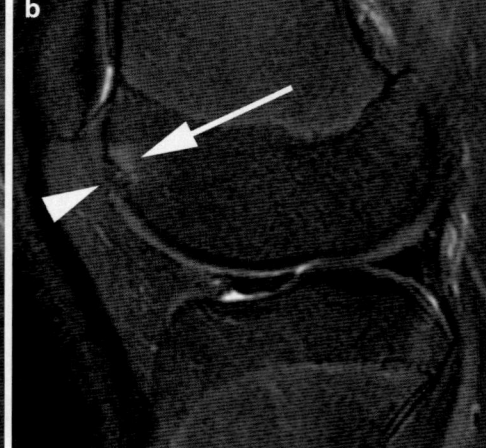

Fig. 8.27 Sagittal T2 FS MR image shows a focal post-traumatic full thickness cartilage defect of the femoral trochlea (*arrow* in **a**). Follow-up MR image (**b**) following microfracture shows filling of the defect with low signal intensity tissue (*arrowhead*). The subchondral bone shows normal postoperative increased T2 signal (*arrow*)

Osteochondral Autologous Transplantation

OAT procedure [46] is a technique whereby one or more cylindrical plugs of subchondral bone and overlying hyaline are harvested from a relatively non-weightbearing area of the joint such as the lateral femoral trochlea (sulcus terminalis or intercondylar region). Following graft harvesting, the site of the osteochondral injury is debrided and tunnels are prepared to receive the harvested osteochondral plugs. Press-fit fixation of the transplanted plugs is utilized without any metal hardware fixation. This technique is most commonly used in the knee where lesions of up to 4 cm² may be treated. The advantage of this technique is that fill of the defect is predominantly hyaline cartilage although the interstices between graft plugs may fill with fibrocartilage.

MR imaging following OAT procedures should be assessed for alignment and orientation of the osteochondral plugs with respect to the host site. On early postoperative MR imaging OAT plugs and the host bone around the osteochondral plugs typically show oedema-like changes, which gradually resolve as the plugs are incorporated into the host bone. Bony incorporation should be visible by 6–9 months and the oedema-like changes typically resolve by 12 months. Persistence of the oedema, development of cysts and cavities may be seen in the setting of poor graft incorporation, and more commonly with proudly positioned graft transplants. The donor site, which is typically located within the same joint, can also be assessed on MRI. The osseous defect initially demonstrates low T1 and high T2 signal intensity before filling with cancellous bone and marrow fat, while the overlying harvest site chondral defect typically fills with fibrocartilage. The plugs should be placed perpendicular to the articular surface with the aim of achieving a congruent surface (Fig. 8.28). As the articular cartilage from the harvest site is typically thinner than the articular cartilage of the host site, the subchondral bone of the plugs may be proud relative to subchondral bone of the host bone but with a congruent cartilaginous articular surface being maintained. Osteochondral plugs which are proud or recessed in relation to the adjacent host cartilage at MRI may be related to technical factors such as under-drilling or over-drilling of the transplantation site at the time of surgery and result in a poorer outcome with more rapid wear of the graft transplant articular cartilage. A normally positioned plug may also undergo subsidence and result in plug recession. Flap tears and articular cartilage fissures represent a poor outcome (Fig. 8.29).

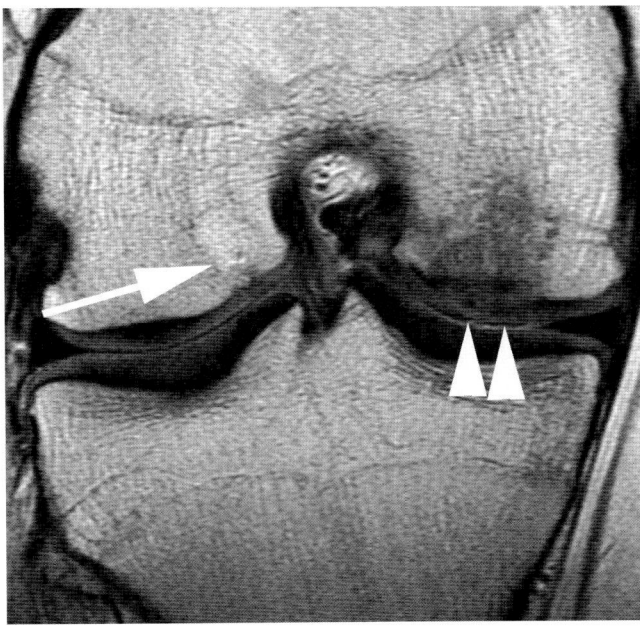

Fig. 8.28 Coronal intermediate-weighted MR image shows a congruent medial femoral condyle articular surface following OAT (*arrowheads*). A barely discernable donor site has filled with fatty marrow (*arrow*) with overlying cartilage fill

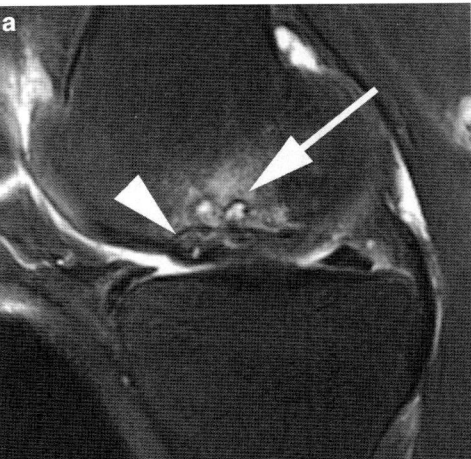 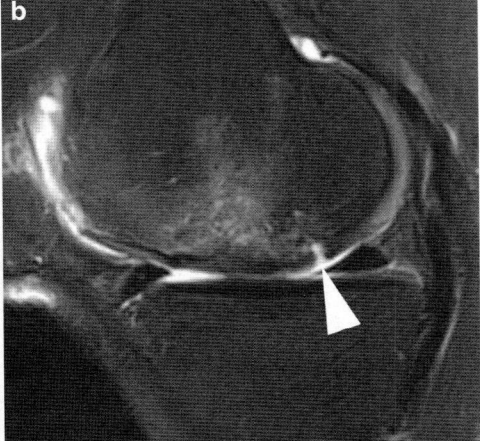

Fig. 8.29 Sagittal T2 FS MR images (**a** and **b**) shows medial femoral condyle mosaicplasty with fluid cleft deep to the articular cartilage (*arrowhead* in **a**) and full thickness fissure posteriorly (*arrowhead* in **b**). There is subchondral cystic change and oedema (*arrow* in **a**)

Autologous Chondrocyte Implantation

ACI is a two-stage repair process usually reserved for treatment of larger full thickness osteochondral defects in excess of 3 cm². During the first stage a biopsy sample of normal articular cartilage is obtained arthroscopically. Cartilage cells from the sample are grown in culture over 4–6 weeks. During the second stage an arthrotomy is performed and the cartilage defect is debrided. An autologous periosteal patch or a bovine cartilage membrane is then sown over the defect. The cultured cells are then injected deep to the patch or membrane [47]. The suspension undergoes proliferation and expansion over the subsequent months. By 6 months the graft begins remodelling and this may continue over 1–2 years. The advantage of the ACI technique is an articular surface consisting of hyaline cartilage but drawbacks include the two-stage nature of the procedure and the long rehabilitation period.

The aim of the procedure is to achieve 100% fill of the previous defect and this should be visible in the first postoperative month [48]. Postoperative assessment of ACI procedures with MRI may be used to assess the defect fill, graft integration and complications such as graft delamination and hypertrophy. MR imaging is capable of demonstrating defect underfilling as areas of generalized or focal thinning. The signal intensity of the graft varies with time. Initially, it has a heterogeneous appearance and may demonstrate fluid signal intensity on T2w images with significant enhancement following intravenous gadolinium. With progressive maturation signal characteristics more closely resemble normal hyaline cartilage and the degree of heterogeneity and enhancement diminishes [48]. The junction between the graft and the native articular cartilage should appear smooth, with the interface poorly visualized or demonstrating a variable degree of linear high T2-signal intensity.

Delamination is a complication of ACI typically seen in the first 6 months whereby there is poor integration of the graft to the underlying bone or the adjacent native cartilage. This is manifested on MR imaging as a linear cleft of fluid signal intensity at the interface of the graft and the adjacent cartilage. Distinguishing features of a delaminating cleft and the normal high signal intensity linear interface include the non-perpendicular nature of the delaminating cleft and extension of the cleft deep to the graft. Indirect MR arthrography may also be helpful in distinguishing between a normal interface and a fissure [45]. Another complication is catching due to hypertrophy of the ACI periosteal, which may occur in up to 26% of patients, typically between the 3rd and 9th months postoperatively. MR imaging demonstrates a graft that is thicker than the adjacent native cartilage and may form a flap over the native cartilage.

Osteochondral Allograft Transplantation

Osteochondral allograft transplantation, utilizing fresh cadaveric grafts, is typically reserved for larger lesions involving articular cartilage and underlying subchondral bone, lesions not suitable for other procedures or which have failed other techniques. The grafts may be fixed with screws or a press-fit technique. Osteochondral allograft signal intensity differs from the host marrow on the initial postoperative examinations but should gradually return to normal. Progression of the marrow signal changes and at the interface may herald poor incorporation and rejection [45]. MR imaging may be used to assess congruency of the graft with the adjacent articular surface (Fig. 8.30). However, the MR appearance of cartilage loss does not appear to correlate with patient symptoms.

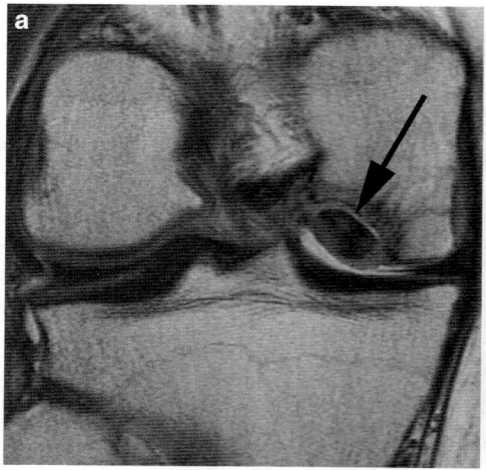
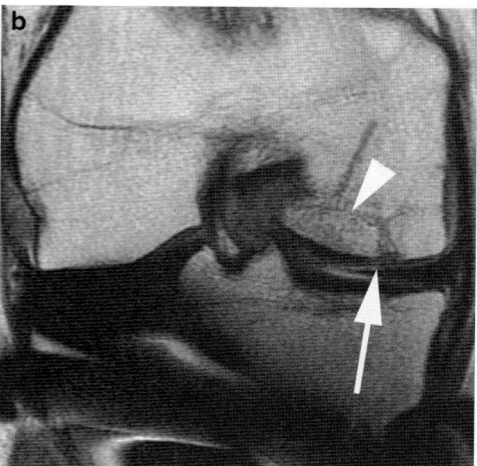

Fig. 8.30 Coronal intermediate-weighted knee MR image (**a**) shows a large unstable medial femoral condyle osteochondral lesion and fluid cleft deep to the lesion (*black arrow*). Postoperative image (**b**) following a press-fit bulk osteochondral allograft shows good graft positioning with congruent cartilage surface (*white arrow*) and normal osseous interface with host bone (*arrowhead*). Artefact is seen from stabilization hardware following an opening wedge tibial osteotomy

Imaging of the Postoperative Shoulder

The utility of MR imaging and MR arthrography are well established in assessment of rotator cuff disease and labral pathology. Morphological alterations, which may be considered as pathological in the virgin shoulder, can be a normal finding following surgery and familiarity with normal postoperative appearances and common surgical techniques are essential. The most common procedures in the shoulder include subacromial decompression, rotator cuff repair and instability surgery.

Subacromial Decompression

Subacromial decompression comprises a series of procedures which include subacromial subdeltoid bursal debridement, partial coracoacromial ligament release or debridement, removal of inferior osteophytes and spurs and flattening of the morphology of the undersurface of the acromion. Subacromial decompression may be combined with distal clavicular resection (Mumford procedure) (Fig. 8.31) or rotator cuff repair, and may be performed as an open technique or arthroscopically. The open procedure involves splitting the deltoid and is commonly performed as part of an open rotator cuff repair.

Postoperative imaging assessment of subacromial decompression typically consists of conventional radiographs, including an outlet view, and MR images. On MR imaging identification of numerous small foci of susceptibility artefact in the subacromial region, best appreciated on gradient-echo images, is a clue to a prior acromioplasty. These are not typically visible on plain radiographs. Conventional radiographs and MR images demonstrate flattening of the undersurface of the anterior acromion and shortening of the acromion with non-visualization of the anterior third (Fig. 8.32). Oedema or marrow fibrosis may be seen along the anterior acromion on MR imaging. If a Mumford procedure has also been performed, widening of the acromioclavicular joint is best appreciated on axial images with the acromioclavicular distance measuring in excess of 1 cm. Oedema, scar tissue and fluid in the subacromial space and into the acromioclavicular interval is also a common finding following subacromial decompression which may not be related to patient symptoms [49, 50] (Fig. 8.33).

Symptoms following subacromial decompression may be evident in up to 20% of patients and have a variety of aetiologies [51]. These include an incorrect initial diagnosis, technical factors during surgery or a complication of surgery [51]. Missed diagnoses include primary shoulder instability, rotator cuff tears, glenohumeral or acromioclavicular arthritis, symptomatic os acromiale or cervical radiculopathy and should be evaluated for on postoperative imaging. Under-resection of the undersurface of the acromion with a residual spur may be seen in up to 50% of cases of treatment failure [51]. The recurrence rate appears to be higher after arthroscopic subacromial decompression. In particular, a residual medial spur is commonly seen after subacromial decompression in patients with a preoperative laterally downsloping acromion. Other postoperative complications include acromial fracture due to over-resection, heterotopic ossification, arthrofibrosis and recurrent subacromial spur formation. Distinguishing a residual spur from a recurrent one is not always possible however, and variable results with evaluation of residual impingement using MR imaging with the visualization of a subacromial spur and indentation of supraspinatus resulting in sensitivities ranging from 64 to 84% and specificities of 82–87% [52, 53].

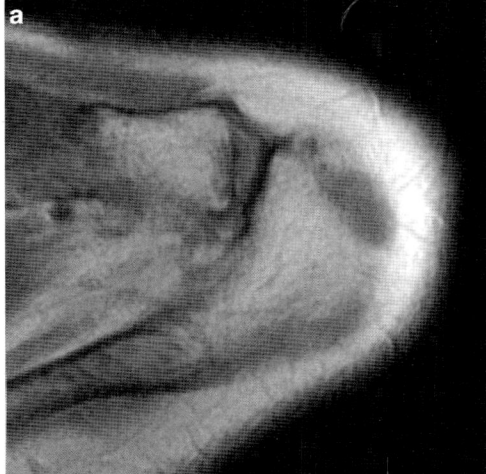
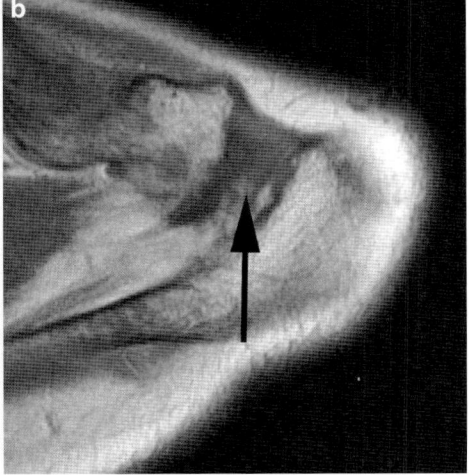

Fig. 8.31 Preoperative (**a**) and postoperative (**b**) axial intermediate-weighted shoulder MR image shows widening of the acromioclavicular joint (*arrow*) following a Mumford procedure

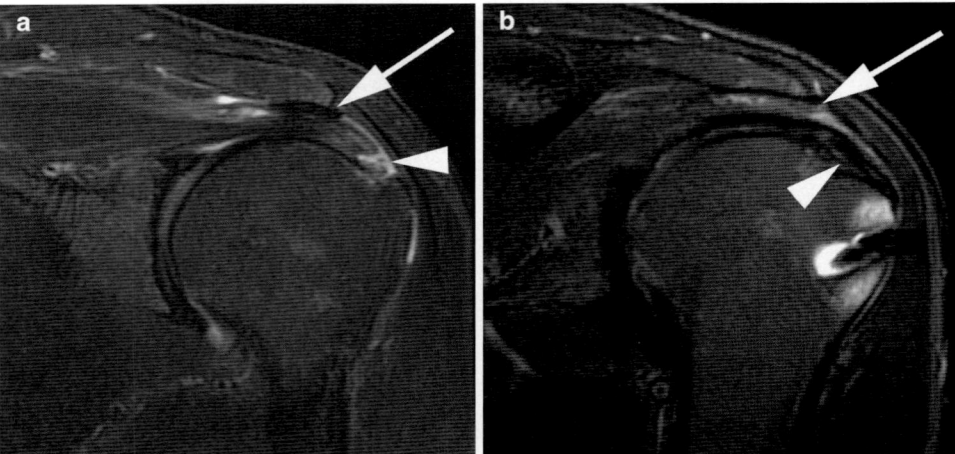

Fig. 8.32 Coronal oblique T2 FS preoperative shoulder MR image (**a**) shows a near full thickness insertional supraspinatus tear (*arrowhead*) and large subacromial enthesophyte (*arrow*). Postoperative image (**b**) shows repair of the rotator cuff tear (*arrowhead*) and acromioplasty with resection of the enthesophyte and undersurface of the acromion (*arrow*)

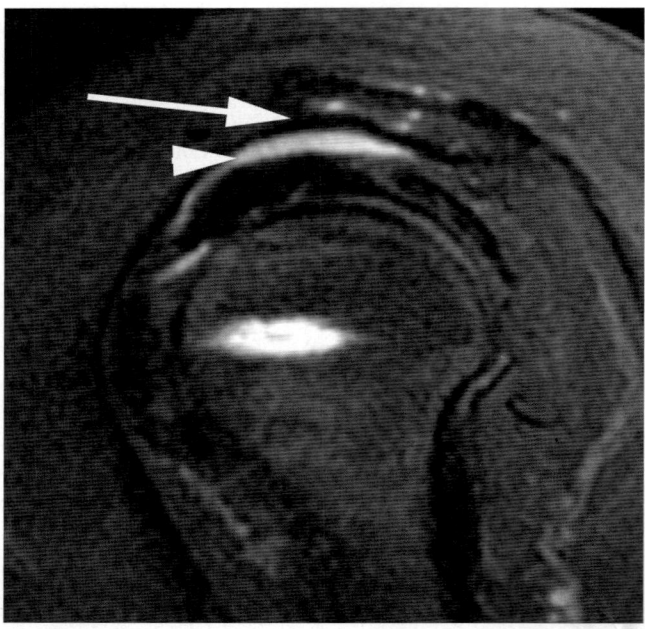

Fig. 8.33 Sagittal oblique T2 FS shoulder MR image following acromioplasty shows flattening of the undersurface of the anterior acromion (*arrow*) with a moderate amount of subacromial fluid (*arrowhead*)

Imaging of the Postoperative Rotator Cuff

Symptomatic low grade partial tears may be debrided whereas partial tears affecting more than half to two-thirds of tendon thickness may be excised and repaired as a full thickness tear. The cuff can be repaired using a side-to-side suturing technique or a tendon-to-bone fixation technique, and can be performed as an open procedure, arthroscopically or as a mini-open procedure. The goal for all techniques is anatomical fixation of the rotator cuff to a bony bed without tension.

Fixation techniques include transossoeus sutures and metallic or bioabsorbable suture anchors or screws. Open techniques have good long-term results, allow direct visualization of the cuff repair and greater access for mobilization of the tendons to produce a tension-free repair. As such, open procedures are often preferable for treatment of large tears. Open technique access is reliant on detachment of the deltoid from the acromion and subsequent suturing of the deltoid back into anatomic position and may be a confounding source of postoperative morbidity.

Arthroscopic repair of rotator cuff tears is widely practised. Advantages include smaller surgical scar, visualization of intra-articular pathology and faster postoperative rehabilitation. The mini-open procedure which combines arthroscopy with a small split between the anterior and lateral heads of the deltoid has many of the advantages of open and arthroscopic repairs.

Pain relief is seen in approximately 90% of patients following rotator cuff repair but over time up to 26% of patients may experience recurrent symptoms. Potential sources of symptoms following repair include residual subacromial impingement, residual or recurrent rotator cuff tears, adhesions and deltoid detachment. A recurrent rotator cuff tear is the most common cause for recurrent pain.

Postoperative MR imaging may show suture artefact in the repaired tendon as well as at the osseous fixation site due to metallic anchors. The humeral head may be mildly superiorly subluxed on conventional radiographs with reduction in the acromiohumeral distance as a result of a combination of resection of the subacromial subdeltoid bursa and capsular tightening [54]. Conventional radiographs are useful for assessing alignment, detecting displacement of metallic suture anchors and other causes of shoulder pain such as acromioclavicular joint degeneration.

Postoperative tendon appearances can be highly variable with less than 10% of asymptomatic cuff repairs meet the normal signal and morphological characteristics of a virgin tendon [49]. Asymptomatic tendon repairs may demonstrate mildly increased signal intensity on intermediate and T2w imaging in about 50% of patients [49]. This is likely due to a combination of suture artefact and granulation tissue. Generalized reduction in tendon thickness and irregularity can also be seen as a normal postoperative finding. In symptomatic patients, comparing MR imaging with arthroscopy, MR imaging has a sensitivity of 84–86% and specificity of 91–92% for detection of full thickness tears using conventional diagnostic criteria of fluid signal extending from the articular surface to the bursal surface or non-visualization of the tendon (Figs. 8.34 and 8.35). Identification of partial tears is highly variable however. A sensitivity and specificity of 83% was observed in two studies whereas a further study was unable to distinguish partial tears from normal postoperative change [52, 53, 55]. However, partial and full thickness tears are also commonly encountered in repaired tendons in asymptomatic patients. Further complicating the diagnostic evaluation is the observation that tears of the rotator cuff in the postoperative setting may demonstrate low signal intensity on intermediate and T2w sequences due to chronic granulation tissue interposed at the tear defect.

MR arthrography may be useful for detection and evaluation of postoperative tears and in particular partial thickness articular-sided tears. In one investigation, MR arthrography had a sensitivity of 86–90% for full thickness tears of supraspinatus with a specificity of 59–89%. The performance for partial thickness tears was only moderate [56] (Fig. 8.36). However, there are several difficulties in using MR arthrography for evaluation of postoperative tears. Water-tightness is

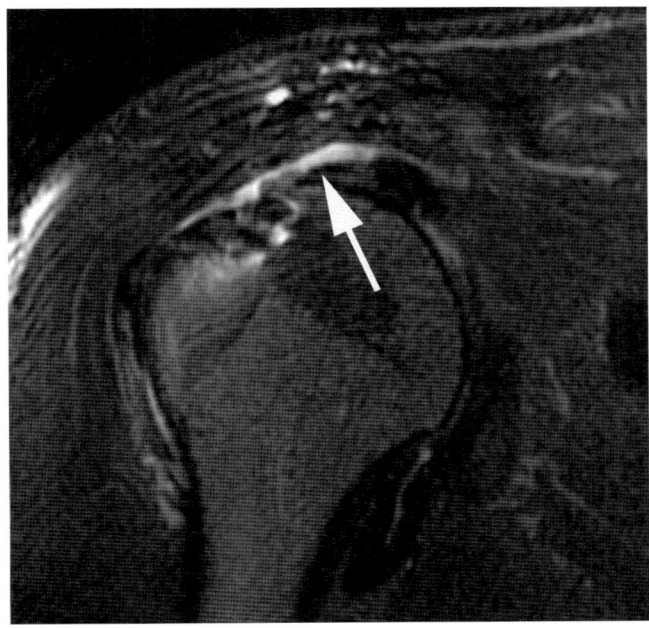

Fig. 8.35 Coronal oblique T2 FS MR image in a patient with previous rotator cuff repair and recurrent symptoms shows complete rupture of the tendon (*arrow*)

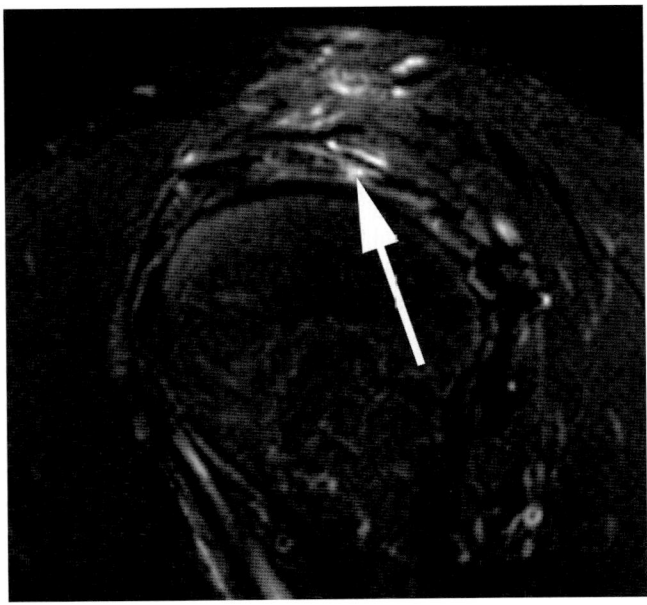

Fig. 8.34 Sagittal oblique T2 FS shoulder MR image following rotator cuff repair in a patient with recurrent symptoms shows a small full thickness defect (*arrow*)

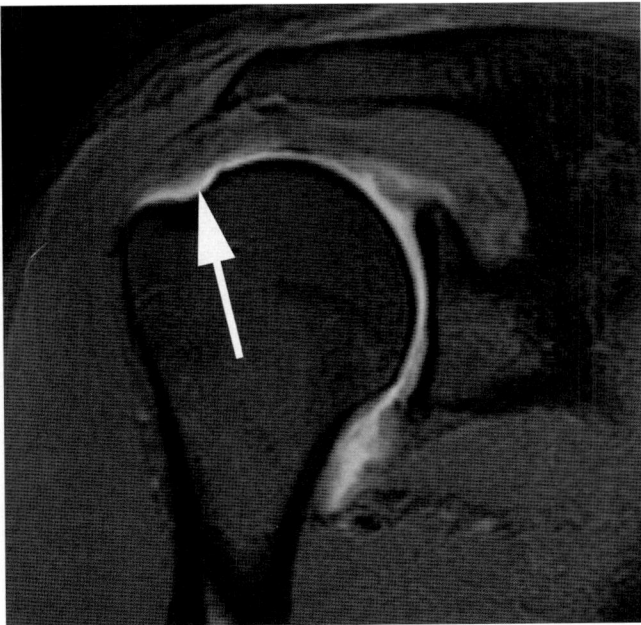

Fig. 8.36 Coronal oblique T1 FS MR arthrographic image following rotator cuff repair shows a high-grade articular supraspinatus tear at its insertion (*arrow*)

not a requirement of successful rotator cuff surgery and as a consequence gadolinium leakage into the subacromial space may be witnessed in functionally normal and asymptomatic repairs [57] (Fig. 8.37). Conversely, intra-articular gadolinium may not extend into the subacromial space despite a full thickness tear. This is typically seen when there is granulation tissue filling the tear gap. It is therefore clear that when assessing potential recurrent tears of the rotator cuff, morphological changes and classic criteria for evaluation of tears can be misleading and close correlation with clinical symptoms and examination is mandatory. The most specific sign of a recurrent tear is that of non-visualization of part of the tendon. Specifically, the size of the defect appears to correlate most closely with patient symptoms. Symptomatic tears or defects are more likely to exceed 11 mm in their largest dimension whereas those with asymptomatic tears and better functional outcome tend to have smaller defects [50]. Use of secondary signs such as fatty atrophy of the muscle belly may also be useful particularly if preoperative or early postoperative examinations are available for comparison.

Ultrasound has potential advantages in imaging of the postoperative rotator cuff due to its dynamic nature and lack of artefact from fixation hardware. Ultrasound has a similar utility to MR imaging in detection of recurrent full thickness tears with a sensitivity of 91%, specificity of 86% and accuracy of 89% in a symptomatic population [58]. A full thickness tear is diagnosed on the basis of non-visualization of the cuff or a defect within the cuff, and a partial thickness tear is considered in the presence of a hypoechoic or mixed echogenicity partial defect seen in two imaging planes. A thinned cuff or mild concavity is considered a normal postoperative finding.

Postoperative imaging may also detect other complications including deltoid dehiscence where there is failure of fixation of the deltoid onto the acromion following an open rotator cuff repair. MR imaging is sensitive and specific for detection of deltoid detachment, may show discontinuity and gap at the site of origin of the deltoid from the acromion with or without associated muscle retraction [53].

Imaging Following Instability Surgery and Labral Repair

Patients with shoulder instability may be treated surgically or conservatively depending on the patient demographics, predisposing factors and the underlying pathological lesion. Surgical treatment of anterior instability is more commonly preformed following traumatic dislocation and can be divided into anatomical and non-anatomical repairs.

Anatomic repairs aim to address the underlying instability lesion, namely the torn capsulolabral complex (Bankart lesion or Bankart variant), without altering the anatomy. With anatomic or Bankart repairs, the anteroinferior labrum is reattached to the glenoid to provide passive constraint of the articulation. Fixation may be achieved using suture anchors, tacks or sutures placed through drill holes, typically from 3 to 5 o'clock. Recurrent symptoms may be evident in up to 10% of patients with open repairs and up to 20% of those who have undergone an arthroscopic procedure. Many surgeons also perform a capsular shift procedure at the same time. Inferior capsular shift is also used in treatment of atraumatic multidirectional instability. This involves a T-shaped incision in the capsule followed by advancement of superior and inferior components of the capsule such that they overlap and result in reinforcement of the inferior capsulolabroligamentous complex.

Direct anatomic labral repairs may also be performed for superior labral anterior posterior (SLAP) tears. While some forms of SLAP tears may be treated with debridement, more advanced lesions, particularly those involving the biceps anchor and causing instability (SLAP 2 and 4), may be repaired using either sutures, anchors or tacks in the superior and posterosuperior glenoid.

Non-anatomic repairs for anterior instability are now rarely performed, unless there has been failed anatomic repair or there is significant glenoid bone loss, as they do not address the underlying lesion and are associated with shoulder function limitation. These procedures can be broadly categorized into those aimed at tightening the subscapularis (Putti–Platt or Magnusson–Stack) and those which aim to prevent anterior displacement of the humeral head by creating

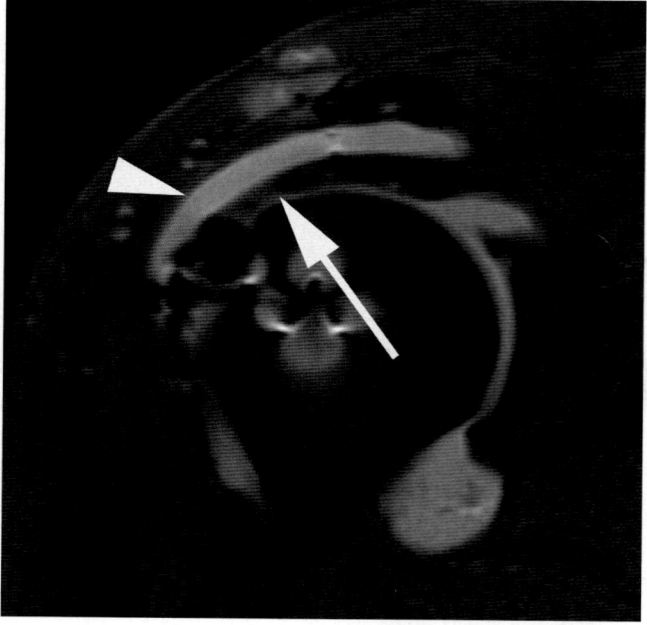

Fig. 8.37 Coronal oblique T1 FS MR arthrogram shows an intact rotator cuff (*arrow*). However, gadolinium is seen in the subacromial bursa (*arrowhead*) suggesting the cuff repair is not watertight

a bony block (bone block osteotomy, Bristow–Helfet or Laterjet procedures).

The Putti–Platt procedure involves incising the subscapularis tendon vertically and advancing the medial stump to the lesser tuberosity and suturing the lateral stump to the soft-tissue of the anterior glenoid cavity thereby effectively tightening the subscapularis and anterior capsule. The Magnusson–Stack procedure has a similar effect and involves releasing the subscapularis tendon and transferring it across the bicipital groove onto the greater tuberosity. These procedures limit external rotation of the humerus but may predispose to posterior subluxation and glenohumeral arthritis. Imaging following non-anatomical soft tissue procedures such as the Putti–Platt and Magnusson–Stack will show internal rotation of the arm, thickening of the subscapularis tendon and a possible persistent labral abnormality. Complications related to overtightening may also be evident with posterior subluxation of the humeral head and glenohumeral osteoarthritis particularly affecting the posterior aspect of the joint (Fig. 8.38).

A variety of bone block osteotomies have been described which utilize bone graft material to reinforce the anterior glenoid and prevent anterior dislocation. Scar tissue, which may also have a role in achieving stability, may be seen anterior to the bone graft on MRI. The Bristow–Helfet and Laterjet techniques involve an osteotomy of the coracoid process distal to the insertion of pectoralis minor and transferring the coracoid tip, including the conjoint tendons of short head of biceps and coracobrachialis, onto the anterior glenoid neck more inferiorly (Fig. 8.39). In the Bristow–Helfet procedure the base of coracoid tip is placed onto the anterior glenoid neck through a slit in subscapularis with the conjoint tendon sutured into the subscapularis. In the Laterjet procedure, the coracoid is laid flat along the anterior glenoid rim and fixed with screws. The main complications of these procedures are the risk of non-union and displacement or migration of the bone block.

Conventional radiography, CT, MR imaging and MR arthrography all have a role in the postoperative evaluation of instability surgery. Conventional radiographs are useful for determining the overall alignment at the glenohumeral joint as well as assessing hardware position. An important

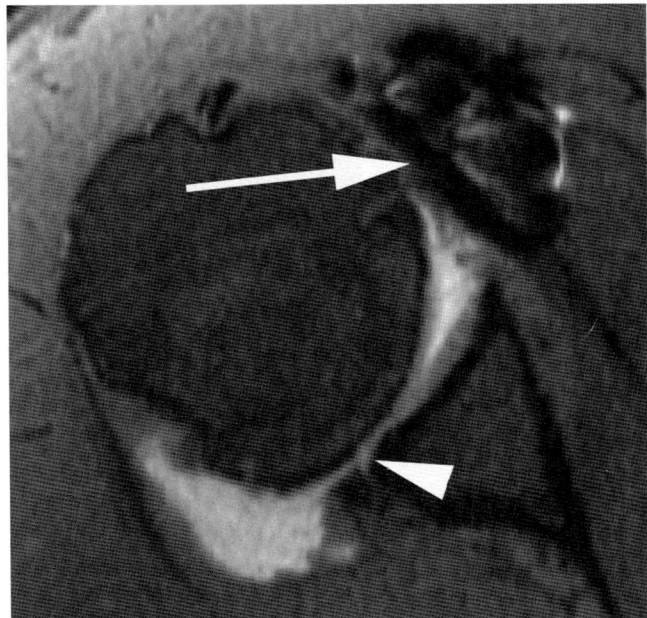

Fig. 8.38 Axial T1 FS MR arthrogram of the shoulder in a patient with prior Putti–Platt procedure shows susceptibility artefact and thickening in the region of the subscapularis (*arrow*). In addition, there is degenerative change and labral tearing posteriorly (*arrowhead*) with posterior subluxation of the humeral head

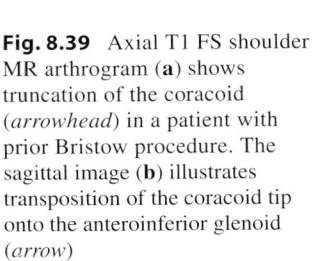

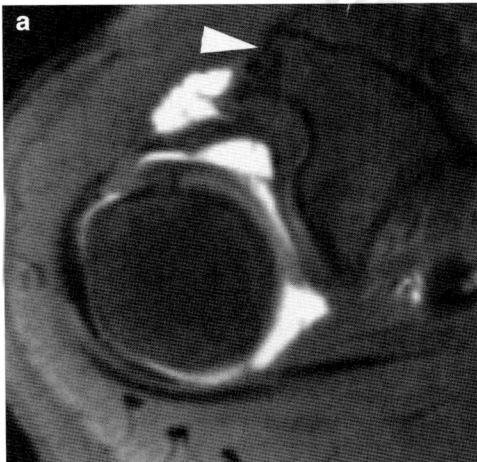

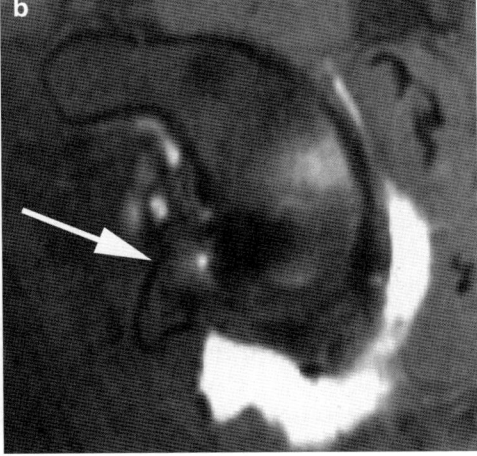

Fig. 8.39 Axial T1 FS shoulder MR arthrogram (**a**) shows truncation of the coracoid (*arrowhead*) in a patient with prior Bristow procedure. The sagittal image (**b**) illustrates transposition of the coracoid tip onto the anteroinferior glenoid (*arrow*)

cause of failed instability surgery is an osseous defect of the glenoid and CT is ideal for assessment of the size of a possible bony Bankart. CT also has a role in evaluation of non-anatomical repairs utilizing bone block osteotomy to evaluate the degree of incorporation of the osteotomy and any potential displacement. Artefact from metal hardware is typically less with CT it may be used to determine the degree of displacement of fixation hardware and the exact relationship of the hardware to the articular surfaces of the joint.

Postoperative imaging evaluation of the labrum principally involves MR imaging and MR arthrography. Artefacts from metallic anchors and screws used in anatomic and non-anatomic repairs may limit visualization of the capsule and labrum on MR imaging. The subscapularis tendon may also appear thickened in cases where an open repair has been undertaken. Normal postoperative labral morphology and signal intensity may be highly variable after direct repair. The labrum may be rounded, truncated or irregular and may be of heterogeneous signal intensity on short TE and T2 sequences [54]. Therefore, labral assessment simply based on morphology and global signal change can be misleading in evaluation of potential recurrent tears. Features suggesting a recurrent tear include the presence of a tear cleft outlined by fluid or gadolinium. As opposed to the situation in the rotator cuff, whereby the repair is not expected to be watertight, the postoperative labrum should be firmly adherent to the glenoid without evidence of clefts through the substance or the base of the labrum.

Injection of intra-articular gadolinium may help in better identifying and delineating a recurrent tear cleft. A further indication of postoperative labral tearing and potential treatment failure is displacement of labral and repair tissue from its expected location along the glenoid rim. In such instance, the labral tissue usually displaces anteriorly or medially (Fig. 8.40). Labral shape and position may be partly influenced by the position of the arm with a medial overhang on internal rotation and an increase in height of the labrum on external rotation [59]. MR arthrography in ABER (Abduction External Rotation) position may also be helpful in assessing the integrity of the Bankart repair. With ABER positioning tension placed on the anterior band of the inferior glenohumeral ligament may cause displacement of an apparently intact labrum and may serve to highlight capsular stripping anteroinferiorly. Using a diagnostic criterion of displaced labral/repair tissue, gadolinium outlined tear cleft and absence, truncation or fragmentation of the labrum as indicative of a recurrent tear, MR arthrography has a sensitivity, specificity and accuracy of 100, 85 and 91.9%, respectively, for identification of anteroinferior labral tears. The corresponding figures for recurrent SLAP tears are 93.8, 85.7 and 89.2% [60]. However, a potential false-negative finding at MR arthrography is the presence of granulation tissue in a tear which prevents imbibition of gadolinium into the tear [54]. Such lesions may be unstable to probing at arthroscopy.

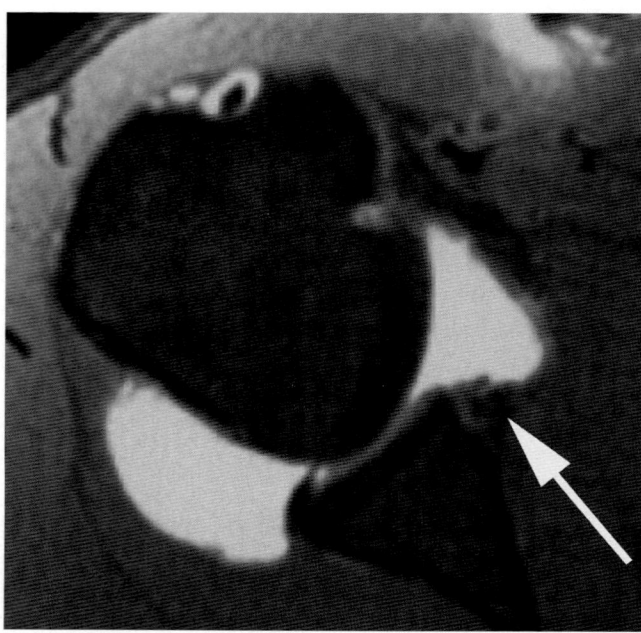

Fig. 8.40 Axial T1 FS shoulder MR arthrogram in a patient with previous Bankart repair and recurrent instability symptoms. There is a recurrent tear of the anteroinferior labrum with anterior and medial displacement of the labrum (*arrow*)

Identification of granulation tissue may be aided by using indirect MR arthrography with administration of intravenous gadolinium, resulting in enhancement of granulation tissue. A study comparing indirect and direct MR arthrography demonstrated an accuracy of 100% for indirect MR arthrography and an accuracy of 67% for direct MR arthrography [61]. The accuracy of MR arthrography in this study was lower than the accuracy of conventional MR imaging, with a higher sensitivity but lower specificity. False-positive cases were related to labral fraying and metal artefact mimicking a tear.

CT arthrography can also demonstrate similar changes to MR arthrography with recurrent tear clefts and displacement of labral tissue but is infrequently performed due to the radiation dose (Fig. 8.41). However, CT with its exquisite bony detail is well suited for assessing the degree of bone loss in patients with a bony Bankart and in those with foreign body reaction around hardware.

In patients who have undergone a capsular shift procedure the capsule may appear normal or may be minimally thickened with a nodular appearance, best appreciated on MR arthrography or in the presence of an effusion. The thickening can be subtle however, measuring between 2 and 4 mm, and is best appreciated when comparative preoperative MR images are available. The aim of capsular shift surgery is to tighten and reinforce the anterior capsule and these changes may be evident on postoperative MR arthrography with respect to the size of the capsule anteriorly and posteriorly. In an unstable shoulder preoperatively the anterior capsular

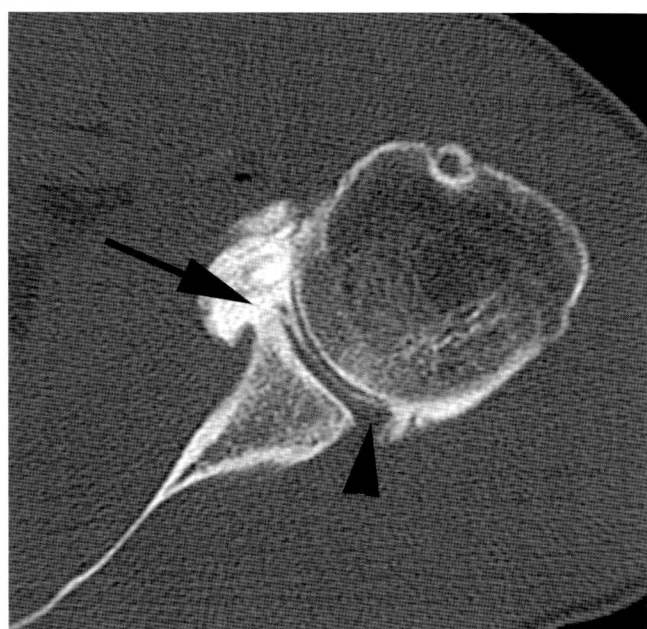 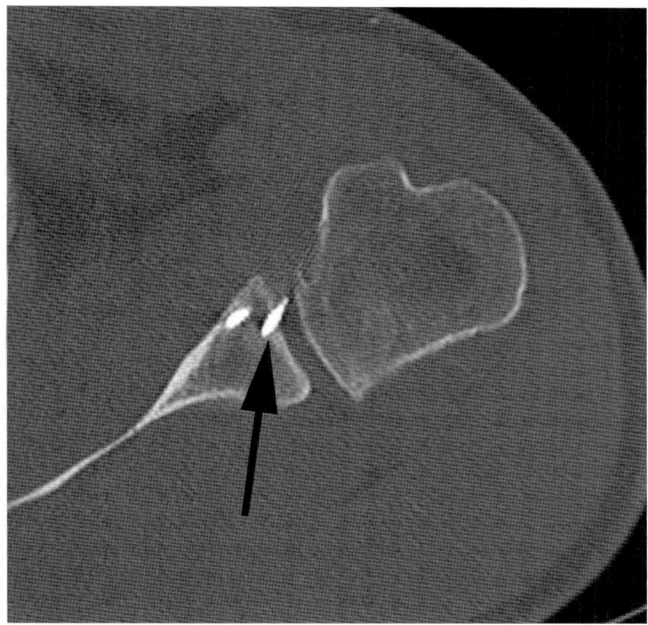

Fig. 8.41 Axial CT arthrogram of the shoulder in a patient with previous labral repair and recurrent tear. The posterior labrum is well visualized (*arrowhead*) but the anteroinferior labrum is deficient (*arrow*)

Fig. 8.42 Axial CT image in a patient with postoperative pain following instability surgery shows multiple anterior glenoid suture anchors with one protruding through the articular surface (*arrow*)

width as measured from the anterior labrum to the capsule may be larger than the posterior capsular width as measured from the posterior aspect of the humeral head to the posterior capsule. Following a capsular shift this situation may be reversed with the posterior capsular width exceeding the anterior capsular width [62]. In addition, a reduction in the size of the rotator interval may be evident. Persistence of a large anterior capsular width and a wide rotator interval may reflect reinjury or an insufficient capsular shift whereas posterior subluxation of the humeral head may reflect overtightening of the anterior capsule, which may lead to posterior instability or secondary degenerative changes posteriorly.

Postoperative imaging may also identify complications related to fixation hardware such as failed and displaced anchors or broken tacks. This may be seen with Bankart repairs as well as repairs of SLAP lesions. If left untreated, displaced hardware may result in chondral damage. CT may be especially useful for displacement of metallic fixation devices (Fig. 8.42). Foreign body reaction may also be seen around components, particularly bioabsorbable fixators, resulting in lucency around the hardware.

Conclusion

Advances in arthroscopic techniques have led to an increase in the number of patients undergoing surgery for sports-related injuries of the knee and the shoulder. Postoperative imaging in these patients may demonstrate the sequelae of surgery as well as residual or recurrent pathologies. Morphological changes, particularly of the menisci, rotator cuff and the glenoid labrum, which could be interpreted as pathological in a preoperative patient, have a different significance in the postoperative setting. In many instances, modification of diagnostic criteria and close clinical correlation are essential for accurate assessment of the postoperative patient.

References

1. White LM, Buckwalter KA (2002) Technical considerations: CT and MR imaging in the postoperative orthopedic patient. Semin Musculoskelet Radiol 6(1):5–17
2. Buckwalter KA, Rydberg J, Kopecky KK, Crow K, Yang EL (2001) Musculoskeletal imaging with multislice CT. AJR Am J Roentgenol 176(4):979–986
3. White LM, Kim JK, Mehta M et al (2000) Complications of total hip arthroplasty: MR imaging-initial experience. Radiology 215(1):254–262
4. Sofka CM, Potter HG (2002) MR imaging of joint arthroplasty. Semin Musculoskelet Radiol 6(1):79–85
5. Deutsch AL, Mink JH, Fox JM et al (1990) Peripheral meniscal tears: MR findings after conservative treatment or arthroscopic repair. Radiology 176(2):485–488
6. De Smet AA, Tuite MJ, Norris MA, Swan JS (1994) MR diagnosis of meniscal tears: analysis of causes of errors. AJR Am J Roentgenol 163(6):1419–1423
7. Farley TE, Howell SM, Love KF, Wolfe RD, Neumann CH (1991) Meniscal tears: MR and arthrographic findings after arthroscopic repair. Radiology 180(2):517–522

8. Lim PS, Schweitzer ME, Bhatia M et al (1999) Repeat tear of postoperative meniscus: potential MR imaging signs. Radiology 210(1):183–188
9. Applegate GR, Flannigan BD, Tolin BS, Fox JM, Del Pizzo W (1993) MR diagnosis of recurrent tears in the knee: value of intraarticular contrast material. AJR Am J Roentgenol 161(4):821–825
10. Arnoczky SP, Warren RF (1983) The microvasculature of the meniscus and its response to injury. An experimental study in the dog. Am J Sports Med 11(3):131–141
11. Smith DK, Totty WG (1990) The knee after partial meniscectomy: MR imaging features. Radiology 176(1):141–144
12. Mariani PP, Santori N, Adriani E, Mastantuono M (1996) Accelerated rehabilitation after arthroscopic meniscal repair: a clinical and magnetic resonance imaging evaluation. Arthroscopy 12(6):680–686
13. Sciulli RL, Boutin RD, Brown RR et al (1999) Evaluation of the postoperative meniscus of the knee: a study comparing conventional arthrography, conventional MR imaging, MR arthrography with iodinated contrast material, and MR arthrography with gadolinium-based contrast material. Skeletal Radiol 28(9):508–514
14. Magee T, Shapiro M, Rodriguez J, Williams D (2003) MR arthrography of postoperative knee: for which patients is it useful? Radiology 229(1):159–163
15. White LM, Schweitzer ME, Weishaupt D, Kramer J, Davis A, Marks PH (2002) Diagnosis of recurrent meniscal tears: prospective evaluation of conventional MR imaging, indirect MR arthrography, and direct MR arthrography. Radiology 222(2):421–429
16. Vives MJ, Homesley D, Ciccotti MG, Schweitzer ME (2003) Evaluation of recurring meniscal tears with gadolinium-enhanced magnetic resonance imaging: a randomized, prospective study. Am J Sports Med 31(6):868–873
17. Hantes ME, Zachos VC, Zibis AH et al (2004) Evaluation of meniscal repair with serial magnetic resonance imaging: a comparative study between conventional MRI and indirect MR arthrography. Eur J Radiol 50(3):231–237
18. Mutschler C, Vande Berg BC, Lecouvet FE et al (2003) Postoperative meniscus: assessment at dual-detector row spiral CT arthrography of the knee. Radiology 228(3):635–641
19. Trattnig S, Rand T, Czerny C et al (1999) Magnetic resonance imaging of the postoperative knee. Top Magn Reson Imaging 10(4):221–236
20. Howell SM, Clark JA, Blasier RD (1991) Serial magnetic resonance imaging of hamstring anterior cruciate ligament autografts during the first year of implantation. A preliminary study. Am J Sports Med 19(1):42–47
21. Boynton MD, Fadale PD (1993) The basic science of anterior cruciate ligament surgery. Orthop Rev 22(6):673–679
22. Vogl TJ, Schmitt J, Lubrich J et al (2001) Reconstructed anterior cruciate ligaments using patellar tendon ligament grafts: diagnostic value of contrast-enhanced MRI in a 2-year follow-up regimen. Eur Radiol 11(8):1450–1456
23. Cheung Y, Magee TH, Rosenberg ZS, Rose DJ (1992) MRI of anterior cruciate ligament reconstruction. J Comput Assist Tomogr 16(1):134–137
24. Howell SM, Knox KE, Farley TE, Taylor MA (1995) Revascularization of a human anterior cruciate ligament graft during the first two years of implantation. Am J Sports Med 23(1):42–49
25. Howell SM, Clark JA (1992) Tibial tunnel placement in anterior cruciate ligament reconstructions and graft impingement. Clin Orthop Relat Res (283):187–195
26. Saupe N, White LM, Chiavaras MM et al (2008) Anterior cruciate ligament reconstruction grafts: MR imaging features at long-term follow-up – correlation with functional and clinical evaluation. Radiology 249(2):581–590
27. Coupens SD, Yates CK, Sheldon C, Ward C (1992) Magnetic resonance imaging evaluation of the patellar tendon after use of its central one-third for anterior cruciate ligament reconstruction. Am J Sports Med 20(3):332–335
28. Simonian PT, Harrison SD, Cooley VJ, Escabedo EM, Deneka DA, Larson RV (1997) Assessment of morbidity of semitendinosus and gracilis tendon harvest for ACL reconstruction. Am J Knee Surg 10(2):54–59
29. Howell SM, Berns GS, Farley TE (1991) Unimpinged and impinged anterior cruciate ligament grafts: MR signal intensity measurements. Radiology 179(3):639–643
30. Simmons R, Howell SM, Hull ML (2003) Effect of the angle of the femoral and tibial tunnels in the coronal plane and incremental excision of the posterior cruciate ligament on tension of an anterior cruciate ligament graft: an in vitro study. J Bone Joint Surg Am 85-A(6):1018–1029
31. May DA, Snearly WN, Bents R, Jones R (1997) MR imaging findings in anterior cruciate ligament reconstruction: evaluation of notchplasty. AJR Am J Roentgenol 169(1):217–222
32. Watanabe BM, Howell SM (1995) Arthroscopic findings associated with roof impingement of an anterior cruciate ligament graft. Am J Sports Med 23(5):616–625
33. Recht MP, Piraino DW, Cohen MA, Parker RD, Bergfeld JA (1995) Localized anterior arthrofibrosis (cyclops lesion) after reconstruction of the anterior cruciate ligament: MR imaging findings. AJR Am J Roentgenol 165(2):383–385
34. Bradley DM, Bergman AG, Dillingham MF (2000) MR imaging of cyclops lesions. AJR Am J Roentgenol 174(3):719–726
35. Horton LK, Jacobson JA, Lin J, Hayes CW (2000) MR imaging of anterior cruciate ligament reconstruction graft. AJR Am J Roentgenol 175(4):1091–1097
36. Rak KM, Gillogly SD, Schaefer RA, Yakes WF, Liljedahl RR (1991) Anterior cruciate ligament reconstruction: evaluation with MR imaging. Radiology 178(2):553–556
37. McCauley TR, Elfar A, Moore A et al (2003) MR arthrography of anterior cruciate ligament reconstruction grafts. AJR Am J Roentgenol 181(5):1217–1223
38. van Trommel MF, Potter HG, Ernberg LA, Simonian PT, Wickiewicz TL (1998) The use of noncontrast magnetic resonance imaging in evaluating meniscal repair: comparison with conventional arthrography. Arthroscopy 14(1):2–8
39. White LM, Kramer J, Recht MP (2005) MR imaging evaluation of the postoperative knee: ligaments, menisci, and articular cartilage. Skeletal Radiol 34(8):431–452
40. Fanelli GC (1993) Posterior cruciate ligament injuries in trauma patients. Arthroscopy 9(3):291–294
41. Christel P (2003) Basic principles for surgical reconstruction of the PCL in chronic posterior knee instability. Knee Surg Sports Traumatol Arthrosc 11(5):289–296
42. Sherman PM, Sanders TG, Morrison WB, Schweitzer ME, Leis HT, Nusser CA (2001) MR imaging of the posterior cruciate ligament graft: initial experience in 15 patients with clinical correlation. Radiology 221(1):191–198
43. Cooper JM, McAndrews PT, LaPrade RF (2006) Posterolateral corner injuries of the knee: anatomy, diagnosis, and treatment. Sports Med Arthrosc 14(4):213–220
44. Steadman JR, Rodkey WG, Briggs KK, Rodrigo JJ (1999) The microfracture technic in the management of complete cartilage defects in the knee joint. Orthopade 28(1):26–32
45. Alparslan L, Winalski CS, Boutin RD, Minas T (2001) Postoperative magnetic resonance imaging of articular cartilage repair. Semin Musculoskelet Radiol 5(4):345–363
46. Matsusue Y, Yamamuro T, Hama H (1993) Arthroscopic multiple osteochondral transplantation to the chondral defect in the knee associated with anterior cruciate ligament disruption. Arthroscopy 9(3):318–321
47. Minas T, Chiu R (2000) Autologous chondrocyte implantation. Am J Knee Surg 13(1):41–50

48. Alparslan L, Minas T, Winalski CS (2001) Magnetic resonance imaging of autologous chondrocyte implantation. Semin Ultrasound CT MR 22(4):341–351
49. Spielmann AL, Forster BB, Kokan P, Hawkins RH, Janzen DL (1999) Shoulder after rotator cuff repair: MR imaging findings in asymptomatic individuals – initial experience. Radiology 213(3):705–708
50. Zanetti M, Jost B, Hodler J, Gerber C (2000) MR imaging after rotator cuff repair: full-thickness defects and bursitis-like subacromial abnormalities in asymptomatic subjects. Skeletal Radiol 29(6):314–319
51. Ryu RK, Burkhart SS, Parten PM, Gross RM (2002) Complex topics in arthroscopic subacromial space and rotator cuff surgery. Arthroscopy 18(2 Suppl 1):51–64
52. Owen RS, Iannotti JP, Kneeland JB, Dalinka MK, Deren JA, Oleaga L (1993) Shoulder after surgery: MR imaging with surgical validation. Radiology 186(2):443–447
53. Magee TH, Gaenslen ES, Seitz R, Hinson GA, Wetzel LH (1997) MR imaging of the shoulder after surgery. AJR Am J Roentgenol 168(4):925–928
54. Rand T, Trattnig S, Breitenseher M, Wurnig C, Marschner B, Imhof H (1999) The postoperative shoulder. Top Magn Reson Imaging 10(4):203–213
55. Gaenslen ES, Satterlee CC, Hinson GW (1996) Magnetic resonance imaging for evaluation of failed repairs of the rotator cuff. J Bone Joint Surg Am 78(9):1391–1396
56. Duc SR, Mengiardi B, Pfirrmann CW, Jost B, Hodler J, Zanetti M (2006) Diagnostic performance of MR arthrography after rotator cuff repair. AJR Am J Roentgenol 186(1):237–241
57. Zlatkin MB (2002) MRI of the postoperative shoulder. Skeletal Radiol 31(2):63–80
58. Prickett WD, Teefey SA, Galatz LM, Calfee RP, Middleton WD, Yamaguchi K (2003) Accuracy of ultrasound imaging of the rotator cuff in shoulders that are painful postoperatively. J Bone Joint Surg Am 85-A(6):1084–1089
59. Kim SH, Yoo JC, Ahn JM (2005) Arthroscopically repaired Bankart lesions and the effect of two different arm positions on immediate postoperative evaluation with magnetic resonance arthrography. Arthroscopy 21(7):867–874
60. Probyn LJ, White LM, Salonen DC, Tomlinson G, Boynton EL (2007) Recurrent symptoms after shoulder instability repair: direct MR arthrographic assessment – correlation with second-look surgical evaluation. Radiology 245(3):814–823
61. Wagner SC, Schweitzer ME, Morrison WB, Fenlin JM Jr, Bartolozzi AR (2002) Shoulder instability: accuracy of MR imaging performed after surgery in depicting recurrent injury – initial findings. Radiology 222(1):196–203
62. Rand T, Freilinger W, Breitenseher M et al (1999) Magnetic resonance arthrography (MRA) in the postoperative shoulder. Magn Reson Imaging 17(6):843–850

Chapter 9
Muscle Injury and Complications

Abhijit Datir and David A. Connell

Introduction

Imaging has established its role as one of the most valuable tools for evaluation of muscle injuries and primarily involves magnetic resonance (MR) imaging and ultrasound (US). MR imaging is widely accepted for sports imaging and has become the standard care for evaluation of the musculoskeletal system. MR imaging is not only operator-independent and provides high-resolution images, but also carries a high degree of sensitivity in detecting soft-tissue abnormalities. The specific role of MR imaging in sports-related muscle injuries is summarized in Table 9.1 [1].

Sonography, on the other hand, requires a substantial level of experience to be used in sports-related muscle injuries because of the technical complexity and the importance of analyzing dynamic studies. However, US offers certain advantages including expense, patient interaction, ease of serial evaluation in following the healing process and the use of colour Doppler for depicting tissue inflammation and vascularity. In experienced hands, US can provide results with sensitivity and specificity comparable to MR imaging in muscle injury imaging [2–4].

Muscle injuries are common in many sport-related activities, especially those involving high-intensity sprinting [5–7]. Muscle strains have one of the highest recurrence rates after return to play [8, 9]. Usually, the fitness evaluation before return to play from most muscle injuries is aimed so that the performance is optimal and the risk of recurrence is minimal. Although, there are no consensus guidelines for safe return to sport following muscle injuries that completely eliminate the risk of recurrence, an early return to play seems to be a plausible strategy, although at a cost of an increased risk of recurrence rate [5].

David A. Connell
Department of Radiology, Royal National Orthopaedic Hospital, Brockley Hill, Stanmore, Middlesex, HA7 4LP, UK
e-mail: david.connell@rnoh.nhs.uk

Imaging Techniques

MR Imaging

MR imaging is the mainstay in the initial diagnosis and evaluation of muscle injury. The radiofrequency coil selected for a particular anatomical area of interest should provide a sufficient field of view with maximum spatial and contrast resolution. Larger coils (such as body coil) provide a poor signal-to-noise ratio than smaller coils (such as surface coil) for a given imaging area. The temptation to cover a large anatomical area may result in missing small muscle tears or poor prognostic information. Phased-array coils are typically used to produce high-quality images with a large FOV by combination of signal from many surface coils. Once selected, the same imaging protocol is usually implemented during follow-up MR imaging, if needed.

The protocols are designed to allow comparison of T1w or proton-density (PD) images with fat-suppressed (FS) T2w images at the same slice location (Fig. 9.1). The high-resolution T1w or PD images are used for anatomic detail and the FS T2w images for delineation of oedema and blood–fluid products. The use of frequency-selective fat-suppression technique helps to differentiate between areas of oedema and increased fat signal on fast spin-echo (FSE) T2w images. However, this technique may results in field inhomogeneity due to poor fat suppression, especially with large field-of-view. Fast short-tau inversion recovery (STIR) techniques are less dependent on field homogeneity and can be used as an alternative to FSE T2w images. The use of intravenous contrast administration is limited and can be used for the evaluation of granulation tissue or scar formation. Although Gradient echo sequences can be used to detect small amount of haemorrhage or achieve dynamic imaging during muscle contraction, these are not routinely employed [10, 11].

Ultrasound

Every attempt should be made to benefit from the patient interaction during US examination including history and physical examination, while allowing the patient to identify the site of maximum symptoms. It should be kept in mind that a history of trauma is not always present in patients with myositis ossificans (MO). A thorough US examination of the symptomatic region with scanning in the longitudinal and transverse planes should be performed. High-frequency linear transducers (9–13 MHz) are usually adequate and can produce good quality diagnostic images. Current technology allows in-plane resolutions of 200–450 µm and section thickness of 0.5–1.0 mm, which exceed that obtainable with MR imaging [12]. An extended field-of-view (FOV) reconstruction of areas up to 60 cm long can provide more anatomic details and are easier to understand for the referring physician. A larger FOV is also helpful in the assessment of muscle strain length or gap following muscle tear. This should always be supplemented with dynamic imaging with active and passive movements of the anatomical part under consideration.

Use of colour Doppler technique should be made in the assessment of regional blood flow and neurovascular bundle (Fig. 9.2). Power Doppler is more sensitive in identifying hyperaemia or neovascularity associated with acute injuries, although it lacks the directional flow information. Tissue harmonic imaging can be used to improve lesion conspicuity [13, 14]. Ultrasound is as sensitive as MR imaging in the acute setting associated with significant oedema and blood–fluid products, but is difficult to assess in subtle, deep-seated and chronic injuries [15].

The role of plain radiography and computed tomography (CT) is quite limited in the evaluation of muscle injuries and are used in specific circumstances such as myositis ossificans.

Table 9.1 Role of MRI in sports-related muscle injury

- High accuracy rate for the diagnosis of specific muscle injury
- Detection of sub-clinical injury and define a period of continued vulnerability
- Distinction between non-operative and surgical conditions
- Accurate pre-operative planning
- Imaging and follow-up of complications like fatty atrophy, scarring, etc.
- Imaging of activity-specific muscle recruitment pattern to tailor exercise and rehabilitation regimens

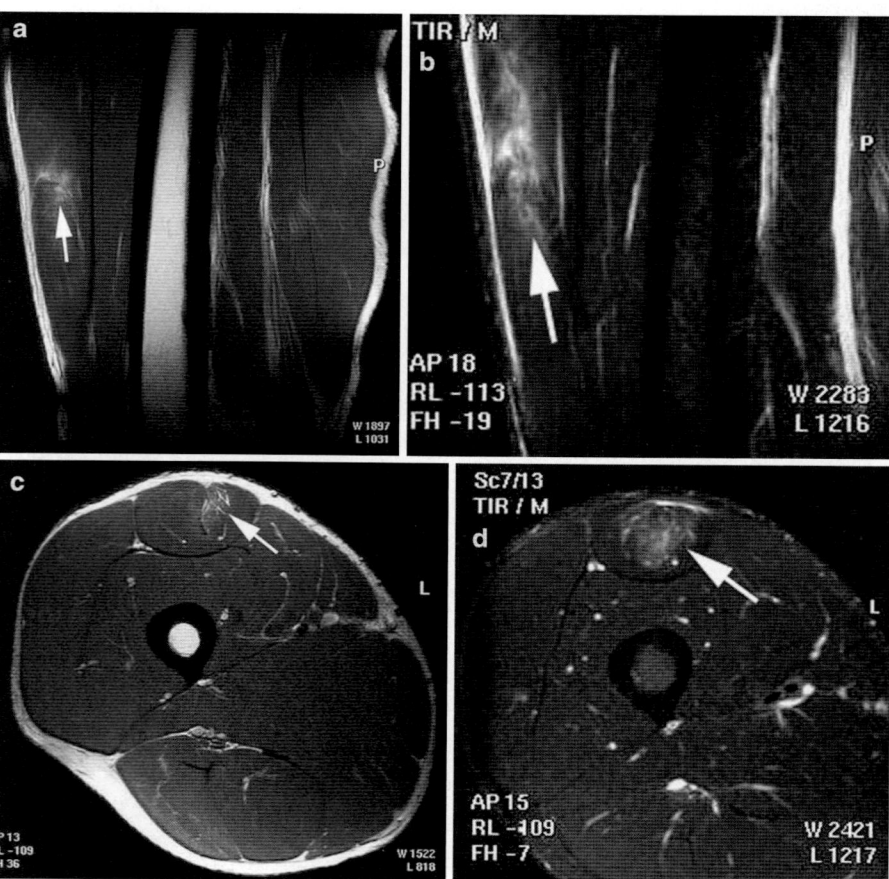

Fig. 9.1 Comparison of sagittal (**a**) and axial (**c**) PD-weighted (PDW) images with corresponding STIR images (**b** and **d**) in a patient with Grade II rectus femoris muscle injury. Anatomical details with depiction of muscle tear are seen on PDW images whereas the extent of oedema and muscle fibre involvement are best seen on STIR images

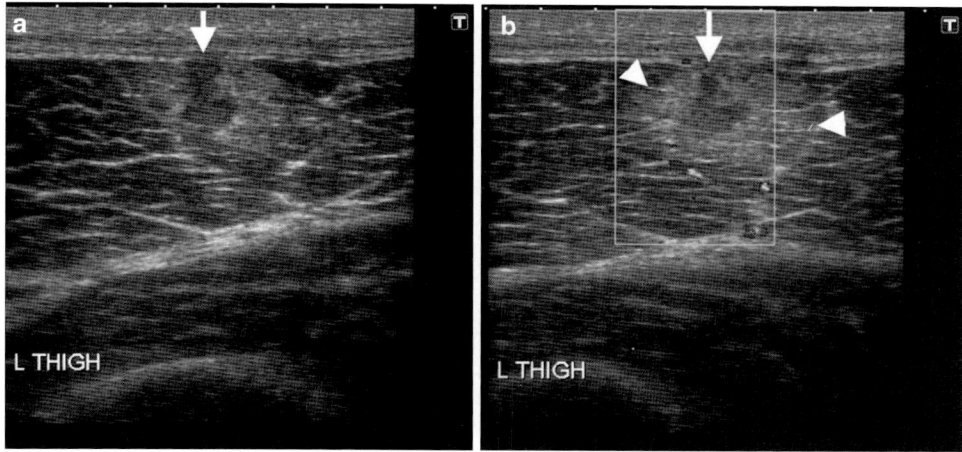

Fig. 9.2 Ultrasound and colour Doppler in muscle injury. Longitudinal views of vastus lateralis muscle showing a partial-thickness superficial surface tear with discontinuity of muscle fibres (*arrows*) with surrounding haematoma formation (*arrowheads*). Associated intramuscular oedema with loss of surrounding normal fibrillary echotexture and increased Doppler signal suggests acute injury

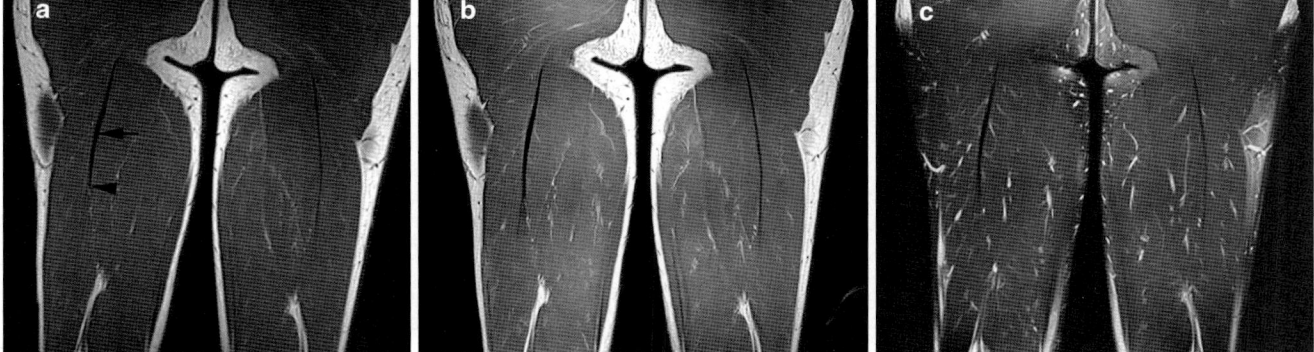

Fig. 9.3 Normal muscle anatomy on MR. (**a**) T1-weighted (**b**) proton-density (**c**) T2 turbo spin echo with fat-suppression images of normal muscles in posterior compartment of the thigh showing intermediate signal intensity with typical feathery appearance due to fat interspersed between muscles and fibres. The tendons are easily identified as discrete linear low-signal structures (*arrow*) in all pulse sequences. *Arrowhead* = MTJ

Anatomy

Simplistically, skeletal muscle can be considered to be composed of two main components, the myofibres and the connective tissue. The myofibres are responsible for the contractile function of the muscle, whereas the connective tissue provides the framework that binds the individual muscle together during contraction. Each myofibre is attached at both ends to the connective tissue of a tendon or the tendon-like fascia at the so-called myotendinous junctions (MTJs).

Microscopically, the myofibre is mainly composed of contractile myofibrils and mitochondria. These are supported by three levels of connective tissue sheaths the endomysium, perimysium and epimysium. The individual myofibre is surrounded by endomysium, which are in turn bound together by perimysium into larger structures called fascicles. Finally, the epimysium surrounds the entire muscle belly (Figs. 9.3–9.5).

In sports-related trauma, the most common site of disruption is at the MTJ, owing to its lower capacity for energy absorption as compared to either the muscle or tendon [16, 17]. At the MTJ, the muscle cells have multiple projections that form intervening recesses, into which collagen fibrils from the tendon insert. This ultrastructural arrangement facilitates increased surface contact between the muscle and tendon, thereby dissipating forces and lessening the risk of injury. The MTJ may be a well-defined discrete area in some muscles or an elongated broad area in others.

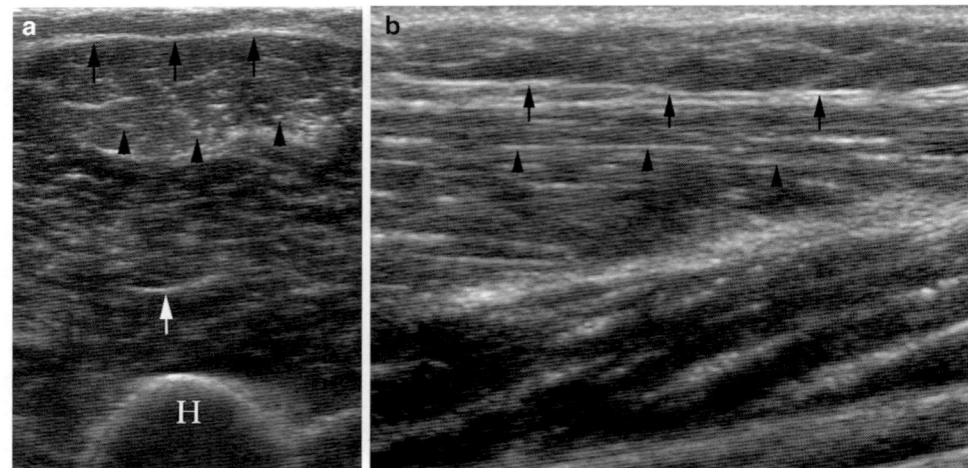

Fig. 9.4 Normal muscle anatomy on US. (**a**) Transverse sonogram shows the epimysium as a bright echogenic band (*black arrows*) and the perimysium as *multiple dots* or *short lines* (*arrowheads*) on a hypoechoic background of muscle fibres. Prominent intramuscular septa (*white arrow*) within the muscle belly. *H* humerus. (**b**) Longitudinal sonogram shows the parallel orientation of perimysium (*arrowheads*) to epimysium (*arrows*), having the typical configuration of a fusiform muscle

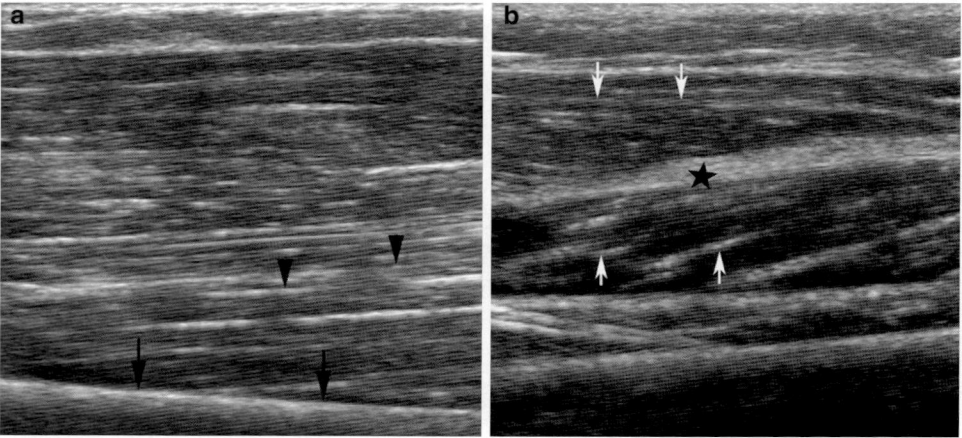

Fig. 9.5 Normal unipennate and bipennate muscles on US. (**a**) Unipennate muscle – US showing obliquely oriented perimysium (*arrowheads*) inserting onto the intermuscular fascia (*arrows*). (**b**) Bipennate muscle – US showing obliquely oriented perimysium (*arrows*) converging on the intramuscular tendon (*star*)

Imaging Characteristics of Normal Muscle

MR Imaging

Normal muscle demonstrates intermediate signal intensity (SI) on both T1w and T2w pulse sequences. On T1w images, the muscle shows a feathery or marbled appearance due to fat interspersed between fibres within a muscle bundle or in between muscle groups. Depending on the amount of interspersed fat, it may be possible to distinguish one muscle group separate from another. The tendons are seen as a discrete linear low SI on all pulse sequences (Fig. 9.3). Low SI tendons may course through a muscle belly (e.g. subscapularis) or may arise near the periphery of a muscle (e.g. biceps brachii) representing the myotendinous junction. Following a traumatic event, there is increase in the water content of the muscle causing T2 prolongation and increased SI on T2w images. This increased water content could be secondary to the increase in the amount of extracellular water or elevated hydrostatic pressures from increased vascularity.

Ultrasound

Normal muscle fibres are arranged in parallel hypoechoic bundles surrounded by echogenic fibrofatty septa in a "pennate" configuration. The perimysium appears as parallel echogenic striations on longitudinal and "dots" on transverse views with muscle fibres forming a hypoechoic background. The epimysium, which represents the outer thick fibrous tissue covering of individual muscle, is seen as highly echogenic, peripheral, linear structure (Fig. 9.4). The orientation of perimysium to the long axis of muscle is oblique in uni/bipennate muscles and parallel in fusiform muscles (Fig. 9.5). Normal tendons demonstrate a hyperechoic fibrillary echotexture because of highly organized collagenous contents. Tendons are strongly anisotropic to ultrasound examination and it is important to position the ultrasound beam perpendicular to its collagen fibres to avoid anisotropy.

Patho-physiology of Muscle Injury

The most important feature distinguishing a healing skeletal muscle from a healing bone injury is that the skeletal muscle heals by a repair process, whereas the bone heals by a regenerative process. The healing of an injured skeletal muscle follows a fairly constant pattern irrespective of the underlying cause (contusion, strain, or laceration) [18]. Three phases are described in this process as summarized in Table 9.2 [19].

On imaging, the appearance of muscle following a traumatic event depends on several factors including, the mode of onset (acute or chronic), type of sporting activity involved, extent of involvement, mechanism (direct or indirect, blunt or penetrating) and severity of injury. Pathologically, a combination of torn muscle fibres, inflammation, oedema and haemorrhage is seen.

Imaging of Muscle Injury: General Considerations

Traumatic muscle injuries can be divided into indirect and/or direct types depending on the basic mechanism involved.

A muscle contusion occurs when a muscle is subjected to a direct sudden, strong compressive force. This typically occurs in contact sports, as opposed to sprinting and jumping activities which are commonly associated with muscle strains [20]. In strains, an excessive tensile force applied across the muscle leads to overstraining of the myofibres and subsequently MTJ rupture. Most contusions involve muscle groups situated close to bones, for example vastus intermedius or brachialis muscles, whereas muscle strain typically affects muscles working across two joints, such as rectus femoris, semitendinosus, gastrocnemius muscles.

Delayed-Onset Muscle Soreness

Delayed-onset muscle soreness (DOMS) refers to muscular pain, soreness and swelling that follow unaccustomed physical exercise. Pathologically, it is thought to result from reversible structural damage at cellular level and may be associated with temporary loss of strength. The onset of symptoms is more insidious as compared with muscle strains; begins about 24 h after activity, peaks at 48–72 h, and resolves by 1 week.

The clinical diagnosis of DOMS is usually straightforward, given the typical history of onset and progression, and imaging is almost never performed for this purpose. However, this entity may be seen occasionally in patients imaged for other reasons and it is important to be aware of DOMS. The imaging findings are non-specific and are the same as for a grade I muscle strain with feathery T2W/STIR SI within the involved muscle groups and peri-fascial oedema in early stages (Fig. 9.6). This may rarely persist up to 80 days and be associated with rhabdomyolysis [21].

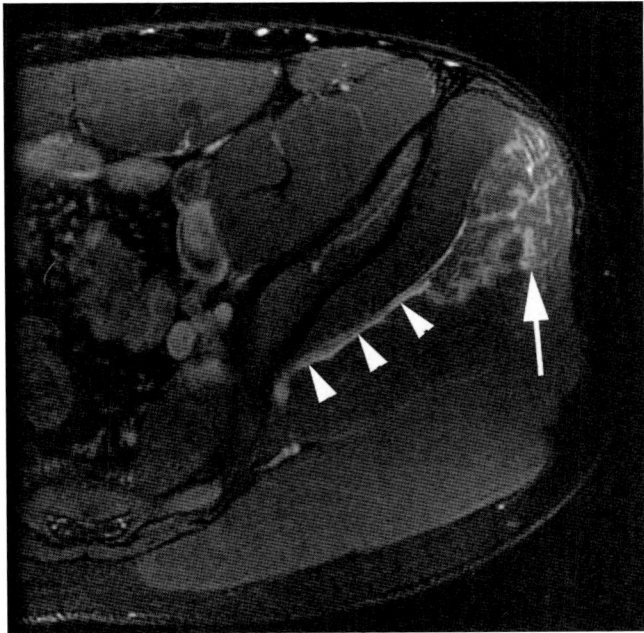

Fig. 9.6 Delayed-onset muscle soreness. Axial MR image showing diffuse oedema of the gluteus medius muscle (*arrow*) and peri-fascial oedema (*arrowheads*)

Table 9.2 The patho-physiology of the muscle injury – *three phases*

Destruction phase	• Rupture of muscle
	• Necrosis of myofibres
	• Haematoma formation
	• Inflammatory cell reaction
Repair phase	• Phagocytosis of the necrotized tissue
	• Regeneration of the myofibres
	• Neo-vascularization
	• Connective tissue scar formation
Remodelling phase	• Maturation of the regenerated myofibres
	• Contraction and re-organization of the scar tissue
	• Functional recovery of the muscle

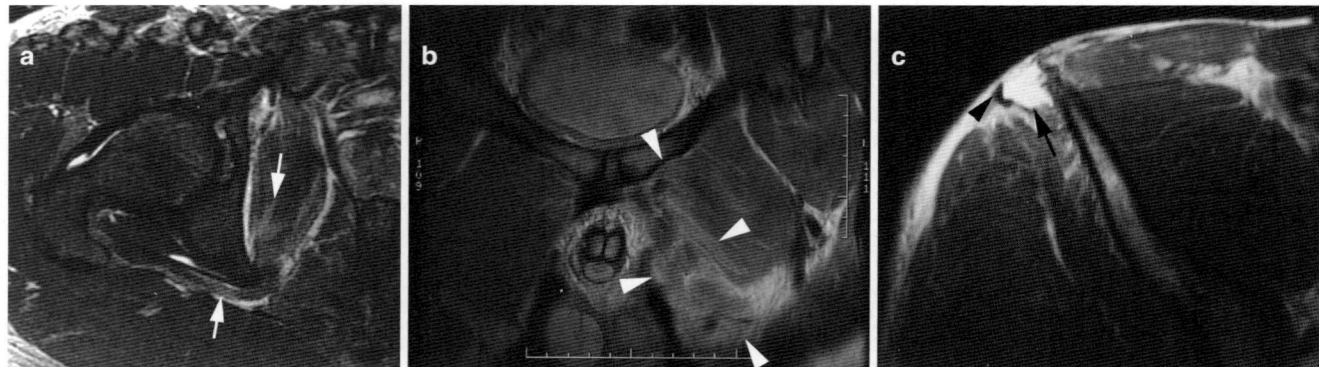

Fig. 9.7 Grading of muscle strain. (**a**) Grade I – axial MR image showing intrasubstance increased signal intensity (*arrows*) involving the obturator internus muscle with peri-fascial oedema but no fibre discontinuity. (**b**) Grade II (high grade) – severe oedema and muscle fibre disruption of the adductor longus (between *arrowheads*) on coronal MR with only few fibres remaining intact. (**c**) Grade III – axial MR image shows complete avulsion and disruption of the attachment of tensor fascia lata (*arrowhead*) from anterior superior iliac spine with gap filled with haematoma (*arrow*)

Muscle Strain

Muscle strains are muscle tears, either partial or complete, and represent the most frequent injury in sports. It typically affects muscle groups that cross two joints, perform primarily eccentric contraction and contain a predominance of fast-twitch (type II) muscle fibres [22, 23]. The most common muscles injured due to strain include the rectus femoris, the hamstrings and the gastrocnemius. It has been demonstrated that interplay of both stretching and contraction is essential to induce this type of injury [24]. Clinically, strain results in acute onset muscle pain and swelling following a period of strenuous physical activity that typically resolve within 2 weeks.

Strains may be classified into three grades (Fig. 9.7).

- Grade I – the most common (75% of cases) and typically associated with a microscopic injury (5% muscle fibre disruption) and no significant loss of muscle strength.
- Grade II – partial-thickness macroscopic tears with continuity of some muscle fibres at the site of injury, associated with some loss of strength. This may be further subdivided into low grade (<1/3rd muscle fibres torn), moderate (1/3rd–2/3rd muscle fibres torn) or high grade (>2/3rd muscle fibres torn) (Fig. 9.8).
- Grade III – characterized by complete disruption of MTJ with/without muscle retraction and associated with significant loss of muscle function. Sometimes, retraction of muscle fibres may result in a palpable defect or a focal mass, mimicking a tumour.

On MR imaging, the findings usually correlate with the clinical grading of injury and are detailed in Table 9.3.

With regard to muscle strain or tear injury, US is most helpful in the acute setting (between 2 and 48 h), during which the sensitivity equals MR imaging primarily because of its ability to detect post-traumatic fluid collections [16]. However, US has two main disadvantages when compared with MR imaging – (1) it underestimates the extent of injury both in longitudinal and cross-sectional dimensions and (2) abnormalities resolve more quickly as acute haematomas resolve.

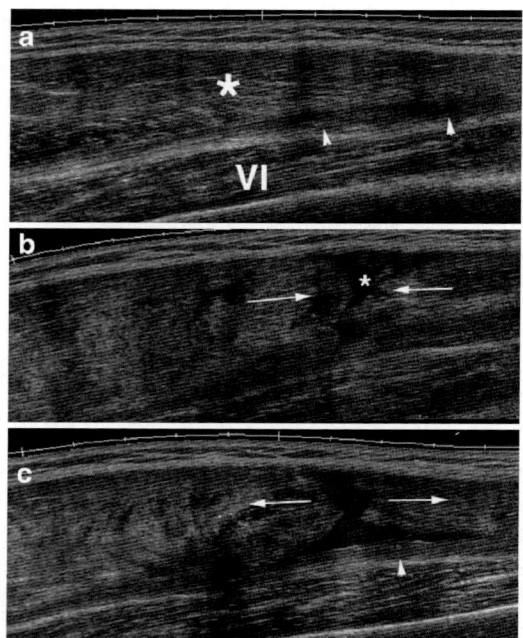

Fig. 9.8 High grade II tear. Longitudinal extended field-of-view sonograms of rectus femoris show (**a**) medially intact muscle (*) and aponeurotic haematoma (*arrowheads*). Vastus intermedius (VI). (**b**) Lateral muscle disruption (*arrows*) with haemorrhage (*). (**c**) During knee flexion the torn muscle margins distract (*arrows*) with inferior haematoma (*arrowhead*)

Table 9.3 MRI grading and appearance in muscle strain

Grade	MR imaging	Additional findings
Grade I	Increased SI on T2W FS/STIR images at the MTJ due to oedema and haemorrhage, tracking along the muscle fascicles producing a feathery pattern	Peri-fascial fluid in 87% of athletes with partial muscle injury
Grade II	Increased SI on T2W FS/STIR images with haematoma formation at the MTJ (typical finding) and peri-fascial oedema; Tendon may thinned, irregular and lax	Focal, stellate-shaped muscle defect may be present; an old second-degree strain may be recognized by the presence of low T2W SI due to haemosiderin, fibrosis and muscle atrophy
Grade III	Complete muscle disruption with haematoma bridging the gap between retracted segments; stage of a haematoma is determined depending on T1W and T2W signal characteristics	Muscle atrophy may begin as early as 10 days after the injury and may be irreversible by 4 months

Grade II and III muscle strains typically take longer to heal mainly because of continued contractions of the injured muscle resulting in repeated microtears and haemorrhage (Figs. 9.1, 9.7 and 9.8). Previous injury is one important risk factor for recurrent muscle injury. It has also been shown that a recent history of strain of one muscle group confers an increased risk of injury to surrounding muscle groups [25]. The role of imaging is not only to confirm the initial clinical diagnosis and define the extent, but also to depict the findings after resolution of clinical symptoms and help define this period of continued vulnerability.

Muscle Haematoma

This may be intermuscular (between two muscle groups) or intramuscular (confined within a single muscle parenchyma).

Intramuscular haematoma are less common, clinically less apparent and takes longer to resolve (6–8 weeks). This describes the free dissection of blood between the muscle fibres, without disrupting the muscle integrity. Due to resultant inflammation, oedema and interstitial haemorrhage following a blunt injury, the entire muscle may become swollen and show a feathery pattern on T2w images due to separation of muscle fibres by intervening blood. T1w images show muscle enlargement or may be normal. This appearance may be difficult to differentiate from grade I muscle strain, and the importance of accurate clinical history for reliable differentiation of the two entities cannot be overemphasized.

Generally the appearance of muscle haematoma on MR imaging is highly variable and age dependent. The MR appearance is primarily determined by the blood product and is summarized in Table 9.4. The MR appearance of muscle haematoma may be complicated by repeated episodes of haemorrhage from recurrent injuries (Fig. 9.9). The use of fat-suppression techniques (e.g. STIR, T2w FS sequences) is useful to differentiate recent haemorrhage from fat, both of which appear hyperintense on T1w images. Sometimes, a resolving haematoma may leave a residual fluid-containing

Table 9.4 Progression of muscle haematoma on MRI

Stage		Blood products	T1 signal	T2 signal
Hyperacute		Oxyhaemoglobin	Intermediate	Hyperintense
Acute		Deoxyhaemoglobin	Intermediate	Hypointense
Subacute	Early	Intracellular methaemoglobin	Hyperintense	Hypointense
	Late	Extracellular methaemoglobin	Hyperintense	Hyperintense
Chronic		Haemosiderin	Hypointense	Hypointense

intramuscular pseudocyst and is most commonly reported to involve the rectus femoris, semimembranosus or semitendinosus muscle [26]. Fluid–fluid levels may also be seen in chronic haematoma. A rare complication of an expanding haematoma is acute compartment syndrome, which may necessitate emergency evacuation. With healing, scarring and fibrosis accompanies muscle regeneration and shows low SI on all pulse sequences (Fig. 9.10). MR imaging can be used to monitor the amount of fibrosis produced and also to predict whether full tensile strength and functional recovery will occur.

Sonographically, focal muscle swelling secondary to oedema and haematoma may be seen in early or low-grade injury. In the first 24 h, focal haematoma may demonstrate variable appearance, from anechoic or hypoechoic to hyperechoic (Fig. 9.2). Over the next 2–3 days, the collection becomes progressively hypo- or anechoic. Following weeks after injury, increased central echogenicity and fluid–debris levels may be identified [27].

Compartment Syndrome

Compartment syndrome may be acute or chronic in nature. Acute compartment syndrome is a potential complication of fracture or severe muscle injury with resultant extensive oedema, haemorrhage and swelling. A sudden increase in intracompartmental pressure may subsequently result in

Fig. 9.9 Intramuscular haematoma. Axial (**a**) and coronal (**b**) MR images show an intramuscular haematoma (*arrows*) at the proximal myotendinous junction of rectus femoris with extensive oedema along the inferior fibres

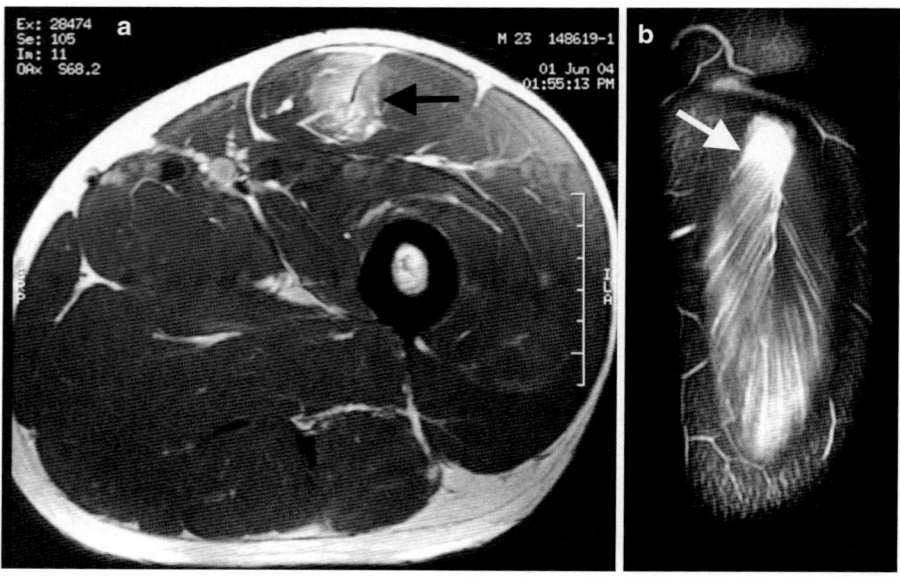

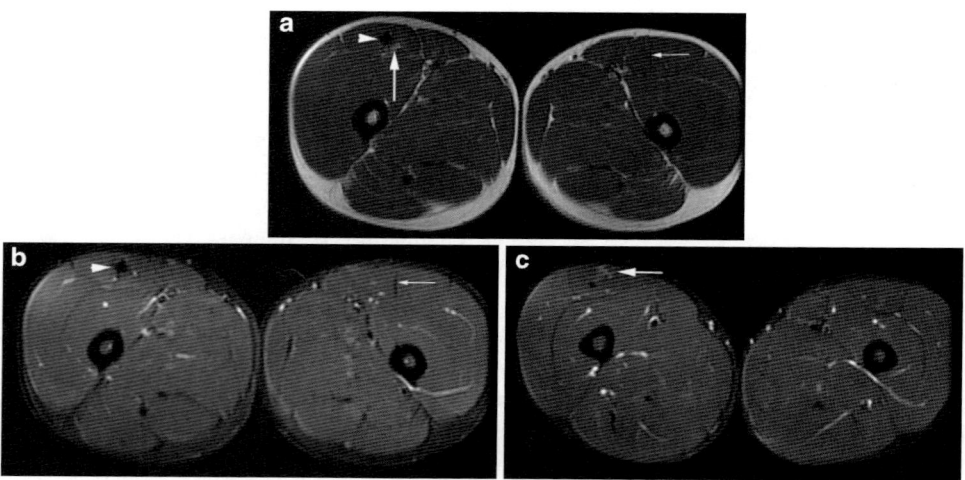

Fig. 9.10 MR image of muscle scarring. Axial (**a**) T1w and (**b**) T2w FS MR images show normal left rectus femoris tendon (*small arrow*), thickened nodular right tendon (*arrowhead*) and adjacent fat replacement (*large arrow*) due to previous injury. (**c**) MR image inferior to b shows oedema (*arrow*) due to low-grade re-tear

decreased tissue perfusion and neuromuscular injury. In athletes, acute compartment syndrome may occur with muscle rupture (e.g. the biceps brachii compartment of the arm and the flexor compartment of the forearm, the superficial posterior or peroneal compartment of the leg) or in the absence of muscle rupture (e.g. the triceps and deltoid muscles of weight lifters). On the other hand, chronic compartment syndrome may be associated with exertional causes (exercise or occupational overuse) or non-exertional causes (e.g. a mass, lesion or infection). In athletes, the lower leg is affected most frequently followed by the thigh, the forearm and the foot. Clinically, acute compartment syndrome presents as a surgical emergency with severe pain disproportionate to the degree of clinical injury, while chronic exertional compartment syndrome presents with aching and tenderness after exercise.

MR imaging findings are non-specific for compartment syndrome and frequently mimicked by muscle strain, DOMS, deep vein thrombosis, cellulitis and lymphoedema. MR imaging generally does not play a role in the diagnostic work-up of acute compartment syndrome; however, can be useful in delineating the anatomic extent of the abnormalities and the degree of muscle loss. In acute cases, the muscle compartment shows increase in size and T2w SI due to oedema [28, 29]. In chronic cases, increased SI on T1w images represents fatty replacement whereas decreased T1w SI may be seen due to fibrosis and dystrophic calcification [30]. Associated findings may include loss of muscle volume due to atrophy and/or fibrosis and fascial thickening. Rarely, chronic compartment syndrome may result in calcific myonecrosis, several decades after trauma. In calcific myonecrosis, the mass is typically comprised of liquefied necrotic muscle with a surrounding thin rim of calcification.

In chronic exertional compartment syndrome, performing the MR examination immediately after a provocative exercise may be helpful. Failure of the oedematous muscles to return to a baseline normal appearance by 15–25 min after the completion of exercise is considered to be diagnostic. US-guided pressure monitoring during exercise may be a helpful investigation tool, especially when the deep posterior compartment of the calf is involved.

On US, diffuse muscle swelling and increased echogenicity may be identified in acute compartment syndrome which becomes more heterogeneous as the condition deteriorates. US may be helpful in detection and percutaneous drainage of fluid collections, if present, to decompress the compartment.

Muscle Herniation

Muscle hernia is a protrusion of muscle through a focal fascial defect. These are common secondary to muscle hypertrophy and increased intracompartmental pressure than traumatic fascial tears. It most commonly occurs in middle and lower leg and involves the tibialis anterior, the extensor digitorum longus and the peroneus brevis/longus. On clinical examination, a small, superficial, soft-tissue mass is palpable that becomes larger and firmer with contraction. These may become incarcerated or result in nerve entrapment.

MR imaging shows generalized outward bulging of muscle with mild peripheral contour irregularity. On dynamic imaging, the focal protrusion may become more pronounced and is a useful technique in inconspicuous cases. Usually, the SI is normal; however, symptomatic hernia may demonstrate increased T2w SI [31].

On US, normal muscle tissue may be seen protruding through a focal epimysial defect (Fig. 9.11). On longitudinal images, perimysium may be seen bulging into the defect. A quick dynamic imaging study may be performed on US with contraction of muscle under evaluation. Care must be taken to avoid exerting excessive probe pressure which may obscure a small muscle hernia.

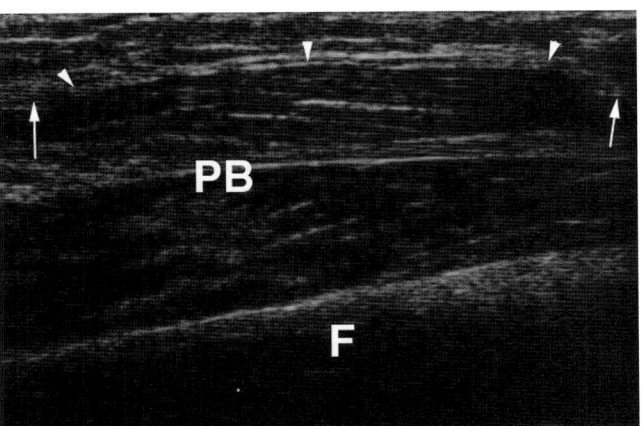

Fig. 9.11 Muscle hernia. Longitudinal sonogram of right leg show fibula (F) and peroneus brevis (PB) muscle hernia (*arrowheads*) breeching the deep fascia (*arrows*)

Imaging of Muscle Injury: Sequelae and Complications

The final outcome of muscle injury can be variable and ideally athletes will return to sports with optimum strength and no further adverse effect(s). Some muscle injuries may result in scar formation which may be from an initial event or repetitive trauma and certainly has the potential to compromise the muscle function. The scar tissue appears as a low SI intensity on all pulse sequences and may be indistinguishable from tendon (Fig. 9.10). The tendon itself may be thickened and irregular. On US, an intramuscular scar appears as a linear or irregular echogenic structure that may be surrounded by a hypoechoic zone or halo, typically found at the MTJ or fascial interface (Fig. 9.12) [27].

Sometimes, the injured muscle undergoes atrophy and fat replacement (*fatty atrophy*) with resultant loss of strength and function. T1w sequence can optimally demonstrate the increased fat content of the muscle with pseudohypertrophy.

Myositis Ossificans

Myositis ossificans (MO) is a well-known sequela of muscle injury often affecting large muscles in extremities [10, 11, 32, 33]. It results in progressive ossification of the involved muscle and usually is secondary to blunt muscle trauma. The most common locations are within the quadriceps in the lower extremity and the brachialis in the upper extremity. However, non-traumatic causes are also implied and may include burns, paraplegia/immobilization. A history of preceding trauma is lacking in 50% of cases and clinically it presents with pain, swelling and progressive loss of function.

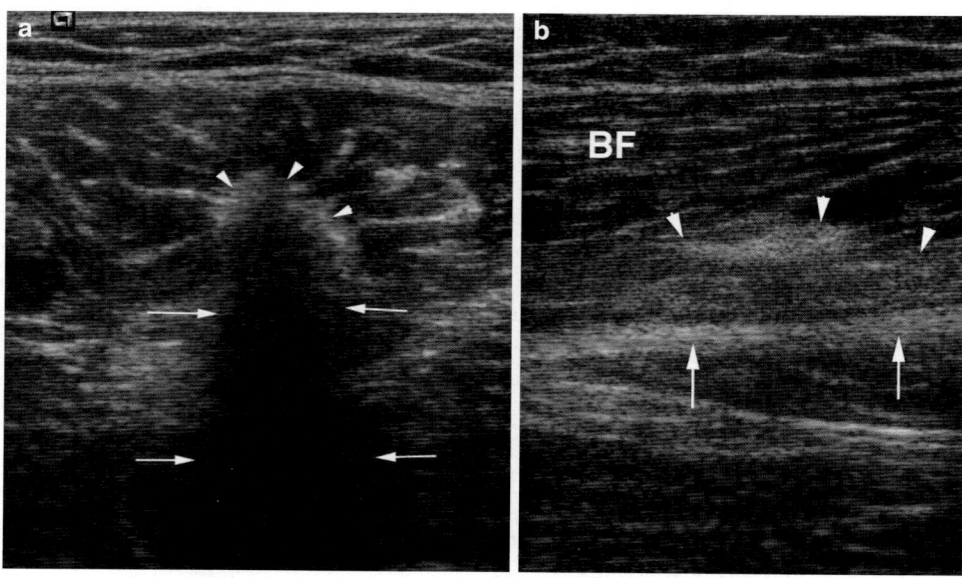

Fig. 9.12 Ultrasound of muscle scarring. (a) Transverse sonogram of left rectus femoris muscle shows loss of normal thin linear tendon structure with replacement by thick echogenic scar tissue (*arrowheads*) with acoustic shadowing (*arrows*). (b) Longitudinal sonogram of right biceps femoris (BF) muscle shows echogenic scarring (*arrowheads*) adjacent to the sciatic nerve (*arrows*)

Fig. 9.13 Myositis ossificans. Axial T2w TSE MR image (**a**) demonstrates a peripheral ring of reduced signal intensity within the quadriceps muscle with associated marked muscle oedema on coronal STIR sequence (**b**). Ultrasound (**c**) shows a curvilinear hyperechoic area of ossification (*arrow*) with posterior acoustic shadowing within the vastus intermedius of thigh, which can be correlated on radiograph (**d**)

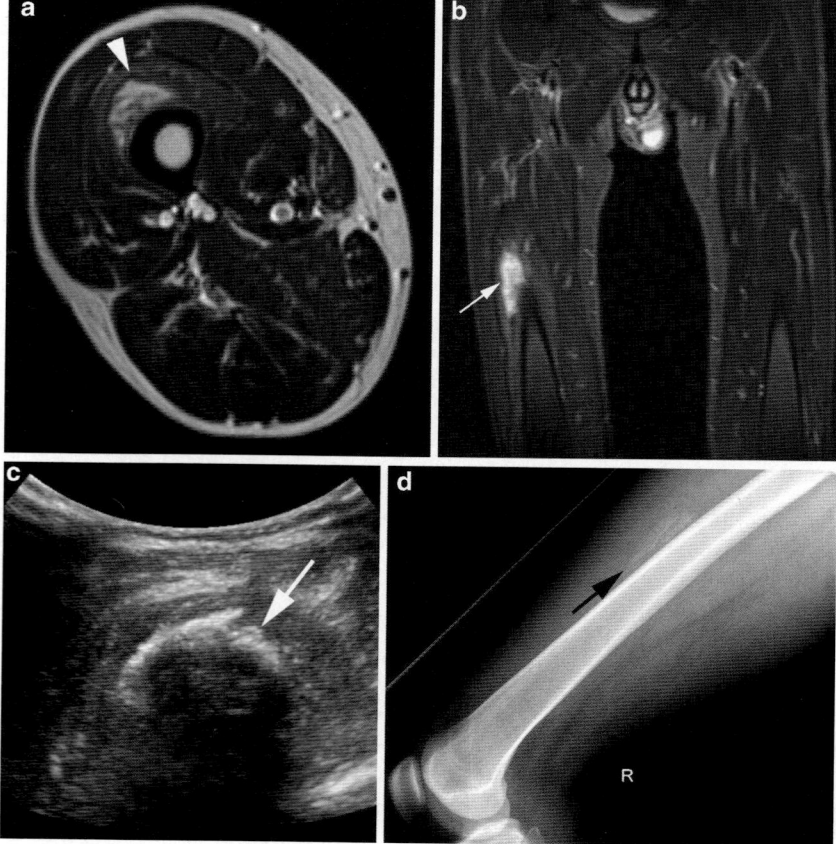

MO presents diagnostic imaging difficulties owing to its variable imaging appearance that can be aggressive and overlap with neoplastic processes. The appearance on MR imaging depends on the age of the lesion and can be described with three stage of evolution – acute (<2 weeks) (Figs. 9.13 and 9.14), subacute (2–8 weeks) and chronic (>8 weeks), as shown in Table 9.5. It is important to remember that the appearances of MO are non-specific and can easily be confused with a soft-tissue sarcoma. Moreover, a percutaneous needle biopsy may fail to demonstrate its true nature if the peripheral mature bone is not sampled and results in erroneous diagnosis of an aggressive lesion. In doubtful cases, a short-term follow-up is recommended to reveal the typical evaluation of this lesion.

US is well suited for detecting the phasic changes of MO, particularly the transition between the non-calcified and calcified stages. In later stages, MO may appear as a hypoechoic or heterogeneous mass, with sheets of echogenic calcification (Fig. 9.13c). Colour Doppler may demonstrate marked vascularity of the rim and central zone. On maturation, acoustic shadowing is seen due to peripheral ossification, often paralleling adjacent bone (Fig. 9.13d) [34].

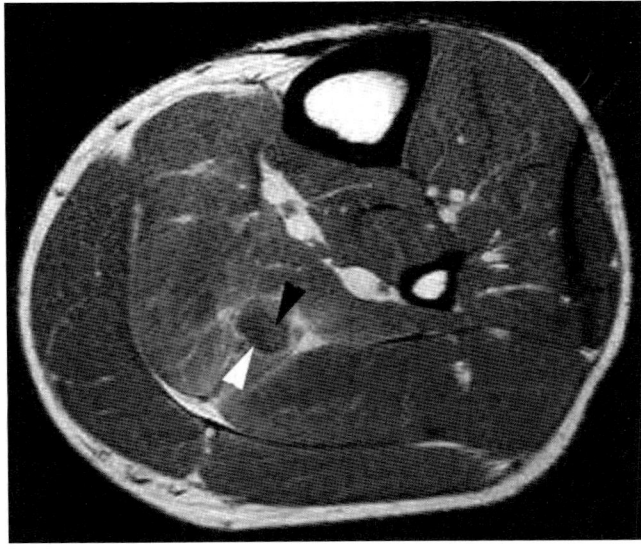

Fig. 9.14 A 28-year-old rugby player with injury to calf 10 days earlier. T1w MR image shows focal contusion with surrounding heterogeneity involving the soleus muscle. Central fat signal intensity (*black arrowhead*) is present with peripheral low signal intensity (*white arrowhead*), which corresponds to the zone of calcification. The features are typical of evolving traumatic myositis ossificans

Imaging of Muscle Injury: Specific Considerations

Appendicular

The most commonly injured muscles in the extremities include the pectoralis major, hamstrings, quadriceps, gastrocnemius, plantaris and adductor muscles.

Pectoralis Major

Although an uncommon sports injury, it is seen more frequently in weight-lifting (particularly in bench-pressing), waterskiing and wrestling. Tears of the pectoralis major muscle tend to occur during powerful eccentric contraction, during which the muscle is subject to concomitant forceful stretching. Partial tears are more common than complete tears (Fig. 9.15). Partial tears typically occur at the MTJ, whereas complete tears occur at the humeral muscle insertion. Rupture of the sternal head occurs more frequently than rupture of the clavicular head. MR imaging is helpful for accurate evaluation of injury and enables identification of patients who would benefit from primary surgical repair [35]. Tendon avulsion from the humeral attachment needs prompt surgical repair, as opposed to a conservative approach for MTJ injuries [36].

Hamstring Muscle Complex

The hamstring muscle complex (HMC) is comprised of semimembranosus, semitendinosus and biceps femoris muscles and are the most commonly injured muscles in sporting activities, especially those involving sudden flexion of the lower extremity (e.g. sprinters, soccer and baseball players). These muscles are important hip extensors and flexors of the knee in the gait cycle. The sudden change in HMC function from a stabilizing role in flexion to rapid activity in extension

Table 9.5 Phasic evolution and MRI features of myositis ossificans

Stage	Lesion characteristics	MRI features
Acute (<2 weeks)	Central area of haemorrhage, necrosis and proliferating fibroblasts surrounded by oedema	• Muscle enlargement and oedema • Isointense on T1W • Hyperintense on T2W/STIR with mass effect
Subacute (2–8 weeks)	Immature osteoid at the periphery with central cystic degeneration	• Best seen on T2W – ring-like pattern of low SI with central hyperintensity • Fluid–fluid levels and adjacent periostitis • Post-contrast rim-enhancement
Chronic (>8 weeks)	Mature bone pattern	• Peripheral hypointensity representing cortical bone • Mixed central SI with fatty changes representing mature trabecular bone

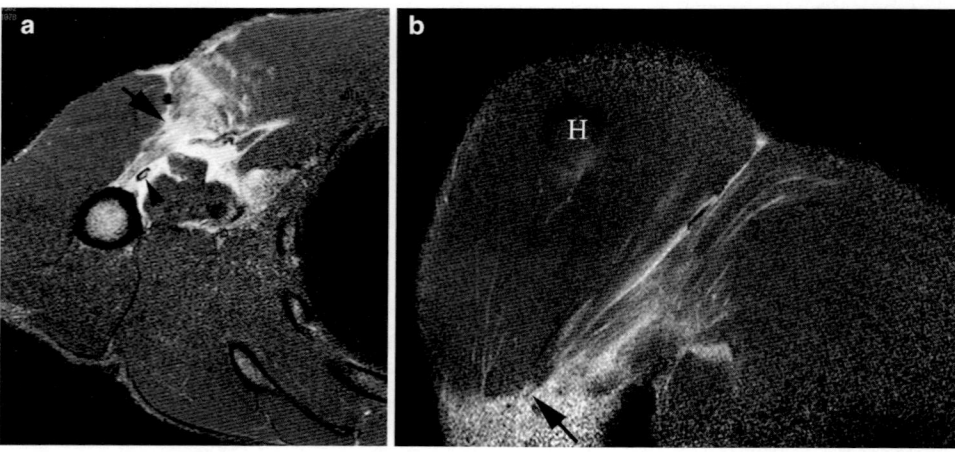

Fig. 9.15 Axial (**a**) and coronal (**b**) STIR MR images showing high-grade partial rupture of pectoralis major typically involving the musculotendinous junction with surrounding fluid and soft-tissue oedema. *Arrowhead* = long head of biceps tendon; *H* humeral head

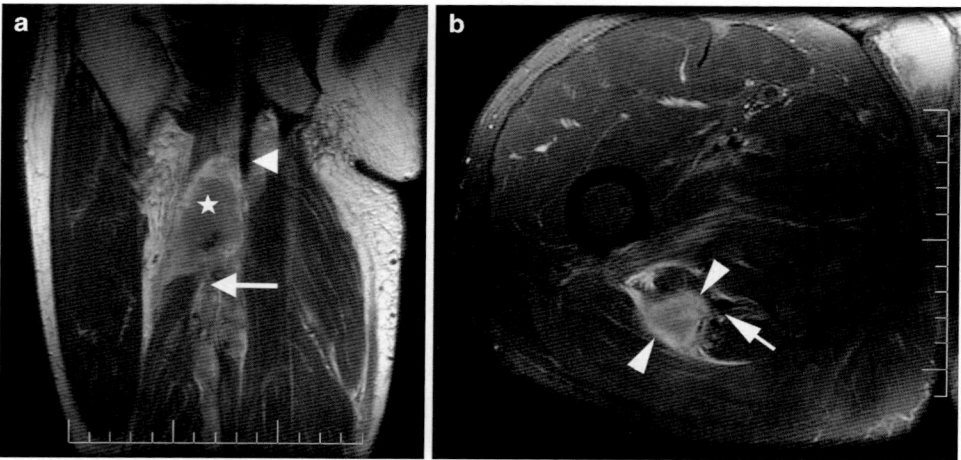

Fig. 9.16 Oblique coronal MR image (**a**) demonstrates a large haematoma (*star*) with retracted fibres of the semitendinosus muscle and the long head of the biceps femoris tendon (*arrow*), features suggestive of an avulsion injury. The semimembranosus muscle (*arrowhead*) is intact. Axial MR image (**b**) shows the haematoma (between *arrowheads*) and disrupted semitendinosus musculotendinous junction (*arrow*)

has been postulated as a cause for injury. Because of their biarticular nature, contraction cannot be localized to one joint, making it crucial for one joint to be stabilized to act on the other. Failure to do so ultimately results in HMC strain. A relative imbalance between the strength of the hamstring and quadriceps muscles, or a significant difference (10% discrepancy) between the two sides of the HMC, have also been suggested as additional biomechanical factors contributing to HMC injury.

In hamstring muscles, the MTJ is represented by a 10–12 cm transition zone rather than being a distinct point. The biceps femoris is the most common individually involved muscle, most injuries being partial tears [16]. In a review of 179 cases with hamstring muscle complex injuries, 80% were shown to involve biceps femoris, with 61% involving the MTJ (Fig. 9.16). MTJ strain in any muscle of the hamstring complex can occur at either end of the muscle (proximal 33%, distal 13%) or within the muscle belly itself (53%) [37]. Multiple muscle involvement may be seen in 30–40% of cases. In an adolescent patient with an unfused ischial apophysis, repeated trauma to the hamstring origin may lead to reactive bone formation.

Quadriceps

Quadriceps injuries are associated with eccentric contraction during vigorous activity in an attempt to control knee flexion (seen in runners and soccer players). The MTJ of the rectus femoris is the most commonly involved site (Fig. 9.9). Different patterns of quadriceps injuries have been described – (1) intramuscular or central tendon (Fig. 9.8), (2) proximal, (3) distal, (4) superficial contusion and (5) pseudotumour [26]. Central tendon injuries have a statistically significant longer time to rehabilitation as compared with peripheral injuries without central tendon involvement (26.8 vs. 9.2 days). This is believed to be secondary to chronic irritation and prolonged healing from the scar formation predisposing to discordant contraction of deep and superficial fibres (Fig. 9.10) [38]. The scar tissue at the injury site may present as a pseudotumour with a painless mass in the anterior thigh [39].

Calf Muscles

Injury most commonly affects the medial head gastrocnemius (86%) and commonly referred to as "tennis leg", with 96% located at the MTJ [40]. Like the hamstring and quadriceps muscles, the gastrocnemius is prone to injury as it spans two joints and has a high proportion of fast-twitch (type II) fibres. These are commonly seen in middle-aged individuals involved in racket sports, skiing or running. Injury to the plantaris tendon can mimic medial gastrocnemius head injury and distinguishing these two entities clinically can be difficult [41]. It is important to have a high clinical suspicion of deep vein thrombosis or thrombophlebitis in athletes presenting with calf pain, as these conditions may occur together or in isolation [42]. The soleus is the second most common calf muscle to be injured (Fig. 9.17). Also, dual injuries of the calf muscle complex occur much more commonly than previously reported and may be of prognostic significance [43].

Adductors

The adductor longus is the most commonly injured muscle (Fig. 9.7b), but other adductors such as adductor brevis, pectineus (Fig. 9.18) and gracilis may be injured. The most common mechanism of injury for this group involves eccentric contraction of the adductors in an attempt to stabilize the hip during contraction of the abductors, as seen in soccer and ice hockey players (Figs. 9.7 and 9.19) [44]. It is of utmost

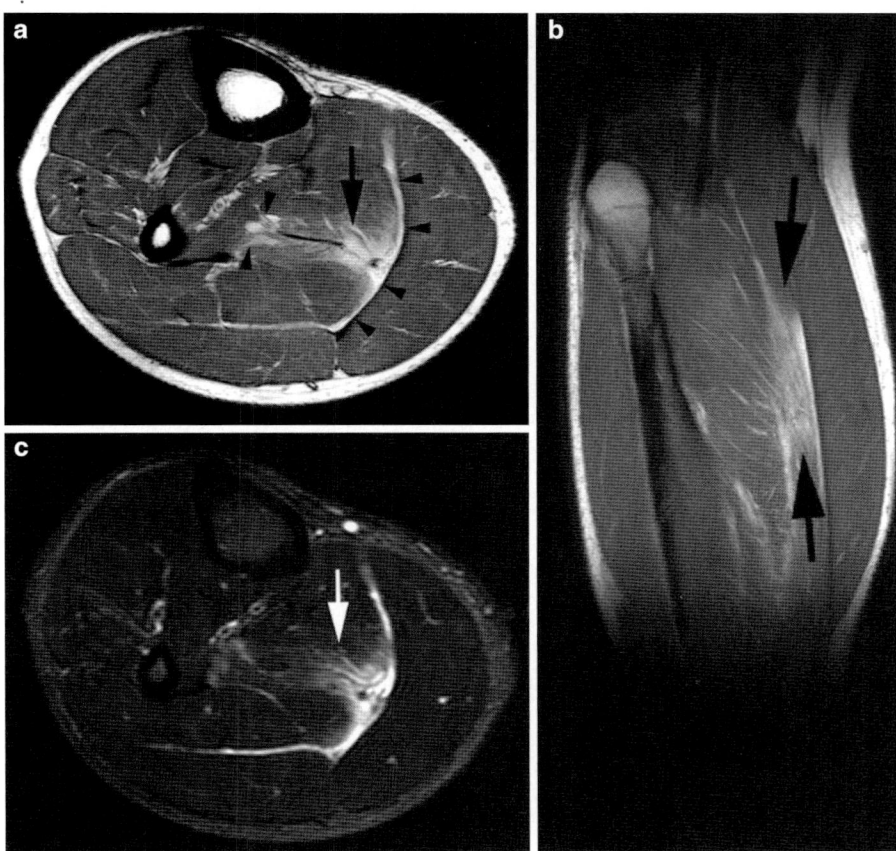

Fig. 9.17 Axial (**a**) and sagittal (**b**) PD-weighted images shows a moderate grade II tear of the soleus (*arrows*) with associated blood/fluid tracking along the fascial planes anteriorly to flexor hallucis longus and posteriorly to medial gastrocnemius (*arrowheads*). Axial PD-weighted fat-suppressed (**c**) image shows the extent of muscle oedema to a better degree

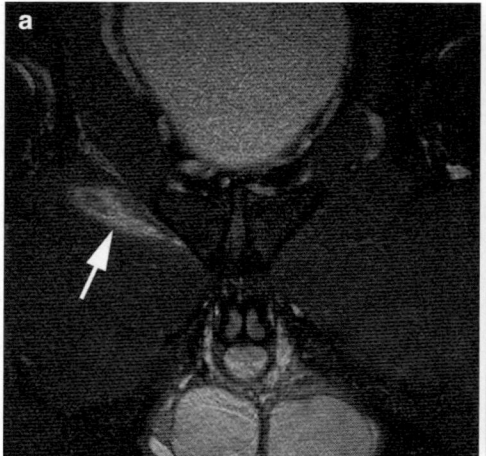
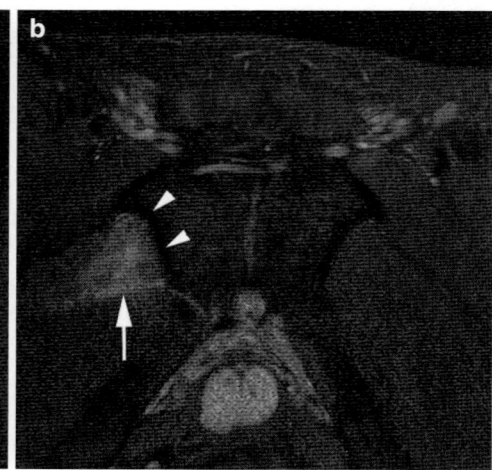

Fig. 9.18 Proton-density-weighted coronal and fat-suppressed axial MR images showing increased signal intensity at the adductor origin, involving the pectineus muscle (*arrow*), in keeping with mild grade II injury. No periosteal (*arrowheads*) oedema or marrow oedema seen, excluding the diagnosis of tenoperiosteal injury

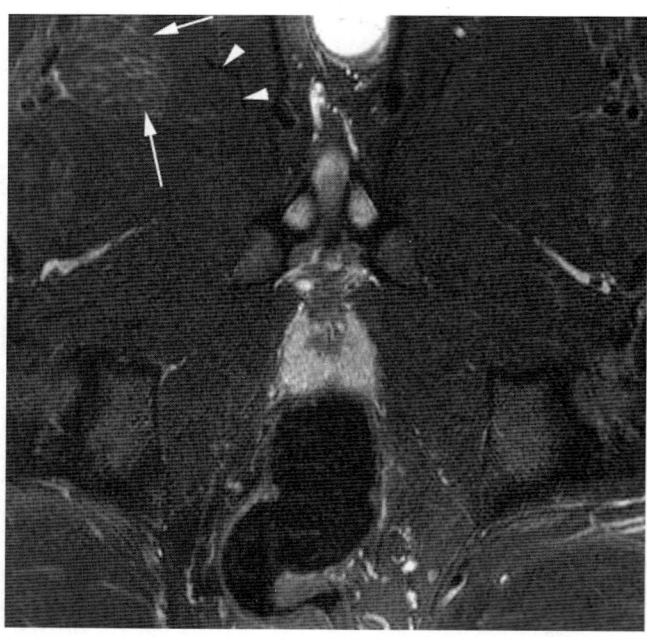

Fig. 9.19 Distal adductor longus tear. Axial oblique T2w FS MR image of the proximal thigh shows a normal right adductor longus proximal myotendinous junction (*arrowheads*) with distal grade II aponeurotic tear (*arrows*)

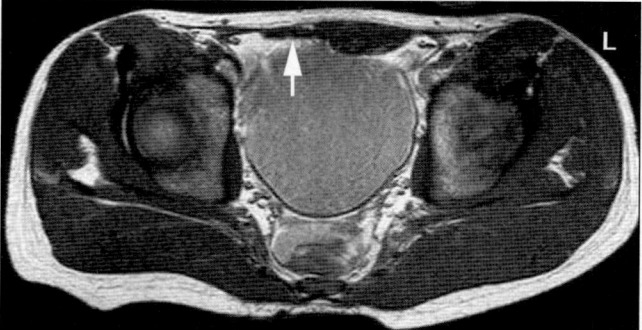

Fig. 9.20 Asymmetry of the rectus abdominis muscles. Axial T1w MR image in an asymptomatic 21-year-old professional footballer shows the right rectus abdominis muscle (*arrow*) to be considerably thinner and smaller in size as compared to the left

Axial

Rectus Abdominis

Rectus abdominis injuries are particularly common in elite tennis players. Eccentric overload, followed by forceful contraction of non-dominant rectus abdominis during the cocking phase of the service motion is the suggested mechanism for this type of injury. Hypertrophy of the contralateral rectus abdominis muscle (the non-dominant arm side) is a common finding in professional tennis players and injuries are most commonly seen involving the distal part (below the umbilicus) of the muscle (Fig. 9.20). Both MR imaging and US are reported to be equally sensitive in the assessment of rectus abdominis injuries, and adequately demonstrate the degree of fibril disruption and retraction [46].

importance to differentiate the routine myotendinous muscle strains of adductor complex from bone–tendon interface injuries or tenoperiosteal injuries. These latter types of injuries are probably sources of chronic pain that do not resolve and more likely associated with chronic groin pain or athletic pubalgia [45].

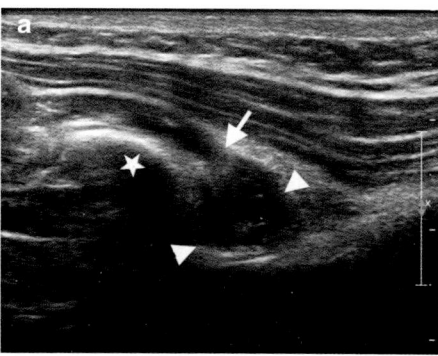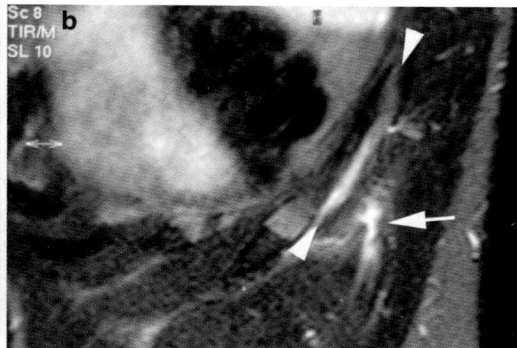

Fig. 9.21 Side-strain injury in a professional cricket player. US image (**a**) shows a disruption of the internal oblique muscle (*arrow*) at the level of 11th rib (*star*) with a small haematoma intervening between the muscle fibres (*arrowheads*). (**b**) Coronal MR image showing haematoma formation (*arrow*) and blood tracking between the fibres of internal and external oblique muscle (*arrowheads*). Associated periosteal stripping and oedema along the rib surface is also noted

Side-Strain

This is a clinical diagnosis characterized by sudden onset of pain and point tenderness over the rib cage and is commonly associated with cricket, javelin throwing, rowing and ice hockey. It is caused by an acute tear of the internal oblique musculature where it inserts into the undersurface of the 9th to 11th rib and is thought to be caused by the sudden eccentric contraction resulting in rupture of muscle fibres. MR imaging can be used for confirming the clinical suspicion of this injury, identify the site and degree of tear as well as to reveal any associated injuries of the thoracic cage. On MR imaging, acute tears are seen as areas of high signal intensity representing oedema and haemorrhage on T1w and STIR images (Fig. 9.21). The periosteal stripping may be seen with haematoma tracking between the myo-fascial coverings of the internal and external oblique muscles [47].

Other Injuries

Other muscle groups are more commonly involved in a particular sport than others, depending upon the type of major activity. For example, in professional baseball players, injuries to the latissimus dorsi and the subscapularis are commonly reported.

Return to Play

In recent years, there have been rising concerns amongst sports physicians, physical therapists and trainers regarding the prognostic factors involved in athlete's return to play. There remains an enormous pressure in professional sporting population to return to play as early as possible, thereby potentially undermining the rehabilitation process. A relative risk of 6.3 has been reported for repeat injury for an 8-week period after initial strain [25]. Even after returning to competition without recurrent injury, it has been shown that player performance rating is reduced in the first 2 weeks of competition [48]. Despite an optimal rehabilitation programme and what is thought to be a sufficient time out of competition, the incidence of repeat injury has been reported to be approximately 30% [5]. It is hoped that these figures will improve with better understanding of prognosis, ability to identify risk factors for repeat injury, an improved understanding of the mechanism of injury, identification of risk management strategies, and improved rehabilitation programmes [49].

With regard to role of imaging in prognostication of sports injury, the severity of injury may be determined in conjugation with the clinical assessment, utilizing specific imaging parameters such as the length, volume or area of injury. The degree of myofibril damage is demonstrated on MR imaging by a proportional increase in dimensions of a strain, as reflected by an increase in the degree of abnormal intramuscular T2w hyperintensity (Fig. 9.22). The length of a muscle injury has been positively correlated with the susceptibility to a recurrent injury [50]. Conversely, a smaller tear is associated with a decreased predicted convalescence period. Also, lack of *any* demonstrable intramuscular signal abnormality on MR imaging does not carry the concomitant increased association for a recurrent strain [51].

Conclusion

The role of imaging in sports-related muscle injury and its associated complications is vital as well as complex. With ever-increasing sporting population, these injuries are

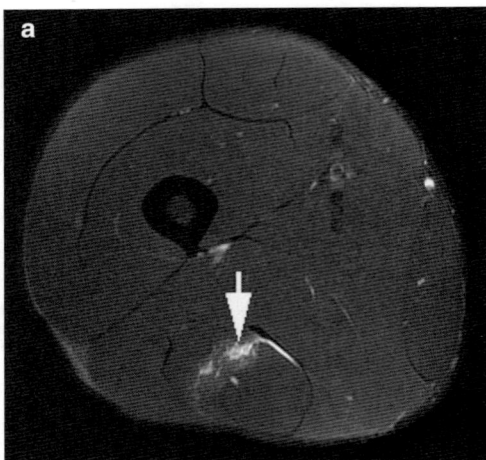 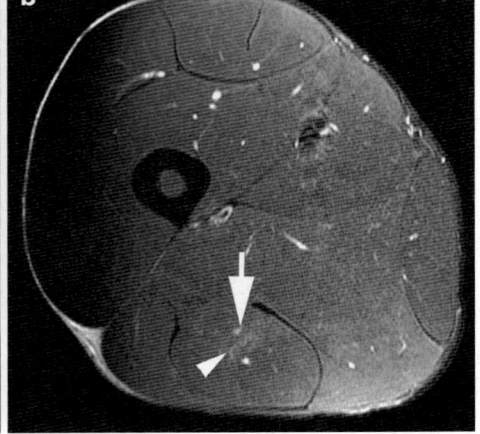

Fig. 9.22 Acute semitendinosus strain in a young athlete. Axial T2w FS images immediately after injury (**a**) shows low-grade epimysial strain with myofibrillar disruption, oedema and blood–fluid products (*arrow*). A follow-up MR image at 4 weeks (**b**) reveals significant resolution of the oedema and blood–fluid products, with only minimal residual hyperintensity (*arrow*) and early granulation tissue formation with intermediate signal (*arrowhead*)

becoming more common. Both MR imaging and US can play a vital role in the diagnosis and management of these injuries, with their own advantages and disadvantages. It is essential to remember that injury usually occurs at the MTJ, which may be intramuscular. The depiction of site, extent and severity of muscle injury can provide decision-making and prognostic information for the elite athlete. With state-of-the-art imaging techniques and precise knowledge, it should be possible to obtain optimal information of the injured region.

Current literature on the prognostication factors for re-injury is rather limited and further research is necessary. With newer rehabilitation and surgical techniques, there is increasing dependence of sport-physicians on imaging modalities. Therefore, a proper evaluation and classification of muscle injury is of considerable importance for early and optimal return of the athlete to the sporting activity.

References

1. Rybak LD, Torriani M (2003) Magnetic resonance imaging of sports-related muscle injuries. Top Magn Reson Imaging 14:209–219
2. van Holsbeeck MT, Kolowich PA, Eyler WR, Craig JG, Shirazi KK, Habra GK, Vanderschueren GM, Bouffard JA (1995) US depiction of partial-thickness tear of the rotator cuff. Radiology 197:443–446
3. Teefey SA, Hasan SA, Middleton WD, Patel M, Wright RW, Yamaguchi K (2000) Ultrasonography of the rotator cuff. A comparison of ultrasonographic and arthroscopic findings in one hundred consecutive cases. J Bone Joint Surg Am 82:498–504
4. Iannotti JP, Zlatkin MB, Esterhai JL, Kressel HY, Dalinka MK, Spindler KP (1991) Magnetic resonance imaging of the shoulder. Sensitivity, specificity and predictive value. J Bone Joint Surg Am 73:17–29
5. Orchard J, Best TM (2002) The management of muscle strain injuries: an early return versus the risk of recurrence. Clin J Sport Med 12:3–5
6. Verrall GM, Slavotinek JP, Barnes PG, Fon GT (2003) Diagnostic and prognostic value of clinical findings in 83 athletes with posterior thigh injury: comparison of clinical findings with magnetic resonance imaging documentation of hamstring muscle strain. Am J Sports Med 31:969–973
7. Heiser TM, Weber J, Sullivan G, Clare P, Jacobs RR (1984) Prophylaxis and management of hamstring muscle injuries in intercollegiate football players. Am J Sports Med 12:368–370
8. Orchard J, Seward H (2002) Epidemiology of injuries in the Australian Football League, seasons 1997-2000. Br J Sports Med 36:39–44
9. Woods C, Hawkins RD, Maltby S, Hulse M, Thomas A, Hodson A (2004) The Football Association Medical Research Programme: an audit of injuries in professional football – analysis of hamstring injuries. Br J Sports Med 38:36–41
10. Boutin RD, Fritz RC, Steinbach LS (2002) Imaging of sports-related muscle injuries. Radiol Clin North Am 40:333–362
11. Nguyen B, Brandser E, Rubin DA (2000) Pains, strains and fasciculations: lower extremity muscle disorders. Magn Reson Imaging Clin N Am 8:391–408
12. Erickson SJ (1997) High-resolution imaging of the musculoskeletal system. Radiology 205:593–618
13. Entrekin RR, Porter BA, Sillesen HH, Wong AD, Cooperberg PL, Fix CH (2001) Real-time spatial compound imaging: application to breast, vascular, and musculoskeletal ultrasound. Semin Ultrasound CT MR 22:50–64
14. Tranquart F, Grenier N, Eder V, Pourcelot L (1999) Clinical use of ultrasound tissue harmonic imaging. Ultrasound Med Biol 25:889–894
15. Connell DA, Schneider-Kolsky ME, Hoving JL, Malara F, Buchbinder R, Koulouris G, Burke F, Bass C (2004) Longitudinal study comparing sonographic and MRI assessments of acute and healing hamstring injuries. AJR Am J Roentgenol 183:975–984
16. Koulouris G, Connell D (2005) Hamstring muscle complex: an imaging review. Radiographics 25:571–586

17. Noonan TJ, Garrett WE (1999) Muscle strain injury: diagnosis and treatment. J Am Acad Orthop Surg 7:262–269
18. Hurme T, Kalimo H, Lehto M, Järvinen M (1991) Healing of skeletal muscle injury: an ultrastructural and immunohistochemical study. Med Sci Sports Exerc 23:801–810
19. Järvinen TA, Järvinen TL, Kääriäinen M, Kalimo H, Järvinen M (2005) Muscle injuries: biology and treatment. Am J Sports Med 33:745–764
20. Crisco JJ, Joki P, Heinen GT, Connell MD, Panjabi MM (1994) A muscle contusion injury model. Biomechanics, physiology, and histology. Am J Sports Med 22:702–710
21. Evans GF, Haller RG, Wyrick PS, Parkey RW, Fleckenstein JL (1998) Submaximal delayed-onset muscle soreness: correlations between MR imaging findings and clinical measures. Radiology 208:815–820
22. Mink JH, Rosenfeld RT (1991) MR views sports-related bony, muscular injuries. Diagn Imaging 13:108–114
23. Palmer WE, Kuong SJ, Elmadbouh HM (1999) MR imaging of myotendinous strain. AJR Am J Roentgenol 173:703–709
24. Garrett WE (1996) Muscle strain injuries. Am J Sports Med 24:S2–S8
25. Orchard JW (2001) Intrinsic and extrinsic risk factors for muscle strains in Australian football. Am J Sports Med 29:300–303
26. Hasselman CT, Best TM, Hughes C, Martinez S, Garrett WE (1995) An explanation for various rectus femoris strain injuries using previously undescribed muscle architecture. Am J Sports Med 23:493–499
27. Fornage BD (2000) The case for ultrasound of muscles and tendons. Semin Musculoskelet Radiol 4:375–391
28. Amendola A, Rorabeck CH, Vellett D, Vezina W, Rutt B, Nott L (1990) The use of magnetic resonance imaging in exertional compartment syndromes. Am J Sports Med 18:29–34
29. Eskelin MK, Lötjönen JM, Mäntysaari MJ (1998) Chronic exertional compartment syndrome: MR imaging at 0.1T compared with tissue pressure measurement. Radiology 206:333–337
30. Verleisdonk EJ, van Gils A, van der Werken C (2001) The diagnostic value of MRI scans for the diagnosis of chronic exertional compartment syndrome of the lower leg. Skeletal Radiol 30:321–325
31. Mellado JM, Pérez del Palomar L (1999) Muscle hernias of the lower leg: MRI findings. Skeletal Radiol 28:465–469
32. De Smet AA, Norris MA, Fisher DR (1992) Magnetic resonance imaging of myositis ossificans: analysis of seven cases. Skeletal Radiol 21:503–507
33. Kransdof MJ, Meis JM, Jelinek JS (1991) Myositis ossificans: MR appearance with radiologic-pathologic correlation. AJR Am J Roentgenol 157:1243–1248
34. Koh ES, McNally EG (2007) Ultrasound of skeletal muscle injury. Semin Musculoskelet Radiol 11:162–173
35. Wolfe SW, Wickiewicz TL, Cavanaugh JT (1992) Ruptures of the pectoralis major muscle. An anatomic and clinical analysis. Am J Sports Med 20:587–593
36. Connell DA, Potter HG, Sherman MF, Wickiewicz TL (1999) Injuries of the pectoralis major muscle: Evaluation with MR imaging. Radiology 210:785–791
37. Koulouris G, Connell DA (2003) Evaluation of the hamstring muscle complex following acute injury. Skeletal Radiol 32:582–589
38. Cross TM, Gibbs N, Houang MT, Cameron M (2004) Acute quadriceps muscle strains: magnetic resonance imaging features and prognosis. Am J Sports Med 32:710–719
39. Temple HT, Kuklo TR, Sweet DE, Gibbons CL, Murphey MD (1998) Rectus femoris muscle tear appearing as a pseudotumor. Am J Sports Med 26:544–548
40. Delgado GJ, Chung CB, Lektrakul N, Azocar P, Botte MJ, Coria D, Bosch E, Resnick D (2002) Tennis leg: clinical US study of 141 patients and anatomic investigation of four cadavers with MR imaging and US. Radiology 224:112–119
41. Helms CA, Fritz RC, Garvin GJ (1995) Plantaris muscle injury: evaluation with MR imaging. Radiology 195:201–203
42. McClure JG (1984) Gastrocnemius musculotendinous rupture: a condition confused with thrombophlebitis. South Med J 77: 1143–1145
43. Koulouris G, Ting AYI, Jhamb A, Connell D, Kavanagh EC (2007) Magnetic resonance imaging findings of injuries to the calf muscle complex. Skeletal Radiol 36:921–927
44. Tyler TF, Nicholas SJ, Campbell RJ, McHugh MP (2001) The association of hip strength and flexibility with the incidence of adductor muscle strains in professional ice hockey players. Am J Sports Med 29:124–128
45. Robinson P, Barron DA, Parsons W, Grainger AJ, Schilders FM, O'Connor PJ (2004) Adductor-related groin pain in athletes: correlation of MR imaging with clinical finding. Skeletal Radiol 33:451–457
46. Connell D, Ali K, Javid M, Bell P, Batt M, Kemp S (2006) Sonography and MRI of rectus abdominis muscle strain in elite tennis players. AJR Am J Roentgenol 187:1457–1461
47. Connell DA, Jhamb A, James T (2003) Side strain: a tear of internal oblique musculature. AJR Am J Roentgenol 181:1511–1517
48. Verrall GM, Kalairajah Y, Slavotinek JP, Spriggins AJ (2006) Assessment of player performance following return to sports after hamstring muscle strain injury. J Sci Med Sport 9:87–90
49. Orchard J, Best TM, Verrall GM (2005) Return to play following muscle strains. Clin J Sports Med 15:436–441
50. Koulouris G, Connell DA, Brukner P, Schneider-Kolsky M (2007) Magnetic resonance imaging parameters for assessing risk of recurrent hamstring injuries in elite athletes. Am J Sports Med 35:1500–1506
51. Schneider-Kolsky ME, Hoving JL, Warren P, Connell DA (2006) A comparison between clinical assessment and magnetic resonance imaging of acute hamstring injuries. Am J Sports Med 34:1008–1015

Chapter 10
Sports-Related Disorders of the Spine and Sacrum

Rob Campbell and Andrew Dunn

Introduction

Modern sports activities are associated with a high incidence of spine pain. Low back pain (LBP) occurs in up to 50% of elite athletes [1]. The majority are under 40 years of age. Most acute spinal injuries are soft tissue related, attributed to muscle and ligament strains, which can be successfully managed with non-invasive therapies.

LBP may not be spine related but secondary to injury at other sites resulting in a breakdown of the bio-mechanical linkage of the spine, pelvis and lower limb. Changes in training regime, running surfaces and even footwear can all be responsible for LBP. It is therefore vital that athletes have a full clinical assessment prior to imaging of the spine.

MRI is the primary imaging modality for diagnosis of most spinal pathology. Fat-suppressed T2W or STIR images are the most sensitive techniques for identifying bone marrow oedema, and should be included in MR protocols for investigation of back pain (Table 10.1). Radiological interpretation should always be informed by clinical findings. Asymptomatic abnormalities such as pars injuries and facet disease in the lower lumbar spine are common in elite athletes [2]. Radiography, CT and SPECT imaging have a limited and specific role in a minority of cases, where MR imaging is normal or required for further evaluation of a bony lesion.

Spinal interventional procedures maybe required as part of the diagnostic or therapeutic management following clinical review. These are often safer and more effectively performed under image guidance.

Anatomy

With the exception of the atlanto-axial articulation, the vertebral segments share a broadly similar morphology throughout the spine. The three-column concept best illustrates the functional and bio-mechanical anatomy of the spine, which is important in understanding the mechanisms of spinal injury and interpreting radiological images.

Anterior and Middle Column

The structures of the anterior and middle column include the vertebral body, the base of the pedicle, the interverbral disc and the supporting ligaments.

Vertebral Body

The vertebrae are formed from up to eight secondary ossification centres which develop at points of ligamentous insertion. The ring apophysis is a raised rim of bone on the periphery of the vertebral body. It is structurally very strong and surrounds the weaker central portion of the vertebral end-plate. This apophysis appears on radiographs by 6 years of age, fusing at 13–17 years.

The lumbar bodies have flat vertebral end-plates. The longitudinal axis of the sacrum is angled 42–45° to the horizontal plane. The spine maintains an upright position by forming the lumbar lordosis to compensate for the sacral angulation. This is achieved by the shape of the lumbo-sacral disc and L5 vertebra which are wedge shaped. The remaining lordotic curve is made up by the other lumbar discs which are slightly compressed posteriorly.

The anterior height of the thoracic vertebral bodies are 2–3 mm less than the posterior height which contributes to the degree of normal thoracic kyphosis (range 25–55°). The cervical end-plates are not flat, but saddle-shaped with an antero-inferior slope and upward curving uncinate joints laterally.

Rob Campbell (✉)
Department of Radiology, Royal Liverpool University Hospital, Liverpool L7 8XP, UK
e-mail: rob.campbell@rlbuht.nhs.uk

Table 10.1 MR protocol for imaging non-specific low back pain

Standard sequences	
Sagittal T1W 3 mm	Thin slices for anatomy of posterior neural arch
Sagittal STIR 4 mm	Identification of bone marrow oedema
Coronal STIR 4 mm	To cover lateral structures, e.g. transverse process and SIJ's
Additional sequences	
In-phase T1W 3D GRE	Anatomy of posterior neural arch with MPR
Oblique sagittal T1W 3 mm	Anatomy of pars interarticularis
Axial T1W and T2W 3 mm	Disc protrusion

Inter-vertebral Disc

The central nucleus pulposus is a semi-fluid mass of proteoglycans and type II collagen fibres which deforms under compression and absorbs axial loading forces. The outer ring of highly ordered collagen fibres called lamellae form the annulus fibrosus. These fibres are predominantly type I collagen which resist radial tension. The lamaellae are thicker anteriorly and laterally. The posterior annulus is the thinnest region and in the cervical spine it is completely deficient with the margin of the disc covered by the posterior longitudinal ligament.

The vertebral end-plates have layers of cartilage of 0.6–1 mm thickness and are encircled by the ring apophysis. The peripheral rim of the annulus is not covered by the cartilaginous end-plate but attaches to the ring apophysis directly by perforating Sharpey's fibres.

Ligaments

The stability of the anterior and middle column is maintained by the anterior longitudinal (ALL) and posterior longitudinal ligaments (PLL). They are composed of type 1 collagen fibres of varying length that span from one to five inter-body joints and attach to the periosteum. The PLL is narrower than the ALL, although the deep fibres spread out laterally to cover the posterior borders of the inter-vertebral discs. The ALL is only loosely attached to the anterior annulus fibrosus. The longitudinal ligaments resist tension and separation of the vertebral bodies in flexion and extension.

Stability of the C1/2 articulation is maintained anteriorly by the apical and alar ligaments which attach to the skull base and odontoid process, and the transverse ligament which extends horizontally from the anterior arch of C1 over the posterior aspect of the odontoid process.

The Posterior Column

The posterior column is formed by the pedicle, transverse process, pars interarticularis, articular processes, laminae and spinous processes.

Facet Joints

The inter-vertebral facet or zygo-apophyseal joints are synovial joints formed by the superior and inferior articular processes. They are lined by hyaline cartilage, enclosed in a fibrous capsule which is loose at the superior and inferior poles of the joint forming sub-capsular pockets. The facet joints stabilise the posterior column by limiting excessive inter-vertebral movement and preventing forward vertebral translation.

The orientation of the articular facets varies throughout the spine depending on their functional role. Facet joints aligned nearer the coronal plane (e.g. lumbar spine), limit forward displacement whereas facets aligned nearer the sagittal plane (e.g. thoracic spine) limit rotation but are less restrictive to forward displacement. The downward slope of the S1 body results in a tendency for the L5 vertebra to slide forwards. This is resisted by the superior articular processes of the sacrum which face directly backwards providing a locking mechanism, and reducing the range of axial rotation.

Pars Interarticularis

The region of the lamina between the superior and inferior articular processes forms the pars interarticularis. The pars is subject to considerable strain as the forces transmitted by the lamina undergo a change of direction into the pedicle [3]. The lumbar pars are oriented near the sagittal plane in the lower lumbar spine and more obliquely in the upper lumbar spine.

Ligaments of Posterior column

The ligamentum flavum, interspinous and supraspinous ligaments are static stabilisers of the posterior column. The ligamentum flavum is short and thick and spans consecutive laminae. It attaches to the anterior aspects of the articular processes forming the anterior capsule of the facet joint. The interspinous ligament runs between the surfaces of the spinous processes. The ventral part of the ligaments blends with the ligamentum flavum. Surprisingly, bio-mechanical studies have shown that the flaval ligament does not significantly limit separation of the spinous processes during flexion [4].

The supraspinous ligament extends across the dorsal surfaces of the spinous processes, blending with the dorsal fibres of the interspinous ligament. It is largely composed of fibres contributed by the dorsal spinal musculature and is not a true ligament.

The Sacro-Iliac Joint

The sacro-iliac joint (SIJ) is oriented vertically and antero-laterally. The antero-inferior two-thirds of the joint are lined by articular cartilage which is thinner on the iliac aspect of the joint. The SIJ is part synovial and part symphyseal similar to the symphysis pubis. The postero-superior portion of the joint is a syndesmosis, stabilised by the inter-osseous ligament. The other static stabilisers of the SIJ are the anterior and posterior SI ligaments and the sacrospinous, sacro-tuberous and ilio-lumbar ligaments.

The SIJ is subject to vertical shear forces as the weight of the trunk is transmitted to the lower limbs. The interlocking contours of the articular surfaces help maintain stability allowing only limited downward gliding and rotational movement under loading [5]. The dynamic stabilisers of the joint include the gluteus maximus muscle which acts perpendicular to the joint line, and the biceps femoris muscle which takes one of its attachments from the sacro-tuberous ligament. The degree of SIJ motion is greater in females than males [6], and decreases with age due to progressive fibrous union.

Biomechanics

Cervical Spine

The function of the atlanto-occipital joint is primarily flexion and extension (range 15–20°). Rotation and lateral flexion of the atlanto-occipital joint is restricted by the depth of the C1 articular facets. The C1/2 articulation produces rotation (range 32–35° in each direction) limited by the alar ligaments. Rotation is facilitated by the bi-convex chondral surfaces of the C1/2 lateral masses. This relationship results in paradoxical C1 flexion and extension with respect to the lower cervical spine (i.e. during cervical flexion the atlas extends) [7].

Axial rotation of the cervical column (C3–7) occurs around a modified axis orientated in a plane which is almost parallel to the plane of the vertebral end-plates [8]. The cervical articular facets are concave, allowing rotation as well as flexion and extension, but lateral flexion is restricted. Flexion and extension are initiated in the lower cervical spine from C4 to C7.

Thoracic Spine

The anterior vertebral bodies provide the primary load-bearing capacity of the thoracic spine. The posterior elements resist tensile forces. The rib cage is a bio-mechanical extension of the spine adding stiffness and resisting rotational forces, particularly during extension and to a lesser degree in flexion and lateral rotation. It acts as an energy-absorbing structure, dissipating axial loads during trauma by an estimated factor of four [9]. Traumatic costo-vertebral dissociation reduces the spine's ability to tolerate normal physiological loads.

Each vertebra is subject to compression, tension and shear forces. The latter are incident through the discs and may occur antero-posteriorly, laterally or by axial torsion. The flexion and compression forces are the most important, and are counter-acted by the tensile forces of the extensor musculature. The vertebra at the apex of the dorsal kyphotic curvature is under the greatest flexion moment being furthest from the vertical line of gravity. Weakness or fatigue of the thoracic extensor muscles leads to an increase in flexion forces on the vertebrae due to imbalance of the opposing tensile forces. Excessive flexion and compression may cause bio-mechanical imbalance during athletic training activities such as rapid acceleration (e.g. weight lifting) and deceleration (e.g. landing from a jump) [10].

Lumbar Spine

The lumbar spine is subject to a wide range of forces and movements, which probably explains the prevalence of LBP.

Axial Compression

Axial compression is exerted on the lumbar spine during weight bearing and by contraction of the longitudinal muscles. The inter-vertebral discs absorb this force with height reduction and radial bulging. Axial compression is greatest at the lumbo-sacral junction where the normal lumbar lordosis transforms some of the axial compressive force into shearing force. Running increases the axial load on the lumbo-sacral junction in excess of three times the body weight above L5 [11].

The exact role of the facet joints in the distribution of axial loading of the spine is unclear. In the relaxed sitting position the facet joints do not bear any axial load. During prolonged standing the disc compresses and the inferior articular processes may impact on the lamina of the vertebra below. Axial loading on the facet joints also occurs during lumbar spine extension. Axial distraction produces strain forces on the annulus, longitudinal ligaments and facet joint capsules, although this is uncommon in most sporting activities.

Flexion

During lumbar spine flexion the lumbar lordosis straightens and may even reverse at L4/5. Vertebral flexion (anterior sagittal rotation) includes an element of forward translation. The facet joints limit the degree of anterior sagittal rotation by absorbing tension in the joint capsule. The inferior articular processes slide over the superior articular processes by up to 5–7 mm. The posterior ligaments also resist flexion. Dividing the dorsal ligaments increases flexion by 5°, and dividing the facet joint capsules allows another 4° of flexion [12].

Lateral Flexion

The biomechanics of lateral flexion are complex and involve interactions between lateral bending and axial rotation. Excessive lateral flexion on the "trailing side" is encountered during the follow-through phase of the modern golf swing, and is associated with unilateral LBP and facet OA [13].

Extension

In extension (posterior sagittal rotation), the vertebrae undergo a small degree of posterior translation. This is limited by tension in the anterior annulus and ALL, and also by buckling of the interspinous ligament which becomes trapped between the spinous processes. Extension may also be limited by impaction of the spinous processes.

The inferior articular processes impact upon the laminae of the vertebra below and this downward force is transmitted into the region of the pars interarticularis. This action may explain the patho-mechanics of lumbar spondylolysis which has a higher incidence in sports that involve hyperextension.

Rotation

Axial rotation of the lumbar spine produces torsion which acts on the inter-vertebral discs and facet joints. The collagen fibres of the annulus orientated in the direction of rotation are under strain, whilst the remainder of the fibres are relaxed. The disc can sustain degrees of rotation up to 3° until microscopic collagen fibre failure ensues, with macroscopic failure occurring at around 12°. Axial rotation is limited anteriorly by the annulus fibrosus and posteriorly by the interspinous and supraspinous ligaments. The facet joints also play a major role in limiting axial rotation. During rotation the contra-lateral articular facets are compressed. The erector spinae, multifidus and quadratus lumborum muscles act as key core stabilisers of the lumbar spine during axial rotation. Poor coordination and fatigue of theses muscles are probable factors of LBP in golfers [14].

Acute Spinal Trauma

Fortunately acute spinal fractures are relatively rare occurrences. They occur most frequently in contact sports such as rugby, American football, and high velocity sports such as skiing and motor sports. Prevention of spinal injuries is a high priority. Whenever an athlete sustains an injury with suspicion of a spinal fracture, they should be immobilised and transferred to hospital for urgent evaluation. Bone and ligamentous injury is evaluated with CT and MR imaging to assess fracture stability, and to exclude multiple fractures.

Prevention of spinal injuries is important for athletes with congenital or acquired spinal abnormality. This particularly applies to athletes with Down's syndrome who have a 15% incidence of atlanto-occipital or atlanto-axial instability.

The Special Olympics Inc. recommendations state that Down's syndrome athletes participating in high-risk activities should be screened with flexion/extension radiographs. An atlanto-dental interval (ADI) of greater than 4.5 mm in children disqualifies the athlete form participating in high-risk activities. This restriction can be waived by the athlete or parent/guardian, and with written certification by two examining physicians. Radiological evidence of instability merits evaluation with MRI. However, this advice is controversial as there is no documented evidence of neurologic injury resulting from participation in sport by "at-risk" individuals [15].

It is also important to distinguish between symptomatic and asymptomatic C1/2 instability. British Gymnastics recommendations do not include radiography for screening Down's syndrome athletes. Participation is dependant upon medical certification that there are no features of progressive myelopathy, that the chin can flex to the chest and there is good muscular control of the head and neck [16]. Advice should be sought from the relevant governing bodies for individuals with disability wishing to participate in sports.

Cervical Spine

Axial loading with the head and neck flexed to approximately 30° results in loss of the normal cervical lordosis and, neutralises the energy-absorbing properties of the spine. This occurs during American Football when a player deliberately strikes another with the crown of the helmet known as a "Spear Tackle." The neck is exposed to a compressive load from the torso producing transient deformation or buckling, which may result in compression burst fractures and spinal cord injury. "Spearing" has been banned as a tackling technique since 1976. Axial loading injury may be sustained during other sports such as rugby during scrum engagement or collapse and following a knee to the head injury [17].

Other mechanisms of injury such as forced hyper-flexion with compression may result in disruption and anterior subluxation of the facet joints and articular process fractures at C2–C7. In rugby players this mechanism of injury is most commonly seen in front row forwards during scrummaging (Fig. 10.1) [17]. This can also cause acute cervical disc extrusion, with or without PLL rupture. The cervical spine can be flexed through greater than 90°, and hyper-flexion alone is rarely implicated as a significant mechanism of injury.

Hyper-extension injuries may be seen during the engaging phase of the rugby scrum. This mechanism produces focal narrowing of the spinal canal producing cord impingement or compression and in severe cases may also lead to fractures of the posterior elements due [18]. The prognosis is poor if neurological injury is sustained.

Thoraco-Lumbar Spine

Fractures of the thoraco-lumbar spine are rarer than cervical spine injuries. Serious spinal injuries may represent up to 10% of all hospital admissions from snow sport-related injuries [19], and often occur around the around the dorso-lumbar junction [19, 20]. Simple wedge fractures are the commonest fracture type [20]. Burst fractures are more frequent in skiers [20], and multiple fractures occur in up to 50% of cases. There are sporadic reports of unusual fractures which reflect the unpredictable mechanisms of injury.

The thoraco-lumbar spine sustains significant flexion-distractions forces during certain sports such as gymnastics, American Football and Rugby, soccer and cricket which may result in either chronic repetitive micro-trauma or acute avulsion and fracturing of the spinal apophyses in the adolescent athlete [21]. Apophyseal avulsion fractures are rare in the mature skeleton [22].

Stress Fractures

Stress fractures of the posterior elements occur during adolescence and early adulthood, and most frequently affect the pars interarticularis. Established fractures of the pars are referred to as spondylolysis, and are most common in activities that involve significant flexion, extension and rotation of the lumbar spine, such as soccer, cricket, gymnastics, rowing and American football [23].

Patients present with LBP, which is worse in extension, and with hamstring pain and tightness. There maybe reduced straight leg raising. Imaging is used to identify and grade stress injuries and to exclude other causes of back pain. The ideal modality for imaging of pars stress fractures remains controversial.

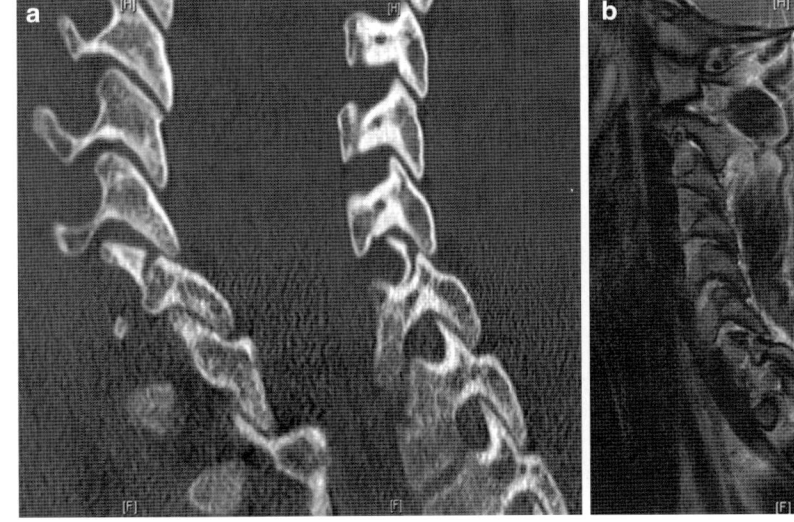
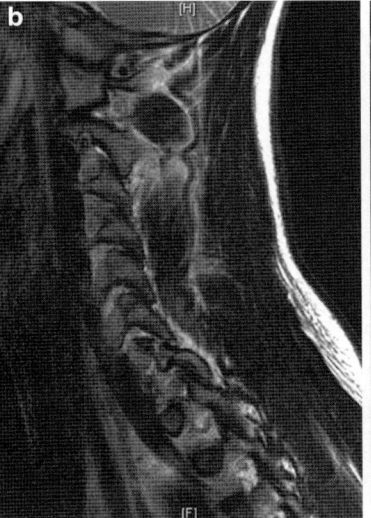
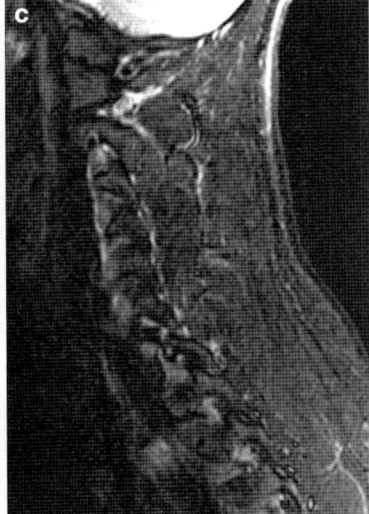

Fig. 10.1 Consecutive para-sagittal CT images (**a**) of a rugby player who sustained a flexion injury of the spine during collapse of a scrum. There is a unilateral facet fracture at C7 with minimal subluxation. The correlative sagittal T2W (**b**) and STIR images (**c**) also show the fracture and associated effusion and haemorrhage within the adjacent facet joints. This is a stable injury

Pars Interarticularis

Pars stress fractures occur most commonly at the L4 and L5 levels. They may be unilateral or bilateral. Unilateral fractures predispose to development of contra-lateral fractures [24]. Multi-level fractures may be encountered, which may be of variable duration. Isolated defects above the L3 level are uncommon.

Radiology cannot reliably distinguish chronic non-union of a stress fracture from developmental pars defects that arise in the first decade of life. However, differentiation of these two lesions is largely academic as it does not influence clinical management.

Imaging

Several radiographic projections of the lumbar spine maybe used for detection of pars defects (i.e. AP and lateral views, oblique lateral views and angled AP views). However, whilst chronic established pars defects may be evident on radiographs, acute stress fractures cannot be reliably detected (Fig. 10.2) [25]. Therefore, radiography should be avoided, except in selected cases, to reduce the radiation dose to the spine of adolescents.

CT is the gold standard for confirming the integrity of the posterior neural arch. Pars defects are identified by the "incomplete ring sign on reversed axial images" (Fig. 10.3) [26], or on oblique axial and sagittal multi-planar reconstructions (MPR). CT is less useful for assessment of the age and grade of stress fractures.

Isotope bone scans are best performed with SPECT imaging to provide the greatest sensitivity and image resolution [25]. Increased uptake is seen in the region of the pars interarticularis in acute stress fractures. However, SPECT cannot exclude chronic pars defects, and cannot distinguish between grade I, II or III lesions (Table 10.2). Combined imaging with CT and SPECT is the gold standard test for diagnosis and grading of pars stress fractures, but involves a large radiation dose, and is difficult to justify for repeated evaluation in patients with recurrent episodes of LBP. Combined CT/SPECT is also limited for detection of other spinal pathology

MRI can accurately demonstrate the normal intact pars, and has been shown to correlate closely with combined SPECT/CT for the diagnosis and grading of stress fractures [27]. This requires the use of appropriate MR protocols which include thin section sagittal T1W images and STIR or fat-saturated T2W imaging (Table 10.1).

Grade 0: Normal Pars

On MR images the intact pars has an intact inferior and superior cortex, with fatty marrow in the medulla. Low signal areas due to partial volume effects or sclerosis may interrupt the normal marrow signal (Fig. 10.4). Diffuse ill-defined low

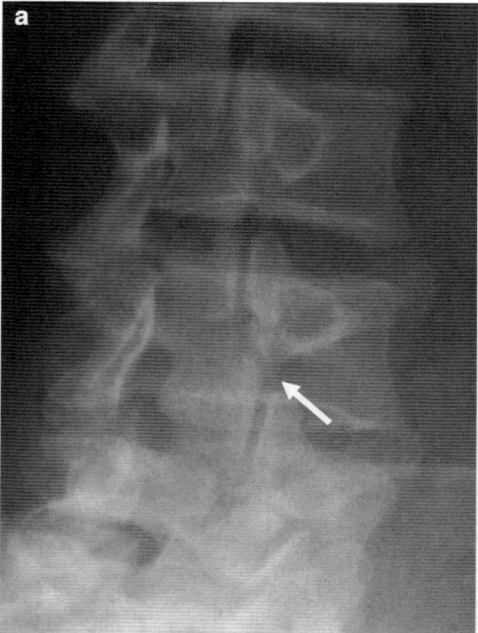
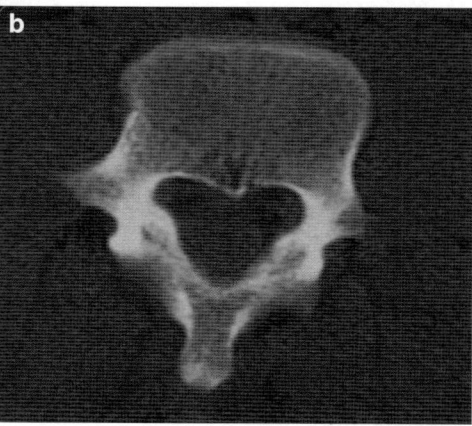

Fig. 10.2 Oblique radiograph of the lumbar spine shows a possible lucent line in the neck of the "scotty dog" (*white arrow*) suggestive of pars defect (**a**). However the corresponding oblique axial CT is normal (**b**)

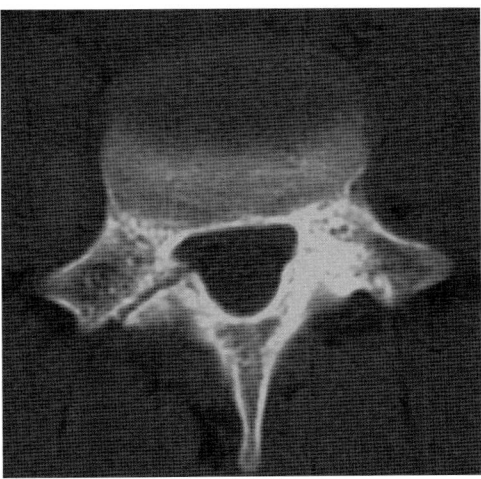

Fig. 10.3 Incomplete ring sign on reversed axial CT with right-sided pars fracture

Table 10.2 Grading of pars stress fractures by stages of development

Grade	
0	Normal intact pars interarticularis
I	Stress reaction (no cortical fracture)
II	Incomplete fracture (typically involves the inferior cortex of pars)
III	Acute complete fracture (with residual osteoblastic activity)
IV	Chronic complete fracture (fracture non-union or developmental defect)

signal is consistent with an intact pars, but a discrete low signal line running transversely across the pars may be a sign of a defect [28].

Oblique pars may need to be viewed over more than one para-sagittal image, particularly in the upper lumbar spine. Oblique sagittal, oblique axial or 3D gradient echo/spin echo MPR images may improve delineation of the pars.

Grade I: Stress Reaction

Stress reaction is identified as marrow oedema on MRI or increased uptake on SPECT without a cortical break on CT (Fig. 10.5). However, the significance of stress reaction is uncertain as it is recognised that isotope uptake may be encountered at asymptomatic sites in athletic individuals [29]. Sclerosis on CT alone is not a reliable sign of a stress reaction.

Grade II: Incomplete Stress Fracture

Pars fractures consistently propagate from the inferior cortex to the superior cortex of the pars [27, 30]. An incomplete fracture is identified as a break in the inferior cortex alone on CT with increased uptake on SPECT or marrow oedema

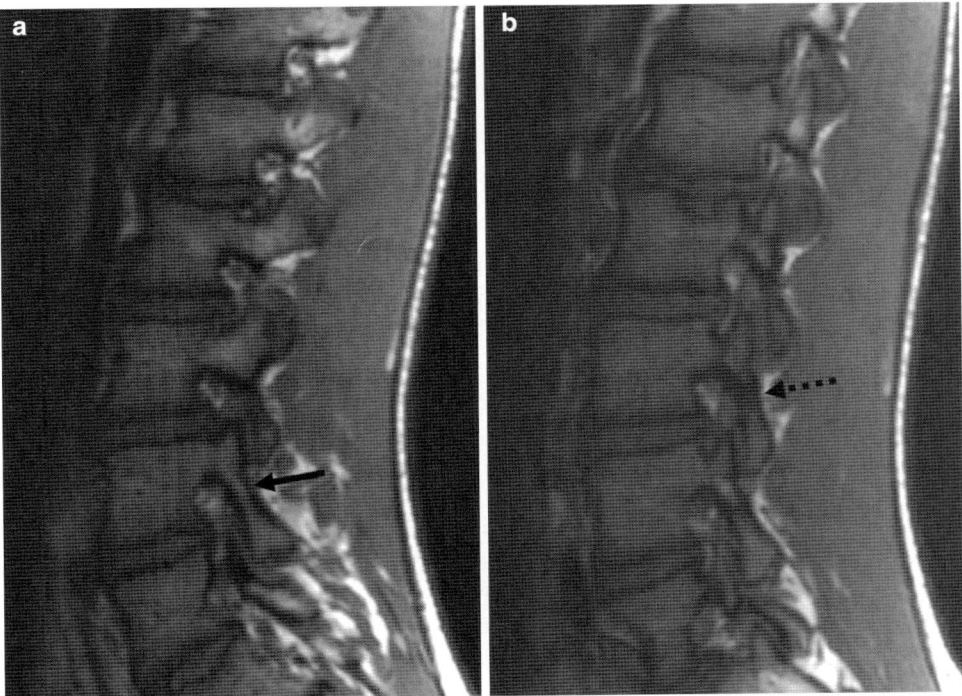

Fig. 10.4 Consecutive para-sagittal T1W images of normal pars (**a** and **b**). The L4 pars has intact cortices with normal uninterrupted fatty marrow signal (*black arrow*). The L3 pars shows an area of low SI consistent with bony sclerosis or partial volume effects (*broken arrow*), but no cortical defect. This finding in isolation is not secondary to stress reaction

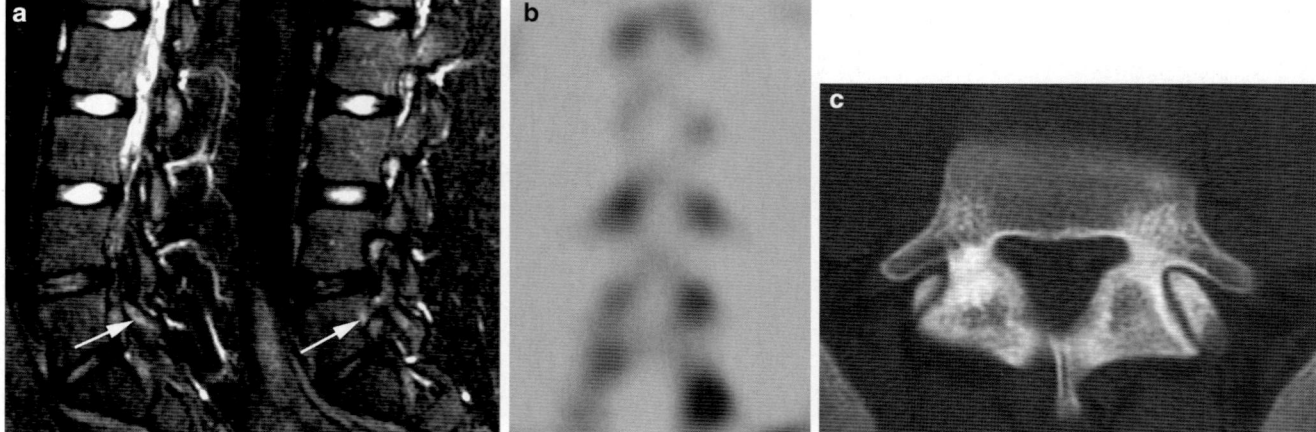

Fig. 10.5 Grade I stress reaction of the pars interarticularis. Consecutive para-sagittal STIR images (**a**) show marrow oedema in the left L5 pars (*white arrows*). There is increased uptake on the SPECT image (**b**), and the oblique axial CT through the same level shows no evidence of fracture (**c**)

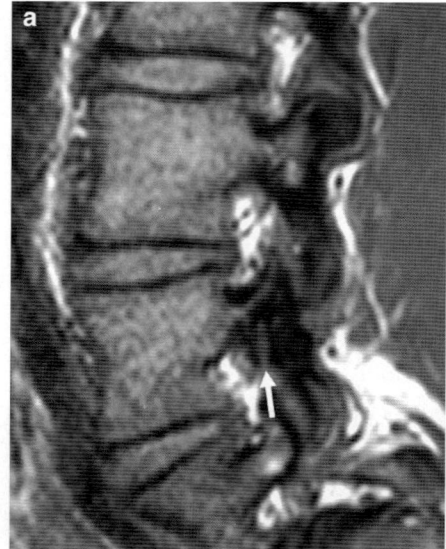
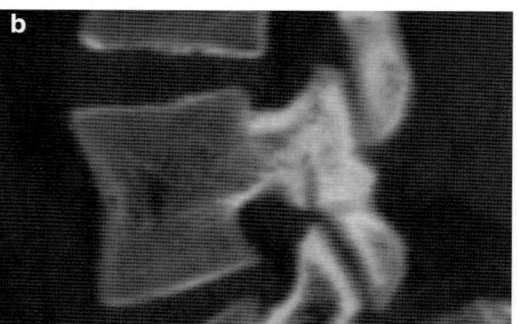

Fig. 10.6 Grade II incomplete stress fracture of the pars interarticularis. There is a cortical break of the inferior margin of the pars on the T1W 3D GRE sequence (**a**). The fracture line propagates superiorly (*white arrow*). The fracture is confirmed on the CT image (**b**). High SI marrow oedema was present on the STIR images (not shown)

on STIR sequences. On MRI the cortical break is best demonstrated on T1-W images (Fig. 10.6). The fatty marrow signal may or may not be interrupted by low signal sclerosis.

Grade III: Complete Active Stress Fracture

The pars fracture is complete when the fracture propagates through the superior cortex. If the fracture is recent there will be persistent increased uptake on SPECT or marrow oedema on STIR images. The cortical breaks are identified on T1-W images as interruption of the normal fatty marrow by an area of intermediate SI, and low signal sclerosis may be present in the adjacent pars (Fig. 10.7).

Grade IV: Complete Inactive Fractures

If the pars fracture progresses to non-union, or if the lesion is developmental, SPECT imaging is normal and there is no marrow oedema on the STIR images (Fig. 10.8). However, the appearances are otherwise the same as grade III fractures. In established non-union, pronounced fatty marrow replacement may be seen in the adjacent pars on either side of the defect.

It is not uncommon to encounter fractures of different grades, particularly with fractures at more than one level. There may be additional features such as fragmentation of the margins of the pars fracture [31], and this is commoner in chronic grade-IV lesions (Fig. 10.17e). Small bony ossicles related to the superior and inferior articular facets have been

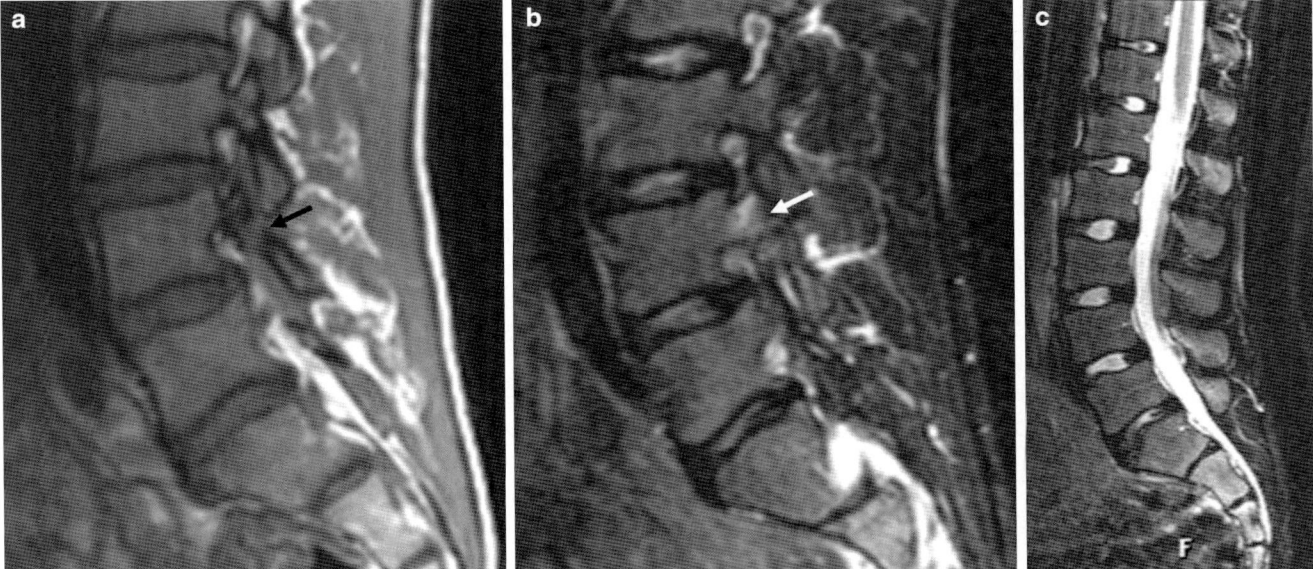

Fig. 10.7 Grade III stress fracture of the pars interarticularis. There is a cortical defect extending through the superior and inferior margins of the pars on the T1W image (**a**), with intermediate SI within the defect (*black arrow*). Reactive marrow oedema is present on the STIR image (**b**) (*white arrow*). The midline sagittal STIR image (**c**) also shows anterior Schmorl node formation without reactive oedema at the L1 and S1 levels

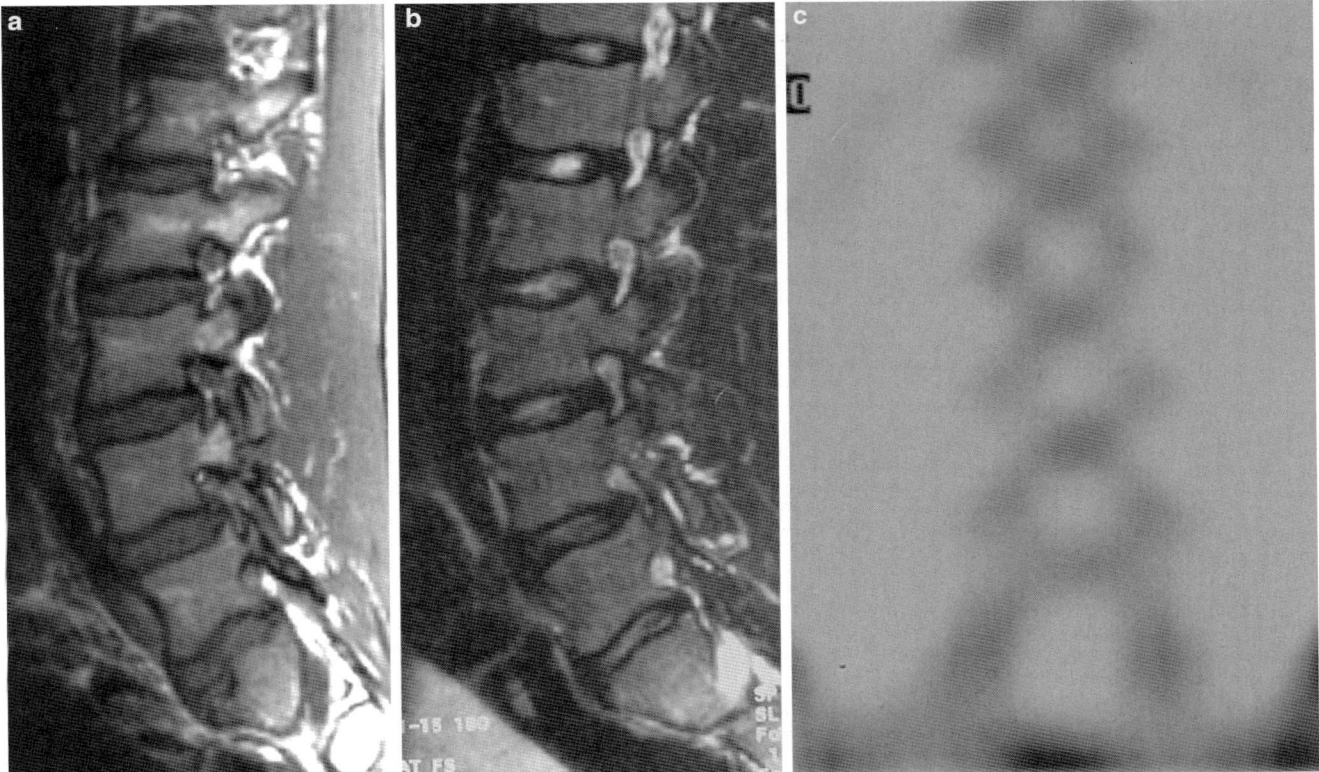

Fig. 10.8 Grade-IV fracture of the L4 pars interarticularis. There is a complete defect of the pars on the sagittal T1W image (**a**). No reactive marrow oedema is present on the STIR image (**b**), although facet joint effusions are present. The SPECT image is normal (**c**)

observed in association with stress fractures of the pars interarticularis, but their significance remains unclear [32]. Isolated stress fractures of the articular processes have been described in gymnasts and ballet dancers.

Fracture Healing

Several parameters predict fracture healing. Incomplete fractures and unilateral fractures are more likely to heal than complete fractures, and bilateral or multi-level fractures. Wide fracture margins, smooth sclerotic margins or bony fragmentation are also poor prognostic indicators. However, one of the most important factors is patient compliance with shutdown of physical activity.

Fractures unite over a variable period of 3–6 months with occasional progressive bony union up to 12 months from diagnosis [30]. CT is the ideal image modality for assessment of fracture union. CT imaging targeted at the affected levels can reduce the radiation dose to the equivalent of a standard radiographic series.

Progressive diffuse sclerosis and obliteration of the fracture line are indicators of fracture healing (Fig. 10.9). Increasing fracture width, fragmentation or increasing delineation of the fracture margins with sclerotic borders indicates non-union (Fig. 10.10). Repeat MR will show loss of marrow oedema over the first 3–6 months but is less accurate than CT in assessing fracture union. SPECT imaging may remain positive for many months after initial diagnosis.

Patient Management

Management is guided by accurate grading of pars stress fractures. The aim is to achieve fracture healing and prevent non-union and complications such as spondylolisthesis.

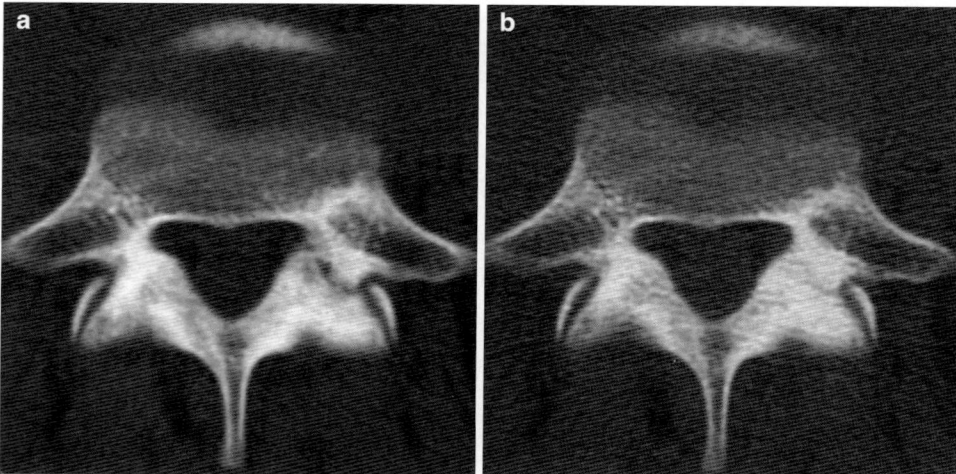

Fig. 10.9 Left-sided grade III pars fracture on reversed axial CT (**a**). Marrow oedema was present on the corresponding STIR MR images (not shown). Follow-up CT (**b**) at 6 months shows near complete bony union

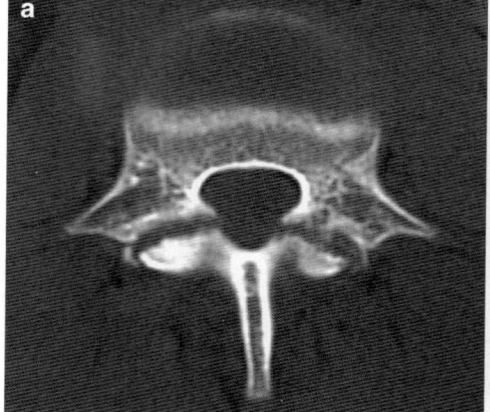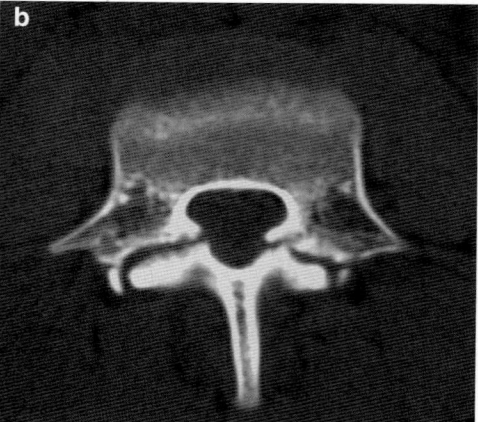

Fig. 10.10 Grade III bilateral pars fractures on oblique axial CT (**a**). The acute fracture margins are ill-defined and irregular with minimal sclerosis. Marrow oedema was present on the corresponding STIR MR images (not shown). Follow-up CT at 6 months shows non-union with smooth sclerotic fracture margins (**b**)

Targeted CT should be performed as a baseline and to distinguish between type I, II and III lesions in the presence of marrow oedema on MR or increased uptake on SPECT.

Grade I stress lesions can be managed by shut down of physical activity until pain symptoms settle followed by spinal rehabilitation. Follow-up imaging and treatment with a brace is not usually required in the majority of cases.

Grade II and III lesions are also treated by shutdown of physical activity and in many cases the use of a spinal brace is advocated. The fractures are assessed by follow-up CT performed at 3 monthly intervals. When back pain has resolved and CT confirms progressive bony union, the patient can commence spinal rehabilitation.

Patients with grade-IV lesions (and grade II/III lesions that progress to non-union) can be rehabilitated and return to normal sporting activities, although athletes with chronic LBP may require specialist treatment.

Pedicle Fractures

Pedicle fractures are much less common than fractures of the pars. They are most commonly seen as insufficiency fractures in association with osteoporosis (Fig. 10.11) or as a complication of spinal surgical fusion.

Bilateral pedicle stress fractures or unilateral pedicle fractures associated with contra-lateral pars fractures may occur in elite athletes [33]. However, the more common pattern of involvement is the propagation of a pars fracture into the pedicle (Fig. 10.12).

The clinical presentation and imaging protocols are the same as pars fractures. They are usually vertically orientated in the coronal plane unlike the horizontal plane of Chance fractures. Bilateral pedicle fractures carry the same risk of non-union and spondylolisthesis as pars fractures, and monitoring of bony healing with CT is important.

Transverse Process Fractures

Acute fractures of the transverse processes are caused by direct impact injuries or violent muscular contraction. However stress fractures can occur without a history of injury. Avulsion injuries are usually the result of torsional forces transmitted through the transverses abdominis and quadratus lumborum muscles at the attachments of the mid lumbar fascia at the L2–L4 levels [34].

Transverse process fractures are usually unilateral and may involve up to three lumbar segments [35]. It is important to differentiate fractures from un-fused transverse apophyses in the adolescent. Unlike transverse process fractures

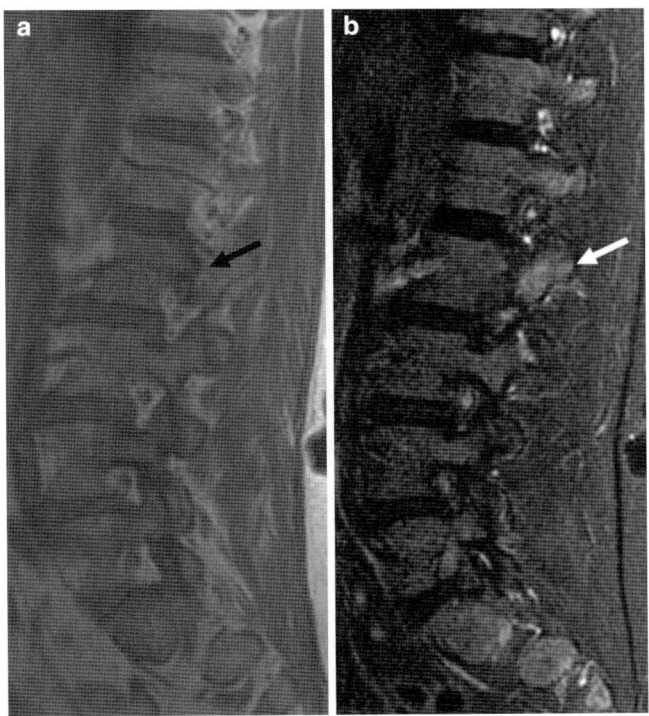

Fig. 10.11 Elderly female runner with recent onset back pain. The sagittal T1W image (**a**) shows a vertical low signal fracture line running though the L2 pedicle (*black arrow*). Reactive marrow oedema is present on the sagittal STIR image (**b**) (*white arrow*). The appearances are consistent with insufficiency fracture and the patient was referred for bone densitometry

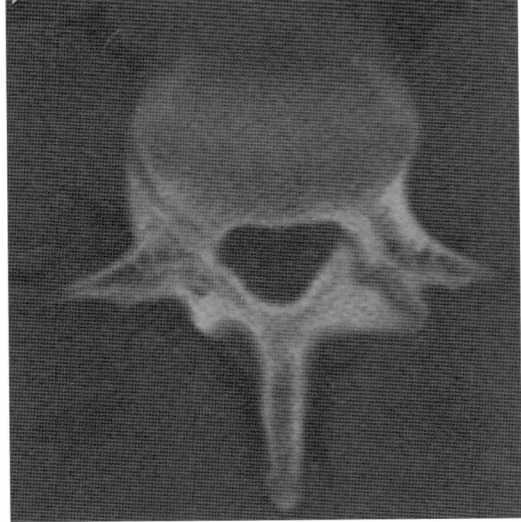

Fig. 10.12 Reverse axial CT of a right-sided stress fracture of the pedicle with a contra-lateral fracture through the left-sided pars interarticularis

occurring with major spinal injuries, associated spinal fractures, visceral injury and neurological complications are rare [35].

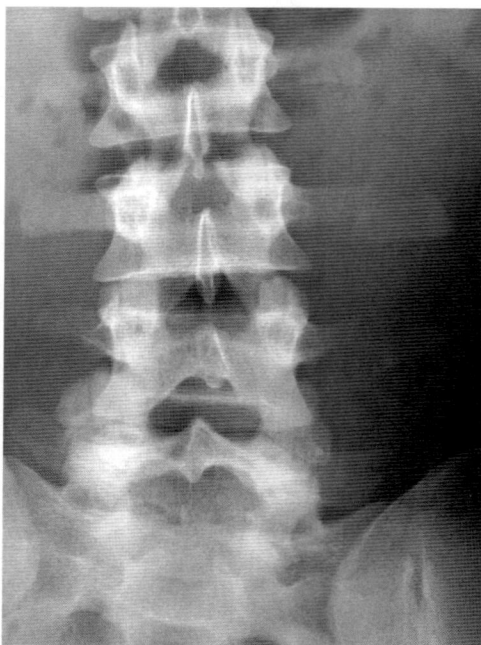

Fig. 10.13 AP radiographs of a professional soccer player presenting with left flank pain following torsional injury. There are acute avulsion fractures of the left L2, L3 and L4 transverse processes

Acute fractures are readily demonstrated on conventional radiographs (Fig. 10.13). In athletes with chronic symptoms, MRI differentiates transverse process from stress fractures of the pars and other causes of LBP (Fig. 10.14). A routine coronal sequence should be performed to fully include the transverse processes within the field of view to identify the presence of bone marrow and adjacent soft tissue oedema (Fig. 10.15) (Table 10.1).

Most transverse process fractures heal with few residual symptoms, and lead to only a few weeks of absence from sporting activity [35]. Follow-up imaging to document bony healing is not usually required.

Lamina and Spinous Process Fractures

Defects of the lamina and spinous process are usually due to acute traumatic fractures and developmental anomalies. Stress fractures may occur in the lower lumbar spine. The mechanism of injury is thought to be similar to pars fractures occurring during hyper-extension of the spine. They may exist in isolation, as an extension of a pars fracture or in association with contra-lateral pars fracture [36].

Isolated fractures of the spinous process occur most frequently in the lower cervical and upper thoracic spine as "clay shoveller" injuries during violent muscle contraction. Fractures of the lumbar spinous process may occur due to acute hyperflexion injury [22], but stress fractures are very rare.

Retro-isthmic lesions of the posterior neural arch are less significant than pedicle or pars fractures because non-union

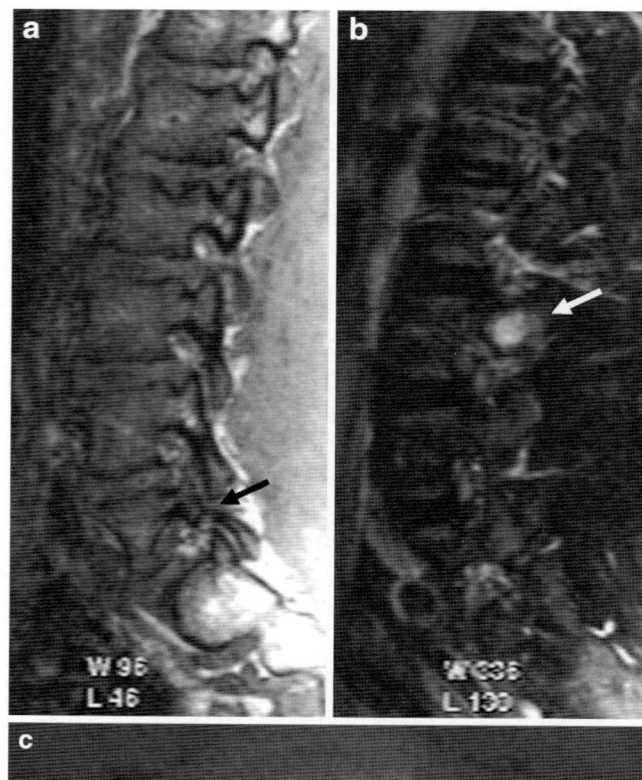

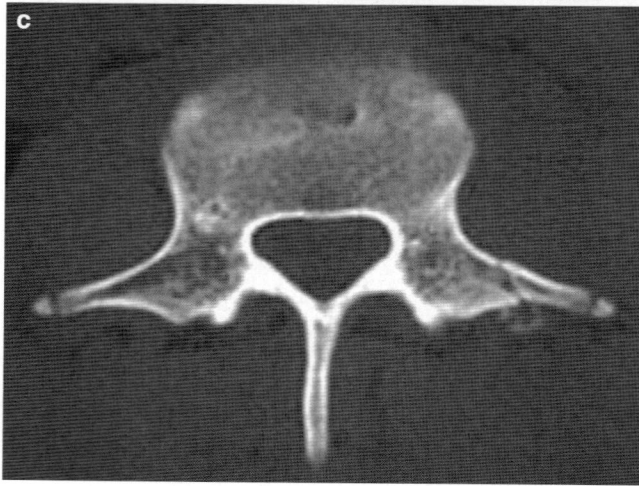

Fig. 10.14 Sagittal T1W image (**a**) shows a L5 pars defect (*black arrow*) in an adolescent footballer. However, this is likely to be an incidental finding as there is reactive marrow oedema at the L3 level (*white arrow*) on the STIR images (**b**). The correlative CT shows a stress fracture of the transverse process with early callus formation (**c**). Note also the bilateral un-fused transverse apophyses

does not predispose to subsequent development of spondylolisthesis. Patients can be rehabilitated when pain settles, and follow-up imaging is not critical.

Sacrum

Stress fractures of the sacrum occur in running athletes. They present with non-specific low back pain or gluteal pain. Rarely, there may be associated radiculopathy [37]. In female patients

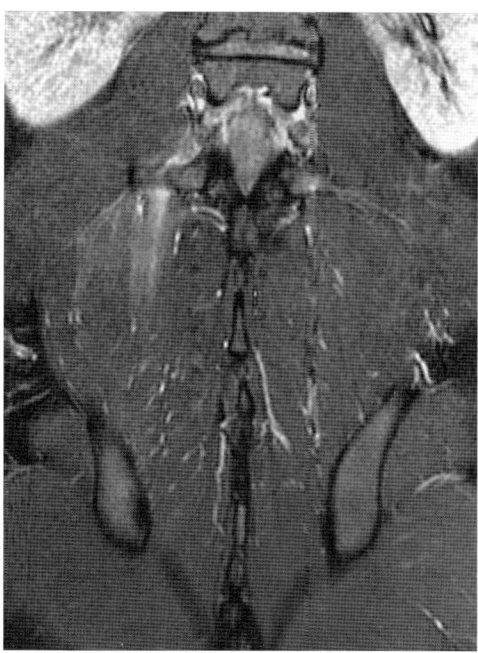

Fig. 10.15 Coronal STIR MR image of an acute traumatic fracture of a right transverse process in a soccer player. There is prominent oedema in the adjacent soft tissues consistent with associated muscle tear resulting from the torsional injury

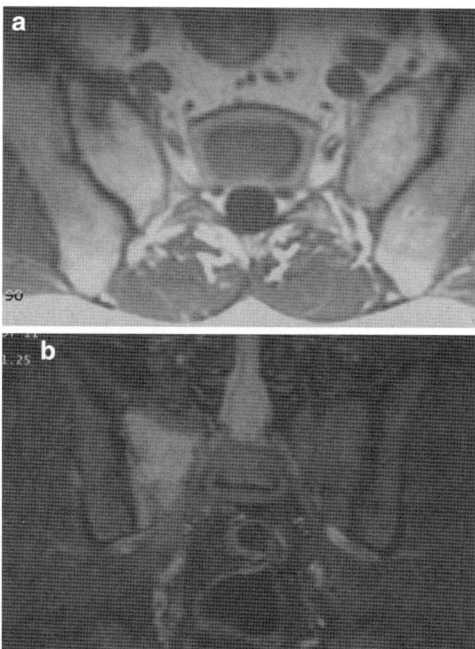

Fig. 10.16 Stress fracture of the right sacral ala in a long-distance runner. The axial T1W image (**a**) shows a low SI vertical fracture line. There is prominent reactive marrow oedema on the coronal STIR image (**b**), and the low SI fracture line is also visible

with a history of amenorrhoea or eating disorders, bone densitometry should be performed to exclude osteoporosis.

The fractures involve the cranial portion of the sacral alar, are oriented in the vertical plane and extend inferiorly to the first or second sacral foramen. Fractures are bilateral in only 16% of cases [38]. This pattern differs from the "H" shaped insufficiency fractures of osteoporosis. There maybe associated stress fractures in other areas of the pelvis.

Radiographs are usually normal. MRI is the ideal modality for confirmation of a sacral stress fracture, although false-negative examinations may occur when performed within the first few days of onset of symptoms [39]. T1W MR images demonstrate a discrete low SI fracture line which is surrounded by an area of less well-demarcated marrow oedema on STIR images (Fig. 10.16). CT may show a sclerotic line running through the cancellous bone, or a break in the cortex of the sacral alar.

Treatment consists of rest and protected non-weight bearing. Patients can usually return to sporting activities within 6 weeks, although many report persistent mild or intermittent pain [40]. MR changes usually resolve by 5–6 months with fatty marrow replacement at the fracture site, although follow-up imaging is not usually required [38].

Spondylolysis and Spondylolisthesis

The terms spondylolysis and spondylolisthesis are often used synonymously with little distinction between the two conditions, particularly when discussing management. Spondylolisthesis is the slipping of a vertebral segment with respect to the adjacent vertebral level, and is classified into five different types.

In young athletes the commonest cause is type I (dysplastic) due to congenital dysplasia of L5 or the sacrum or type II (isthmic) associated with a defect in the pars interarticularis. Type II listhesis is due to either a grade-IV fracture of the pars or a developmental defect. Approximately one quarter of symptomatic spondylolysis are associated with listhesis [41]. Spondylolisthesis may also be due to chronic degenerative facet disease.

The degree of spondylolisthesis is assessed on lateral radiographs or sagittal MRI using Myerding's classification (grade I <25%; grade II 25–50%; Grade III 50–75%; grade IV 75–100%; grade V >100% (spondyloptosis) (Fig. 10.17). MRI demonstrates associated disc degeneration and disc bulging. In type II spondylolisthesis, there is progressive loss of height of the exit foramina, eventually resulting in compression of the exiting nerve root. Associated focal disc protrusions are rare. In degenerative listhesis, a combination of chronic disc bulging, facet arthropathy and ligament hypertrophy leads to central canal stenosis.

The significance of spondylolysis and listhesis needs to be considered carefully, as both conditions are prevalent as asymptomatic findings in the general population. It is important to exclude other potential causes of back pain, and remember that acute pars fractures may occur in association with chronic defects at other levels.

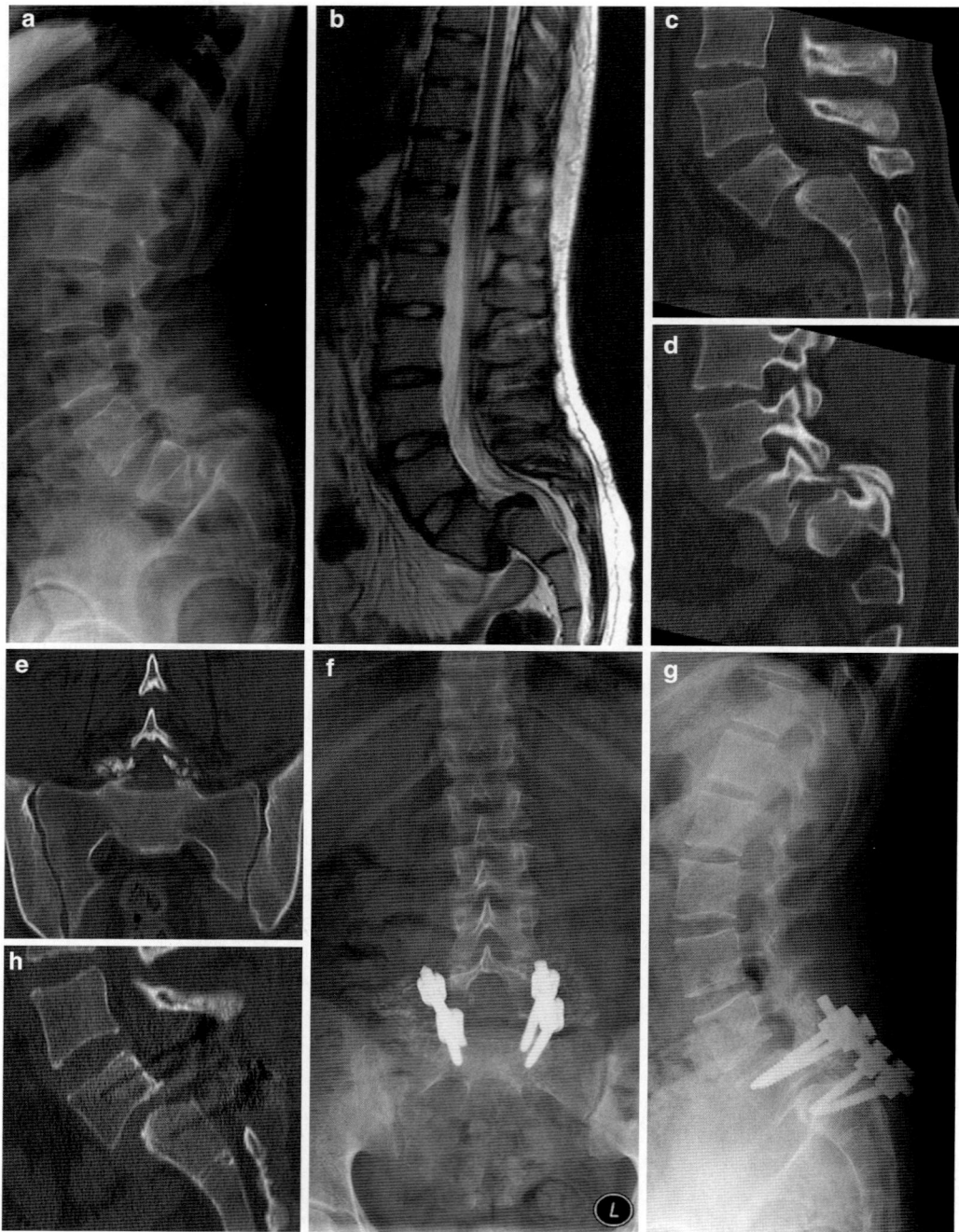

Fig. 10.17 Lateral radiograph (**a**), sagittal T2W image (**b**) and sagittal CT reformat (**c**) in an adolescent with back pain and neurogenic symptoms. There is a grade-IV lytic spondylolisthesis at L5/S1 with secondary disc degeneration. Intra-discal gas is present on the CT (**c**). There is doming of the antero-superior surface of the S1 vertebral body. Para-sagittal (**d**) and coronal (**e**) CT reformats show the pars defect and the associated bony fragmentation. The post-operative AP (**f**) and lateral (**g**) radiographs show the presence of pedicle screw fixation and bone graft material. There is significant reduction of the listhesis which is best demonstrated on the sagittal CT image (**h**)

Management of symptomatic spondylolysis and spondylolisthesis is usually non-operative with a period of rest, which may be supplemented by spinal bracing, followed by rehabilitation [40]. Patients with chronic LBP and spondylolysis may be candidates for spinal fusion. Diagnostic pars block with local anaesthetic or discography are used as part of the pre-surgical assessment (Fig. 10.18) [42], and steroids may provide short-term pain relief. The exact role of the pars defect as a pain generator is unclear, although there are reactive nerve fibres and neuropeptides present which may explain the pain relief response to pars block [43].

Progressive slip is associated with early return to sporting activities in up to 38% of young athletes [44]. Predictive factors include wedging of the L5 vertebra and rounding of the

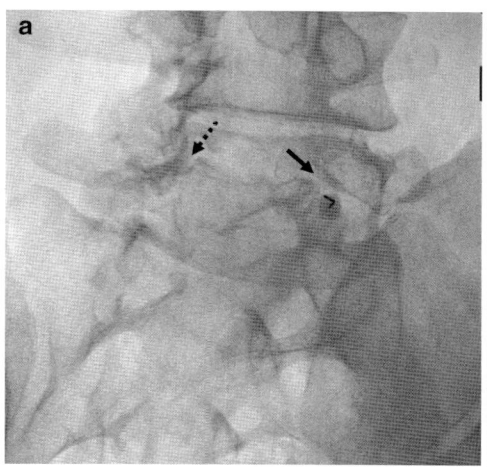 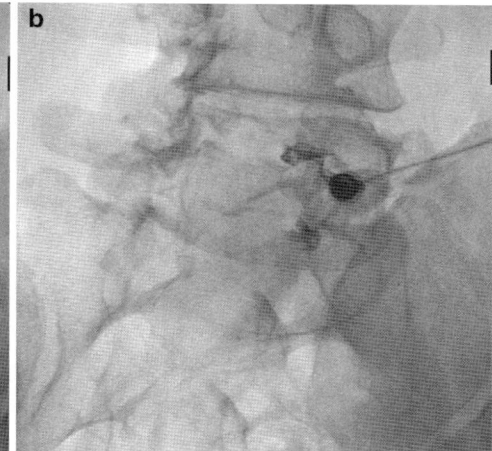

Fig. 10.18 Flouroscopic guided pars block in a patient with chronic LBP and grade I lytic spondylolisthesis. The spinal needle is present within the left pars defect on the oblique view (*black arrow*) (**a**). The contra-lateral pars defect is also seen (*broken arrow*). Injection of contrast (**b**) confirms needle localisation. There was period of complete relief of LBP for a few weeks, and the patient subsequently had a spinal fusion procedure

superior end-plate of the S1 vertebra (Fig. 10.17c), although this may be the result rather than the effect of the spondylolisthesis [40]. Sacral kyphosis may also predict progressive spondylolisthesis. In high grade listhesis, standing lateral radiographs are acquired to assess the sagittal spino-pelvic balance and distinguish between balanced and unbalanced listhesis for treatment planning [45].

Follow-up imaging with lateral radiographs should be considered in young patients managed non-operatively with grade II listhesis or higher, and those with high-risk sporting activities with excessive spinal flexion or axial loading (Fig. 10.19). Surgical options include spinal fusion, decompression and direct pars repair (Fig. 10.17f–g). Indications for operative treatment include, persistent back pain, neurological deficit, progressive slip or grade III slip or higher at presentation [40].

Inter-vertebral Disc Disease

Abnormalities of the inter-vertebral disc are common findings on MR imaging, particularly in the lumbar spine. They are frequently asymptomatic and the radiologist should be cautious about attributing symptoms of LBP to disc disease.

Annular Fissures and Discal Herniation

Under compression the nucleus pulposus deforms, absorbing and distributing pressure radially to the annulus. Nuclear pressure is transmitted to the vertebral end-plates. Compressive

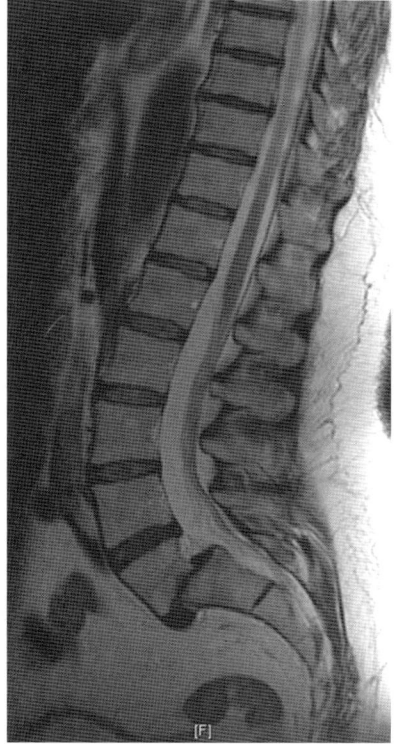

Fig. 10.19 Sagittal T2W MR image of the lumbar spine in an adolescent female show jumper. There is a grade II lytic spondylolisthesis at L5/S1 with hyper-kyphotic sacrum and lordotic lumbar spine. Surgery was not performed as the LBP settled spontaneously. However, follow-up imaging is required in this case because of the unbalanced listhesis, and the associated risk of high axial loading during her sporting activities

forces may be distributed through the disc asymmetrically during flexion, extension and lateral flexion, with tensile forces acting on the opposing annulus. Deficiencies of the posterior annulus arise due to transverse fissures which progress with age but it is unclear whether these reflect normal development or micro-trauma from repetitive axial rotation. Macroscopic focal deficiencies of the annulus are best referred to as fissures rather than tears, as the term "tear" necessarily implies a traumatic aetiology.

Annular fissures are evident on T2W MR images as "high intensity zones." Associated changes of disc dehydration and degeneration maybe absent. These fissures can rupture completely under compression to produce a herniation or extrusion of the nucleus pulposus (Fig. 10.20). Acute disc herniations are high SI on T2W and intermediate SI on T1W MR images. Chronic protrusions are low SI on T1W and T2W sequences.

Although annular fissures, herniations, sequestrations and accelerated disc degeneration are usually considered to be more significant in adolescents and young adults, asymptomatic annular fissures and disc herniations are prevalent in the general population between 20 and 50 years of age [46].

Lumbar disc herniation in adolescent athletes tends to be centrally located and often presents with non-specific LBP (Fig. 10.20). Discogenic radiculopathy due to an extruded fragment of nucleus pulposus is thought to trigger the release of local inflammatory mediators such as phospholipase A2, causing nerve root inflammation and swelling. Radiculopathy is less commonly encountered in the athletic population, with a reported incidence of 11% in young athletes vs. 48% in the general population [47]. However, discogenic back pain is probably under-reported in athletes, as many at elite level may be unwilling to risk the loss of playing time, sponsorship or scholarship opportunities.

Lumbar disc herniation is often successfully managed conservatively with spontaneous resolution over time and usually responds well to anti-inflammatory therapy. Athletes may report earlier recovery times than non-athletic patients. Effective temporary pain relief of LBP can be achieved with epidural steroid injection by blocking inflammatory mediators [1]. Blind Epidural injection often results in incorrect needle placement, and safe and effective epidural injections can be achieved with either fluoroscopic or CT guidance (Fig. 10.21).

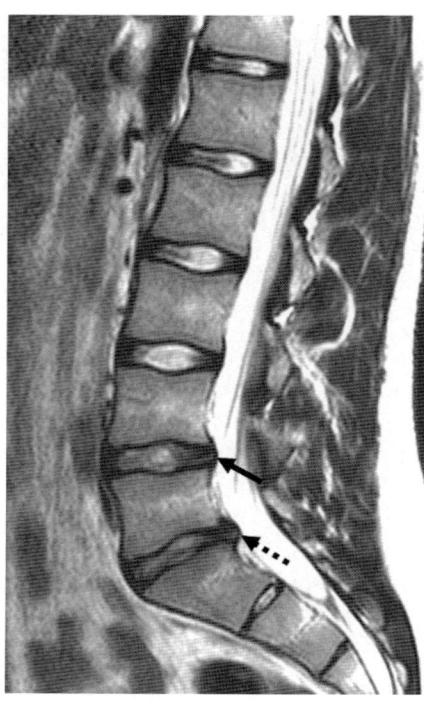

Fig. 10.20 Sagittal T2W MR image in an adolescent with low back pain, but no radicular symptoms. There is early disruption of the nucleus pulposus at L4/5 and L5/S1 with loss of signal, and there is early disc space narrowing at L5/S1. An annular fissure is present at L4/5 with a HIZ (*black arrow*). A similar appearance with a fissure and a small central protrusion is present at L5/S1 (*broken arrow*)

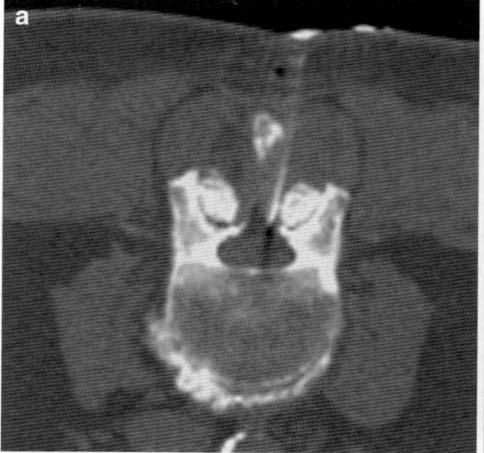 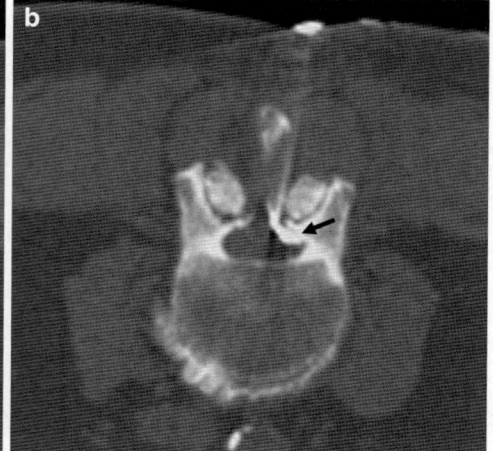

Fig. 10.21 Therapeutic epidural injection for an elderly running athlete with LBP associated with multi-level lumbar disc disease and spondylosis. The spinal needle is passed between the lamina (**a**), and epidural space localisation is confirmed by a small volume of contrast agent (*black arrow*) (**b**)

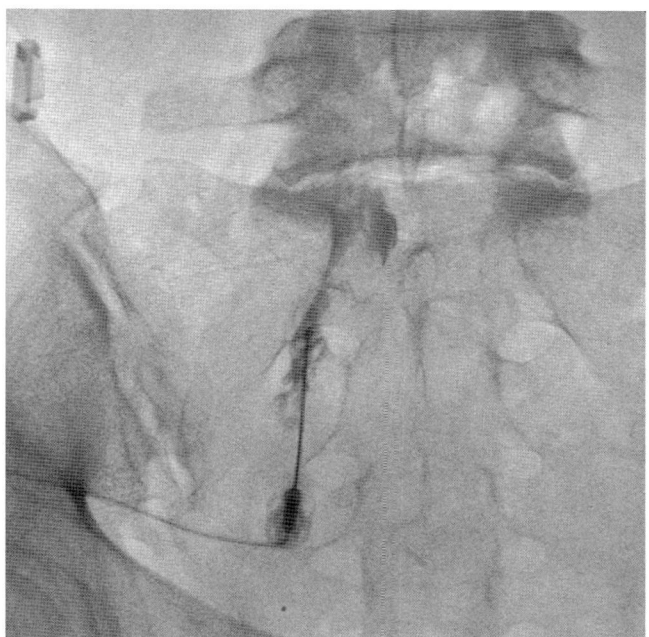

Fig. 10.22 Fluoroscopic-guided S1 nerve root injection performed as a therapeutic procedure in a patient with an acute paracentral disc protrusion at L5/S1. Contrast outlines the nerve root sleeve, and extends proximally to the level of the L5/S1 disc space, confirming correct needle localisation without vascular filling, prior to steroid and anaesthetic injection

The role of diagnostic selective nerve root block (SNRB) as a treatment for lumbar radiculopathy is controversial. There is only moderate evidence to support the use of SNRB as a treatment for radicular symptoms [48], but it maybe an effective adjunct to conservative management for patients in whom surgery would otherwise be clinically indicated due to intractable pain (Fig. 10.22) [49].

Disc Degeneration

The inter-vertebral disc undergoes a process of dehydration and desiccation which is often considered a normal ageing process. It is widely recognised that disc degeneration is more prevalent in athletes [50], but associated LBP is less common than in non-competitive control groups [51]. The role of the annulus fibrosus as a resistor of axial rotation may contribute to the increased incidence of painful degenerative disc disease in golfers. However a large proportion of the golfing population are over the age of 50 years, in whom asymptomatic degenerative disc disease is just as common [52].

Patterns of disc degeneration may vary with sporting activity. Soccer players tend to have lower lumbar disc degeneration whilst global involvement of the lumbar discs is seen in weight lifters [51]. By comparison accelerated disc degeneration is not seen in competitive runners.

T2W MR images demonstrate loss of normal high SI of the nucleus pulposus, disc space narrowing and loss of differentiation with the outer annulus which is often deficient leading to broad-based disc bulging (Fig. 10.20). Ultimately Modic changes develop in the vertebral end-plates with oedema, fatty replacement or sclerosis.

Most patients with mechanical back pain can be managed conservatively with spinal rehabilitation and anti-inflammatory agents. The presence of disc degeneration on MRI is not necessarily an indicator of discogenic pain, and MR imaging is used to exclude other causes of back pain in cases of failed rehabilitation. Pain reproduction with discography is regarded as the gold standard for diagnosis of discogenic pain in patients with intractable LBP undergoing assessment for spinal fusion or other interventional procedures.

Vertebral End-Plate and Ring Apophysis

Abnormalities of the vertebral end-plate and ring apophysis are usually due to degenerative disc disease or Scheuermann's disease. Acute ring apophyseal avulsion injuries and intraosseous disc herniation may result in appearances similar to Scheuermann's disease. Discitis and inflammatory spondyloarthropathy are less frequently encountered, but should be considered when disco-vertebral abnormalities are identified.

Scheuermann's Disease

Scheuermann's disease affects juveniles with cartilaginous node (Schmorl nodes) formation at the vertebral end-plate and thoracic kyphosis. Although various aetiological factors have been implicated, it is likely that it is a stress-related spondylodystrophy resulting from traumatic growth arrest and end-plate fracture occurring during the heightened vulnerability phase of the adolescent growth spurt. Repetitive vertebral loading and flexion compression forces in sports such as gymnastics may have a role in the causation of vertebral wedging and thoracic hyper-kyphosis. The incidence of Scheuermann's disease is as high as 41% in elite athletes as opposed to 10% of non-sporting controls [53].

Scheuermann's disease is often asymptomatic. However, patients may present during puberty with postural deformity, aching pain and fatigue often occurring during or after exercise. There may be an exaggerated lordosis of the thoracic or lumbar spine. Alternatively, symptoms may first appear in adulthood with the onset of secondary degenerative changes. There is an increased prevalence of vertebral end-plate disease in athletes with back pain compared to asymptomatic groups [54].

Scoliosis also occurs in up to 80% of athletes with asymmetric load on the trunk such as javelin throwers and tennis players, but the curvature is usually small and does not cause back pain [54].

Imaging

Sorenson's criteria for diagnosis of Scheuermann's disease are: kyphosis of 40° and vertebral wedging of 5° over at least three contiguous vertebral levels (Fig. 10.23). However, this classification does not account for vertebral end-plate disease that occurs without associated vertebral body wedging. Vertebral end-plate abnormalities with Schmorl node formation and disc space narrowing that do not otherwise fulfil Sorenson's criteria have been observed to be more prevalent in athletic adolescents (Fig. 10.24) [55].

Radiographs demonstrate irregular vertebral end-plates with radiolucent depressions of varying sizes. Reactive sclerosis may be present at the margin of the nodes. There is variable vertebral wedging, kyphosis, disc space narrowing and osteophytosis. Anterior Schmorl nodes may lead to separation of the ring apophysis. On MRI disc material is seen within the cartilaginous nodes. The nodes are high SI on T2W images unless there is associated disc degeneration. Low SI at the margin of the nodes represents reactive sclerosis. The disc spaces are narrowed, but the T2 signal of the inter-vertebral disc is maintained early in the disease. As secondary disc degeneration develops there may be Modic type vertebral end-plate changes of oedema, fatty replacement and sclerosis.

Juvenile Lumbar Osteochondrosis

Juvenile lumbar osteochondrosis affects the lower thoracic and lumbar spine [55, 56]. It is probably a variant of Scheuermann's disease. Patients present during adolescence. Boys are affected more commonly than girls, and there is a higher incidence in competitive athletics. Back pain is often severe.

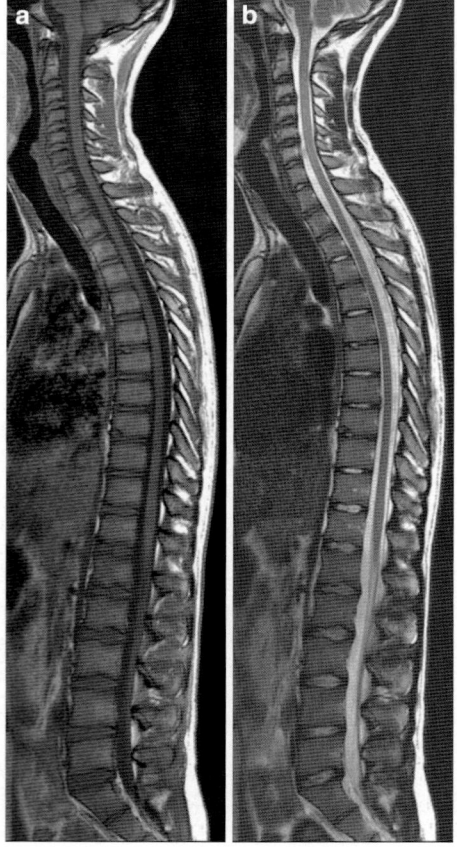

Fig. 10.24 Sagittal T1W (**a**) and T2W (**b**) MR images of a young athlete with back pain. There are minor multi-level VEP abnormalities with Schmorl node formation in the dorsal and upper lumbar spine. There is also early secondary disc degeneration at some affected levels. However, there is no vertebral wedging or kyphosis present, and these findings do not fulfil Sorensen's criteria for Scheuermann's disease

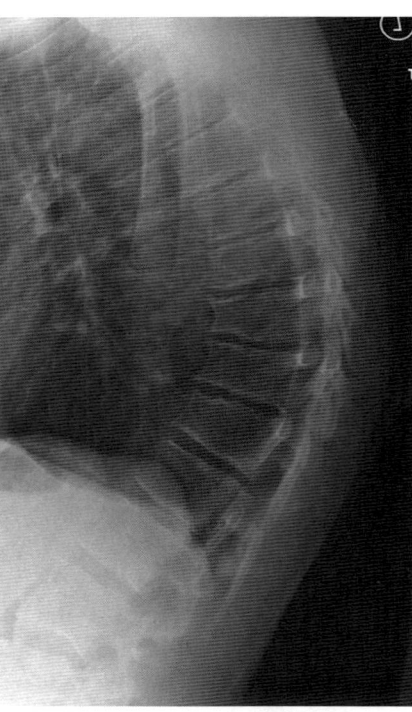

Fig. 10.23 Lateral radiograph of a patient with back pain and Scheurmann's disease. There is vertebral body wedging over three contiguous levels associated with kyphosis. There are also VEP abnormalities and early secondary disc degeneration and spondylosis

Schmorl nodes, disc space narrowing and increased A-P diameter of affected vertebral bodies are seen on radiographs and MR imaging. There may be associated narrowing of the spinal canal at the level of the inter-vertebral disc [56]. Kyphotic deformity is usually absent. There is a higher incidence of pars defects in adolescents with lumbar Scheuermann's disease, and the pars interarticularis should be carefully scrutinised on MR imaging for the presence of spondylolysis (Fig. 10.25).

Acute Traumatic Lesions of the Vertebral End-Plate

Acute traumatic intra-osseous disc herniation and ring apophyseal avulsion may occur as due to compression or flexion injuries [57]. Back pain may be severe. Differentiation from non-traumatic cartilaginous Schmorl nodes or chronic injuries can be difficult on radiographs. Marrow oedema adjacent to apophyseal separation on MR images suggests an acute or symptomatic lesion (Fig. 10.26). There may be associated changes of more widespread lumbar Scheuermann's disease (Fig. 10.17c).

Apophyseal injuries usually occur anteriorly. Posterior ring avulsion is less common, but has a high association with sciatica in adults (Fig. 10.27) [58]. Ring apophyseal injury associated with adolescent disc herniation often causes more severe symptoms [59]. Large lesions are associated with chronic back pain. In adulthood, failure of fusion of the apophysis is seen as a limbus vertebra, which is often an asymptomatic lesion (Fig. 10.28).

Facet Joint Pain

The zygo-apophyseal or facet joints are a source of chronic spinal pain in around 15% of the general population, the majority of which have facet osteoarthrosis (OA). Facet joint synovitis, or facet syndrome, is a condition that presents with painful acute or sub-acute inflammation of the facet joint without degenerative changes. It typically affects younger athletes, such as gymnasts, baseball pitchers and cricket bowlers, with posterior element overuse syndrome due to high torsional forces across the facet joints. [60]. Symptoms are identical to facet OA. MRI imaging demonstrates facet joint capsular oedema, effusion and sub-chondral marrow oedema on T2W and STIR images (Fig. 10.29). Marginal bone formation and capsular hypertrophy are present in facet OA.

Non-interventional, conservative management of facet joint-related pain includes physiotherapy, chiropractic manipulation and oral anti-inflammatory medications. Interventional therapeutic procedures include intra-articular

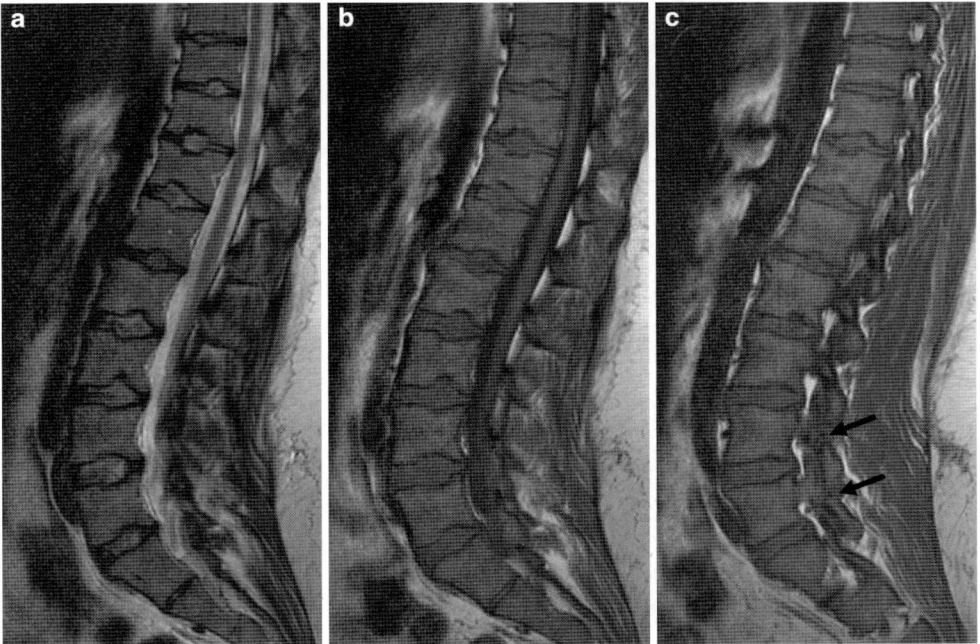

Fig. 10.25 Adolescent male presenting with lumbar Scheuermann's type disease, pars defects with LBP. Sagittal T2W (**a**) and T1W (**b**) image show multi-level Schmorl node formation within the lumbar spine, with loss of disc height at some levels. Disc hydration is largely preserved. The spinal canal is narrowed inferiorly. The para-sagittal T1W image (**c**) shows chronic pars defects at the L4 and L5 levels (*black arrows*)

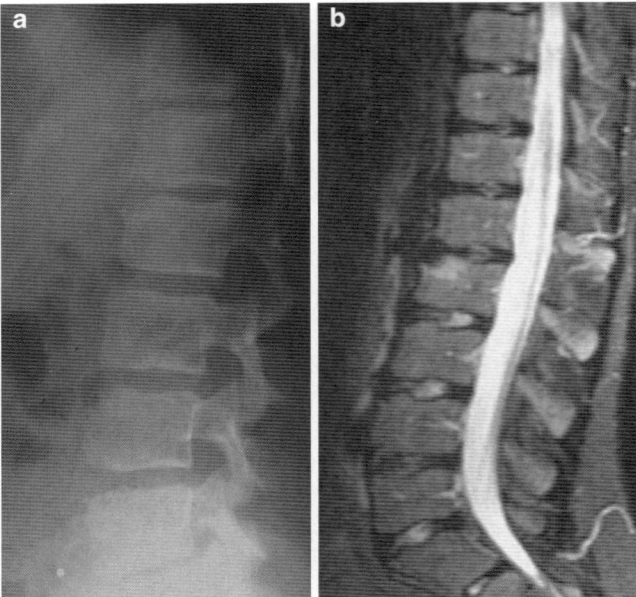

Fig. 10.26 Lateral radiograph (**a**) of an adolescent with minor central Schmorl node formation in the upper lumbar spine, but with a prominent defect in the antero-superior margin of the L2 vertebral body. It is not clear whether this is an acute ring avulsion injury or a more long-standing Schmorl node. The presence of marrow oedema on the sagittal STIR MR image (**b**) is more suggestive of an acute ring apophyseal separation and suggests this is likely to be the symptomatic lesion

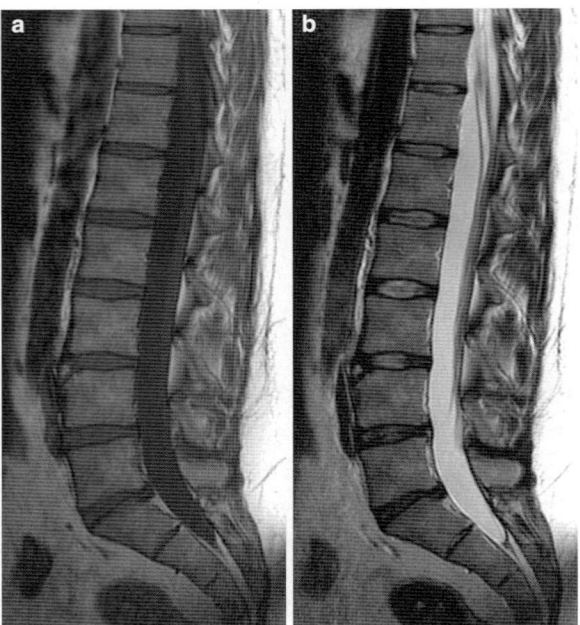

Fig. 10.28 Sagittal T1W (**a**) and T2W (**b**) MR images of a young adult athlete with back pain. There is a limbus vertebra at the upper anterior margin of the L4 vertebral body. This is likely to be an asymptomatic finding. The disc degeneration and annular fissures at L4/5 and L5/S1 are more likely pain generators

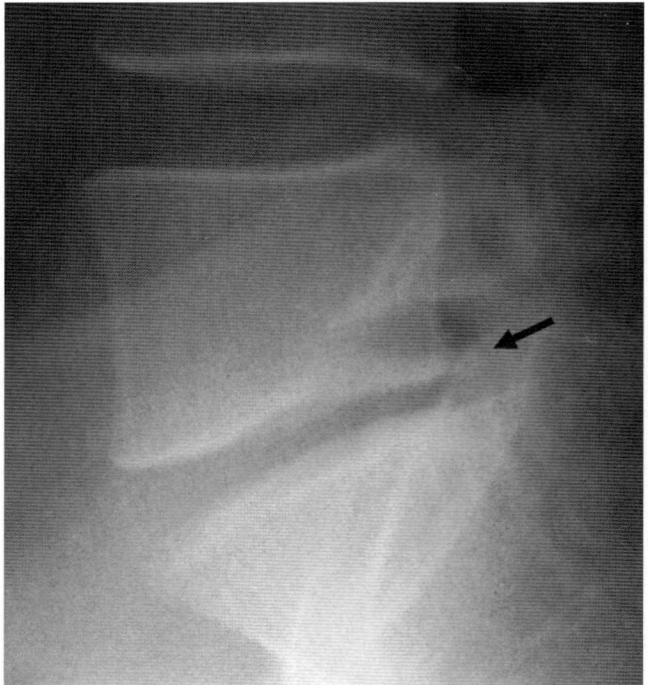

Fig. 10.27 Lateral radiograph of an adult with chronic radicular symptoms. There is a posterior ring apophyseal avulsion (*black arrow*). Moderate compression of the traversing nerve root was present on MRI

facet joint injections, medial branch blocks and medial branch radiofrequency (RF) neurolysis or ablation. There is conflicting evidence regarding the effectiveness and indications of these techniques [61], but the majority of the evidence is based on patients' with degenerative facet OA.

Diagnostic anaesthetic intra-articular facet joint injections (FJI) can be used to determine the source of back pain. Cortico-steroids are added to treat associated synovitis. FJI is performed under fluoroscopic or CT guidance, and intra-articular needle placement is confirmed by injection of contrast media. Although FJI may be useful for localising painful facet joints in the cervical and lumbar spine, the clinical effectiveness for pain relief is limited [62]. There is only moderate evidence for short and long-term pain relief with FJI in the lumbar spine [61].

The facet joints are innervated by the medial branches of the dorsal rami of the spinal nerve roots. The medial branches run over the superior surface of the transverse process where they divide supplying the facet joints above and below their respective level.

Medial branch blocks (MBB) are an alternative method of achieving pain relief for facet joint syndrome. They are performed by selectively anaesthetising the medial branches from above and below the painful facet joint by direct injection of local anaesthetic. The needle is placed at the base of the

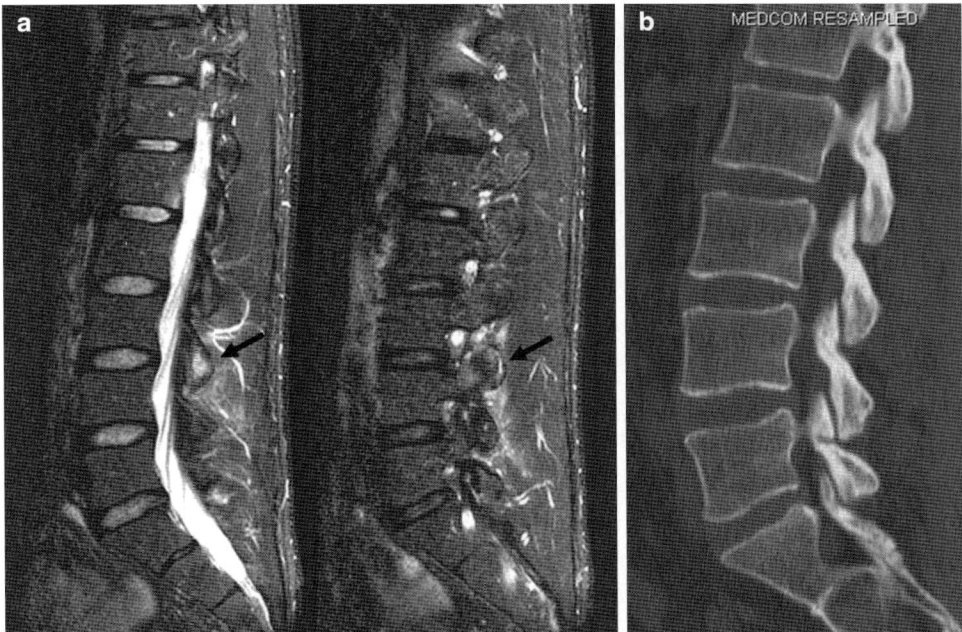

Fig. 10.29 Consecutive sagittal STIR MR images (**a**) in a young adult athlete with LBP, and facet joint syndrome. There is high SI marrow oedema in the articular processes at L3/4 with surrounding soft tissue oedema (*black arrows*). A sagittal CT reformatted image (**b**) excludes a stress fracture or other intrinsic bony lesion. There is no established OA change. Symptoms resolved with a facet joint injection

posterior margin of the transverse process. MBB can be performed under fluoroscopic guidance or ultrasound guidance. There is no evidence to suggest that the addition of steroid provides any additional benefit [63]. A positive response to medial branch block may be an indication for RF ablation of the medial branches for persistent facet joint pain.

Sacro-Iliac Joint Pain

SIJ dysfunction is a term used where there is no demonstrable pathology. Joint instability associated with abnormal muscle recruitment maybe a mechanism for SIJ pain. Load across the joint associated with weak or inappropriate gluteus maximus action combined with compensatory contraction of biceps femoris may lead to an increase in soft tissue strain and pain [64]. Delayed EMG activity occurs in the obturator internus, multifidus and gluteus maximus muscles in symptomatic patients compared with control groups [65].

Pain over the posterior sacrum and SIJ is associated with vertical loading, and clinical tests include pain aggravated by active straight leg raising and the "stork" test (standing hip flexion of the leg contra-lateral to the side of pain). Pain may also radiate into the thigh, groin, abdomen and calf.

SIJ dysfunction is a self-limited process. Radiographs are usually normal. However, abnormal stresses across the SIJ in athletic individuals may result in bony resorption, erosion and reactive sclerosis. Long-distance runners and soccer players are particularly affected [66], similar changes may be present in the symphysis pubis. The mechanism for the osseous changes is possibly due to synovial hyperplasia and hyperaemia leading to bone resorption. Alternatively, repetitive stress and micro-fractures may lead to a reparative response [67]. A similar effect may be seen following pregnancy where the hormone relaxin leads to ligamentous laxity in preparation for delivery. A triangle of reactive sclerosis termed osteitis condensans ilii, may develop and is most prominent on the iliac side of the inferior aspect of the SIJ.

Older athletes with chronic SIJ instability may progress to OA associated with anterior osteophyte formation which may bridge the joint margin. However, this is a common finding associated with ageing and not necessarily associated with SIJ symptoms.

Imaging

Interpretation of radiographs of the SIJ's is difficult because of the complex orientation of the joint surfaces. There is significant inter and intra-variation for diagnosis of sacro-iliitis. CT or MRI is recommended for detection of early SIJ pathology when conventional radiographs are normal or equivocal, and helps to distinguish a stress-related process from inflammatory sacro-iliitis and other SIJ disorders.

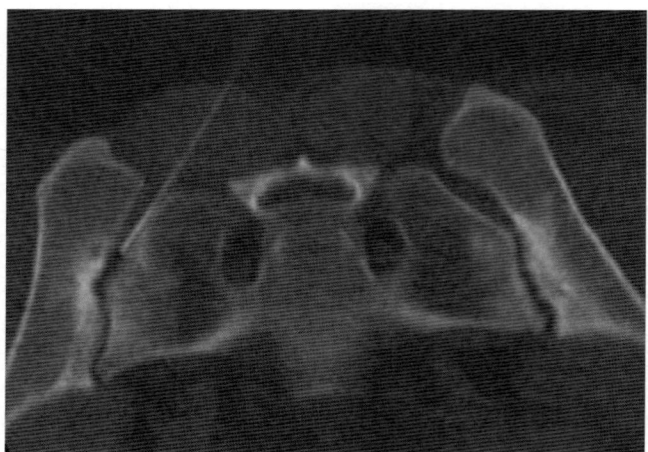

Fig. 10.30 Prone CT image of a young female runner with stress-related changes in both SIJ's. There is linear sub-chondral sclerosis which is largely confined to the iliac side of the joint and is not associated with erosive disease. The scan has been performed as part of a CT-guided joint injection. A 22G spinal needle is seen within the left SIJ

CT is both sensitive and specific for diagnosis of early bone erosion and sclerosis [68]. The iliac aspect of the joint is often affected in early disease due to the thinner articular cartilage. Sclerosis is usually discrete, linear and well-defined. Unilateral or bilateral involvement may occur (Fig. 10.30). MR imaging has the advantage of demonstrating SIJ synovitis and sub-chondral marrow oedema. STIR images are more sensitive for detection of early marrow oedema than fat-suppressed T2W images [68]. Sub-chondral marrow oedema is identified as ill-defined areas of high SI adjacent to areas of low SI sclerosis in evolving disease.

MR imaging and CT are probably equally effective in detection of early sacro-iliac disease, although neither MRI nor CT are sensitive or specific for diagnosis of SIJ dysfunction [69]. Radiological features that help distinguish an inflammatory process include prominent erosive change, joint space widening, ill-defined sclerosis, high SI within the joint line, or enhancement within the joint line following contrast administration [70].

SIJ dysfunction is confirmed by a positive pain relief response from injection of cortico-steroids and local anaesthetic [69], and helps to distinguish SIJ pain from other causes of LBP such as facet syndrome or disc disease. SIJ injection can be performed under fluoroscopic guidance, but CT-guided injection is just as effective and can be combined with diagnostic imaging as a single procedure (Fig. 10.30). SIJ injection may provide at least short-term pain relief in up to 88% of patients with non-inflammatory pain [71]. However, CT demonstration of sclerosis, erosion and joint space narrowing has only 58% sensitivity and 69% sensitivity for predicting pain relief from intra-articular injection [72].

Summary

MR imaging is recommended as the primary imaging modality for investigation of athletes presenting with back or radicular pain. It is imperative to employ fluid-sensitive sequences such as STIR or fat-saturated T2W images in the MR protocol to optimally demonstrate the presence of bone marrow oedema which is often the hallmark of physical injury to the spine. When bony injury is suspected, targeted CT should be obtained to help accurately grade the injury and act as a baseline for monitoring the healing response.

The radiologist must be aware that asymptomatic findings are common even in adolescents and young adults, and should always correlate the image findings with the results of the clinical history and physical examination.

Image-guided intervention can provide useful short-term pain relief for many conditions and can be used to select patients for definitive surgical procedures in some cases.

References

1. Trainor TJ, Trainor MA (2004) Etiology of low back pain in athletes. Curr Sports Med Rep 3(1):41–46
2. Alyas F, Turner M, Connell D (2007) MRI findings in the lumbar spines f asymptomatic, adolescent, elite tennis players. Br J Sports Med 41(11):836–841, discussion 841
3. Bogduk N (1997) The lumbar vertebrae. In: Clinical anatomy of the lumbar spine and sacrum. Churchill Livingstone, New York, pp 1–12
4. Hukins DW, Kirby MC, Sikoryn TA, Aspden RM, Cox AJ (1990) Comparison of structure, mechanical properties, and functions of lumbar spinal ligaments. Spine 15(8):787–795
5. Slipman CW, Lipetz JS, Plastaras CT, Jackson HB, Vresilovic EJ, Lenrow DA et al (2001) Fluoroscopically guided therapeutic sacro-iliac joint injections for sacroiliac joint syndrome. Am J Phys Med Rehabil 80(6):425–432
6. Cohen SP (2005) Sacroiliac joint pain: a comprehensive review of anatomy, diagnosis, and treatment. Anesth Analg 101(5): 1440–1453
7. Van Mameren H, Drukker J, Sanches H, Beursgens J (1990) Cervical spine motion in the sagittal plane (I) range of motion of actually performed movements, an X-ray cinematographic study. Eur J Morphol 28(1):47–68
8. Penning L, Wilmink JT (1987) Rotation of the cervical spine. A CT study in normal subjects. Spine 12(8):732–738
9. Andriacchi T, Schultz A, Belytschko T, Galante J (1974) A model for studies of mechanical interactions between the human spine and rib cage. J Biomech 7(6):497–507
10. Goldstein JD, Berger PE, Windler GE, Jackson DW (1991) Spine injuries in gymnasts and swimmers. An epidemiologic investigation. Am J Sports Med 19(5):463–468
11. Cappozzo A (1983) Force actions in the human trunk during running. J Sports Med Phys Fitness 23(1):14–22
12. Twomey LT, Taylor JR (1983) Sagittal movements of the human lumbar vertebral column: a quantitative study of the role of the posterior vertebral elements. Arch Phys Med Rehabil 64(7):322–325
13. Gluck GS, Bendo JA, Spivak JM (2008) The lumbar spine and low back pain in golf: a literature review of swing biomechanics and injury prevention. Spine J 8(5):778–788

14. van Dieen JH, Cholewicki J, Radebold A (2003) Trunk muscle recruitment patterns in patients with low back pain enhance the stability of the lumbar spine. Spine 28(8):834–841
15. Tassone JC, Duey-Holtz A (2008) Spine concerns in the Special Olympian with Down syndrome. Sports Med Arthrosc 16(1): 55–60
16. Gymnastics B Atlanto-axial information pack. www.british-gymnastics.org
17. Fuller CW, Brooks JH, Kemp SP (2007) Spinal injuries in professional rugby union: a prospective cohort study. Clin J Sport Med 17(1):10–16
18. Shelly MJ, Butler JS, Timlin M, Walsh MG, Poynton AR, O'Byrne JM (2006) Spinal injuries in Irish rugby: a ten-year review. J Bone Joint Surg Br 88(6):771–775
19. Franz T, Hasler RM, Benneker L, Zimmermann H, Siebenrock KA, Exadaktylos AK (2008) Severe spinal injuries in alpine skiing and snowboarding: a 6-year review of a tertiary trauma centre for the Bernese Alps ski resorts Switzerland. Br J Sports Med 42(1):55–58
20. Donald S, Chalmers D, Theis JC (2005) Are snowboarders more likely to damage their spines than skiers? Lessons learned from a study of spinal injuries from the Otago skifields in New Zealand. N Z Med J 118(1217):U1530
21. Shaskan G, Simons SM (2008) Thoracic apophyseal avulsion fracture in an adolescent football player. Curr Sports Med Rep 7(1): 33–34
22. Jones A, Andrews J, Shoaib A, Lyons K, Ahuja S, Howes J et al (2005) Avulsion of the L4 spinous process: an unusual injury in a professional rugby player: case report. Spine 30(11):E323–E325
23. Gundry CR, Fritts HM Jr (1999) MR imaging of the spine in sports injuries. Magn Reson Imaging Clin N Am 7(1):85–103
24. Sairyo K, Katoh S, Sasa T, Yasui N, Goel VK, Vadapalli S et al (2005) Athletes with unilateral spondylolysis are at risk of stress fracture at the contralateral pedicle and pars interarticularis: a clinical and biomechanical study. Am J Sports Med 33(4):583–590
25. Papanicolaou N, Wilkinson RH, Emans JB, Treves S, Micheli LJ (1985) Bone scintigraphy and radiography in young athletes with low back pain. AJR Am J Roentgenol 145(5):1039–1044
26. Langston JW, Gavant ML (1985) "Incomplete ring" sign: a simple method for CT detection of spondylolysis. J Comput Assist Tomogr 9(4):728–729
27. Campbell RS, Grainger AJ, Hide IG, Papastefanou S, Greenough CG (2005) Juvenile spondylolysis: a comparative analysis of CT SPECT and MRI. Skeletal Radiol 34(2):63–73
28. Saifuddin A, Burnett SJ (1997) The value of lumbar spine MRI in the assessment of the pars interarticularis. Clin Radiol 52(9): 666–671
29. Matheson GO, Clement DB, McKenzie DC, Taunton JE, Lloyd-Smith DR, Macintyre JG (1987) Scintigraphic uptake of 99mTc at non-painful sites in athletes with stress fractures. The concept of bone strain. Sports Med 4(1):65–75
30. Dunn AJ, Campbell RS, Mayor PE, Rees D (2008) Radiological findings and healing patterns of incomplete stress fractures of the pars interarticularis. Skeletal Radiol 37(5):443–450
31. Hollenberg GM, Beattie PF, Meyers SP, Weinberg EP, Adams MJ (2002) Stress reactions of the lumbar pars interarticularis: the development of a new MRI classification system. Spine 27(2):181–186
32. Lalam R, Cassar-Pullicino VN, Kumar DS, Fotiado A, Tins B, Tyrrell PNM (2008) Ossicles of the lumbar articular facets: normal variant or spondylolytic variant? In: Proceedings of the scientific session of the international skeletal society, New Delhi
33. Parvataneni HK, Nicholas SJ, McCance SE (2004) Bilateral pedicle stress fractures in a female athlete: case report and review of the literature. Spine 29(2):E19–E21
34. Barker PJ, Urquhart DM, Story IH, Fahrer M, Briggs CA (2007) The middle layer of lumbar fascia and attachments to lumbar transverse processes: implications for segmental control and fracture. Eur Spine J 16(12):2232–2237
35. Tewes DP, Fischer DA, Quick DC, Zamberletti F, Powell J (1995) Lumbar transverse process fractures in professional football players. Am J Sports Med 23(4):507–509
36. Wick LF, Kaim A, Bongartz G (2000) Retroisthmic cleft: a stress fracture of the lamina. Skeletal Radiol 29(3):162–164
37. Aylwin A, Saifuddin A, Tucker S (2003) L5 radiculopathy due to sacral stress fracture. Skeletal Radiol 32(10):590–593
38. Ahovuo JA, Kiuru MJ, Visuri T (2004) Fatigue stress fractures of the sacrum: diagnosis with MR imaging. Eur Radiol 14(3): 500–505
39. Fredericson M, Moore W, Biswal S (2007) Sacral stress fractures: magnetic resonance imaging not always definitive for early stage injuries: a report of 2 cases. Am J Sports Med 35(5):835–839
40. Bono CM (2004) Low-back pain in athletes. J Bone Joint Surg Am 86-A(2):382–396
41. Fredrickson BE, Baker D, McHolick WJ, Yuan HA, Lubicky JP (1984) The natural history of spondylolysis and spondylolisthesis. J Bone Joint Surg Am 66(5):699–707
42. Wu SS, Lee CH, Chen PQ (1999) Operative repair of symptomatic spondylolysis following a positive response to diagnostic pars injection. J Spinal Disord 12(1):10–16
43. Eisenstein SM, Ashton IK, Roberts S, Darby AJ, Kanse P, Menage J et al (1994) Innervation of the spondylolysis "ligament". Spine 19(8):912–916
44. Muschik M, Hahnel H, Robinson PN, Perka C, Muschik C (1996) Competitive sports and the progression of spondylolisthesis. J Pediatr Orthop 16(3):364–369
45. Mac-Thiong JM, Labelle H, Parent S, Hresko MT, Deviren V, Weidenbaum M (2008) Reliability and development of a new classification of lumbosacral spondylolisthesis. Scoliosis 3:19
46. Weishaupt D, Zanetti M, Hodler J, Boos N (1998) MR imaging of the lumbar spine: prevalence of intervertebral disk extrusion and sequestration, nerve root compression, end plate abnormalities, and osteoarthritis of the facet joints in asymptomatic volunteers. Radiology 209(3):661–666
47. Micheli LJ, Wood R (1995) Back pain in young athletes. Significant differences from adults in causes and patterns. Arch Pediatr Adolesc Med 149(1):15–18
48. DePalma MJ, Bhargava A, Slipman CW (2005) A critical appraisal of the evidence for selective nerve root injection in the treatment of lumbosacral radiculopathy. Arch Phys Med Rehabil 86(7): 1477–1483
49. Narozny M, Zanetti M, Boos N (2001) Therapeutic efficacy of selective nerve root blocks in the treatment of lumbar radicular leg pain. Swiss Med Wkly 131(5–6):75–80
50. Ong A, Anderson J, Roche J (2003) A pilot study of the prevalence of lumbar disc degeneration in elite athletes with lower back pain at the Sydney 2000 Olympic Games. Br J Sports Med 37(3):263–266
51. Videman T, Sarna S, Battie MC, Koskinen S, Gill K, Paananen H et al (1995) The long-term effects of physical loading and exercise lifestyles on back-related symptoms, disability, and spinal pathology among men. Spine 20(6):699–709
52. Boden SD, Davis DO, Dina TS, Patronas NJ, Wiesel SW (1990) Abnormal magnetic-resonance scans of the lumbar spine in asymptomatic subjects. A prospective investigation. J Bone Joint Surg Am 72(3):403–408
53. Blazek O, Streda A, Cermak V, Skallova O (1986) The incidence of morbus Scheuermann in sportsmen. J Sports Med Phys Fitness 26(1):55–59
54. Sward L (1992) The thoracolumbar spine in young elite athletes. Current concepts on the effects of physical training. Sports Med 13(5):357–364
55. Blumenthal SL, Roach J, Herring JA (1987) Lumbar Scheuermann's. A clinical series and classification. Spine 12(9):929–932
56. Tallroth K, Schlenzka D (1990) Spinal stenosis subsequent to juvenile lumbar osteochondrosis. Skeletal Radiol 19(3):203–205

57. McCall IW, Park WM, O'Brien JP, Seal V (1985) Acute traumatic intraosseous disc herniation. Spine 10(2):134–137
58. Yang IK, Bahk YW, Choi KH, Paik MW, Shinn KS (1994) Posterior lumbar apophyseal ring fractures: a report of 20 cases. Neuroradiology 36(6):453–455
59. Chang CH, Lee ZL, Chen WJ, Tan CF, Chen LH (2008) Clinical significance of ring apophysis fracture in adolescent lumbar disc herniation. Spine 33(16):1750–1754
60. Helbig T, Lee CK (1988) The lumbar facet syndrome. Spine 13(1):61–64
61. Boswell MV, Colson JD, Sehgal N, Dunbar EE, Epter R (2007) A systematic review of therapeutic facet joint interventions in chronic spinal pain. Pain Physician 10(1):229–253
62. Barnsley L (2002) Steroid injections: effect on pain of spinal origin. Best Pract Res Clin Anaesthesiol 16(4):579–596
63. Manchikanti L, Damron K, Cash K, Manchukonda R, Pampati V (2006) Therapeutic cervical medial branch blocks in managing chronic neck pain: a preliminary report of a randomized, double-blind, controlled trial: clinical trial NCT0033272. Pain Physician 9(4):333–346
64. Hossain M, Nokes LD (2005) A model of dynamic sacro-iliac joint instability from malrecruitment of gluteus maximus and biceps femoris muscles resulting in low back pain. Med Hypotheses 65(2):278–281
65. Hungerford B, Gilleard W, Hodges P (2003) Evidence of altered lumbopelvic muscle recruitment in the presence of sacroiliac joint pain. Spine 28(14):1593–1600
66. Brolinson PG, Kozar AJ, Cibor G (2003) Sacroiliac joint dysfunction in athletes. Curr Sports Med Rep 2(1):47–56
67. Tuite MJ (2008) Sacroiliac joint imaging. Semin Musculoskelet Radiol 12(1):72–82
68. Puhakka KB, Jurik AG, Egund N, Schiottz-Christensen B, Stengaard-Pedersen K, van Overeem Hansen G et al (2003) Imaging of sacroiliitis in early seronegative spondylarthropathy. Assessment of abnormalities by MR in comparison with radiography and CT. Acta Radiol 44(2):218–229
69. Tuite MJ (2004) Facet joint and sacroiliac joint injection. Semin Roentgenol 39(1):37–51
70. Bollow M, Hermann KG, Biedermann T, Sieper J, Schontube M, Braun J (2005) Very early spondyloarthritis: where the inflammation in the sacroiliac joints starts. Ann Rheum Dis 64(11):1644–1646
71. Fortin JD, Dwyer AP, West S, Pier J (1994) Sacroiliac joint: pain referral maps upon applying a new injection/arthrography technique. Part I: Asymptomatic volunteers. Spine 19(13):1475–1482
72. Elgafy H, Semaan HB, Ebraheim NA, Coombs RJ (2001) Computed tomography findings in patients with sacroiliac pain. Clin Orthop Relat Res (382):112–118

Chapter 11
Ultrasound-Guided Sports Intervention

Philip J. O'Connor

Introduction

There has been a significant increase in use of ultrasound (US) in the assessment of sports injury worldwide. Awareness of the value of high-resolution musculoskeletal ultrasound has lead to increasing interest by both radiologists and clinicians in using ultrasound to perform guided interventions in sports injury patients [1–4].

The principles of ultrasound-guided intervention are simple with both the technical aspects of performing a procedure and the clinical decision-making process important. In general, it is the decision about what treatment option to follow that is the most important part of ultrasound-guided intervention, similar to the surgical adage "it is the decision not the incision that has most impact."

There are a wide range of interventions available including diagnostic injections to determine the origin of symptoms or therapeutic interventions targeted on a variety of tissues. The evidence base and science underlying these interventions is generally weak especially in elite sportsmen and women. This mainly results from the difficulties in performing randomised controlled trials in this patient group. Much of the available evidence comes from either animal work (e.g. from horse racing) or translating results from non-elite sometimes older athletes such has occurred with much of the tendon intervention. These procedures are however still widely performed to apparent good success in terms of patient satisfaction and as such warrant discussion in this chapter.

Philip J. O'Connor (✉)
Department of Musculoskeletal Radiology, Leeds Teaching Hospitals, Chapeltown Road, Leeds LS7 4SA, UK
e-mail: philip.o'connor@leedsth.nhs.uk

Needle Placement

Principles

1. The needle approach should be carefully planned.

    "You put needles in with your head and not your hands!"
    The needle must reach the target site safely and accurately

Safely

Avoiding where possible sensitive structures such as viscera, tendons, neurovascular bundles. This requires planning of the access route for the needle before marking the puncture site and requires the operator to think three dimensionally and pre-visualise the needle track through the patient's tissues.

Accurately

This requires good visualisation of the needle throughout it course.

Needle tracking is best achieved with the needle parallel to the probe surface when the surface of the needle has maximal sound reflecting potential (Fig. 11.1a–c). Getting the needle as close to parallel as possible is usually achievable for musculoskeletal sports interventions even for deep structures such as hip injections. Tilting the probe can help convert a steep oblique approach into a shallow oblique or near-parallel approach (Fig. 11.2a, b).

Deciding on the Puncture Site and Needle Path

The patient is positioned appropriately so that both the patient and the operator are comfortable and the target site for the needle tip is optimally visualised. It is useful to mark

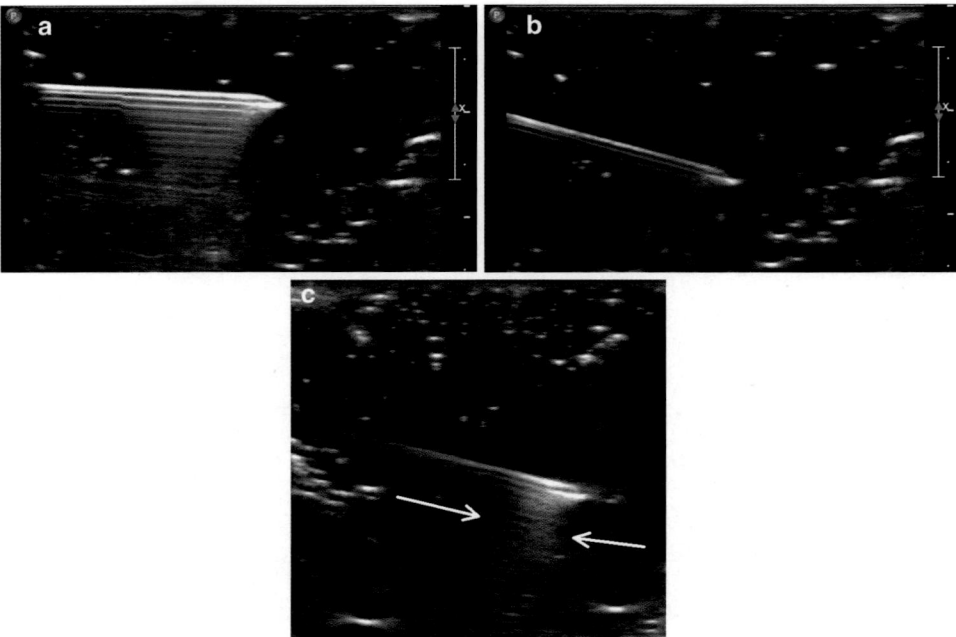

Fig. 11.1 With the needle near to parallel, the conspicuity of the needle increases (**a**) in comparison with an oblique approach (**b**). **c** shows the typical reverberation artefact seen from the bevel even when scanned obliquely (*arrow*)

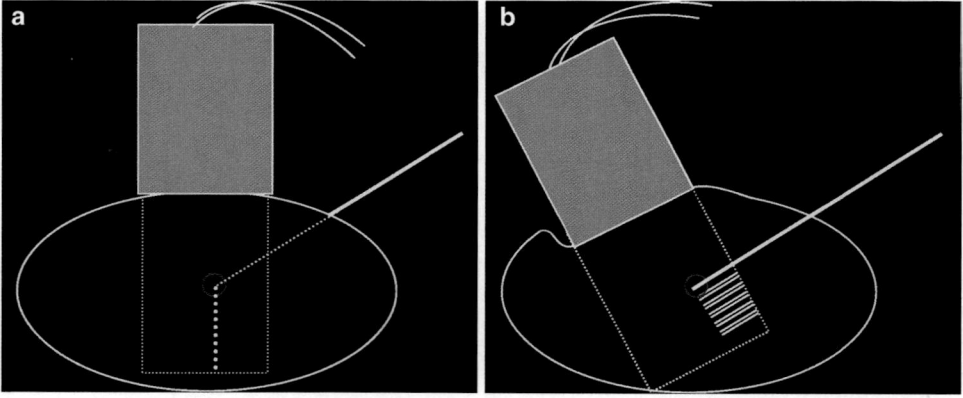

Fig. 11.2 A standard oblique approach (**a**) can be converted into a near-parallel approach by tilting the scanning angle (**b**)

the site of the probe for later reference and then the site of puncture is marked. When it comes to the injection, it is often helpful to penetrate the skin prior to positioning the probe so it is helpful to indicate the direction the needle needs to travel with a line or arrow on the skin rather than a dot.

For best visualisation of the needle, the needle track should be parallel (or close to parallel) to the probe face. The site of needle entry is therefore usually a few centimetres away from the probe margin but this will vary with the depth of the injection target. Use the centimetre markers on the edge of the ultrasound screen to estimate the ideal puncture distance from the probe (Fig. 11.3). Puncturing the skin some distance from the target (and probe) will require a longer needle than would be used for a more direct approach.

The use of an arrow or line when marking helps direct the needle so the operator can part insert the needle in the correct direction before beginning scanning.

Aseptic technique is used throughout with the skin preparation and a probe cover, with particular care when a joint injection is being undertaken. In general, introduce your needle without any syringe attached, this aids needle manipulation and results in better positioning, once you have achieved good needle position ideally you want to preserve it.

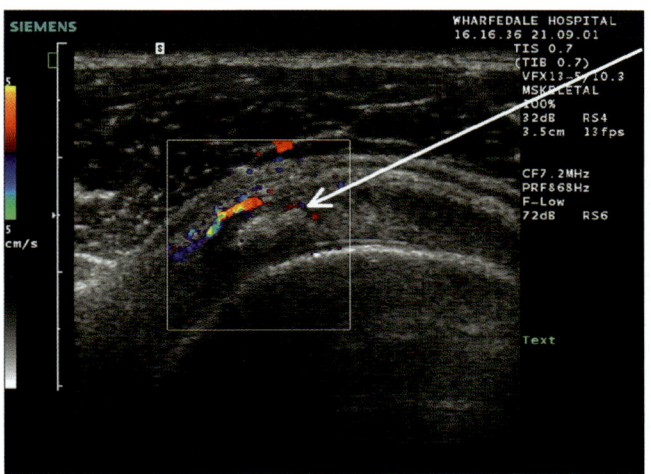

Fig. 11.3 When deciding the right distance from the probe to puncture the skin use the centimetre markers on the screen. Here in a patient with calcific tendonitis you can see the ideal approach (*arrow*) would require puncture approximately 1 cm lateral to the probe edge

It is difficult to connect a syringe directly onto the end of your needle and then scan and inject without significantly changing its position. This is not so important when the needle is up against bone but very important when injecting in soft-tissues. The use of a pre-flushed connector is useful and should be non-leuer lock and preferably short giving the operator the best chance for directly visualising the needle tip during the injection itself.

For accurate positioning it is important to know the exact position of the needle tip when positioning your needle. To achieve this you need to keep the needle in longitudinal alignment with the transducer, failure to do so will introduce cross-cut or volume averaging artefacts which can result in poor or inadequate positioning.

Cross-cut artefact is where the needle and probe are not parallel with only a portion of the needle visualised at any one time.

The portion of needle may or may not include the needle tip, to avoid cross-cut artefact the radiologist needs to be aware:

1. When they are not visualising the full length of needle appreciating the differing appearance of the needle bevel from the shaft (Fig. 11.1).
2. Cross-cut can sometimes be caused by needle deviation within the patient especially when using flexible narrow-gauge needles rather than failure of probe needle alignment.

The entire length of the needle is best seen when the probe face and needle are in longitudinal alignment. In this position, regardless of angle, the bevel normally gives off reverberation artefact. The closer to parallel the approach, the stronger the reverberation artefact. Identification of the bevel helps avoid cross-cut artefact.

There are other techniques to improve needle visualisation without altering the angle between probe and needle. Electronic beam steering on modern machines allows the user to angle the beam from a linear transducer to bring the needle near to parallel to the "effective" transducer surface. Small backward and forward movements increase visibility of needle. This is particularly important if targeting at depth when needle visualisation is usually more difficult. The use of power Doppler and tapping the end of the needle to produce a shock wave and power Doppler signal within the needle can also help improve visualisation.

Controlling and altering the path of your needle is important. Either the probe or the needle is moved, but not both at the same time. Visualising the bevel and particularly the direction of the bevel can also help with positioning. The needle is preferentially directed away from the bevel direction as the needle passes through tissues, the thinner the needle the more prominent is this effect. Spinal needles have a notch in the stilette indicating the direction of the bevel. Bending the needle in the opposite direction to that required is a useful way of redirecting the thin flexible spinal needles used for deeper injections. More superficial injections are normally performed with 21G, 23G or 25G needles of varying length. Five-centimetre 21G needles are available commercially; these are very useful for slightly deeper injection such as the symphysis pubis or shoulder joints. These shorter needles are less flexible than spinal needles and are somewhat harder to readjust en route. If the needle is not following close to the correct path with these shorter needles it is better to start afresh and modify your puncture site rather than trying to accommodate suboptimal positioning. Once the needle is in place, it important to be able to inject and scan the needle tip without altering needle position. This requires the use of an injection short connecter, in general a non-leuer lock connecter is best. The needle tip should be watched throughout the start of the injection. If you are injecting a joint space or cavity such as a bursa the injectate should flow away from the tip of the needle. If the injection collects around the tip of the needle the injection is not correctly sited and the needle repositioned. The bevel can also be used to glide off the surface of cartilage for joint injections or the bursal aspect of the rotator cuff for bursal injections, this is particularly useful when the joint is dry or the bursa being injected is thin.

Common Pitfalls and Solutions

1. Inadequate planning before the procedure.
   Action: no one plans to fail, they just fail to plan. Take longer setting up and considering your needle path.

Plan to get the needle as near to parallel as possible, the better you see the needle the better the intervention.

2. Needle not visualised.
   Action: Look at your hands not the screen. The needle needs to be re-oriented with respect to the probe. Move your probe or the needle, avoid moving both at the same time. Tilt probe to be as near to parallel as possible and use small backward and forward movements of the needle to improve needle conspicuity.

3. Needle tip not directed towards target.
   Action: Different action for superficial and deep injections. For superficial injections have a low threshold for re-siting the puncture point, there is normally little room to compensate for poor initial set up. In deeper injections, adjustment of the needle path can usually be achieved without changing the puncture point.

4. Injection against extreme resistance.
   Action: This happens in US-guided joint injections when the needle tip is in solid tissue rather than a cavity. Adjustment of needle tip position is required; do not persevere with the injection in these circumstances.

5. Unsure of exact needle tip position.
   Action: If even after point 2 further confirmation of needle tip position is required before injection. For non-arthrographic studies a small amount of room air can be injected, air has much greater ultrasound conspicuity than fluid though avoid using too much air injection as it limits beam penetration and can obscure the injection site. Use air injection when you are pretty sure that you are in the right place but need a bit of extra confidence/confirmation. If you are unhappy with the procedure and cannot visualise your needle tip do not inject.

Once you understand how to introduce your needle, visualise your needle and have control of needle positioning during injection you can start to think about what interventions can be undertaken. These broadly involve injecting something, taking something out, or performing an intervention with the needle itself.

Interventions

Injections can split into diagnostic and therapeutic.

Diagnostic Injections

These involve the injection of long or short-acting local anaesthetic to determine the origin of a patient's symptoms. Patients are required to keep a symptom log post-injection and, if their pain is of an episodic nature or related to specific activity, test themselves out to determine whether the pain is worse, unaltered, improved or gone. These injections can be into bursae such as the subacromial or greater trochanteric bursa or joints. Lidocaine is the short-acting agent of choice with effects lasting 30–45 min. Longer-acting agents are bupivocaine and ropivacaine which have anaesthetic effects for 5–6 h post-injection. When injecting joints do not use bupivocaine as recent reports of potential cartilage toxicity have resulted in it not being recommended for intra-articular use.

Therapeutic Interventions

These can be divided into three main types:

1. Steroid injection; undertaken for a variety of reasons in sports practise
2. Tendon interventions
   a. Dry needling
   b. Autologous blood, spun platelet-rich plasma or stem cell injection
   c. Calcium aspiration
3. Haematoma aspiration; normally performed for muscle tears

Steroid Injection

The injection of long-acting steroids is common place in sports medicine practise. It has specific uses although it tends to be somewhat overused. Long-acting steroids such as triamcinolone has anti-inflammatory effects that are of value in shrinking down tissues which have an activated inflammatory cascade (such as synovitis, thickened bursae), an antifibroblastic action (as a result triamcinolone has been used to inhibit Keloid formation around scars) and a neurolytic action preventing aberrant nerve stimulation [5–7].

These complex modes of action need to be considered before performing guided steroid injection. Probably the most important is the antifibroblastic effect with steroid injection associated with anecdotal and experimental evidence of tendon damage. As a result, steroid injection is not recommended by the author in or around tendons where there is evidence of pre-existing tendon damage. Tendon sheath or paratenon injection can be performed when there is no ultrasound evidence of tendinopathy. When patients have evidence of tendon damage, the understanding of the potential for progressing to a torn tendon is necessary for informed consent.

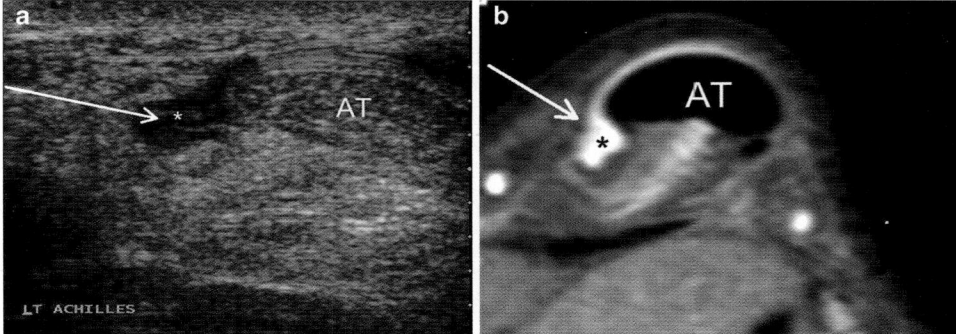

Fig. 11.4 Transverse scan of Achilles paratendonitis with needle insertion (*arrow*) normally performed from the medial side to avoid the sural nerve when possible

Paratenon injection is most useful in the Achilles tendon and is best used in combination with bupivocaine stripping or distension of the tendon sheath. This has value as adhesions are an aetiological factor in Achilles paratendonitis as well as short-term overuse normally seen at the beginning of the season on resumption of training. The paratenon injection is normally performed at the site of pain with a needle inserted into the thickened paratenon using transverse medial approach (Fig. 11.4). After this a relatively high volume of bupivocaine mixed with steroid is injected, often 10–15 ml of injectate is used. Following this procedure a minimum of 2 weeks rest is required before returning to full sporting activity.

One way of considering steroid is to treat it as a form of long-acting local anaesthetic. They are therefore of value in self-limiting conditions to control symptoms. An example of this would be a patient with calcific tendonitis of the shoulder, this is an acutely painful condition that in the majority of cases resolves. The patient normally has secondary impingement and associated bursitis, bursal steroid injection is an excellent initial therapeutic option with review after 6 weeks at which time aspiration and wash out of the deposit can be considered if the patient remains symptomatic. Steroids can also be of value in reducing symptoms sufficiently to allow a course of effective physiotherapy. Shoulder impingement syndrome is an excellent example where subacromial bursal steroid injection facilitates effective rehabilitation.

Steroids can also be used to shrink down inflamed tissues that can be causing mechanical impingement. This is seen in specific areas where there is tissue thickening in an enclosed mobile space, examples are the AC joint, posterior ankle impingement and anterolateral ankle impingement.

Injection for impingement syndromes of the ankle is common and effective.

Intra-articular steroid injections can be of value in patients with synovitis with the most common sites being the hip, knee and shoulder. Intra-articular injection can be performed by placing the needle tip within a visible joint effusion or by placing the needle tip adjacent to articular cartilage. In the hip, this is best approached from a lateral oblique approach (also see Chap 2). A posterior approach with internal rotation positioning is used to visualise the humeral head articular cartilage in the shoulder with the cartilage of the trochlear groove the best approach for the knee though effusions are normally a simpler target in patients requiring knee injections.

Tendon Interventions

Dry needling and autologous blood injection are used in the treatment of tendinopathy [8–13]. The theory behind these injections is to release blood products into a tendon inducing a healing cascade. It is now accepted that tendinopathy is a stress-related response probably resulting from stress-induced protein kinase production causing cell damage leading to apoptosis and increase in glycoprotein matrix. Enzyme production is greater with increased amplitude of stress and increased temperature. There is no inflammatory cascade stimulated as part of this process, the term tendinitis is a misnomer and should not be used. Paratendinitis is a true inflammatory process and is correctly named and has differing aetiology. The use of steroids is as a result appropriate in Achilles paratendonitis though only when the adjacent tendon shows little or no evidence of tendinopathy.

Dry needling involves running a needle multiple times through an area of tendinopathy targeting the vessels within the tendinopathic area. Power Doppler examination of the relaxed tendon best demonstrates vascularity. Demonstration of the vessels is also important as they have a close relationship to symptoms and are an indicator of active and clinically significant tendinopathy.

Dry needling and autologous blood should only be performed for refractory cases who fail conservative management. Dry needling with or without autologous blood works best for localised disease with diffuse tendinopathic change more difficult to effectively cover from percutaneous puncture sites.

The entheses are the areas best treated, particularly the proximal patellar tendon and the common extensor origin at the elbow. Needling the tendons themselves can be quite painful and good local anaesthesia and patience is required for these tendon interventions (ideally a 30-min appointment time required). Dry needling is performed normally through a single puncture angling the needle from superficial to deep through the entire tendon. Local anaesthetic should be injected on the superficial aspect of the tendon and with each pass some local will be carried into the tendon (Fig. 11.5). Injection of local into the tendon itself may well be required, the procedure should be pain free, achieving this allows for more effective needling. Power Doppler should be used to identify any persisting vessels with needling of these areas continued until little or no flow remains in the tendon. Tendons with only low-grade vascularity may require injection of autologous blood. This can be assessed to some extent during the procedure by watching for back bleeding down the needle during dry needling. Only low-grade vascularity and a lack of back bleeding are indicators that autologous blood injection should be considered. The autologous blood is usually drawn up only once dry needling and good needle positioning has been achieved. This is to avoid any delay between drawing up of the injectate and injection to avoid clotting. The dry needling ensures good distribution of the injectate through the tendon. This has to be assessed in real time as fresh autologous blood is virtually isoechoic with diseased tendon.

The post-procedure advice to the patient is important, players should be advised to rest post-procedure for a minimum of 2 weeks with no return to full sporting activity/training until 6 weeks. A common error is for players to continue with an eccentric programme post-procedure, this will not allow effective healing to occur. I explain the post-procedure care as being akin to healing of an operative incision or cut, you wouldn't keep moving it everyday to check whether it was healing, would you!

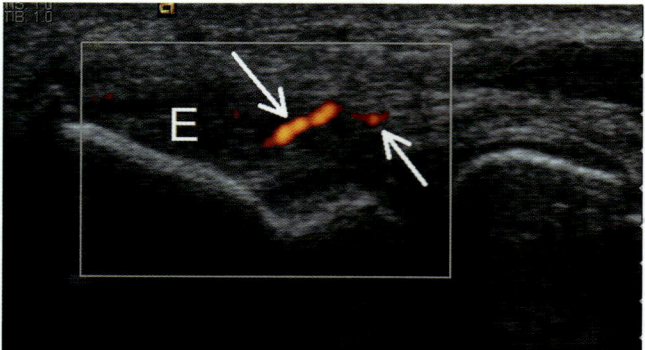

Fig. 11.5 Tennis elbow patient with thickened common extensor origin (E) and increased vascularity (*arrows*). These vessels and the hypoechoic portion of the tendon are the target for dry needling and autologous blood injection

Muscle Intervention

Haematoma Aspiration

Aspiration of muscle haematoma in sports injury is relatively common in sports medicine practise. The aim is to minimise the gap that required to infill during healing, it is most commonly performed in muscle contusion with vastus intermedius most frequently treated.

Aspiration cannot be performed until the haematoma has sufficiently liquidised, this does not occur until at least 10 days post-injury.

This can be assessed with ultrasound by assessing the echotexture and compressibility of the haematoma (Fig. 11.6a–c). Altering probe pressure shows the amount of free movement of the fluid. Aspiration should be performed under strict sterile conditions with skin prep, gloves and probe cover. The aspiration should be performed with a 19- or 20-gauge needle with the haematoma aspirated to dryness.

Specific Injections

Some specific injections and injection techniques require further discussion

Subacromial Bursal Injection

Deciding who to inject can be difficult, look for the "step" sign in the subacromial bursa as it becomes entrapped under the coracoacromial ligament during abduction to indicate impingement (Fig. 11.7). Comparing bursal appearances with the contralateral side can also be of value (Fig. 11.8) [14].

The patient is seated comfortably with the arm behind the back with the back of the hand touching the small of the back. The bursa is identified and an appropriate point of entry is chosen. The bevel can help localise the needle with the cavity of the bursa. With the bevel facing the tendon the needle will glance off the surface of the supraspinatous into the bursa. The hardest bursae to inject are the very thick bursae where it is difficult to know the exact site of the bursal cavity, in general the cavity of the bursa is close to the surface of the supraspinatous. With an appropriately sited injection the injectate flows away from the needle tip completely. It is important to be able to inject and scan at the same time to observe the needle tip during injection. This is very difficult with a syringe attached directly to the needle, the use of a short non-leuer lock connector is of great value; it allows you to scan,

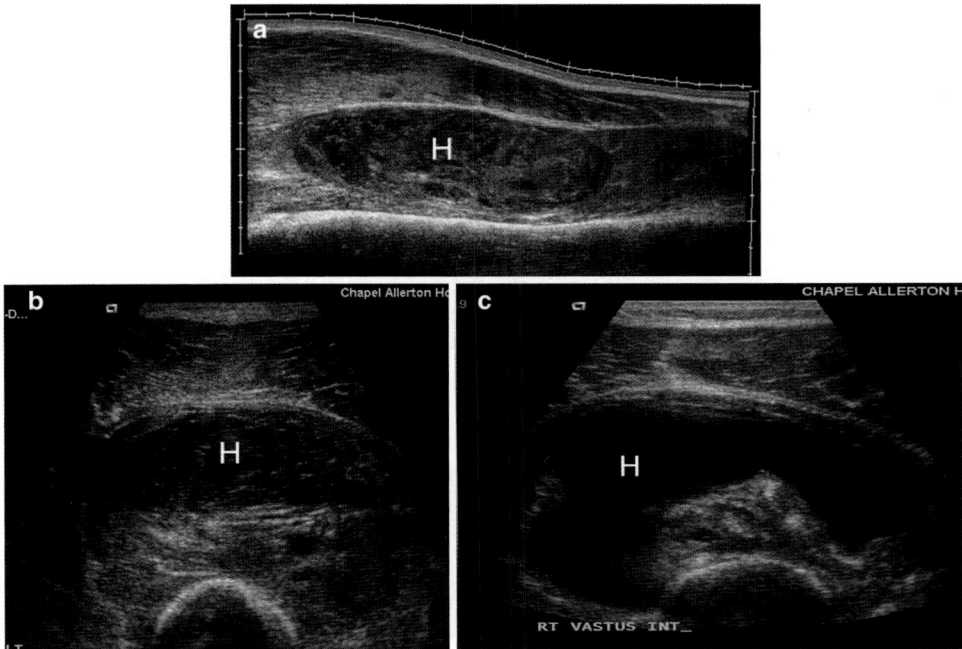

Fig. 11.6 Patient with large contusion of vastus intermedius with haematoma (H). Longitudinal (**a**) and transverse (**b**) on day 1 show complex haematoma with internal structure. By day 10 (**c**) the haematoma has cleared of internal echoes and would be amenable to aspiration

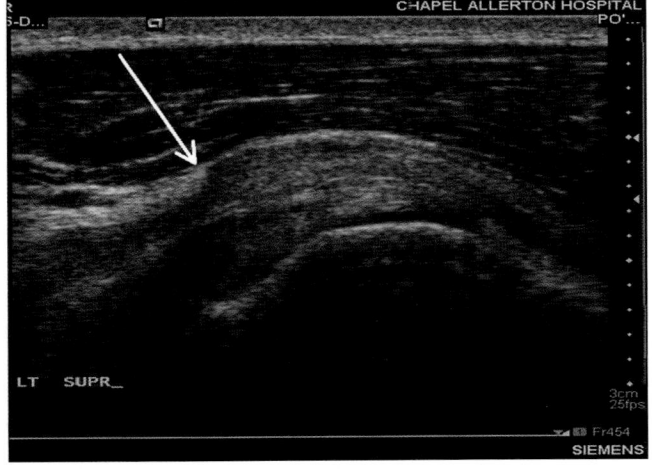

Fig. 11.7 Longitudinal scan of the supraspinatous and subacromial bursa in a patient with impingement showing the step sign of the coracoacromial ligament indenting the subacromial bursa (*arrow*)

inject and observe the needle tip without moving the needle position. The injection should be without resistance with little or no injectate seen collecting around the needle tip. If the injectate pools around the needle tip it is not in the bursa and requires repositioning. Inject a minimum of 5 ml lignocaine–bupivocaine mix for diagnostic injections with the addition of 40 mg depomedrone or triamcinolone for therapeutic injections.

Symphysis Pubis and Acromio-Clavicular Joint Injection

These joints have more in common than you might think, structurally they are similar and the approach to injection is similar.

Osteitis pubis is common in many sports especially soccer. The combination of steroid injection with appropriate rehabilitation has been shown to be effective in treating soccer-related osteitis pubis [15] (see also Chap 2).

The ultrasound probe is positioned to scan along the long axis of the symphysis/AC joint in an antero-posterior (i.e. sagittal) plane till the gap between the lateral clavicle and the acromion/pubic bodies is identified. The joint will appear as a hypoechoic and oval. The needle is then inserted from above the probe (symphysis) or anterior (ACJ) at approximately 3 cm away from the probe to allow a near-parallel or oblique approach (Fig. 11.9).

Pitfall: sometimes the AC joint can be very degenerated with narrow joint space and osteophytosis, make sure the arm is unsupported at the patient's side to open up the joint space.

Fig. 11.8 Longitudinal scan of the supraspinatous and subacromial bursa in a patient with impingement. (**a**) The symptomatic side shows marked bursal thickening (*) with the contralateral asymptomatic side showing no bursal thickening (**b**)

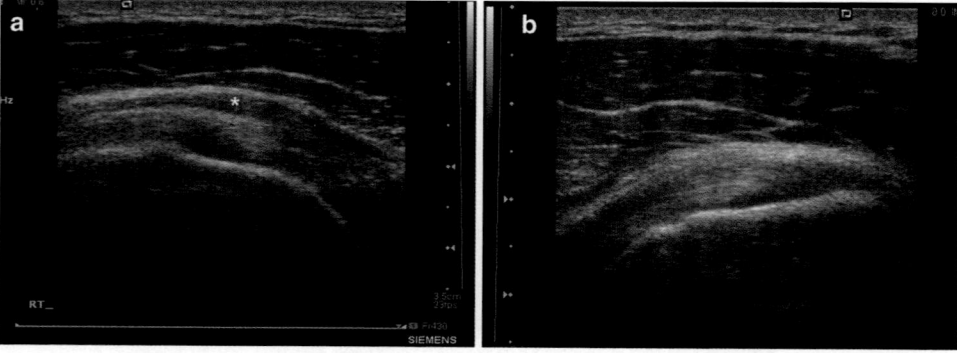

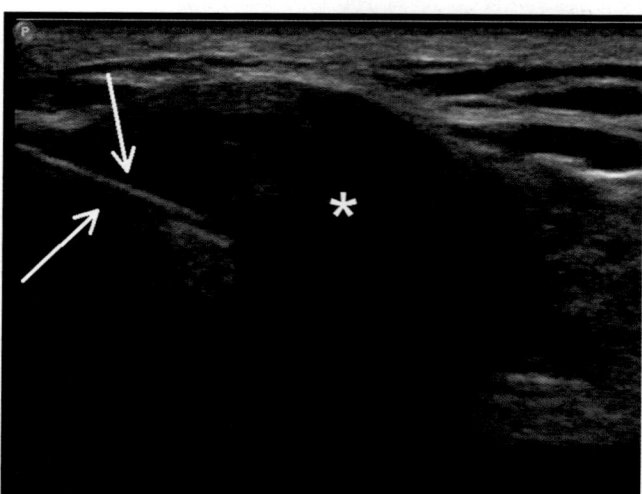

Fig. 11.9 AC joint injection with the joint space visualised sagittally as a hypoechoic oval (*) and the needle inserted anteriorly (*arrow*)

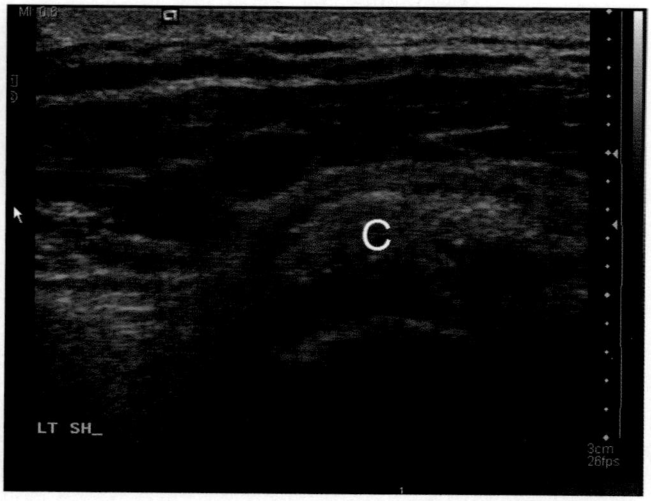

Fig. 11.10 Longitudinal scan of the supraspinatous in a patient with acute calcific tendonitis. The calcific deposit (C) is well defined, slightly hyperechoic compared to the surrounding cuff with no distal acoustic shadowing

US-Guided Barbotage for Calcific Tendinitis

Calcific tendinitis results from the deposition of calcium hydroxyapatite within or close to tendons. It is particularly common around the limb girdle with the shoulder most commonly affected. Calcific tendonitis is of unknown aetiology and can be treated effectively with barbotage [16–19]. This essentially consists of puncturing and aspirating acute calcific deposits with repeated puncture and wash out of more mature solid calcifications [16]. The initial US gives some indication as to whether the deposit will aspirate [20]. Acute deposits show low-grade hyper-echogenicity compared to the surrounding tendon with no distal acoustic shadowing (Fig. 11.10). More mature deposits are brighter with clear posterior acoustic shadowing, they are also often fragmented (Fig. 11.11).

The bursa and cuff in these patients is very sensitive, it wise to at least initially perform this procedure with the patient lying down. Local anaesthetic infiltration needs to be

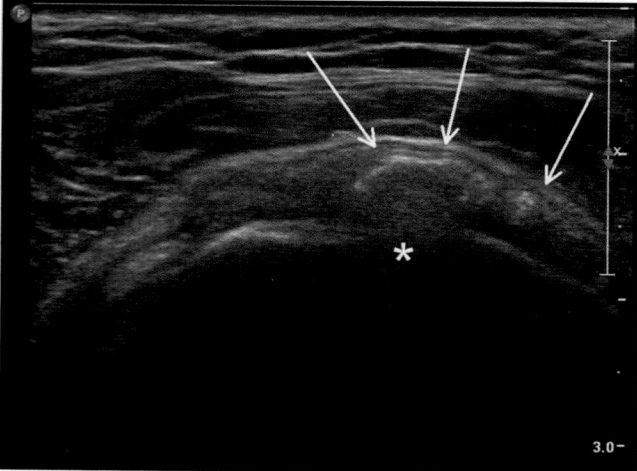

Fig. 11.11 Longitudinal scan of the supraspinatous in a patient with chronic calcific tendonitis. The calcific deposit (*arrows*) is very bright compared to the surrounding cuff, fragmented and has distal acoustic shadowing evidenced by the lack of cortex visualisation in the underlying bone (*)

performed into the skin, bursa and tendon with sufficient time left for this to take full effect. Once needle placement has been achieved within the deposit lignocaine is then injected into the deposit to wash out or lavage the cavity. A pumping action works well with lignocaine passing into and out of the tendon carrying out the calcium into the syringe. In well-formed calcification, it is often not possible to aspirate even through a 19G needle, dry needling of the deposit in these cases should be performed with further wash out of the deposit. This works in two ways, it can work to stimulate scar formation within the tendon and secondly it makes a communication between the bursa and the calcific cavity allowing wash out of the deposit into the bursa.

After either of these approaches the final part of barbotage is to inject 40 mg of depomedrone or triamcinolone into the subacromial bursa, this helps combat any acute flare up of subacromial bursitis.

Results are in the order of 70% good response rate with this approach, this figure is significantly higher if the calcification does not cast posterior acoustic shadowing and is greater than 1 cm [16]. The above principles can be extended to treat calcific tendinitis at other sites [21].

Injection at Ischial Tuberosity (Hamstring Origin)

The patient lies prone with the injection approach from the medial aspect of the common hamstring origin scanning in the transverse plane. Ultrasound can demonstrate changes with hypoechoic thickening of the tendon the most frequent finding. MR is, however, the most appropriate modality for determining the site and type of hamstring intervention to be performed. A tear of the hamstring origins should be allowed to heal without intervention. Tendinopathy would require dry needling [21] with paratendonitic inflammatory change targeted by local steroid infiltration.

Plantar Fasciitis Injection

The diagnosis of plantar fasciitis is in general clinical with normally little requirement for diagnostic imaging.

Patients present with heel pain over the inferomedial aspect of the heel worse after rest easing with exercise. This history is characteristic especially a history of the pain being most severe first thing in the morning, if this is not present be suspicious you are not dealing with plantar fasciitis. Night pain or a history of unusual exercise should make one think of bone pathology, this can be checked by looking for pain with calcaneal squeeze testing. If this is present radiography and or MR will be required for further assessment. The radiological assessment is best performed with ultrasound, radiographs for assessing the presence or absence of plantar spurs are not indicated. Diagnosis can be made on ultrasound which demonstrates tendinopathic change in the plantar fascia. This is most commonly seen in the medial band of the proximal plantar fascia with typical changes of hypoechogenicity and increased thickness. A fascia measuring over 5 mm is highly suggestive of fasciitis with the measurement best taken at the thickest point of the plantar fascia.

This is normally at the level of the distal origin of the plantar fascia from the calcaneus with the proximal 2–3 cm most commonly involved, more distal involvement is more commonly seen following rupture rather than fasciitis.

Comparison with the contra lateral plantar fascia can be of value in cases where there is diagnostic doubt. When there is still diagnostic difficulty or in recalcitrant cases MR can be of value in diagnosis and in demonstrating inflammatory change to help guide injection placement.

Therapeutic approaches include guided steroid injection, dry needling and autologous blood injection [1, 4, 22, 23].

The preferred injection technique is a posterior approach using a 5-cm 21-gauge needle with liberal use of local anaesthetic. This approach allows access to both the tendon and its superficial and deep aspects of the proximal tendon over the entire length of tendon normally involved in fasciitis (Fig. 11.12).

The injection of long-acting steroids is a common treatment for plantar fasciitis. The effects in plantar fasciitis could be both neurolytic or anti-inflammatory and given the MR inflammatory change is seen deep and superficial to the plantar fascia steroid injection around rather than within the plantar fascia should be most effective. Following this procedure, a minimum of 2 weeks rest is required before returning to sporting activity.

It is difficult to determine with ultrasound the ideal site for injection, the author prefers injection of the superficial aspect of the fascia with a relatively small volume injection

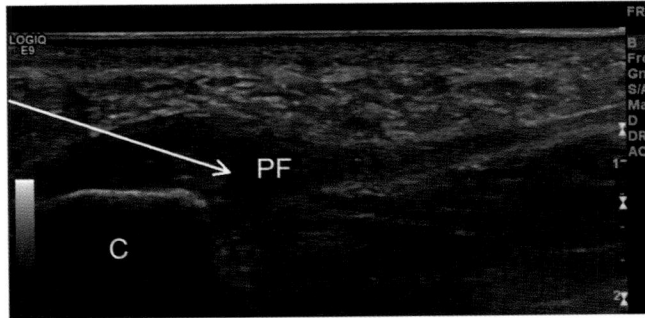

Fig. 11.12 Longitudinal scan of the plantar fascia origin from the calcaneus (C). The plantar fascia is grossly thickened and hypoechoic (PF). The posterior needle approach used for guided intervention is shown by the *white arrow*

to avoid spread into the adjacent heel fat pad. Use only 40 mg triamcinolone and 1 ml 1% Lignocaine for the whole injection and position the needle as close to the tendon as possible.

Dry needling involves running a needle through a diseased tendon numerous times to release blood products into the tendon. This is performed from a posterior approach with local anaesthetic applied to the skin and on the superficial aspect of the plantar fascia. The plantar fascia is very sensitive and local anaesthetic injection into the fascia itself will be required. The amount of bleeding occurring can be assessed during the procedure by the presence or absence of back bleeding down the needle bore. If there is no back bleeding then autologous blood injection can be performed. This is undertaken with the needle positioned in the centre of the plantar fascia and injection of 1 ml autologous blood drawn up normally from the patients arm just before injection. Any delay may result in clotting impairing injection and effective spread of the injection within the tendon. Dry needling and autologous blood injection can be combined with steroid injection over its superficial aspect.

As with steroid injection rest after the procedure is advised with treatment taking up to 6 weeks to have full effect. With this approach, audits in our department show a success rate of 80% for symptom resolution at 12 months for secondary care and recalcitrant cases.

References

1. Sofka CM, Collins AJ, Adler RS (2001) Use of ultrasonographic guidance in interventional musculoskeletal procedures: a review from a single institution. J Ultrasound Med 20:21–26
2. Cardinal E, Beauregard CG, Chhem RK (1997) Interventional musculoskeletal ultrasound. Semin Musculoskelet Radiol 1:311–318
3. Cardinal E, Chhem RK, Beauregard CG (1998) Ultrasound-guided interventional procedures in the musculoskeletal system. Radiol Clin North Am 36:597–604
4. Adler RS, Sofka CM (2003) Percutaneous ultrasound-guided injections in the musculoskeletal system. Ultrasound Q 19:3–12
5. Smith JR, Gomez NH (1970) Local injection therapy of neuromata of the hand with triamcinolone acetonide. A preliminary study of twenty-two patients. J Bone Joint Surg Am 52:71–83
6. Pataky PE, Graham WP 3rd, Munger BL (1973) Terminal neuromas treated with triamcinolone acetonide. J Surg Res 14:36–45
7. Robbins TH (1977) The response of tender neuromas and scars to triamcinolone injections. Br J Plast Surg 30:68–69
8. Taylor MA, Norman TL, Clovis NB, Blaha JD (2002) The response of rabbit patellar tendons after autologous blood injection. Med Sci Sports Exerc 34:70–73
9. Edwards SG, Calandruccio JH (2003) Autologous blood injections for refractory lateral epicondylitis. J Hand Surg Am 28:272–278
10. Suresh SP, Ali KE, Jones H, Connell DA (2006) Medial epicondylitis: is ultrasound guided autologous blood injection an effective treatment? Br J Sports Med 40:935–939, discussion 939
11. Connell DA, Ali KE, Ahmad M, Lambert S, Corbett S, Curtis M (2006) Ultrasound-guided autologous blood injection for tennis elbow. Skeletal Radiol 35:371–377
12. James SL, Ali K, Pocock C et al (2007) Ultrasound guided dry needling and autologous blood injection for patellar tendinosis. Br J Sports Med 41:518–521, discussion 522
13. Zhu J, Hu B, Xing C, Li J (2008) Ultrasound-guided, minimally invasive, percutaneous needle puncture treatment for tennis elbow. Adv Ther 25:1031–1036
14. Farin PU, Jaroma H, Harju A, Soimakallio S (1990) Shoulder impingement syndrome: sonographic evaluation. Radiology 176:845–849
15. Schilders E, Bismil Q, Robinson P, O'Connor PJ, Gibbon WW, Talbot JC (2007) Adductor-related groin pain in competitive athletes. Role of adductor enthesis, magnetic resonance imaging, and entheseal pubic cleft injections. J Bone Joint Surg Am 89:2173–2178
16. Farin PU, Jaroma H, Soimakallio S (1995) Rotator cuff calcifications: treatment with US-guided technique. Radiology 195:841–843
17. Bradley M, Bhamra MS, Robson MJ (1995) Ultrasound guided aspiration of symptomatic supraspinatus calcific deposits. Br J Radiol 68:716–719
18. Farin PU, Rasanen H, Jaroma H, Harju A (1996) Rotator cuff calcifications: treatment with ultrasound-guided percutaneous needle aspiration and lavage. Skeletal Radiol 25:551–554
19. Lin JT, Adler RS, Bracilovic A, Cooper G, Sofka C, Lutz GE (2007) Clinical outcomes of ultrasound-guided aspiration and lavage in calcific tendinosis of the shoulder. HSS J 3:99–105
20. Farin PU, Jaroma H (1995) Sonographic findings of rotator cuff calcifications. J Ultrasound Med 14:7–14
21. Housner JA, Jacobson JA, Misko R (2009) Sonographically guided percutaneous needle tenotomy for the treatment of chronic tendinosis. J Ultrasound Med 28:1187–1192
22. Tsai WC, Hsu CC, Chen CP, Chen MJ, Yu TY, Chen YJ (2006) Plantar fasciitis treated with local steroid injection: comparison between sonographic and palpation guidance. J Clin Ultrasound 34:12–16
23. Kalaci A, Cakici H, Hapa O, Yanat AN, Dogramaci Y, Sevinc TT (2009) Treatment of plantar fasciitis using four different local injection modalities: a randomized prospective clinical trial. J Am Podiatr Med Assoc 99:108–113

Index

A
Abduction external rotation (ABER), 196
Abductor pollicis longus (APL), 164
ACI. *See* Autologous chondrocyte implantation
Adhesive capsulitis, 123
Ankle and foot injury
    Achilles tendon (AT)
        paratendinitis, 70–71
        tears, 71–72
        tendinopathy, 69–70
    anterior tibialis tendon (ATT), 80–81
    flexor hallucis longus (FHL) tendon, 81–82
    great toe
        hallux rigidus, 84–85
        turf toe, 83–84
    impingement syndromes
        anterior ankle, 64–65
        anterolateral (ALI), 63–64
        anteromedial ankle, 65–66
        posterior ankle (PAI), 65–68
    ligamentous
        lateral, 56–58
        Lisfranc, 60–61
        medial, 58–60
        syndesmotic/high ankle sprains, 62–63
    mechanical (non stress) fractures
        biomechanics of injury, 49
        calcaneous, 50
        pilon, 49–50
        talar/snowboarder's, 50–52
    osteochondral injuries (OCI), 55–56
    peroneal tendons
        brevis tendon tear/rupture, 74–75
        longus tendon tear/rupture, 75–76
        painful os peroneum syndrome (POPS), 76–77
        retinacular injuries, 75–76
        tenosynovitis, 73–74
    plantar fascia, 82–83
    stress fractures
        calcaneal, 53
        metatarsal, 53–54
        navicular, 53
        proximal fifth metatarsal, 54
        sesamoids, 54–55
    tibialis posterior tendon (TPT), 77–79
Anterior ankle impingement, 64–65
Anterior cruciate ligament (ACL), 2, 11–15. *See also* Postoperative imaging, sports medicine
Anterior labroligamentous periosteal sleeve avulsion (ALPSA) lesion, 123–124
Anterior talofibular ligament (ATFL) injury, 57–58
Anterior tibialis tendon (ATT), 80–81
Arthrofibrosis, 183, 184
Athletic groin pain (pubalgia)
    anatomy, 41–42
    biomechanics and core stability, 40
    clinical problem, 42–43
    imaging, 43
    inguinal *vs.* parasymphyseal, 43, 44
    injection technique, 45
    management, 45
    ultrasound role, 45
Autologous chondrocyte implantation (ACI), 190

B
Bankart lesions
    IGHL
        failure locations, 118
        and variants, 117–118
    variant, 194
Barton's fracture, 155
Blummensaat's line, 181, 182
Bone-patellar tendon-bone (BPTB), 179
Bristow–Helfet, Laterjet techniques, 195

C
Capitate fracture, 156
Carpal tunnel syndrome, 166
Carpometacarpal fracture (CMC), 170
Cartilage repair procedures
    autologous chondrocyte implantation (ACI), 190
    marrow stimulation, 188
    osteochondral allograft transplantation, 190
    osteochondral autologous transplantation (OAT), 189
Cervical spine, biomechanics, 221
Chauffeur's fracture, 155–156
Chronic repetitive trauma. *See* High-energy single injury
CMC. *See* Carpometacarpal fracture
Colles' fracture, 155
Computer tomography (CT)
    ankle and foot injury, 50, 61, 62, 65
    elbow injuries, 129
    glenohumeral instability, 120
    osseous stress injury, 93
    shoulder injury, 110, 120
Cruciate ganglion cysts, 15–16
Cyclops lesions, 183

D

Degenerative joint disease, 134–136
Delayed-onset muscle soreness (DOMS), 205
Deltoid ligament injury, 59–60
De Quervain's stenosing, 164
DIPJ. *See* Distal interphalangeal joint
Direct MR arthrography, drawbacks, 179
DISI. *See* Dorsal intercalated segment instability
Distal clavicular resection. *See* Mumford procedure
Distal interphalangeal joint (DIPJ), 169
Distal radial styloid fracture. *See* Chauffeur's fracture
Distal radioulnar joint (DRUJ), 163
DOMS. *See* Delayed-onset muscle soreness
Dorsal impingement, distal radius, 165
Dorsal intercalated segment instability (DISI), 159
DRUJ. *See* Distal radioulnar joint

E

Elbow injury
    acute (*see* Epicondylitis)
    anatomy and biomechanics, 127–128
    chronic (*see* Epicondylosis)
    epidemiology, 127
    imaging
        CT, 129
        MR imaging, 129
        musculoskeletal ultrasound, 129–130
Epicondylitis
    distal biceps injury, 138–140
    fractures, 138–139
    triceps injury, 139–140
Epicondylosis
    degenerative joint disease, 134–136
    lateral epicondylosis, 130–131
    medial epicondyle apophysitis, 133–135
    medial epicondylosis, 130–132
    medial ulnar collateral ligament injury, 131–133
    nerve entrapments, 137–138
    osteochondritis dissecans, 134–136
Extensor pollicis brevis (EPB), 164
Extrinsic ligaments, 147

F

Facet joint pain, 237–239
FAI. *See* Femoroacetabular impingement
Fast-spin echo (FSE), 176
Fatigue fracture, aetiology, 89–90
FDP. *See* Flexor digitorum profundus
FDS. *See* Flexor digitorum superficialis
Femoroacetabular impingement (FAI)
    appearances of, 32–34
    and labral abnormalities, 30–32
Finger pathology
    Bennett's fracture, 169
    Boxer's fracture, 170
    Boxer's Knuckle, 168
    mallet finger
        distal interphalangeal joint (DIPJ), 169
        proximal interphalangeal joint (PIPJ), 169
    pulley disruption, 167, 168
    tenosynovitis, 167
    trigger finger (*see* Stenosing tenosynovitis)
    ulna collateral ligament injury of thumb
        gamekeeper's thumb, 170
        Stener lesion, 170
        volar plate injury, 169
Finklestein's test, 164
Flexor digitorum profundus (FDP), 150
Flexor digitorum superficialis (FDS), 150
Flexor hallucis longus (FHL) tendon, 81–82
Footballer's ankle. *See* Anterior ankle impingement
Fracture dislocations, carpometacarpal joints
    carpometacarpal fracture (CMC), 170
    punching injury, 170
FSE. *See* Fast-spin echo

G

Galeazzi fracture, 155
Ganglion cysts, 185
Glenohumeral instability, IGHL
    Bankart lesions
        failure locations, 118
        and variants, 117–118
    CT arthrography, 120
    imaging and arthrography, MR, 118–120
    non-traumatic multidirectional instability, 118
    posterior labral injury, 118
    types and imaging modalities, 116–117
Glenohumeral internal rotation deficit (GIRD), 107
Glenolabral articular disruption (GLAD) lesions, 118
Golfers elbow, 130–132
Greater arc, wrist, 144
Guyon's canal, 149, 150
Gymnast's wrist. *See* Dorsal impingement, distal radius

H

Haematoma aspiration, 248
Haglund's syndrome, 67–68
Hammer hand syndrome, 165, 166
Hamstring muscle complex (HMC), 211–212
Hand
    tendon anatomy
        adductor aponeurosis, 170
        flexor digitorum profundus (FDP), 150
        flexor digitorum superficialis (FDS), 150
        metacarpophalangeal joint (MCPJ), 168
        proximal interphalangeal joint (PIPJ), 169
    wrist injury, 143–170
Hernias
    bulging and pre-hernia complex, 46
    femoral hernias, 46
    imaging modalities, 45
High-energy single injury, 163
High-risk stress fracture, 100
Hip internal derangement. *See also* Pelvis and groin injuries
    athletes management, 35
    biomechanics and anatomy, 29–30
    femoroacetabular impingement, 30
    imaging, 31
    labral abnormalities and femoroacetabular impingement, 30
    magnetic resonance techniques, 31
    osteochondral lesions, role of, 32–33
    post-operative imaging, 35–36
HMC. *See* Hamstring muscle complex
Hoffa's disease and impingement, 21
Hoffa's fat pad, 176–177
Hypothenar hammer syndrome. *See* Hammer hand syndrome

I

IGHL. *See* Inferior glenohumeral ligament
Iliotibial band (ITB) friction syndrome, 20–21
Imaging techniques, muscle injury
    appendicular
        adductors, 211
        calf muscles, 213
        hamstring muscle complex (HMC), 211–212
        pectoralis major, 211, 212
        quadriceps, 206, 208, 212–213
    axial
        rectus abdominis, 214
        side-strain, 215
    clinical grading, 206–207
    compartment syndrome, 207–209
    haematoma, 207, 208
    herniation, 209
    MR imaging, 203, 204
    normal muscle, 204–205
    sequelae and complications, 208–210
    ultrasound, 204–205
Impingement syndromes
    anterior ankle, 64–65
    anterolateral (ALI), 63–64
    anteromedial ankle, 65–66
    posterior ankle (PAI), 65–68
Inferior glenohumeral ligament (IGHL), 105
Inflammatory arthropathy, 164
Instability surgery and labral repair, imaging
    abduction external rotation (ABER), 196
    Bristow–Helfet, Laterjet techniques, 195
    torn capsulolabral complex (*see* Bankart lesion/variant)
Interference screw fixation, 186
Intersection syndrome, 165
Inter-vertebral disc disease
    annular fissures and discal herniation, 233–235
    disc degeneration, 234, 235
Intraarticular loose bodies. *See* Degenerative joint disease
Ischial tuberosity (hamstring origin), 251
Isometric graft positioning, 181, 182
Itercondylar notch roof. *See* Blummensaat's line

J

Joint compartments, wrist anatomy
    carpometacarpal, 145–146
    distal radioulnar, 145
    intermetacarpal, 146
    midcarpal, 144, 145
    pisotriquetral, 145
    radiocarpal, 144–145

K

Keinbock's disease, 143
Killer turn, 186
Knee injuries
    bone and articular cartilage injury
        cartilage and osteochondral injury, 25–26
        cartilage repair, 26
    collateral ligaments and posterior corner injuries
        anatomy, 2–3
        imaging appearances, 16
        LCL and posterolateral corner, 17–18
        MCL, 16–17
    tendinopathy and overuse injuries (*see* Tendinopathy and overuse injuries)
    cruciate ligaments
        ACL, 12–13
        anatomy, 2
        conventional radiographs and CT, 11
        injury grading, 10–11
        MR imaging, 11–12
        PCL, 13–14
        post-operative imaging, 14–15
    menisci
        anatomy, 1
        imaging (*see* Magnetic resonance imaging)
        parameniscal cyst, 10
        post-operative surgery, 10–11
    patellofemoral syndrome
        anatomy, 23
        causes of, 22–23
        chronic patella maltracking, 23–24
        transient patellar dislocation, 23

L

Lacerating injury, 164
Lateral collateral ligament (LCL), 3, 16–18
Lateral epicondylosis. *See* Tennis elbow
Lesser arc, wrist, 144, 145
Ligament injury
    scapholunate, 156–158
    triquetrolunate ligament tears, 157–159
Ligamentization, 180
Lister's tubercle, 149
Little leaguer's elbow, 133–135
Lower extremity stress injuries
    femur, 97–98
    fibular stress injury, 99
    foot, 99–100
    imaging, 97
    pelvis, 97
    pubic rami and symphysis, 97
    tibial stress syndrome, 98
Lumbar spine, biomechanics
    axial compression, 221–222
    extension, 222
    flexion, 222
    lateral flexion, 222
    rotation, 222
Lunate angulation *vs.* lunate dislocation, 154

M

Magnetic resonance imaging (MRI), 184
    advantages and disadvantages, 115–116
    ankle and foot injury, 53, 55, 59–62, 64–84
    classification and tears appearances
        horizontal tears, 6
        longitudinal tears, 6–8
        meniscocapsular and meniscal root injury, 8
        radial tears, 8
        system, 93
    discoid meniscus, 4
    elbow injury, 129
    glenohumeral instability, 118–120
    normal meniscus, 3–4
    osseous stress injury, 93–94
    persistent meniscal vascularisation, 4

Magnetic resonance imaging (MRI) (cont.)
   shoulder injury, 110–113, 118–120
   STIR and T2 fat-suppressed images, 94
Marrow stimulation, 188
MCPJ. See Metacarpophalangeal joint
Medial collateral ligament (MCL), 2, 9–10, 16, 23
Medial epicondyle apophysitis. See Little leaguer's elbow
Medial epicondylosis. See Golfers elbow
Medial plica syndrome, 22
Medial ulnar collateral ligament injury, 131–133
Meniscal cysts, 9–10
Meniscal imaging
   conventional and CT arthrography, 9
   conventional radiography, 8
   ultrasound, 8
Metacarpophalangeal joint (MCPJ), 168
Midcarpal instability. See Non-dissociative instability
MO. See Myositis ossificans
MRI. See Magnetic resonance imaging
Mumford procedure, 191
Muscle injury and complications
   acute semitendinosus strain, 216
   anatomy, 203–204
   appendicular
      adductors, 211
      calf muscles, 213
      hamstring muscle complex (HMC), 211–212
      pectoralis major, 211, 212
      quadriceps, 206, 208, 212–213
   axial
      rectus abdominis, 214
      side-strain, 215
   clinical grading, 206–207
   compartment syndrome, 207–209
   haematoma, 207, 208
   herniation, 209
   imaging techniques
      MR imaging, 201, 202
      ultrasound, 202–203
   normal muscle imaging characteristics
      MR imaging, 203, 204
      ultrasound, 204–205
   patho-physiology of
      delayed-onset muscle soreness, 205
      muscle strain, 202, 206–207
   sequelae and complications
Muscle intervention, 248, 249
Myositis ossificans (MO), 209–211
Myotendinous junctions (MTJs), 203, 208, 214

N
Needle placement, US-guided intervention. See also Ultrasound (US)
   accurately, 243, 244
   cross-cut artefact, 245
   pitfalls, 245–246
   principles, 243
   puncture site, 243–245
   safely, 243
Nerve anatomy, 150
Non-dissociative instability, 160

O
OAT. See Osteochondral autologous transplantation
Osgood–Schlatters disease, 22

Osseous stress injury
   anatomy, 89
   biomechanics, 89
   differential diagnosis, 101
   fatigue fracture aetiology, 89–90
   imaging
      bone scintigraphy, 92–93
      computed tomography (CT), 93
      MR imaging, 93–94
      radiography, 91
      ultrasound, 91–92
   risk factors, 90
   site-specific stress injury
      lower extremity, 97–100
      upper extremity, 94–96
Os styloideum, 144
Osteochondral autologous transplantation (OAT), 189
Osteochondral injuries (OCI), 55–56
Osteochondritis dissecans, 134–136

P
Painful os naviculare syndrome (PONS), 79
Patellofemoral syndrome
   anatomy, 23
   causes of, 22–23
   chronic patella maltracking, 23–24
   transient patellar dislocation, 23
Pelvis and groin injuries
   athletic groin pain (pubalgia)
      anatomy, 41–42
      biomechanics and core stability, 40
      clinical problem, 42–43
      imaging, 43
      inguinal vs. parasymphyseal, 43, 44
      injection technique, 45
      management, 45
      ultrasound role, 45
   hernias
      bulging and pre-hernia complex, 46
      femoral hernias, 46
      imaging modalities, 45
   hip and soft tissues, ultrasound-guided injection, 35–36
   hip internal derangement
      athletes management, 35
      biomechanics and anatomy, 29–30
      femoroacetabular impingement, 30
      imaging, 31
      labral abnormalities and femoroacetabular impingement, 30
      magnetic resonance techniques, 31
      osteochondral lesions, role of, 32–33
      post-operative imaging, 35–36
   pelvic muscle and tendon injury
      abdominal muscles, 40–41
      adductor group
      gluteal muscles, 39
      hamstring group, 38–39
      iliopsoas tendinopathy and snapping, 37
      imaging, 36
      quadriceps and sartorius, 37–38
      tensor fascia lata, 38
Perthe's lesion, 117–118
PIPJ. See Proximal interphalangeal joint
Plantar fasciitis, 82–83
Plantar fasciitis injection, 251–252
Posterior cruciate ligament (PCL), 2, 7, 12–16

Posteromedial ankle impingement (PAI) syndrome, 67–69
Postoperative imaging, sports medicine
  cartilage repair procedures
    autologous chondrocyte implantation, 190
    marrow stimulation, 188
    osteochondral allograft transplantation, 190
    osteochondral autologous transplantation, 189
  instability surgery and labral repair
    Bristow–Helfet and laterjet techniques, 195
    multiple anterior glenoid suture, 197
    Putti–Platt procedure, 195
    superior labral anterior posterior (SLAP), 194
  knee ligaments
    anterior cruciate ligament (ACL), 179–186
    collateral ligament repairs, 187–188
    posterior cruciate ligament (PCL), 186–187
  knee, meniscal surgery
    computer tomography, 179
    MR imaging, 176–179
  optimisation of, 175–176
  shoulder
    rotator cuff, 192–194
    subacromial decompression, 191–192
Proximal interphalangeal joint (PIPJ), 169
Pubalgia. See Athletic groin pain (pubalgia)
Putti–Platt procedure, 195

Q
Q angle, patellofemoral syndrome, 23
Quadriceps tendon disease, 20

R
Radioscaphoid arthritis, 152
Retinacular injuries, 75–76
Rotator cuff
  tears
    classification of, 109
    partial thickness, 109
    rotator interval, 109–110
  tendinopathy
    external impingement, 106–107
    internal impingement, 107–108

S
Sacro-iliac joint (SIJ), 221
Scaphoid fractures
  radioscaphoid arthritis, 152
  scintigraphy, 152
Screw head. See Lacerating injury
Short-tau inversion recovery (STIR), 157, 201
Shoulder injury
  acromioclavicular joint (ACJ), 123–124
  adhesive capsulitis, 123
  anatomy
    biceps tendon and rotator interval, 105–106
    rotator cuff, 103–104
    static stabilisers, 104–105
  glenohumeral instability
    CT arthrography, 120
    imaging and arthrography, MR, 118–120
    lesion and variants, Bankart, 117–118
    non-traumatic multidirectional instability, 118
    posterior labral injury, 118
    types and imaging modalities, 116–117
  imaging
    advantages and disadvantages, MR, 115–116
    CT, 110
    imaging and arthrography, MR, 118–120
    postoperative rotator cuff, 116
    radiographs, 110
    ultrasound, 113–115
  nerve entrapments, 124
  rotator cuff tears
    classification of, 109
    partial thickness, 109
    rotator interval, 109–110
  rotator cuff tendinopathy
    external impingement, 106–107
    internal impingement, 107–108
  SLAP lesions
    imaging, 121–122
    types of, 121
Signal conversion, 177
SIJ. See Sacro-iliac joint
Site-specific stress injury
  lower extremity, 97–100
  upper extremity, 94–96
SLAP. See Superior labral anterior posterior tears
Smith's fracture, 155
Soft tissue anatomy, ligaments
  extrinsic, 147, 148
  intrinsic/interosseous, 146–147
Spine and sacrum physical-related disorders
  anterior and middle column, anatomy
    inter-vertebral disc, 220
    ligaments, 220
    vertebral body, 219
  biomechanics
    cervical spine, 221
    lumbar spine, 221–222
    thoracic spine, 221
  facet joint pain, 237–239
  inter-vertebral disc disease
    annular fissures and discal herniation, 233–235
    disc degeneration, 234, 235
  lamina and spinous process fractures, 230
  pedicle fractures, 229
  posterior column, anatomy
    facet joints, 220
    ligaments of, 220–221
    pars interarticularis, 220
  sacro-iliac joint (SIJ), 221
  spinal trauma, acute
    cervical spine, 221
    thoraco-lumbar spine, 223
  spondylolysis and spondylolisthesis, 231–233
  stress fractures
    fracture healing, 228
    pars interarticularis, imaging, 224–228
    patient management, 228–229
  transverse process fractures, 220, 229–231
  vertebral end-plate and ring apophysis
    acute traumatic lesions, 232, 237, 238
    juvenile lumbar osteochondrosis, 236–237
    Scheuermann's disease, 235–236
Sports injuries, imaging in children, 163
Stenosing tenosynovitis, 167–168
Steroid injection, 246–247
STIR. See Short-tau inversion recovery

Stress fractures, spine and sacrum
    lamina and spinous process fractures, 230
    pars interarticularis
        complete active stress fracture, grade III, 226, 227
Stress fractures, spine and sacrum (*cont.*)
        complete inactive fractures, grade IV, 226–228, 232
        fracture healing, 228
        incomplete stress fracture, grade II, 225–226
        normal pars, grade 0, 224–225
        patient management, 228–229
        stress reaction, grade I, 225, 226
    pedicle fractures, 229
    SI fracture line, 231
    transverse process fractures, 220, 229–231
Subacromial bursal injection, 248–250
Superior labral anterior posterior (SLAP) tears, 194
Superior labral anterior to posterior (SLAP) lesion
    imaging, 121–122
    types of, 121
Symphysis pubis and acromio-clavicular joint injection, 249, 250

T
Tendinopathy and overuse injuries
    bursae, 22
    Hoffa's disease and impingement, 21
    iliotibial band friction syndrome, 20–21
    patellar tendinopathy, 18–20
    plica, 21
    quadriceps tendon disease, 20
    semitendinosus, 20
    traction enthesopathy, adolescent, 22
Tendon interventions, 247–248
Tendon, soft tissue anatomy
    extensor
        abductor pollicis longus (APL), 164
        extensor pollicis longus, 149
    flexor, 149–150
Tennis elbow, 130–131
Tenosynovitis, wrist
    De Quervain's stenosing
        abductor pollicis longus (APL), 164
        extensor pollicis brevis (EPB), 164
        extensor carpi ulnaris (ECU), 164–165
        transverse sonogram, 164
TE sequences, 177
TFCC. *See* Triangular fibrocartilage complex
Tibialis posterior tendon (TPT), 77–79
Tibial tunnel, 182
Torn capsulolabral complex. *See* Bankart lesion/variant
Triangular fibrocartilage complex (TFCC)
    anatomy, 147–148
    injury types, 160–162
Trigger finger. *See* Stenosing tenosynovitis
Triple phase bone scintigraphy (TPBS), 92

U
Ulna abutment syndrome, 162
Ulnar collateral ligament (UCL) injury, 169–170
Ultrasound (US)
    advantages and disadvantages, 115–116
    ankle and foot injury, 70, 71, 76, 79, 82–83
    calcific tendinitis, barbotage for, 250–251
    diagnostic injections, 246
    ischial tuberosity (hamstring origin), 251
    needle placement
        accurately, 243, 244
        cross-cut artefact, 245
        pitfalls, 245–246
        principles, 243
        puncture site, 243–245
        safely, 243
    osseous stress injury, 91–92
    plantar fasciitis injection, 251–252
    shoulder injury, 113–115
    subacromial bursal injection, 248–250
    symphysis pubis and acromio-clavicular joint injection, 249, 250
    therapeutic interventions
        muscle intervention, 248, 249
        steroid injection, 246–247
        tendon interventions, 247–248
Upper extremity stress fractures
    chest wall, 96
    forearm, 94–95
    hamate, 96
    hand, 95
    humerus, 94
    lunate, 95–96
    metacarpals and phalanges, 96
    scaphoid, 95
    shoulder girdle, 94

V
Vertebral end-plate and ring apophysis
    acute traumatic lesions of, 232, 237, 238
    juvenile lumbar osteochondrosis, 236–237
    Scheuermann's disease, 235–236
Volar intercalated segment instability (VISI), 159–160

W
Wrist
    anatomy
        joint, 144–146
        osseous, 143–144
    biomechanics, 151
    ganglia
        post-gadolinium scanning, 167
        seed ganglia, 166
    instability
        carpal, 159
        dorsal intercalated segment, 159
        dynamic, 160
        non-dissociative, 160
        ulna translocation, 160
        volar intercalated segment, 159
    joint compartments, anatomy
        carpometacarpal, 145–146
        distal radioulnar, 145
        intermetacarpal, 146
        midcarpal, 144, 145
        pisotriquetral, 145
        radiocarpal, 144–145
    pathology
        fracture dislocation, 153–154
        hamate fracture, 152–154
        scaphoid fractures, 152, 153
    tenosynovitis, characterization, 164

Printed in the United States of America